Neurology of Cognitive and Behavioral Disorders

SERIES EDITOR:

Sid Gilman, M.D., F.R.C.P.
William J. Herdman Professor of Neurology
University of Michigan Medical Center

CONTEMPORARY NEUROLOGY SERIES

NEUROLOGY OF COGNITIVE AND BEHAVIORAL DISORDERS

ORRIN DEVINSKY, M.D.

Professor of Neurology, Neurosurgery, & Psychiatry
New York University School of Medicine
Director, Comprehensive Epilepsy Centers
New York University, New York, NY
Saint Barnabas Medical Center, Livingston, NJ
Staten Island University Hospital, Staten Island, NY

MARK D'ESPOSITO, M.D.

Professor of Neuroscience and Psychology
Director, Henry H. Wheeler, Jr., Brain Imaging Center
Helen Wills Neuroscience Institute
 & Department of Psychology
University of California, Berkeley

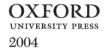

OXFORD
UNIVERSITY PRESS

2004

OXFORD
UNIVERSITY PRESS

Oxford   New York
Auckland   Bangkok   Buenos Aires   Cape Town   Chennai
Dar es Salaam   Delhi   Hong Kong   Istanbul   Karachi   Kolkata
Kuala Lumpur   Madrid   Melbourne   Mexico City   Mumbai   Nairobi
São Paulo   Shanghai   Taipei   Tokyo   Toronto

Published by Oxford University Press, Inc.
198 Madison Avenue, New York, New York, 10016
http://www.oup-usa.org

Library of Congress Cataloging-in-Publication Data
Neurology of cognitive and behavioral disorders /
[editors], Orrin Devinsky, Mark D'Esposito.
p. cm. — (Contemporary neurology series : 68)
Includes bibliographical references and index.
ISBN 0-19-513764-7
1. Mental illness—Etiology. 2. Neuropsychology
3. Brain—Diseases—Complications.
I. Devinsky, Orrin. II. D'Esposito, Mark.
III Series.
RC454.4.N488 2003   616.89'071—dc21   2003048639

The science of medicine is a rapidly changing field. As new research and clinical experience broaden our
knowledge, changes in treatment and drug therapy do occur. The author and publisher of this work have checked
with sources believed to be reliable in their efforts to provide information that is accurate and complete, and in
accordance with the standards accepted at the time of publication. However, in light of the possibility of human
error or changes in the practice of medicine, neither the author, nor the publisher, nor any other party who has
been involved in the preparation or publication of this work warrants that the information contained herein is in
every respect accurate or complete. Readers are encouraged to confirm the information contained herein with
other reliable sources, and are strongly advised to check the product information sheet provided by the
pharmaceutical company for each drug they plan to administer.

9 8 7 6 5 4 3 2 1

Printed in the United States of America
on acid-free paper

To my family,
Deborah, Janna, and Julie,
and to my mentors,
Dick Gershon, Norman Geschwind, Jerry Posner, and Oliver Sacks.

O.D.

To my family,
Judy, Zoe, and Zack,
and to my mentors,
Mick Alexander and Marty Albert.

M.D'E.

Preface

Understanding the anatomy and function of cognition and behavior challenges neuroscience and neurology. Unraveling the mechanisms and discovering effective treatment of cognitive and behavioral disorders are demanding goals. Correlating the signs and symptoms with the brain's pathological anatomy—the clinical–pathological method that allowed Broca, Wernicke, Dejerine, and Liepmann to define the neurobehavioral syndromes—returned to prominence as behavioral neurology was reborn in the second half of the twentieth century. The classic topics of aphasia, apraxia, alexia, agnosia, neglect, and other disordered behaviors were reintroduced as side streams in neurology. Over the subsequent decades, these and other topics, such as memory disorders and prosodic, executive, and emotional dysfunction, attracted greater interest. Behavioral neurology moved from the fringes of medicine (in the 1970s, it had occupied the last hour of the American Academy of Neurology meetings) toward the mainstream. In this book, we integrate modern insights of cognitive neuroscience with traditional approaches to behavioral neurology.

Our view of the mind evolves. Twenty years ago, the brain was viewed as a serial processor. The visual neuroscientist perceived an image as passing from the retina to the lateral geniculate to the primary visual cortex, where it then passed from simple to complex to hypercomplex cells. At the same time, the behavioral neurologist viewed a visual image as passing from the visual association cortex in the occipital cortex to "higher-order," visually dominant multimodal association cortices in the temporal and parietal lobes, where it was further analyzed and associated, permitting reading, facial recognition, and other functions. The concept of parallel processing and a modular mind, operating in concert with serial processing, was a paradigm shift. Similarly, consciousness, a nearly forbidden topic in neuroscience 20 years ago, is now vigorously considered, although our knowledge remains nascent. A clear picture of brain function will likely require many more paradigm shifts in our understanding of it.

Recent decades have witnessed an explosion of new technologies for exploring mental function, the era of molecular neurogenetics, and the realization that neurochemical, neuroelectric, degenerative, and even destructive processes can be treated. Functional imaging provides unpredicted views into the operation of the healthy brain and the impact of disease on the mind. A huge portion of our genome is dedicated to brain function, yet only 1%–2% of our genes differ from those of a chimpanzee. Duplication and modification of critical genes and alterations in the sequence of gene activation during the past five million years may underlie many unique aspects of the human brain. Molecular neurogenetics will offer deep insights into brain function and disease, yet it is a field that remains largely unmined; it receives little attention in this book. The abundance of new information and the consequent changes in the perception of brain function have revitalized cognitive and behavioral neuroscience.

Two important features distinguish this book. In addition to relying heavily on images to convey our story, we also focus on therapies for cognitive and behavioral disorders. Diagnosis is essential for treatment. We encourage readers to copy the Appendices on the Mental Status Examination (pp. 49–51) and use them in their practice.

While reviewing the traditional neurobehavioral topics in the modern era and delving into their cognitive and functional underpinnings, we keep sight of the individuals behind the disorders and, insofar as efficacious remedies are available, offer hope of improving their lives.

Until we know more about the anatomy and mechanisms of brain function in cognitive and neurobehavioral disorders, the recent increased interest in understanding "quality-of-life" issues marks a critical step in the care and management of affected patients. Since there are no single pills to fix many of the most vexing disorders our patients face, we must depend on the expertise of our colleagues in other disciplines, such as rehabilitation medicine, speech therapy, psychology, neuropsychology, and psychiatry. Mostly, we must depend on our humanity and compassion.

Our own professional interests, functional imaging, and epilepsy not only provide lessons about brain function and brain disorders but also highlight the exciting developments in their understanding and treatment. Advances harbor both challenges and dangers. As functional imaging studies proliferate and address new cognitive domains ranging from self-recognition to dreaming to consciousness, we must remain vigilant to methodological limitations and overinterpretation of results. In epilepsy, we continue to miss therapeutic opportunities and "the forest for the trees." For example, depression is prevalent in patients with difficult-to-control seizures and may more severely impair quality of life than seizure control. However, neurological care often focuses exclusively on seizure frequency and severity, and effective therapy that can dramatically improve a patient's life may be overlooked.

We hope this book serves to stimulate greater interest in both the mysteries of the human mind and the treatment of its disorders.

New York, New York   O.D.
Berkeley, California   M.D'E.

Acknowledgments

This book reflects the generous suggestions and critical commentary of our friends and colleagues. During the process of accumulating data, writing and editing the chapters, and creating the illustrations, we asked for their help and benefited enormously from the advice of Michael P. Alexander, William B. Barr, John J. Barry, Joan C. Borod, Gary Brendel, Nouchine Hadjikhani, Mark Hallett, Michael A. Koffman, Rachel Laff, Deepak N. Pandya, Heather D. Rubin, Oliver W. Sacks, Cornelia Santschi, Clifford B. Saper, Melanie B. Shulman, Anuradha Singh, and Brent Vogt, Anjanette Naga, Shawna Cutting, Margarita Hernandez, and Andrea C. Foust provided invaluable help in coordinating the overall project. Images tell stories and describe anatomy much better than words, and Tomo Narashima's outstanding illustrations form a vital element of our work. B.J. Hessie's critical editing focused our ideas and ordered our words. Fiona Stevens, Senior Editor at Oxford University Press, and Sid Gilman, Series Editor for Contemporary Neurology Series, guided us through the long journey from conception to publication. To all, our deepest gratitude.

Contents

Neurology of Cognitive and Behavioral Disorders

Chapter 1

Neuroanatomy and Assessment of Cognitive–Behavioral Function

The assessment of cognitive and behavioral functions provides a benchmark for gauging and tracking these functions over time and assists in understanding the nature of normal and abnormal physiology, the mechanisms underlying these processes, and rational plans for treating cognitive and neurobehavioral disorders. Our exploration into how the brain and mind mediate behavior begins with neurobehavioral assessment, which traditionally focuses on abnormal or deficient performance. Understanding the mechanisms of neurobehavior is better served by also studying normal and superior performance. The explosion of information from newer technologies such as positron emission tomography and functional magnetic resonance imaging (fMRI), expands our knowledge of the processes and networks underlying behavior.

This chapter presents an approach toward bedside observation and full mental status test-ing of patients with cognitive and neurobehavioral dysfunction and surveys the formal assessment of neuropsychological functioning. An overview of neuroanatomy is presented first because an accurate diagnosis depends on linking the findings of neurobehavioral assessment to the anatomical location of the abnormality. Other chapters focus on the detailed examination of each cognitive domain.

OVERVIEW OF BRAIN ANATOMY

The major gyral and sulcal patterns of the human cerebral cortex vary among different populations and individuals (Fig. 1–1). Parceling cortical areas has fascinated anatomists ever since Meynert[1] suggested in 1868 that distinct cytoarchitectural regions serve different functions. Exner,[2] in 1881, and Vogt and Vogt,[3] in

1

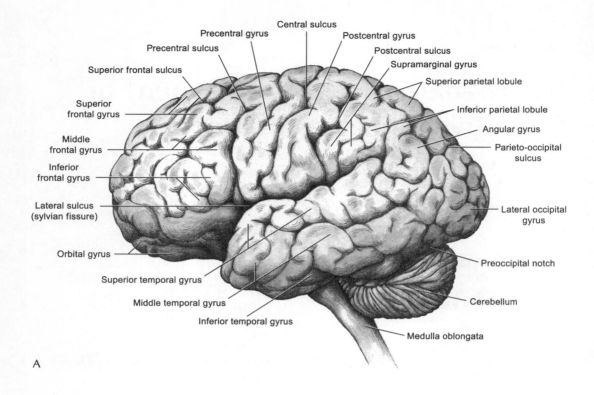

A

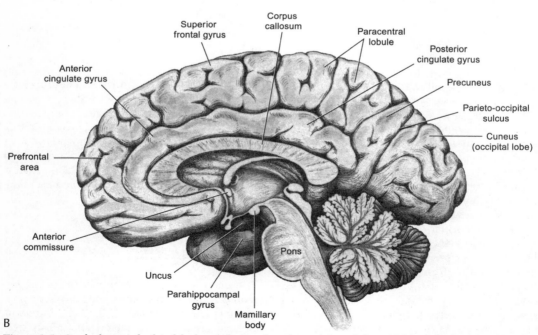

B

Figure 1–1. Cerebral gyri and sulci of the human brain in lateral view (*A*), medial view (*B*), and inferior (basal) view (*C*).

2

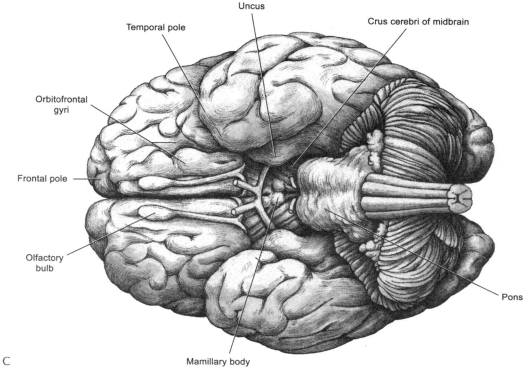

Uncus

Temporal pole

Crus cerebri of midbrain

Orbitofrontal gyri

Frontal pole

Olfactory bulb

Pons

C

Mamillary body

Figure 1–1. *Continued.*

1919, identified several hundred discrete areas; but these ambitious attempts at localization found little support. Brodmann's[3a] map of 47 areas in the cerebral cortex (Brodmann's areas, BAs) remains popular and useful today (Fig. 1–2). Its divisions are based on the architectural patterns of cells and fibers and on the patterns and sequences of myelination, vasculature, and pigmentation. Brodmann did not map the enormous expanse of cortex buried in sulcal banks. In addition, individual variations prevent confident assignment of BAs to anatomical areas identified on MRI. Electrical stimulation, fMRI, and lesional studies provide a complementary functional classification of cortical areas. New techniques and markers, such as tracers for defining connections, cytochrome oxidase staining patterns, membrane antigens, receptors, neurotransmitters, and neuropeptides, also help to define the functional zones.

In 1927, von Economo[4] distinguished five major cortical types based on regional varia-

tions in the cortical thickness and the densities and sizes of granule and pyramidal cells in the various layers (Fig. 1–3). These types of cortex, which encompass the entire cortical mantle, are classified as homotypic (six layers are easily distinguished) and heterotypic (idiotypic, prominent structural variability obscures the six-layered architecture). The homotypic cortical regions are association areas, composing most of the cerebral cortex, and comprise three of the five major cortical types (Fig. 1–3). The heterotypic cortex is limited to specialized regions: agranular (e.g., precentral gyrus, primary motor cortex) and granular (koniocortex, e.g., primary sensory cortex). A modern integration of structural and functional data distinguishes four basic cortical types in a hierarchy of structural complexity: limbic, higher-order (heteromodal) association, modality-specific (unimodal) association, and idiotypic (primary sensory or motor) (Fig. 1–4).

The limbic areas, representing the simplest level of structural complexity (Fig. 1–4), are

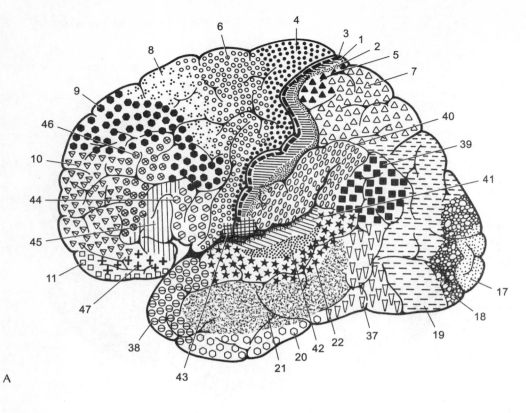

A

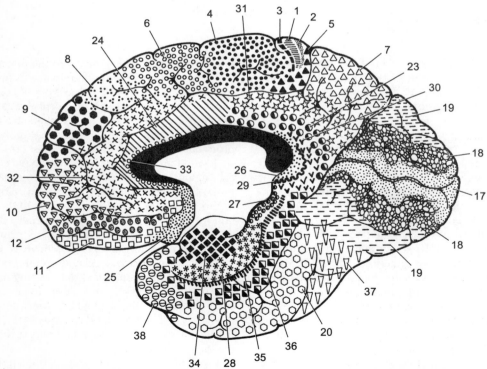

B

Figure 1–2. Brodmann's map of cortical cytoarchitectural organization of the human brain in lateral view (*A*) and medial view (*B*).

4

composed of the basal forebrain (including the septal nuclei, substantia innominata, and parts of the amygdala complex), amygdala, hippocampus, parahippocampal gyrus, temporal pole, insula, the cingulate complex (including the retrosplenial, cingulate, and paraolfactory areas), and the posterior orbitofrontal cortex.

The basal forebrain and amygdala are transitional in location and architecture between subcortex and cortex. The hippocampal formation is a three-layered cortex containing the hippocampus with prominent pyramidal cells (cornu ammonis, CA1–4) and the dentate gyrus with prominent granule cells, one of the few

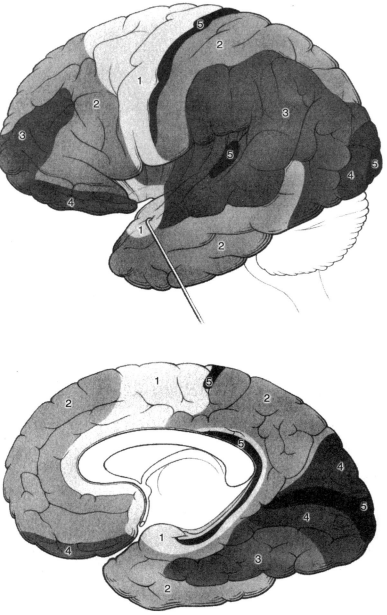

A

Figure 1–3. Von Economo's classification of human cortical types. *A:* Topographic distribution of different cortical types (lateral and medial views).

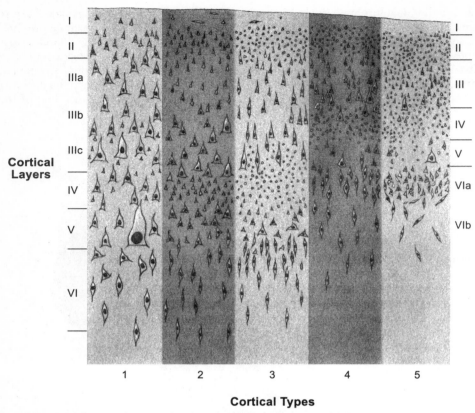

Cortical Layers

Cortical Types

B

Figure 1–3. *Continued. B:* Nissl preparation showing cellular architecture of different cortical types. *(1)* Heterotype agranular (e.g., motor cortex); *(2)* homotype cortex (frontal, parietal, and temporal association cortex); *(3)* homotype cortex (frontal and parietal association cortex); *(4)* homotype granular cortex ("polar" cortex, frontal and occipital lobes); and *(5)* heterotype granular cortex (primary sensory areas).

nonprimary sensory cortices with this feature. At the hippocampal fissure, the subiculum and entorhinal cortex of the parahippocampal gyrus contain a gradual transition from a three- to a six-layered cortex. The transition of these cortical regions is shown in Figure 1–5. We refer to the cingulate, posterior orbitofrontal, anterior insula, parahippocampal gyrus, and temporal pole as *limbic cortical areas.* Although these areas are often classified as *paralimbic,*[5] Papez[6] introduced the term *paralimbic* in 1956 to identify the medial frontal area lying anatomically and architecturally between anterior cingulate (limbic) and frontopolar (association) cortices.

Homotypic cortex, the next level of structural complexity, is divided into modality-specific (unimodal) association cortex and higher-order (multimodal or heteromodal) association cortex. Unimodal association cortex is

found within all four lobes: *(1)* unimodal visual association cortex is in the extrastriate occipital and inferior temporal regions, *(2)* unimodal somatosensory association cortex is in the superior parietal lobule, *(3)* unimodal auditory association cortex is in the superior temporal gyrus, and *(4)* unimodal motor association cortex is just anterior to primary motor cortex. Heteromodal association cortex is found in three areas: *(1)* prefrontal cortex, *(2)* posterior parietal lobe, and *(3)* the posterior portion of the temporal lobe.

Heteromodal association cortex receives input from multiple sensory and motor association cortices and performs higher-order analysis, integration, and synthesis of sensorimotor data. It is cognitive and synthetic rather than sensorimotor and analytical. These cortical areas are not tied to one sensory modality or motor function. Reciprocal connections between

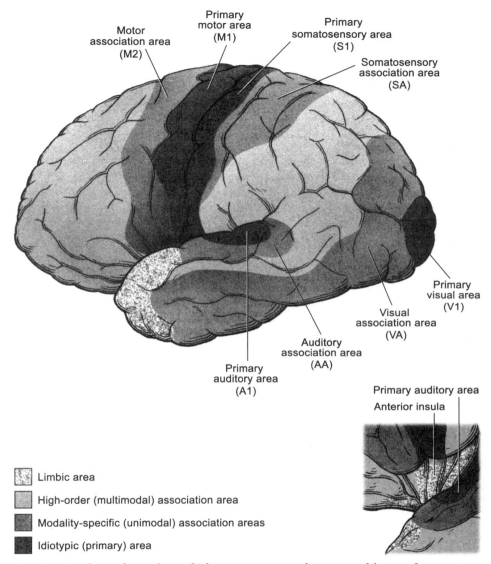

Figure 1–4. Functional map of cortical areas (limbic, primary motor and sensory, modality-specific association, and heteromodal) of the human brain in lateral view *(A)* with insula (inset), medial view *(B)*, and coronal views *(C)*. *(continued)*

heteromodal cortex and limbic areas help to assess the motivational and emotional relevance of stimuli and complex situations, providing the pathway for conceptual ideas to modify mood and affect. The connections from limbic areas to heteromodal association cortex also enable emotions to modify cognitive processes. For example, feelings of fear or paranoia can trigger intent scanning of the visual field in search of threatening stimuli.

Heterotypic cortex, the highest level of structural complexity, is composed of the agranular, macropyramidal primary motor, and granular primary sensory (somatosensory, visual, and auditory) cortices. Primary motor areas, as well as secondary and cingulate motor areas, send efferents in the corticospinal tract to control skeletal muscle activity. The motor association areas are analogous to secondary sensory areas and are important in the initia-

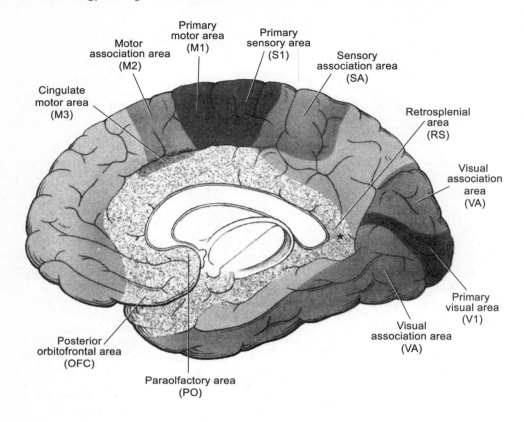

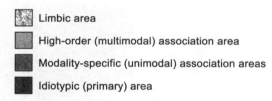

B   * Located in the banks of the callosal sulcus

Figure 1–4. *Continued.* PFC, prefrontal cortex; CG, cingulate gyras; OF, orbitofrontal cortex; MA, motor association area; TP, temporal pole; PO, paraolfactory area; PHG, parahippocampal gyrus; MTL, medial temporal lobe; SMG, supramarginal gyrus; ITL, inferior temporal lobe; MPO, medial parieto-occipital gyrus; SPL, superior parietal lobule; AG, angular gyrus.

tion of movement. These functions include regulation of motor exploration; ocular scanning, located in the frontal eye fields (BA 8); motor programs for speech, located in Broca's area (BA 44, 45); and complex hand movements, such as piano playing. In addition, motor-specific association areas are probably involved in initiation, learning, planning, and inhibition of complex movements.

The primary sensory areas are the first cortical areas to receive modality-specific (e.g., visual and auditory) input. While the thalamus processes and relays sensory data, primary sensory areas perform elaborate categorization and analysis of sensory input. Sensory input is organized by modality-specific criteria. For example, somatosensory input is organized by body part, visual input by visual field topography, and auditory input by tone and spatial location. Secondary sensory areas lie adjacent to primary areas and are intermediate between primary and unimodal-specific sensory areas in both cytoar-

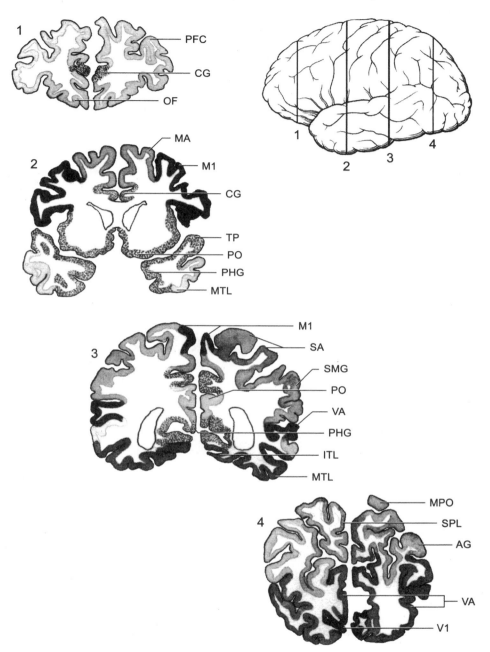

Figure 1–4. *Continued.*

chitecture and function. Secondary and unimodal association cortices contain additional somatotopic representations of the sensory[7,8] and motor[9] functions. During evolution, duplication of cortical areas (e.g., motor, visual) may have provided the substrate for secondary, specialized sensorimotor areas, analogous to the basic evolutionary mechanism of gene duplication.[10] Unimodal-specific sensory association areas perform additional analysis and processing of sensory information and communicate this higher-order information to heteromodal association cortex.

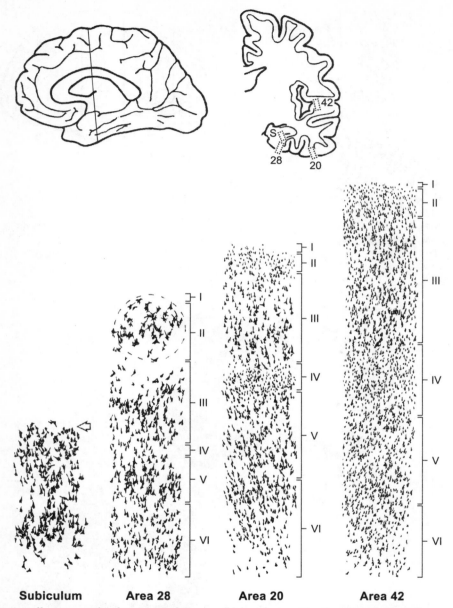

Figure 1–5. Different cortical architecture in the temporal lobe. The transition from three-layered allocortex to perial-locortex to proisocortex (perirhinal cortex, not shown) to six-layered isocortex. Boxes in the coronal section show areas sampled. Brackets indicate boundaries between different layers (Roman numerals). The junction between the molecular and pyramidal cell layers of the subiculum is demarcated with an arrow. In area 28, an island of layer II star pyramidal neurons is shown with a dashed line to emphasize that it is not a continuous layer. In addition to differentiation of the external pyramidal layers in the temporal cortices, the large pyramidal neurons are progressively reduced in size.

Macroscopic Anatomy

Macroscopically, the cerebral cortex consists of four distinct lobes: (1) frontal lobe, (2) parietal lobe, (3) temporal lobe, and (4) occipital lobe.

The frontal lobe lies anterior to the central sulcus and includes the primary motor cortex (BA 4), premotor or secondary motor area (BA 6, 8), supplementary motor area (medial portion of BA 6), frontal eye fields (BA 6, 8), Broca's area (BA 44, 45), and prefrontal cortex. The extensive prefrontal cortex includes the dorsolateral superior, middle, and inferior frontal gyri (BA 9, 10, 46, 47), orbital gyri (BA 11, 12), and anterior cingulate gyri (BA 24, 25, 32).

The parietal lobe lies behind the central sulcus. The primary somesthetic cortex (BA 1, 2, 3) is situated on the posterior bank of this sulcus, with the somesthetic association cortex (BA 5, 7) lying immediately behind it. The secondary somesthetic cortex (BA 43) is a small area located in the most anterior and inferior region of the parietal lobe. The posterior parietal lobe is divided into superior (BA 7) and inferior (BA 39, 40) lobules. The inferior parietal lobule is divided into the supramarginal and angular gyri.

The temporal lobe lies inferior to the sylvian fissure, and its posterior and superior aspects are continuous with the occipital and parietal lobes. The lateral temporal lobe is divided into superior, middle, and inferior gyri (BA 20, 21, 22, 37, 38, 41, 42). The primary auditory cortex, or Heschl's gyrus (BA 41), and auditory association cortex (BA 42, 22), which includes Wernicke's area, lie in the posterosuperior aspect. The remainder of the lateral temporal lobe is association cortex, much of which has connections with visual, auditory, and limbic areas. The temporal pole (BA 38) is limbic cortex. The medial temporal lobe is part of the limbic system and includes the amygdala, hippocampus, and parahippocampal and fusiform gyri.

The occipital lobe lies posterior to the temporal and parietal lobes and consists mainly of visual cortex: primary visual, or striate, cortex (BA 17) and visual association cortex (BA 18, 19).

The various disorders associated with damage to the primary and association cortex in each of these four cerebral lobes are summarized in Tables 1–1 to 1–4.

Cortical Connections

The 50-100 billion neurons in the human brain are linked by a network of trillions of synapses. These connections permit both serial and parallel processing between cells within a vertical column, in cortical areas involved in a local functional system, and in more extensive cortical and subcortical networks. Early maps on myelinogenesis[11] provided a blueprint for phylogenetic development of the cortex (Fig. 1–6). A selective increase in frontal lobe size is often suggested as

the basis for intellectual differences between humans and the great apes. However, the size of the frontal cortices and the proportions of their major areas are similar among great apes and humans.[12] In primate evolution, white matter increases exponentially relative to gray matter.[10] The human frontal lobe has a greater proportion of white matter underlying prefrontal cortex.[13] We owe our intellect to having more extensive connections, as well as more neurons.

Cortical columns are vertically organized around layers III, V, and VI pyramidal cells, with their apical dendrites extending to layer I and their basal dendrites extending to layer VI. Pyramidal cell axons are the major output of the cortical column, with most intracortical fibers arising from layer III. Inputs arrive from the thalamus (mainly to layer IV) and distant cortical regions (mainly to layers I–III). Neighboring cortical areas connect reciprocally. In the sensory system, "forward" connections (e.g., from V1 to V2, V2 to V4) originate mainly in layer III and terminate in layers III and IV. The "backward" reciprocal connections originate in layers V and VI and terminate in various layers of the preceding area. Reciprocal connections between prefrontal and parietal association cortices arise in layer III. Connections between successive and nonsuccessive steps in sensory processing allow simultaneous synthesis and analysis in widely distributed regions. Figure 1–7 shows selected corticocortical connections in the chimpanzee.

The thalamus provides a blueprint for cortical anatomy and connections. In mammalian evolution, thalamic size correlates with the neocortical surface.[15] The projection fields of thalamic nuclei closely correspond to cortical cytoarchitecture, suggesting that thalamocortical afferents partly determine neocortical cytoarchitectonic differentiation.[15] Thalamocortical afferents arise from thalamic sensory relay and associational nuclei (Fig. 1–8). The sensory relay nuclei include the medial (auditory), lateral (visual) geniculate, and ventral posterior (somatosensory) nuclei. Thalamic association nuclei receive input from other subcortical and cortical areas and send fibers to association cortex: parietal, temporal, and occipital cortices (pulvinar–lateral posterior complex), frontal cortex (dorsomedial nucleus), motor cortex (ventral lateral), and limbic cortex (anterior and dorsomedial nuclei). All neocortical areas receiving thalamic input send reciprocal fibers to the thalamus (from layer VI neurons).

Table 1–1. Disorders Associated with Frontal Lobe Lesions

Primary motor cortex
  Weakness (maximal in distal muscles, fine
    movements)
  Increased tone (spasticity)
Motor association cortex
  Weakness (maximal in proximal muscles)
  Increased tone (spasticity)
  Buccofacial and limb apraxia, left side
  Callosal apraxia (white matter fibers), left side
  Grasp reflex
Supplementary motor area
  Grasp reflex
  Impaired rapid alternating movements
  Transient transcortical motor aphasia, left side
  Transient impairment of motor initiation
Broca's area, left hemisphere
  Broca's aphasia (with permanent disorder, lesion
    extends to subcortical white matter)
  Aphemia, a nonaphasic defect of hypophonia
    and dysarthria
  Dysprosody (also occurs with right-sided lesions)
Prefrontal area
  Left side
    Inability to plan and execute multistep
      processes
    Transcortical motor aphasia
    Apraxia
    Depression
  Right side
    Left-sided extinction and neglect
    Blunted and labile affect, depression
    Disinhibition
    Impairment of sustained attention
    Impersistence (reduced motor attention)
    Motor neglect
    Impaired affective prosody

    Reduced gestural expression
    Reduplication syndromes (e.g., Capgras
      syndrome)
    Alien hand sign
  Bilateral
    Abulia or catatonia
    Depression
    Impaired working memory
    Inability to plan and execute multistep
      processes
    Dysprosody
    Disinhibition and loss of social graces
    Incontinence
    Confabulation
    Perseveration
    Delusions
  Bilateral, dorsolateral
    Executive dysfunction and impaired working
      memory
      Concrete thought
      Impaired generation of solutions to novel
        problems
      Impaired planning and regulating of
        adaptive and goal-directed behavior
    Apathy
  Bilateral, orbitofrontal
    Impaired "theory of mind" (ability to make
      inferences about other people's
      mental states)
    Disinhibition of motor activity (hyperactivity)
    Disinhibition of instinctual behavior
    Impaired self-monitoring (failure to appreciate
      the consequences of one's actions)
    Emotional lability, with euphoria or dysphoria
    Increased aggressiveness
    Increased appetite and weight gain

RECIPROCAL AND REDUNDANT INPUTS AND OUTPUTS

Cerebral inputs and outputs are often reciprocal. Primary sensory and sensory association areas are reciprocally connected. Reciprocal connections also extend between sensory areas and limbic areas, linking information about the outside world (exteroception) and the internal state (interoception and emotion). Reciprocal connections also link sensory association cortices with motor areas, providing, for example, the basis for directing movement and feedback to adjust trajectory.

Cerebral inputs and outputs are often redundant. For example, visual input passes from lateral geniculate to primary *and* secondary visual cortices. The amygdala projects not only to the autonomic-drive behavior centers in the hypothalamus but also to brain stem areas such as the dorsal motor nucleus of layer X, which receives a large hypothalamic projection. Overlapping projections from sensory, limbic, and motor areas likely serve, in part, to allow an area to know where its input originates. For example, higher visual association areas could receive input from area 17 or 18 or other visual association areas. The simultaneous input from the lateral geniculate allows these areas to correlate the cortically derived input with more peripherally derived "raw" data.

Table 1–2. **Disorders Associated with Temporal Lobe Lesions**

Primary auditory cortex (Heschl's gyrus)
 Unilateral lesions, no hearing impairment
 Bilateral lesions, cortical deafness (rare)
Auditory association cortex (Wernicke's area)
 Left side
  Wernicke's aphasia
  Conduction aphasia
 Right side
  Impaired music perception
  Sensory dysprosodia
 Bilateral
  Auditory agnosia
Lateral temporal (nonauditory) cortex
 Anomia
 Impaired visual learning
 Retrograde amnesia
 Agitated delirium, right side
 Impairment of associating auditory and visual
  stimuli with emotional valence

Posterior inferior temporal visual association
 cortex
 Visual agnosia
  Prosopagnosia
  Achromatopsia (lesion often extends to inferior
   occipital lobe)
  Impaired color naming, dominant hemisphere
   (lesion often extends to inferior
   occipital lobe)
Medial temporal (limbic) cortex
 Impaired long-term memory (verbal, greater on
  left; visuospatial, greater on right)
 Decreased or increased aggression
 Emotional disorders
 Depression
 Mania (usually right basal lesions)
 Hallucinations or illusions
 Klüver-Bucy syndrome (bilateral anterior
  lesions)

The brain stem, cerebellum, subcortical nuclei, and cortex have multiple representations of the same functional systems that are reciprocally connected. Functionally related areas connect in series and parallel with one another. Thus, analysis of information, cognition, planning, and execution of motor behavior is both hierarchical and simultaneous. Behavior expresses the brain's synchronized activity, reflecting the simultaneous activation and inhibition of multiple areas. The line between *localized* and *holistic* reflects our logic, not our brain organization.

Table 1–3. **Disorders Associated with Parietal Lobe Lesions**

Primary somatosensory cortex
 Impaired cutaneous and proprioceptive (joint
  position) sensation
 Impaired ability to localize pain and
  temperature sensations
Secondary somatosensory cortex
 Impaired fine sensory discrimination (changes
  in weight, texture, temperature; two-point
  discrimination)
Parietal association cortex
 Left side°
  Agraphia
  Acalculia
  Finger agnosia
  Right–left disorientation
  Alexia, with agraphia
  Conduction aphasia
  Anomic aphasia
  Constructional apraxia

 Impaired proverb and similarities–differences
  interpretation
 Apraxia, ideomotor
 Extinction and neglect of right-sided stimuli
  (uncommon)
 Right side
  Extinction and neglect of left-sided stimuli
  Visuospatial disorders
  Topographic (spatial) and geographic
   disorientation (lesion often extends to
   anterior occipital lobe)
  Constructional apraxia
  Dressing apraxia
  Impersistence
 Bilateral
  Balint's syndrome (oculomotor apraxia,
   simultagnosia and optic ataxia; superior
   lesions, often extending to anterior occipital
   lobe)

°The first four disorders are associated with Gerstmann's syndrome, and the first nine disorders are associated with angular gyrus syndrome.

Table 1–4. **Disorders Associated with Occipital Lobe Lesions**

Primary visual (striate) cortex
  Contralateral homonymous hemianopia,
    unilateral lesions
  Cortical blindness, bilateral lesions
Visual association cortex
  Left side
    Alexia (lesion extends to splenium of corpus
      callosum)
    Color anomia (lesion may extend to inferior
      temporal lobe)
    Right-sided achromatopsia (lesion may extend
      to inferior temporal lobe)
	Right side
	  Palinopsia
	  Left-sided hemiachromatopsia (lesion may
	    extend to inferior temporal lobe)
	Bilateral, inferior
	  Visual agnosia (lesion usually extends to
	    temporal lobes, fusiform and lingual gyri)
	  Prosopagnosia (lesion usually extends to
	    temporal lobes, fusiform and lingual gyri)
	Bilateral, superior
	  Balint's syndrome (oculomotor apraxia,
	    simultagnosia, optic ataxia; lesion usually
	    extends to parietal lobes)

SPECIFIC AND DIFFUSE BRAIN CONNECTIONS

Brain connections are organized into specific and diffuse groups. Discrete, channel-specific connections mediate distinct neurobehavioral functions. Cell groups with related functions are often interconnected. For example, the visual radiations link lateral geniculate nucleus and striate cortex (V1) with great precision. Major cortical fibers providing specific connections include associational (intracortical)

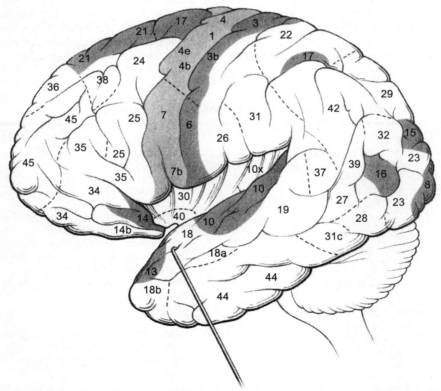

A

Figure 1–6. Flechsig's map of myelogenesis: the sequence of human cerebral areas that undergo myelination. *A:* Lateral view.

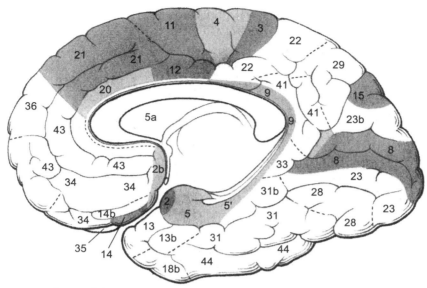

B

Figure 1–6. *Continued. B:* Medial view. Shaded areas are myelinated at birth. Numbers show temporal sequence of cortical area myelination (1, earliest; 45, latest).

fibers that interconnect cortical areas within the same hemisphere, commissural (callosal and other) fibers that interconnect the two hemispheres (usually homologous areas), and projection fibers that connect cortex to subcortical areas, brain stem, and spinal cord. Others include the arcuate fibers that connect adjacent gyri.

Specific connections also project from subcortical and brain stem areas to influence the cortex and spinal cord. Specific fibers have selective connection patterns, with terminations on discrete, vertical columns and lamina. For example, connections between parietal and frontal heteromodal association cortices are organized into discrete, vertically oriented

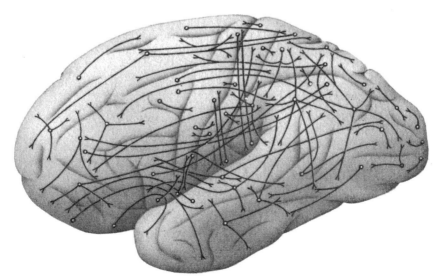

Figure 1–7. Map of corticocortical connections identified by physiological neuronography in the chimpanzee. (From Bailey and von Bonin.[14])

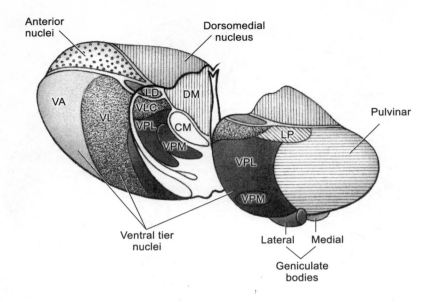

A

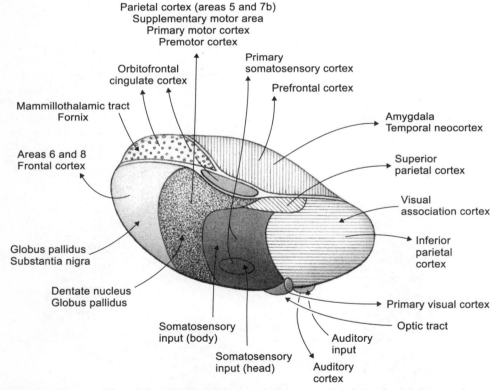

B

Figure 1–8. *A:* Projections from thalamic nuclei to lateral cerebral cortex. *B:* Projections from thalamic nuclei to medial cerebral cortex. *C:* Thalamic nuclei. *D:* Main afferent and efferent connections of thalamic nuclei. VA, ventral anterior; DM, dorsomedial; LP, lateral posterior; VL, ventral lateral, VLC, ventral lateral caudal; VPL, ventral posterolateral; VPM, ventral posteromedial; CM, centromedian; DM, dorsomedial; LD, lateral dorsal.

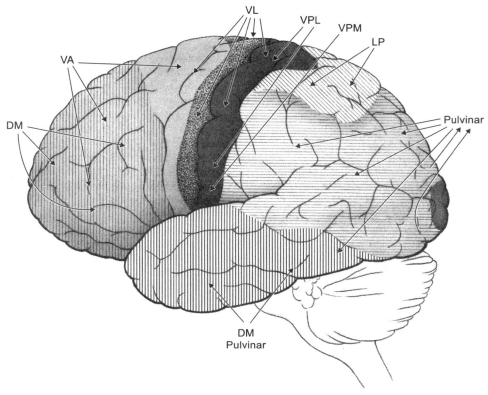

C

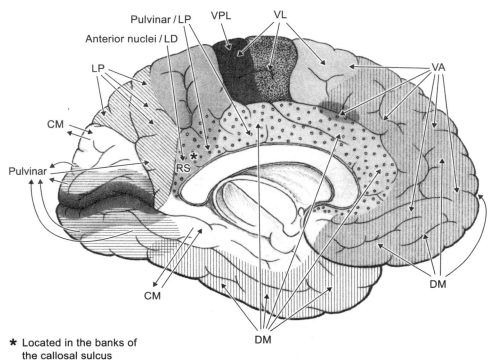

* Located in the banks of
D   the callosal sulcus

17

columns. All cognitive functions rely on these specific pathways.

The diffuse projection systems arise in subcortical nuclei, which widely disseminate a specific neurotransmitter throughout the brain. These neurotransmitters are important for arousal (e.g., norepinephrine), attention (e.g., norepinephrine, acetylcholine), motivation (e.g., dopamine), and mood (e.g., serotonin) (see Chapter 4). These subcortical–to–cortical aminergic and γ-aminobutyric acid (GABA) fibers arise from distinct subcortical nuclei: raphe nuclei (serotonin), locus ceruleus (norepinephrine), substantia nigra and ventral tegmental area (dopamine), hypothalamus (histamine), and basal forebrain (acetylcholine and GABA). In addition, a cholinergic pathway from the brain stem reticular formation stimulates the thalamus, which in turn gives rise to a pathway carrying excitatory amino acids to activate the cortex. These diffuse modulatory pathways do not receive balanced reciprocal projections from the cortex. Thus, although neurotransmitters such as acetylcholine and norepinephrine influence widespread cortical areas, the basal forebrain and locus ceruleus receive input from a small set of limbic areas. These limbic areas can thereby swiftly alter global cortical states.

Diffuse projections modulate the information-processing states and efficiency of specific systems. Cognition requires wakefulness and arousal. A tired, unmotivated, and inattentive person learns poorly. Thus, failure to activate the state-dependent diffuse projections impairs otherwise intact cortical networks. Deficiencies in the single-neurotransmitter diffuse systems contribute to neurobehavioral disorders such as parkinsonism (dopamine), obsessive–compulsive symptoms and depression (serotonin), and impaired memory (acetylcholine). However, disorders rarely result from deficiencies of a single neurotransmitter. For example, Parkinson's and Alzheimer's diseases are associated with greater neuronal loss in the locus ceruleus than in the substantia nigra and nucleus basalis.[9a] Excessive activity in these diffuse systems can also cause neurobehavioral problems ranging from paranoia and psychosis (dopamine) to mania (dopamine and norepinephrine). Drug therapies affect specific neurotransmitter-receptor systems and can help to treat disorders of the diffuse, but not the specific, cortical connection systems.

SUBCORTEX

The brain stem, diencephalon, and basal ganglia are early phylogenic versions of the brain. The hierarchy of subcortical and cortical areas reflects evolutionary advances, but cortical areas remain critically tied to and dependent on subcortical sites. Similarly, the development of multiple cortical maps for motor and sensory function reflects a major mechanism in evolution: replication of single body parts (in this case, brain areas) due to genetic mutation. These duplicated parts gradually diverge structurally and functionally over time. Allman[10] offers a revealing analogy:

. . . during a visit to an electrical power-generation plant . . . in operation for many decades, and I noticed that there were numerous systems for controlling the generators. There was an array of pneumatic controls, an intricate maze of tiny tubes that opened and closed various valves; there was a system of controls based on vacuum tube technology; and there were several generations of computer-based control systems. All these control systems were being used to control processes at the plant . . . the older systems were still in use . . . [because] the demand for continuous generation of power was too great to allow the plant to be shut down for the complete renovation. . . . The brain, like the power plant, can never be shut down and fundamentally reconfigured. . . . All the old control systems must remain in place, and new ones with additional capacities are added and integrated . . . to enhance survival. (pp 40, 41)

The subcortex controls arousal, the internal milieu, initial filtering of and orientation to sensory stimuli, coordinated stereotypic response patterns (e.g., "fight or flight"), and execution of complex behaviors, including instinctive responses. Subcortical areas powerfully modulate attention and mood and can also "learn" some "cortical" cognitive and behavioral functions through automization. For example, the basal ganglia and cerebellum are important in procedural knowledge (see Chapter 7), and left-sided thalamic lesions can cause aphasia (see Chapter 6). Subcortical lesions can profoundly disrupt the organism's behavior despite a normal or near-normal neocortex (Table 1–5). For example, a patient with a hypothalamic hamartoma may violently beat a relative despite understanding that doing so is wrong as the cortex cannot inhibit subcortical directives,[16,17] a man with progressive supranuclear palsy is intellectually slowed and functions poorly at work,[18] and a thalamic or

Table 1–5. **Disorders Associated With Subcortical Lesions**

Disorder	Lesion Site
Amnesia	Hippocampus, fornix, basal forebrain (septum, hypothalamus), diencephalon (mamillary bodies, dorsomedial and anterior nuclei)
Aphasia	Basal ganglia, thalamus
Attentional impairment	Midline brain stem and diencephalon, hypothalamus, striatum
Delirium	Thalamus, multiple subcortical gray or white matter areas
Depression	Subcortical white matter (? more with left anterior), caudate nucleus, substantia nigra, ventral tegmental area
Dysarthria	Pyramidal and extrapyramidal motor centers and pathways, cerebellum, motor language areas, subcortical white matter, thalamus, lower motor neurons
Emotional disturbance	Limbic system, basal ganglia, hypothalamus, thalamus, medial forebrain bundle, brain stem nuclei (synthesize biogenic amines)
Frontal lobe syndrome	Bilateral striatum, brain stem nuclei (synthesize biogenic amines)
Mutism	Bilateral cingulate, medial forebrain bundle, diencephalon
Unilateral neglect: usually left side of environment with right-sided lesion	Subcortical white matter, striatum, thalamus

pericapsular stroke can disrupt, usually transiently, language function.[19,20]

Cortical and subcortical anatomy and physiology are intricately interwoven. Lesions in cortical or subcortical areas with rich interconnections cause strikingly similar clinical findings in humans and other species. Bilateral destruction of striatal areas that strongly connect with prefrontal regions causes a frontal lobe syndrome.[21] Right-sided thalamic and striatal lesions of areas connected with right-sided parietal association cortex cause left-sided neglect.[22–24] Bilateral lesions of the hippocampus, mamillary bodies, or thalamic mediodorsal nuclei cause severe long-term memory loss.[25] Akinetic mutism results from large bifrontal lesions involving cingulate and supplementary motor areas, as well as from subcortical lesions in the medial forebrain bundle, which carries ascending catecholaminergic fibers to the frontal lobes.[26,27]

MENTAL STATUS EXAMINATION

Localization of Cognitive–Behavioral Function

The neurologist's law—localize the lesion—also applies to mental function but with some

modification. In cognitive neurology, the area of neural dysfunction, as well as the pathogenesis, must be determined. The components of the mental status examination are separable and can be individually tested and correlated with the anatomical localization. However, localization is an integrative process: anatomical sites in which a lesion may cause specific behavioral changes are systematically explored, and findings from the medical history and neurological examination are synthesized with functional neuroanatomy to identify the pathological focus or foci. For example, synthesis of the diverse mental, neurological, and medical signs and symptoms in an anxious, diaphoretic patient with tachycardia, brisk reflexes, tremor, exophthalmos, and thyromegaly easily leads to a diagnosis of hyperthyroidism.

The approach to localization of complex behavior, such as a language deficit, is similar to that of other neurological disorders. In evaluating arm weakness, for example, the neurologist systematically explores the motor system, beginning with the most peripheral portion (i.e., muscle) and ending with the most central portion (i.e., primary and association motor cortex). Incorrect localization often results from placing the lesion too centrally and failing to consider more peripheral sites, such as the neuromuscular junction, or intermediate sites, such as the plexus or spinal cord. Similarly, in evaluating behavioral changes, it is wise to begin more peripherally before moving to the cortex or subcortical structures. Speech problems may be caused not only by left perisylvian cortical lesions but also by drugs, metabolic disorders, vocal cord lesions, or recurrent laryngeal nerve palsies. Likewise, impaired visual recognition may result not only from a lesion of the visual association cortex but also from eye and optic nerve injuries, as well as psychiatric disorders.

Consider signs and symptoms in the context of the associated deficits. For example, dysarthria accompanied by diplopia and facial numbness suggests a brain stem lesion, but dysarthria accompanied by nonfluent speech with phonemic paraphasias (spoken sound substitution errors such as "slat" instead of "slack" or "boot" instead of "book") and right-sided weakness of the face and arm usually indicates a lesion in the left frontal lobe. Computed tomography and MRI of the brain have permitted almost immediate correlation of clinical and anatomical data, allowing refinement of the localization process. However, overly precise localization of cognitive function is a common pitfall.

The limitations of the localization process remain one of the most durable controversies in cognitive neurology. One the one hand, the extreme view conceptualizing an equipotential cerebral cortex is ludicrous.[28] On the other hand, complex behaviors are more difficult to quantify and localize accurately than elementary neurological functions (e.g., muscle strength); personality cannot be mapped to a small cube of frontal lobe, and affect cannot be assigned to a parcel of temporal lobe. Another potential pitfall in the localization process is the assumption that when a function is disrupted, the area in which the lesion is found subserves that function. As Jackson[29] admonished in 1878, lesions and deficits—not functions—can be localized on the cerebral map. The intellectual leap between lesion site and function site is not trivial. A behavioral disorder emerging after the infliction of a focal lesion is attributable, in part, to preserved areas of the brain. In rejecting the cerebellar "braking" theory to explain dysmetria after cerebellar lesions (the cerebellum was considered to inhibit overshooting and undershooting), Walsh[30] provided an insightful metaphor for misunderstanding brain function:

Consider an automobile transmission with a gear tooth knocked off, causing a "clunk" when the drive shaft turns slowly and a vibration at faster speeds. One might conclude that the gear tooth serves to prevent "clunks" and vibrations, supported by the resolution of these abnormalities after the tooth is replaced. The gear teeth, however, transmit power from the drive to the shaft.

A useful theoretical aid in achieving the balance between too precise localization and overgeneralization is the network approach of directed attention. Using principles outlined by nineteenth and twentieth century neurologists, Mesulam[31,32] constructed an important model for such cognitive processes as language, memory, and visuospatial function. The network theory postulates that complex behaviors are subserved not by isolated centers but by sets of distributed regions that form integrated functional systems. These functional systems, in turn, are determined by neural interconnections. Mesulam[33] summarized the general principles of the network approach as follows: (1) complex functions are represented within distributed interconnected sites that collectively constitute an integrated network for each function; (2) individual cerebral areas contain the neural substrate for several sets of behaviors and may, therefore, belong to several partially overlapping networks; (3) lesions confined to a single region are likely to result in multiple deficits; and (4) different aspects of the same complex function may be impaired because of damage to one of several cortical areas or their interconnections.

This network approach can be helpful in localizing such neurobehavioral functions as subcortical aphasia, particularly in defining the nature of the deficits or predicting the extent of recovery. Although language functions are located primarily in the left hemisphere, subcortical areas important for activation and coordination of cortical functions are interconnected with language areas. Thus, subcortical lesions can disrupt language functions.[19] However, since other subcortical and cortical areas may "replace" the work done by the damaged subcortical areas, subcortical aphasia may be transient.

Finally, the precision with which specific behaviors and behavioral deficits, and therefore a function, can be localized depends on many factors, including age, handedness, the time course and nature of the pathological process, and previous brain insults. For example, a slow-growing, massive right frontotemporal glioma in a young woman may be associated over months with only subtle personality changes, and a small Wernicke's area infarct in an elderly woman can devastate language comprehension in a minute.

Always Test Mental Status

The mental status examination has an undeservedly bad reputation and should never be omitted from the bedside assessment of the patient. It is as inappropriate to omit the mental status examination as it is to ignore testing of muscle strength or reflexes. The mental status examination assesses cerebral cortex functioning. Without it, an assessment of the nervous system is incomplete. Indeed, a mental status evaluation is equally as important as the rest of the neurological examination and can be critical to the correct interpretation of other findings. For example, delirium and brisk doll's eyes are likely signs of hepatic encephalopathy, and the recent onset of memory impairment, olfactory hallucinations, and fever suggests herpes simplex encephalitis. In addition, to mistake aphasia for dementia because language was not systematically tested is as grave as mistaking motor neuron facial weakness for Bell's palsy because upper extremity drift and reflex asymmetries were not sought. The following case report illustrates this problem:

A 70-year-old woman, a multimillionaire, was admitted to an inpatient neurology service with the diagnosis of dementia. She had been well until 18 months earlier when the New York City police discovered her wandering the streets in the middle of the night; she appeared "psychotic." She was admitted to a nearby hospital and treated with chlorpromazine. She was discharged without medication and remained "confused and bizarre." She was followed up for 18 months by an attending neurologist, and was again admitted to the hospital, this time to exclude possible intentional poisoning by a relative for financial gain. Her speech was pressured, fluent, and well-articulated but peppered with neologisms and paraphasias and made no sense. When asked "Where are you," she replied "Where are, where are . . . yes, well of course I was. . . . " "Is it true that helicopters in South America eat their young?" she was asked. "Those children . . . always eating," she replied. The question "Do two pounds of flour weigh more than one?" brought the response "Flour, I love flowers."

This woman had Wernicke's aphasia, not dementia. Screening of language function with testing of comprehension would have revealed the correct diagnosis 18 months earlier.

Recent advances in our understanding of brain–behavior relationships and the recognition that neurobehavioral disorders often occur and are treatable mandate that physicians routinely examine cognition and behavior. Unfortunately, many neurologists mistakenly regard the mental status examination as difficult, ambiguous, time-consuming, better left in the hands of a psychiatrist or psychologist, and, worst of all, irrelevant. It is, or should be, none of the above. One needs only to read a detailed neuropsychological evaluation or watch a lengthy, obsessive language examination to conclude that a resident or practicing neurologist has no time to be fussing over higher cortical functions. However, with experience, an examiner can complete a good bedside assessment of mental status in 15–20 minutes.[34,35] In some instances, by the time the patient's medical history has been taken, the examiner may need only to supplement the observations with a few tests. The essentials of the diagnosis and classification of cognitive disorders are straightforward and can be mastered with practice.

Cognitive–Behavioral Observation

The observation and history of the patient's behavior are the most important aspects of the mental status examination. Diagnostic and therapeutic opportunities are often missed because important clues are never observed or sought. An adolescent with labile emotions and paranoia whose upper lip is drawn tightly over the teeth and whose mouth is open with a fixed smile may have Wilson's disease, as well as primary psychiatric disease. A patient whose dinner plate is clean on the right side but barely touched on the left side may have a lesion of the right parietal lobe and left-sided neglect. Similarly, lack of motor and verbal spontaneity suggests depression or a frontal lobe or subcortical disorder.

Behavioral observation begins with the introduction of the patient and continues throughout the interview and mental status testing. How does he or she greet you (eye contact, speech)? Is he or she distracted by novel stimuli? Is the mood appropriate for the situation? Observing how the patient presents, appears, and behaves provides crucial information about brain functioning. Simple observation reveals signs of many neurobehavioral syndromes, such as masked facies in Parkinson's disease, shaving only on the right side of the face (left-sided hemispatial neglect) in right hemisphere stroke, or fluent paraphasic speech in Wernicke's aphasia. A patient's behavior is also a mitigating factor that profoundly affects the interpretation of test scores. For instance, if a patient is drowsy from medication, scores on all cognitive tests must be interpreted very cautiously to avoid overdiagnosing impairment. Thus, before formal cognitive testing, quickly run through a series of behavioral observations (Table 1–6).

Behavioral problems are easily overlooked for several reasons: (1) most people tend to minimize problems, especially behavioral ones; (2) some patients are not fully aware of their problem; (3) the physician's time with the patient is often limited; and (4) behavioral problems are often intermittent or situation-dependent. These barriers to behavioral assessment can be overcome. Interviews with family or friends, who have the advantage of more extensive and diverse contact with the patient, or with nurses and ancillary medical personnel, such as physical therapists, may reveal vital behavioral information or important insights.

An alert patient who provides a clear and organized account of the present illness usually does not have a major neurobehavioral disorder. However, important exceptions to this assumption do exist, and this is where physicians most often err. In fact, a patient who seems normal on first appearance may suffer from serious cognitive or emotional disorders. Even standard intelligence quotient (IQ) testing may fail to uncover major cognitive impairment. A famous patient, H.M., had bilateral temporal lobectomies and was left with a severe, permanent loss of anterograde long-term memory; but his postoperative IQ was 13 points higher than before surgery.[36] The patient with memory loss may confabulate, filling in memory gaps with the best or most plausible answer.

Table 1–6. **Behavioral Observation of the Patient**

General appearance	Emotional contact: engaged and interested,
Degree of illness, distress, or pain	withdrawn
Age: apparent age vs. chronological age	Anxiety, anger, suspiciousness
Body habitus: obese, anorexic, wasting	Appropriateness of behavior
Facial expression	Affect
Hygiene: skin, hair, teeth, feet, grooming	Normal
Dress: cleanliness, appropriateness	Labile, with prominent fluctuations
Motor activity	Apathetic and unconcerned
Spontaneity (motor, verbal): delay in initiation	Inappropriate (e.g., talks about sad subject but
Level of motor activity: hyperactivity vs.	acts elated)
bradykinesia, akathisia	Mood
Asymmetry of movement: facial expression,	Normal (includes mild sadness or happiness)
extremities	Dysphoric: depression, anxiety, irritability
Abnormal movements	Euphoric: pathological elation, as in mania
Dystonic posture	Labile: broad and excessive mood fluctuations
Tics	Thought and ideation
Tremors	Loose associations: unable to maintain a
Facial grimaces, dyskinesias	coherent stream of thought
Level of consciousness	Paranoid ideation (suspiciousness)
Hyperalert	Illusions (misperceptions of stimuli)
Alert	Hallucinations
Somnolent (lethargic)	Delusions (false beliefs)
Obtunded	Language
Stuporous	Spontaneous speech: clarity, rate, volume, prosody
Comatose	Spontaneous language: fluency, paraphasias,
Interpersonal relatedness	neologisms, word finding
Eye contact	Perseveration or palilalia (pathological repetition)

Corroborate details if memory impairment is suspected. Patients with psychiatric impairments may be aware of their problems (e.g., delusions, paranoia, depression, obsessions, and compulsions) but attempt to hide them. The decision to survey specific symptoms in these patients must be based on behavioral observations and medical history from the patient and others. However, questions about sensitive issues, such as suspiciousness, must be phrased in a nonjudgmental way.

APPEARANCE

Assess the patient's appearance, including the degree of distress, physical appearance, apparent versus chronological age, dress and makeup, and cleanliness and hygiene. Observe motor behavior for spontaneity, adventitious movements, bradykinesia, simple or complex tics, and akathisia.

LEVEL OF CONSCIOUSNESS

Describe the patient's level of consciousness (alertness, wakefulness) in accepted terms and by examples. Consciousness is separated into six levels:

1. *Hyperalertness* includes excessive arousal, motoric hyperactivity, increased sympathetic activity, and distractibility; it may be seen in patients with mania, acute psychosis, agitation, and anxiety.
2. *Alertness* is the normal state of wakefulness.
3. *Somnolence,* or *lethargy,* is a drowsy state in which a person will fall asleep if not stimulated. Recognizing lethargy is important because it may foreshadow a progressive decline of consciousness or may be the initial behavioral change in treatable, but potentially lethal, disorders, such as subdural hematoma. Because lethargy is accompanied by a decrease in attention and cognitive function, the assessment of higher cognitive functions, such as memory and visuospatial skills, in a lethargic patient is unreliable. Do not attempt to assess cognitive functions in a patient whose level of consciousness is below lethargic.
4. *Obtundation* is a pronounced tendency to fall asleep, and frequent and vigorous stimulation is required to maintain wakefulness.
5. *Stupor* is suppressed consciousness in which the patient can be aroused only with constant, vigorous, noxious stimulation. The patient never rises above a lethargic or obtunded condition.
6. *Coma* is the absence of arousal, either spontaneous or evoked. The eyes remain closed, and noxious stimuli provoke no response other than primitive withdrawal movements at best. Acute coma often evolves into a vegetative state, a subacute or chronic condition characterized by sleep–wake cycles and spontaneous eye opening without cognitive or affective functions.[37] Whether the vegetative state is classified as a chronic coma or a noncomatose condition of arousal without awareness is a matter of semantics.

The Glasgow Coma Scale,[38] a system for classifying comatose patients, is based on three categories of response (Table 1–7). The coma scale correlates closely with the outcome: the lower the total score, the worse the long-term prognosis for functional recovery. In coma, it is also extremely important to assess the pupillary responses, ocular movements, and respiration.[39]

Coma must be distinguished from akinetic mutism, the locked-in syndrome, and catatonia. In *akinetic mutism,* the patient appears to be awake and the eyes may follow the examiner, but he or she lacks spontaneous motor and verbal responses.[40] Akinetic mutism may follow bilateral damage to the frontal lobes, including the cingulate and orbital gyri and the septal area,[41] and small lesions of the paramedian reticular formation in the diencephalon and midbrain.[42] The *locked-in syndrome* is characterized by tetraplegia and mutism, with preserved cognition, due to deefferentation of lower cranial nerves and truncal and appendicular muscles caused by infarction of the ventral pons or midbrain.[39] Patients can usually communicate by blinking or moving their eyes volitionally. *Catatonia* is characterized by a dramatic decrease in spontaneous movements and activity and reactivity to the environment. Catatonia is also often accompanied by resistance to movement and cataleptic rigidity. It can have either organic or psychiatric causes.[43]

Table 1–7. **Glasgow Coma Scale**

  I. Eye opening
   1. None
   2. To pain
   3. To speech
   4. Spontaneous
 II. Motor response
   1. No response
   2. Extension
   3. Abnormal flexion
   4. Withdrawal
   5. Localizes pain
   6. Obeys commands
III. Verbal response
   1. No response
   2. Incomprehensible
   3. Inappropriate
   4. Confused
   5. Oriented

Source: From Jennett and Teasdale.[38]

Merely classifying consciousness according to the six levels does not fully describe the behavioral diversity seen in practice, and more complete information is often required to identify changes in the patient's condition. Alertness is a sign of normal consciousness. If the patient is not alert, provide additional descriptive information and define the maximal level of behavioral responsiveness and the intensity of stimulation required for arousal. For example, "The patient is stuporous; he responds to moderate sternal rubbing with eye opening and grunting, and with more vigorous stimulation, he pulls the examiner's hand away. Within 30 seconds after cessation of stimulation, he is unresponsive to voice." In addition, indicate the level of consciousness and other mental functions by recording the patient's responses (e.g., "drowsy, does not know the date") instead of recording negative statements (e.g., "patient is not alert").

OTHER COGNITIVE–BEHAVIORAL ASPECTS

Some other important aspects of behavior also warrant observation. Assess interpersonal relatedness, as indicated by eye contact, degree of engagement, and evidence of hostility or suspiciousness. Observe *affect,* the overt manifestation of emotions. Elevated affect is marked by overly demonstrative emotions, as seen in manic episodes. Normal affect is the expression of emotion consonant with the intensity and content of stated mood and thought, such as smiling when discussing happy events or crying appropriately when discussing grief experiences. Inappropriate affect is the expression of emotions discordant with reported mood, such as giggling when discussing a loved one's death. Restricted or blunted affect is diminished expression of emotion; flat affect is a near absence of mood manifestations (e.g., absence of a smile or frown, emotional prosody in speech). Assess mood (internal feeling state of the patient) by querying the patient; common mood states include anxiety, depression, and fear.

Observation of language may be revealing as spontaneous discourse complements formal mental status testing of linguistics. Assess the mechanical aspects of speech production, such as clarity, rate, volume, and prosody of speech. *Dysarthria* is slurred, inarticulate speech production. An accelerated rate of speech may be seen in Parkinson's disease and may even have a "festinating" quality, mimicking the gait disturbance. *Hypophonia* (reduced volume) is also seen in movement disorders such as Parkinson's disease. *Aprosodia* (disruption of the melodic intonation accompanying speech) is typically seen after injury of the right hemisphere, but also occurs after left frontal lesions. Observe language, the linguistic aspects of communication, for spontaneous word-finding difficulty and circumlocution. Be attentive to the production of paraphasic errors, consisting of whole-word (verbal or semantic) or phoneme (literal or phonemic) substitutions, perseverations, echolalia, palilalia, and neologisms.

Anomalies of thought and ideation may be revealed in the patient's spontaneous discourse and response to questions. Loose associations, in which connections between thoughts are loose and tangential, are found in many neurological conditions, as well as in the formal thought disorders of psychosis. Unexpected delays in responding to questions may reflect problems with attention, comprehension, or mental processing speed; lack of knowledge; or an attempt to deceive. Delusions, paranoia, and distrust may accompany neurological disorders such as reduplicative paramnesia. *Illusions,* distortions of real percepts, and *hallucinations,* creation of percepts that are not there, may occur in some of the epilepsies or after stroke or surgery. In many cases, symptoms such as hallucinations are not spontaneously reported but uncovered only with specific questions.

Testing Cognitive–Behavioral Abilities

The bedside mental status examination is an essential part of the general neurological examination (Appendix A). The goal is a brief functional survey of all areas of the cerebral cortex. Although this may seem a daunting task, the objective can be accomplished by assessing a limited number of cognitive abilities (Appendix B). Even a comprehensive examination can be completed in a short period of time. A common flaw in the performance of the mental status examination is the asking of many questions that probe only a limited number of cognitive domains, usually memory and language, while other cognitive domains, such as visuospatial skills and executive function, are ignored. Structured mental status examinations are summarized in Table 1–8. Scales such as the Mini-Mental State Examination (MMSE), which focus on a test score rather than the nature of the deficits, cannot replace a bedside mental status examination.[46] The mental status examination determines whether all regions of the cerebral cortex are functioning; the MMSE is only useful for deriving a general impression of the patient's cognitive status. Moreover, the MMSE does not test executive function, which can lead, for example, to a missed diagnosis in a patient with severe frontal lobe dysfunction whose test scores on the MMSE are within the range of normal.

The mental status examination should proceed within a hierarchical framework (Appendices A and B). This is necessary because the assessment of certain functions is critically dependent on the integrity of other functions. *Praxis*, the ability to perform a motor movement to a verbal command, can only be assessed after comprehension because normal comprehension is required for praxis. Memory cannot be tested before attention because patients must be attentive for meaningful memory assessment. The mental status examination should test the cognitive abilities of attention, language, memory, visuospatial function, and executive function. Observation while taking the patient's medical history will provide a sense of his or her status regarding attention, language, and memory.

ATTENTION

Assess attention by observing the patient's ability to focus on the questions asked and noticing the responses to distracting environmental stimuli. Attention can be formally tested in several ways. Direct tests of attention include asking the patient to count backward from 20 or to state the months of the year backward. If the patient is inattentive, any impairment exhibited in other cognitive domains may not represent localized brain damage.

LANGUAGE

As tests of language, include as a minimum the assessment of fluency, naming, repetition, and comprehension. Fluency is tested by asking any open-ended question and assessing the patient's ability to produce an effortless, spontaneous, grammatical phrase. The technical definition of fluency is the number of utterances in an unbroken string; the utterances may be words, paraphasic errors, neologisms, clangs, or any other verbal output. For instance, a patient who says "I gripach the zanbo flench aftrot jenning the talsop pleet" is fluent, even though the output contains neologisms and paraphasias. Dysfluent language is the markedly impoverished output typically seen in Broca's aphasia, such as "I . . . I . . . no . . . but, no . . . see!" Naming is tested by asking the patient to name objects encountered more often (e.g., a watch) and less often (e.g., a buckle). If visual agnosia is suspected, ask the patient to describe an object or to identify it in another modality (e.g., examiner jingles a set of keys). Repetition is tested by asking the patient to repeat short and long phrases (e.g., "No ifs, ands, or buts" or "The boxer gets ready for the championship bout"). Comprehension is tested by asking the patient a series of yes-or-no questions (e.g., "Am I wearing glasses?" or "Can you eat soup with a fork?") or pointing to individual objects within a group of objects placed on a table. After this exercise, the test can be made more difficult (e.g., "Point to the object that I use to start my car." or "With the pen, touch the comb"). Praxis bridges the gap between language and motor functions. It is tested by asking the patient to perform buccofacial movements (e.g., "Puff out your cheeks")

Table 1–8. **Structured Mental Status Examinations**

Examination	Skills Assessed	Population Examined	Maximum Score	Timing (min)
Mental Status Questionnaire[44]	Orientation, personal and general information	Mainly geriatric patients	10 (10 items)	5–10
Short Portable Mental Status Questionnaire[45]	Orientation, serial 3s, personal and general information	Mainly geriatric patients	Sum of errors with correction for educational background (10 items)	5–10
Mini-Mental State Examination[46]	Orientation, immediate and delayed verbal memory, language, serial 7s, three-step praxis, copying geometric design	Broad range of neurological, medical, and psychiatric populations	30 (11 items)	5–10
Cognitive Capacity Screening Examination[47]	Orientation, concentration, immediate and delayed verbal memory, language, serial 7s, verbal concept formation, digit span, arithmetic	Mainly medical patients with delirium	30 (30 items)	5–15
Blessed Information-Memory Concentration Test[48]	Orientation, concentration, immediate and delayed memory	Mainly geriatric patients	33 (28 items)	10–20
Blessed Information-Memory Concentration Test (Short Form)[49]	Orientation, concentration, immediate and delayed memory	Mainly geriatric patients	28 (6 items)	3–6
Neurobehavioral Cognitive Status Examination[50]	Orientation, attention, comprehension, repetition, naming, construction, memory, calculation, similarities, judgment	Mainly medical patients with delirium	10 domains (screen and metric approach)	5–30
Mattis Dementia Rating Scale[51,52]	Attention, initiation and perseveration, construction, conceptual memory	Mainly geriatric patients with dementia or delirium	144 (5 domains)	30–45

and limb movement (e.g., "Pretend to salute"). If a language disturbance is suspected, test reading and writing ability.

MEMORY

Memory can be tested in many different ways, and there are many types of memory function. Short-term memory, the ability temporarily to hold on to information, is tested with a digit span (normal performance is six or seven digits). Long-term memory includes both anterograde and retrograde memory. Test anterograde memory by asking the patient to learn five words (e.g., cat, apple, table, purple, bank). After a distracted delay period of approximately 1 minute, ask the patient to re-call them. If the patient fails to recall the words, give simple cues (e.g., "One of the words was a color") or multiple-choice cues (e.g., "Was it blue, green, or purple?") to as-sess whether the problem is limited to a re-trieval deficit. Test retrograde memory by as-sessing the patient's knowledge of recent public or personal events.

VISUOSPATIAL FUNCTION

Test visuospatial function by asking the patient to copy a simple geometric design (for exam-ples, see Appendix B). If neglect is suspected, ask the patient to bisect a line on the page. If the line is bisected toward the right and left-sided hemianopia, rather than neglect, is sus-pected, place the line in the patient's right vi-sual field. A patient with hemianopia will correct the mistake, but a patient with neglect will not. Another method of testing for neglect is to place many short lines in various orienta-tions on a sheet of paper and ask the patient to cross them all off. Patients with neglect fail to cross off some lines on half of the page (see Chapter 4, Fig. 4–3).

EXECUTIVE FUNCTION

Although executive function is difficult to as-sess at the bedside, several easily performed tests may be revealing. Phonemic fluency (e.g., "Generate as many words as possible in 1 minute that start with the letter F") and cate-gory fluency (e.g., "Generate names of ani-mals") are markedly reduced in a patient with executive dysfunction. For example, a patient who is a high-school graduate will generate 12 or more items. A patient with impaired execu-tive functions will have a clearly disorganized approach toward this test, exhibit persevera-tion, and give out-of-category answers (e.g., hamburger). To test perseveration, ask the pa-tient to copy an alternating pattern of loops. To assess the ability to shift a set, ask the patient to recite the alphabet alternating with numbers (a, 1, b, 2, c, 3 . . .). To test problem-solving ability, place a coin in one hand held behind your back and ask the patient to guess which hand it is in. By alternating the choices be-tween hands in a sequential fashion and letting the patient know the correct answer after each guess, he or she should be able to solve the pat-tern within a few guesses. To assess response-inhibiting ability, ask the patient to put up one finger when you put up two, and not to put up any fingers when you put up one finger.

NEUROPSYCHOLOGICAL TESTING

Like the bedside mental status examination, neuropsychological testing assesses the cogni-tive and behavioral manifestations of brain dys-function. Neuropsychological testing is a more detailed expansion of the bedside mental sta-tus assessment, with measures of validity and reliability. Normative values for each neu-ropsychological test are derived from a refer-ence group of neurologically healthy persons. A patient's scores may be examined for the de-gree of deviation from normal or for differ-ences between his or her own tests (*scatter*), which are used in assessing specific strengths and weaknesses and in determining patterns of lateralization and localization of cortical dys-function. Several textbooks[53-55] provide exten-sive information on the administration, nor-mative values, and use with patient populations of the different neuropsychological tests.

Neuropsychological tests are sensitive to dis-ruptions in cerebral functioning and may iden-tify damage to systems that is not evident from neurophysiological or neuroradiological stud-ies. The assessments can help to determine the laterality and intrahemispheric localization of brain dysfunction associated with injuries such as contusions, hemorrhage, tumors, and seizure foci, as well as to identify diffuse dys-function in disorders such as Alzheimer's dis-ease. Neuropsychological testing accomplishes this lateralization and localization by quantify-ing changes in sensory or motor functions and by revealing patterns of higher cortical func-tions (e.g., language, visuospatial abilities, ver-bal memory, nonverbal memory) mediated by specific brain networks. Table 1–9 summarizes neuropsychological tests.

The results of neuropsychological testing can help to identify potential problem areas as well as particular talents or strengths. Testing re-sults also predict many areas of everyday func-tioning, although the prediction of executive, social, and emotional functions in the real world remains limited. This information is use-ful for understanding a patient's ability to co-operate with treatment and care, for making treatment and vocational recommendations, and for planning cognitive remediation. Quantifying cortical functioning also helps to track a patient's progress over time and detects patterns of improvement or decline that can guide treatment and intervention.

Patients are referred for neuropsychological testing to obtain an in-depth assessment of cognitive and behavioral function. Typically, referrals are made to clarify a differential diagnosis (e.g., dementia versus depression, neurological versus psychiatric disorder, consistency with a particular syndrome), to quantify the breadth and degree of deficits (e.g., to obtain a baseline for later longitudinal studies, to assess the impact on daily functions, for forensic assessment or to judge mental competence), to localize brain dysfunction before and after neurosurgery, and to confirm functional localization in the absence of radiological confirmation or to determine consistency with radiological studies.

The neuropsychological evaluation reflects a synthesis of information on the patient's medical history, behavioral observation during the interview and testing, and interpretation of the test scores. Composite batteries of multiple discrete tests from clinical and research studies have largely replaced the fixed neuropsychological batteries (e.g., Halstead-Reitan, Luria-Nebraska). A typical battery consists of tests tapping the same cognitive domains (attention, language, visuoperception, memory, and executive function) that are surveyed in a bedside mental status examination, except that each domain is tested in greater depth. Moreover, other behavioral and cognitive features that are difficult to test at the bedside, such as intelligence and personality, can also be assessed.

Table 1–9. **Neuropsychological Tests for Assessment of Cognitive Function**

1. Symptom validity testing
   a. Rey's 15-Item Test:[54] immediate recall of 15 simple items
   b. Rey's Dot Counting Test:[54] rapid counting of organized and disorganized dot arrays
   c. Portland Digit Recognition Test:[56] forced choice recognition of digit sequences
   d. Test of Memory Malingering:[57] forced two-choice recognition of pictorial stimuli
2. Estimated premorbid intelligence
   a. Regression-based formula using age, education, occupation:[58] limited by regression to the mean; less accurate for outer ranges of intelligence
   b. Highest subtest score in current testing generalized to average premorbid score
   c. Vocabulary Subtest of Wechsler Adult Intelligence Scale–Revised (WAIS-R):[59] may provide better estimate of premorbid and current IQ than adult reading test
   d. North American Adult Reading Test-Revised (NART-R) and National Adult Reading Test:[59,60] may not validly estimate IQ in patients with neurological disorders with suspected language impairment
   e. Peabody Picture Vocabulary Test–3[61,103]
   f. Performance on prior standardized academic tests (e.g., Scholastic Aptitude Test)
3. General cognitive and intellectual abilities
   a. Wechsler Preschool and Primary Scale of Intelligence–III (WPPSI-III):[62] IQ test for preschool children, aged 3–7 years
   b. Wechsler Intelligence Scale for Children–III (WISC-III):[63] IQ test for children and adolescents, aged 6–16 years
   c. Wechsler Adult Intelligence Scale–III (WAIS-III):[64] IQ test for older adolescents and adults, aged 16–89 years
   d. Wechsler Abbreviated Scale of Intelligence (WASI):[65] provides brief estimates of IQ for children and adults, aged 6–89 years
   e. Raven Standard Progressive Matrices (RSPM):[66] nonverbal measure of intellectual functioning
   f. NEPSY:[67,68] composite battery for assessment of children, aged 3–12 years
   g. Repeatable Battery for the Assessment of Neuropsychological Status:[69] brief battery for assessing discrete functions in adults, aged 20–89 years
   h. Kaufman Brief Intellligence Test:[70] derives IQ estimate from vocabulary test and reasoning test
4. Academic achievement
   a. Wide Range Achievement Test–3 (WRAT-3):[71] brief measures of reading, spelling, and arithmetic
   b. Wechsler Individual Achievement Test–2nd Edition (WIAT-2):[72] comprehensive battery of reading, mathematics, and language skills

(Continued on following page)

Table 1-9.—continued

   c. Woodcock-Johnson-III Tests of Achievement (WJ-III):[73] broad coverage of various academic skills
   d. Gray Oral Reading Test, 3rd Edition (GORT-3):[74] standard measure of reading skills and comprehension
   e. Test of Written Language, 3rd Edition (TOWL-3):[75] formal measure of writing mechanics and composition

5. Attention and concentration
   a. Wechsler Memory Scale-3:[76] simple attentional processes (e.g., counting, serial addition)
   b. Wechsler Intelligence Batteries:[62,63,65] complex attentional process (e.g., Digit Span, Arithmetic subtest)
     (1) Digit Span
       Forward: simple attentional processes
       Backward: attentional control processes
     (2) Trail Making Test Part A[77]
       Sequential processing for attention
     (3) Paced Auditory Serial Addition Test (PASAT)[78]
       Measure of attentional capacity and information processing speed
     (4) Corsi Block Span[79]
       Nonverbal measure of spatial attention
   c. Symbol Digit Modalities Test:[80] graphomotor test of sustained attention and processing speed
   d. Continuous Performance Test:[81] computerized measure of sustained attention and vigilance
   e. Mesulam-Weintraub Cancellation Test:[33] letters on a page are aligned horizontally or randomly; patient is instructed to put a line through the target letter; identifies hemispatial neglect
   f. Behavioral Inattention Test:[82] battery for assessing inattention and spatial neglect, relevant to everyday problems

6. Memory and learning
   a. Wechsler Memory Scale–III (WMS-III):[76] most commonly used battery for assessment of auditory and visual memory functions
   b. Memory Assessment Scales:[83] comprehensive battery of various memory tests
   c. Recall of the Rey-Osterrieth Complex Figure:[84,85] immediate and delayed recall of details from complex figure
   d. Brief Visuospatial Memory Test–Revised (BVMT-R):[86] standardized design learning format, including delayed recall and recognition
   e. Autobiographical Memory Inventory:[87] structured interview for assessment of remote autobiographical events
   f. Boston Remote Memory Test:[88] identification of famous faces and remote public events
   g. Pyramid and Palm Trees Test:[89] systematic test of semantic knowledge; assesses access to detailed semantic representations from words and pictures
   h. Pursuit Rotor Test:[90] assessment of procedural memory
   i. Rey Auditory Verbal Learning Test:[91] learning and retention of a 15-word list presented over five trials
   j. California Verbal Learning Test:[92] another serial learning paradigm using a 16-word categorized list
   k. Biber Figure Learning Test:[93] another form of a visual design learning test
   l. Buschke Selective Reminding Test:[94] verbal learning test administered in novel selective reminding format
   m. Hopkins Verbal Learning Test–Revised:[95] brief verbal learning paradigm using 12 words presented over three trials
   n. Benton Visual Retention Test:[96,97] retention of visual designs under various conditions
   o. Design Learning Test:[98] learning a sequence of designs presented over repeated trials

7. Language
   a. Boston Diagnostic Aphasia Examination (BDAE):[99] comprehensive battery of various language skills affected by aphasia
   b. Multilingual Aphasia Examination:[100] language battery consisting of various standardized tests
   c. Western Aphasia Examination:[101] standardized language battery
   d. Boston Naming Test:[102] frequently used measure of confrontation naming to pictures
   e. Peabody Picture Vocabulary Test–3:[103] assessment of vocabulary through pointing to pictures

(Continued on following page)

Table 1–9.—*continued*

f. Benton Sentence Repetition Test:[100] test of the ability to repeat sentences of increasing length
g. Token Test:[104,105] most commonly used paradigm for assessing auditory comprehension
h. Semantic Fluency Tests:[99] generation of word lists from semantic categories (e.g., animals, fruits, and vegetables)
i. Pyramids and Palm Trees Test:[89] formal test of semantic knowledge
j. Test of Written Language, 3rd Edition (TOWL-3):[75] formal measure of writing mechanics and composition

8. Visuospatial and visuoconstructive abilities
   a. Rey Complex Figure Test (RCFT):[84,85] copy of a complex geometric design
   b. Beery-Buktenica Developmental Test of Visuomotor Integration (VMI):[106] assessment of drawing simple to more complex geometric designs
   c. Benton Visual Retention Test:[96,107] measure of visual perception, visual memory, and visuoconstructive skills
   d. Hooper Visual Organization Test (HVOT):[108] mental assembly of fragmented drawings
   e. Judgment of Line Orientation Test:[109] commonly used measure of spatial perception
   f. Facial Recognition Test:[110] matching unfamiliar faces transformed by angle and lighting
   g. Visual Object and Spatial Perception Battery (VOSP):[111] comprehensive battery of tests for assessment of spatial and perceptual abilities

9. Executive function
   a. Wisconsin Card Sorting Test:[112] commonly used measure of hypothesis testing and set shifting
   b. Category Test:[113] standard measure of problem solving and mental flexibility
   c. Trail Making Test:[77,114] measure of mental flexibility, psychomotor speed, and attention
   d. Stroop Color Naming Test:[115] measure of mental speed and response inhibition
   e. Verbal Fluency (CFL, FAS):[100] patient generates as many words as possible in one minute with different letters (i.e., C, F, L or F, A, S)
   f. Controlled Oral Word Association Test (COWAT):[100] measure of verbal initiation and letter fluency
   g. Ruff Figural Fluency Test:[116] measure of nonverbal initiation and design fluency
   h. Gotman-Milner Design Fluency Test:[98] measure of nonverbal initiation and design fluency
   i. Luria's Tests of Sequencing and Praxis:[117] informal measures of motor planning, graphomotor sequencing, and response inhibition
   j. Executive Control Battery:[118] many of Luria's procedures administered in standardized format
   k. Go–No Go Tasks:[119] assess response inhibition
   l. Tests to assess planning and organization
      (1) Rey Complex Figure Test[84,85]
      (2) Block Design Test from WAIS-3[64]
      (3) California Verbal Learning Test[92]
      (4) Rey Auditory Verbal Learning Test[91]
   m. Tower of London Test:[120] assessment of organization and planning abilities
   n. Cognitive Estimation Test:[121] verbal assessment of common sense judgment
   o. Behavioural Assessment of the Dysexecutive Syndrome (BADS):[122] test battery to assess disorders of planning, organization, problem solving, and attention
   p. Frontal Assessment Battery (FAB):[123] bedside test of frontal lobe function; subtests on conceptualization, mental flexibility, motor programming, sensitivity to interference, inhibitory control, and environmental autonomy

10. Sensory and motor function
    a. Sensory Perceptual Examination:[124] standardized assessment of various sensory and tactile functions
    b. Boston Parietal Lobe Battery:[125] qualitative assessment of components of Gerstmann's syndrome (writing, calculation, finger naming, right–left confusion)
    c. Hand Dynamometer:[114] grip strength meter to quantify strength in each hand
    d. Finger Oscillation (Tapping) Test:[114] measure of fine motor control as assessed through finger oscillation speed
    e. Grooved Pegboard Test:[126,127] test of manual speed and complex motor coordination
    f. Purdue Pegboard Test:[128] pegboard test of manual speed
    g. Tactile Performance Test (TPT):[114] test of tactile perception and memory
    h. Edinburgh Handedness Inventory:[129] formal questionnaire assessment of hand preference

Many factors affect performance on neuropsychological testing. Cultural and linguistic issues strongly influence test results. Motivation, like attention, is essential for normal cognition and behavior. Motivation is closely linked with mood as well as sustained attention. Slowed psychomotor speed, confusion, or impaired comprehension may falsely suggest impaired motivation or cooperation. In assessing motivation, note diminished spontaneity of motor and verbal behavior. Lack of spontaneity suggests apathy or abulia, common intrinsic causes of reduced motivation. Unmotivated patients often fail to respond to questions, provide abbreviated and incomplete responses, or respond with a shoulder shrug or "I'm not sure." The examiner must persist, further explaining the test or encouraging the patient to answer the question or follow the command, or patiently wait for the delayed response. Poor motivation, from either intrinsic factors, such as mood disturbances, or extrinsic factors, such as referral for testing by others, can lead to misdiagnosis and artificially lower the scores. For instance, many demented patients are referred by relatives and are not motivated for testing. Their poor performance underestimates their actual capabilities unless they are encouraged throughout the testing. Anxious or depressed but cognitively normal patients may become overwhelmed in the testing situation and perform very poorly. Finally, patients with possible secondary gain (e.g., lawsuits, disability) may deliberately underperform and exaggerate their deficits, from either conscious and intentional malingering or an unconscious motivation to perform poorly.

Underperformance, Exaggeration, and Malingering

Neuropsychological tests are designed to detect underperformance, exaggeration, or frank malingering (Table 1–9). Some of these tests present putatively difficult tasks that are actually quite simple and that even moderately demented patients can perform without much difficulty. For example, the Rey 15-Item Memory Test[91,130] displays 15 items in five rows of three elements each (e.g., A, B, C; 1, 2, 3 . . .) for the patient to recall. Given the structured stimuli and the use of immediate recall with no distraction, even patients with severe memory disorders perform reasonably well. Malingerers give odd responses such as "A, C, 3, 1" with few elements or elements not organized by groups of three. The Rey Dot Counting Test[84,131] displays cards with dots to be counted rapidly; the first set of dots is ungrouped (random), and the second set is grouped (20 dots in five groups of four each). Malingering patients will make mistakes on this easy task and will take as long counting the grouped dots as they did the ungrouped dots.

Some tests for assessing underperformance use statistical probability to determine if a patient's performance is worse than chance alone. For instance, in the Portland Digit Recognition Test,[56] a short digit span is presented and followed, after a short distraction task, with recognition of the previously displayed span versus a foil span. Malingering patients perform worse than chance (e.g., 30% correct) on this two-item, forced-choice task without recognizing the implausibility of their performance. Similar forced-choice testing can detect symptoms such as sensory loss. For example, a patient is asked to answer "yes" or "no" after the examiner either touches or does not touch the anesthetic zone, while the patient's eyes are closed. If the examiner touches the zone 50% of the time and the patient guesses wrong on more than half of the answers, then it is likely that he or she consciously perceives the stimulus (or the lack thereof) and then gives the opposite response. The Test of Memory Malingering[57] is a visual recognition test with forced choices to help discriminate between malingered and true memory impairments. Whenever a patient is referred for forensic assessment or financial gain is involved, some of these malingering tests should be administered.

Intelligence

Most neuropsychological assessments will include intelligence testing. Although the concept of "intelligence" may be of questionable validity, some estimates of global cognitive ability are useful for analyzing the deviation of specific cognitive areas from an average, or baseline, level of functioning. This deviation model helps to identify relative strengths and weaknesses in various cognitive domains, thereby facilitating localization hypotheses, as well as treatment planning and recommendations for return to work, vocational counseling, or other activities.

Estimating premorbid intelligence permits an analysis of whether various intellectual abilities have declined. These estimates are sometimes no more than impressionistic guesses of categorical levels of functioning, based on education or occupation (e.g., "superior" or "below average" intelligence), with little empirical support but intuitive sense. Quantitative formulas that derive estimates of premorbid intelligence from regression equations, based on age, education, and occupational category, have more empirical support than heuristic guessing. These formulas are susceptible to error, especially at the outer ranges of intelligence.[58] Other estimates are based on the pattern of test scores obtained on the concurrent intelligence tests, with the assumption that premorbid intelligence is at least at the level of the highest subtest score obtained in the current testing. Either the vocabulary subset of the Wechsler Adult Intelligence Scale–Revised (WAIS-R) or the Peabody Picture Vocabulary Test–Revised may be a more valid estimate of premorbid intelligence than reading tests, which are less accurate predictors outside of the average range and may not accurately estimate intelligence in patients with neurological disorders and suspected language impairment.[59-61] Yet another method is to examine the patient's performance on standardized tests from school (e.g., Iowa Tests) or admissions boards (Scholastic Aptitude Test, Graduate Record Examination, Law School Admission Test, or Medical College Admission Test). No one technique is definitive, but estimated premorbid functioning is helpful in interpreting actual test scores.

The most widely accepted intelligence test batteries are the Wechsler scales.[63,64] Currently, three scales, each for a different age range, are available. The Wechsler Preschool and Primary Scale of Intelligence (WPPSI) is used for children younger than 6 years. The Wechsler Intelligence Scale for Children–III (WISC–III) is used for children ages 6–16 years. The Wechsler Adult Intelligence Scale–III (WAIS–III) is used for persons older than 16 years. The WAIS–III replaces the WAIS–R,[132] which was used from 1981 to 1997. Some neuropsychologists continue using the WAIS–R when comparison with prior test

results or interpretation of the test profile depends on validation with the WAIS–R. For example, the extended Halstead-Reitan Neuropsychological Test Battery[133] cannot be fully interpreted without use of the WAIS–R. Neuropsychologists must await future research on the validation and normalization of the Halstead-Reitan Battery with the WAIS–III.

The WISC–III and WAIS–III generate scores on the Full Scale, Verbal Scale, and Performance Scale IQs. The Full Scale IQ is a composite of scores from the Verbal Scale and Performance Scale subtests. In addition to these three IQ scores, four indexes, based on factor analytic methods, are calculated: (1) Verbal Comprehension, (2) Perceptual Organization, (3) Attention and Concentration, and (4) Speed. There are 14 subtests in a battery. Each subtest usually begins with easy items and progresses to increasingly more difficult items, with cut-off criteria that help to keep the patient from becoming too discouraged.

The Verbal Scale IQ is derived from seven subtests:

1. The Information subtest is a series of questions tapping the store of general factual knowledge, such as "Who painted the Mona Lisa?" (This and the following examples are not actually from the battery but are representative of the test difficulty.)
2. The Vocabulary subtest asks for definitions of words of increasing difficulty (e.g., *summer, voracious*).
3. The Similarities subtest assesses verbal concept formation by asking the patient to define similarities between pairs of words (e.g., *cat–dog, honest–deceitful*).
4. The Comprehension subtest is more diverse, assessing proverb interpretation and common-sense judgment by questions such as "Why should people obey traffic laws?" and "What does 'Don't cast pearls before swine' mean?"
5. The Digit Span subtest assesses attention, concentration, and rote immediate recall by digit spans forward and backward.
6. The Arithmetic subtest assesses calculation ability by presenting oral arithmetic problems, such as "How much is 3 dollars plus 7 dollars?" and "If nine men are needed to complete a job in 4 days, how many men would be needed to complete the job in half a day?"
7. The Symbol Search subtest, which is op-

tional, assesses simultaneous visual processing and scanning with a strong attentional load.

The Performance Scale IQ is also derived from seven subtests:

1. The Picture Completion subtest assesses visual discrimination by the presentation of pictures in which the patient must identify the most important missing detail.

2. In the Picture Arrangement subtest, the patient must perform visual thematic sequencing and reasoning by arranging a series of randomly ordered cartoon strip frames in the correct order to make a sensible story.

3. The Block Design subtest assesses nonverbal concept formation and visuoconstructional ability by having the patient copy complex colored geometric patterns using blocks that have two white, two red, and two white/red faces.

4. The Digit Symbol subtest assesses psychomotor speed, sequencing, learning, and visual scanning by having the patient write the symbol corresponding to numbers according to a key presented at the top of the response sheet.

5. The Matrix Reasoning subtest presents a series of matrix sequence reasoning problems that assess perceptual identification, nonverbal reasoning, and abstraction.

6. Object Assembly, an optional subtest, is a required subtest on the WAIS–R; it assesses visuoconstructional abilities and visual synthesis by having the patient assemble jigsaw puzzle pieces to make an object.

7. In Symbol Search, another optional subtest, perceptual accuracy, scanning, attention, and speed are assessed by requiring the patient to match two geometric symbols on the left to a series of five symbols on the right.

Most of the Performance Scale subtests are timed, with either time limits on responses or credits for rapid responses.

Because it takes patients 1–1.5 hours to complete these intelligence batteries, some neuropsychologists use short-form estimates of the Wechsler scales. These estimates utilize either combinations of only a few but complete subtests or half of the items from several subtests. These estimates are reasonably valid for estimating the general range of intellectual functioning but are not the actual IQ score. They were derived from the WAIS–R and are not yet validated for the new WAIS–III. The Wechsler Abbreviated Scale of Intelligence (WASI)[65] provides IQ estimates based on a smaller number of subtests and can be administered in 20–30 minutes, in contrast with the WAIS–III, which requires 80–90 minutes to administer.

The Raven Standard Progressive Matrices[66] is a nonverbal measure of intellectual function. The test is most valuable for assessing patients with language disorders and those from other linguistic backgrounds.

The NEPSY, a commonly used neuropsychological battery for children ages 3–12, assesses five domains:

1. Attention and executive functions (inhibition, self-regulation, monitoring, vigilance, selective and sustained attention, maintenance of response set, planning, flexibility in thinking, and figural fluency).

2. Language (phonological processing abilities, receptive language comprehension, expressive naming under confrontation and speeded naming conditions, verbal fluency, and the ability to produce rhythmic oral motor sequences).

3. Sensorimotor functions (sensory input at the tactile level, fine motor speed for simple and complex movements, the ability to imitate hand positions, rhythmic and sequential movements, and visuomotor precision in controlling pencil use).

4. Visuospatial processing (ability to judge position and directionality and to copy two-dimensional geometric figures and reconstruct three-dimensional designs from a model or picture).

5. Memory and learning (immediate memory for sentences; immediate and delayed memory for faces, names, and list learning; and narrative memory under free and cued recall conditions).

Normative data are available to assess children with congenital or acquired brain disorders.[67,68] Like the WISC-III, the NEPSY is used for planning treatment, special education, and long-term follow-up care. The test was developed for both sexes and different racial groups, using brightly colored, attractive materials to maintain a child's interest.

Intelligence can also be assessed by several briefer or self-administered tests. The Repeatable Battery for the Assessment of Neuropsychological Status[69] was developed to identify and characterize cognitive decline in older adults and to screen neuropsychological function in younger patients. The battery takes 20–30 minutes to administer and yields scaled scores for five cognitive domains. The Kaufman Brief Intelligence Test[70] derives an IQ from a vocabulary test and a matrix reasoning test. The Shipley Institute of Living Scale[134] derives a conceptual quotient, from which an IQ may be estimated, from self-administered vocabulary and series problem subtests.

Several other intelligence batteries exist but are used infrequently. The Stanford-Binet Intelligence Test, the original intelligence battery, was widely used before the 1950s, when it was largely supplanted by the Wechsler scales. It is now used primarily for testing very young children or severely retarded patients who cannot complete the Wechsler scales.[135]

Academic Achievement

Many neuropsychological examinations include an assessment of academic achievement, especially in patients with learning disabilities or attention-deficit disorder. Achievement tests assess what a patient has learned, and aptitude tests, which constitute most of the neuropsychological battery, assess what a patient is capable of performing. Achievement tests are psychometrically sophisticated and validated on very large normative samples. Scores are typically provided in grade equivalents or some type of standard score relative to age categories. The Wide Range Achievement Test–3 is a typical battery.[136] It includes three subtests: (1) spelling (written spelling to orally presented words), (2) arithmetic (written), and (3) reading (oral reading, without comprehension). Few neuropsychologists administer entire academic achievement batteries but instead give a few subtests targeting one or more specific presenting problems. Other achievement tests include the Wechsler Individual Achievement Test-2,[72] The Woodcock-Johnson-III Tests of Achievement,[73,137] and tests of reading and writing (Table 1–9, item 4).

Attention

The first step in neuropsychological assessment is an examination of the many different aspects of attention. Mental control tasks from the Wechsler Memory Scale–III,[76] including counting and serial addition tasks, quantify simple attentional processes. The Digit Span and Arithmetic subtests of the Wechsler intelligence batteries are used for tapping more complex attention. Backward digit or spatial span assesses attentional control better than the simpler attention assessed by forward spans. Sequential processing, such as drawing lines to sequentially connect randomly dispersed numbers on Part A of the Trail Making Test,[77] tests both psychomotor speed and attention. Sustained attention and vigilance are best assessed with more complex tasks, such as the Paced Auditory Serial Addition Test,[78] which requires sequential serial addition, or a computerized continuous performance test, which requires key presses to select target stimuli displayed on a computer monitor over a lengthy (usually more than 5 minutes) period of time. Other measures assess spatial attention (Corsi Block Span),[79] sustained attention and processing speed in a graphomotor test (Symbol Digit Modalities Test),[80] and sustained attention and processing speed on a computerized measure (Continuous Performance Test).[81]

Hemispatial neglect can be identified with informal drawing tests, as well as cancellation and bisection tasks. Drawing a daisy in a flower pot, a bicycle, or a clock face will elicit left-sided hemispatial neglect. Neglect is also tested in tasks of cancellation and bisection. Cancellation tests present an array of letters, numbers, or symbols in which the patient must cancel, or strike through, all items matching a target. The Mesulam–Weintraub Cancellation Test[33] presents two versions of letter cancellation; in one, the letters are aligned horizontally, and in the other, the letters are displayed randomly on the page. An analogous form presents simple geometric figures aligned horizontally or randomly displayed on the page. The Behavioral Inattention Test assesses visuospatial neglect with tasks that tap everyday skills relevant to visual neglect.[82] The test may provide insight into difficulties patients experience in everyday life from hemispatial neglect. In a task of line bisection, line segments of different lengths and angles are preprinted on a sheet of paper; the patient must make a slash mark at the exact midpoint of each line. The line is measured with a ruler to determine if the midpoint mark is displaced from the exact center, which can arise from hemispatial neglect.

Memory and Learning

Memory and learning functions are only cursorily examined in bedside mental status testing. For example, the patient's ability to recall three objects or phrases after a delay of 5 minutes may identify gross memory disorders (as well as anxious and inattentive patients with normal memory), but the test is inadequate for detecting neurological disorders with subtle memory impairment, such as early Alzheimer's disease, sequelae of head trauma, postconcussion syndrome, and temporal lobe seizures.

Several batteries for testing memory contain subtests that assess different memory processes. The current standard battery is the Wechsler Memory Scale–III (WMS–III).[76] The Memory Assessment Scales[83] is less often used. The WMS-III is based on a large normal sample in conjunction with the WAIS–III, which permits a direct comparison of IQ and memory. The WMS–III surveys verbal memory, visual memory, and learning as well as a wide range of abilities related to memory, including attention and concentration.

Episodic memory, both verbal and nonverbal, is assessed by three subtests of the WMS–III:

1. The Logical Memory subtest is used to test verbal memory. Two paragraphs are read aloud (one at a time) to the patient, who is asked to repeat them. A half-hour later, the patient again is asked to recall the paragraphs.
2. The Visual Reproduction subtest is used to evaluate nonverbal memory. Four cards with simple geometric stimuli are used; the patient is shown one card at a time and asked immediately to draw the geometric figure from memory, and then, after 30 minutes, he or she is asked to draw the figures again.
3. The Figural Memory subtest is used to test nonverbal memory; the patient must identify a series of geometric figures among a group of foil designs for immediate recognition.

Another test of episodic memory is the Rey Complex Figure Test,[84,85,138] in which the patient copies an unusual and detailed geometric figure and then draws immediate and delayed renditions of it.

Tests of remote memory are not commonplace in neuropsychological testing because psychometric tests are not widely available and are not a part of the WMS–III. Nevertheless, assessment of remote memory can provide valuable information on many neurological disorders. Remote memory of one's own past (i.e., autobiographical knowledge) can be assessed with the Autobiographical Memory Interview.[87] The patient is tested for knowledge of events in his or her own life and for a number of personal facts (e.g., grade school attended), and this information is checked against information obtained from someone who knows the patient well. Because the test of autobiographical knowledge is difficult to validate and administer, other tests of remote memory rely on testing a patient's knowledge of past "public" rather than "personal" events. For example, the Boston Remote Memory Test[88] assesses a patient's ability to remember past events and to recognize photographs of famous people from the 1920s to the 1980s. The Pyramid and Palm Trees Test,[89] described later, assesses semantic knowledge.

Tests of procedural memory are not commonly administered as part of a standard neuropsychological battery. A common test is the Pursuit Rotor Test.[90] In this motor skill learning test, the patient holds a stylus over a target (a rotating light source) and keeps the stylus on the target until it stops rotating. If the stylus is held properly over the target, a tone is emitted. The time on the target over successive trials is measured.

Learning is often used synonymously with memory, but the two processes are partly distinct in terms of cognitive demands and network localization. Memory is usually regarded as the recall of previously presented information, with that information appearing on only one occasion without repetition. Learning also involves recall (retrieval), but the memories for later retrieval are encoded deeper by multiple learning trials of the same material. Hence, memory is incidental recall, and learning is deliberate memorization over repeated exposures.

Several verbal learning tests are currently used in neuropsychological batteries. Each has unique advantages and disadvantages, and there is no "gold standard" test of verbal learning. The Rey Auditory Verbal Learning Test (RAVLT)[91] involves the oral presentation of a 15-word list for immediate recall. Five trials of immediate recall of the list are followed by an immediate recall trial of a different, distracter, list. The patient is then asked to recall the original list. Discrepancies between the various trials are used to assess retroactive and proactive interference effects, as well as learning over repeated trials and immediate recall. There is also a 20-minute delayed recall trial of the original list and a recognition trial, including foils from the distracter trial as well as foils related semantically or phonetically to the original target words. The test assesses verbal learning, interference effects, immediate verbal recall, delayed verbal recall, and verbal recognition. The California Verbal Learning Test (CVLT)[92] uses a similar procedure, but the list contains 16 words organized by four words in each of four categories (fruits, spices, tools, clothes). After the immediate and delayed free recall trial, the patient is given a cued recall of the semantic category (e.g., "Tell me all the spices"). The test is also scored for clustering strategies, as well as acquisition, recall, and recognition. A children's version of the CVLT is also available.[139] Nonverbal learning tests are less commonly employed. One such test, the Biber Figure Learning Test,[93] is similar to the RAVLT but consists of only 10 items, each composed of two geometric figures. After the presentation of all 10 items, the patient is asked to draw them from memory for five learning and recall trials. There is also an immediate recognition condition following the five learning trials and a 20-minute delayed recall and recognition condition.

The Buschke Selective Reminding Test[94] assesses verbal learning with a novel selective-reminding format. Modifications of this selective-reminding format are used to assess retrieval from long-term memory. Several other tests assess different dimensions of learning: verbal (Hopkins Verbal Learning Test–Revised),[95] visual designs (Benton Visual Retention Test),[96,97] and design sequences (Design Learning Test).[98]

Language

Neuropsychological assessment of language, much like the bedside mental status examina-

tion, usually includes testing of speech mechanisms, fluency, naming, repetition, comprehension, reading, writing, and praxis. Aphasia batteries used for formal testing of language ability include the Boston Diagnostic Aphasia Examination,[125] the Multilingual Aphasia Examination,[100] and the Western Aphasia Examination.[101] These batteries facilitate the classification of aphasia syndromes, such as Broca's or Wernicke's aphasia.

Speech and fluency are tested in a manner similar to that of the bedside mental status examination. For example, fluency is typically assessed by counting the number of utterances in an unbroken string and may be elicited in spontaneous discourse or in response to open-ended questions. Word retrieval is most often assessed with visual confrontation naming. In the Boston Naming Test,[102] the patient has to name 60 pictures, ranging from easy (e.g., bed) to very difficult (e.g., yoke). The test includes phonetic and semantic cueing paradigms to differentiate absence of the item from the patient's lexicon or perceptual misidentification from true word finding difficulty. The Peabody Picture Vocabulary Test[140] assesses vocabulary through pointing to pictures, tapping several levels of difficulty for single-word comprehension. For the assessment of repetition, the patient may be asked to repeat increasingly longer and more difficult sentences, as in the Benton Sentence Repetition Test,[100] or to repeat phonetically complex sentences that elicit paraphasic errors, as in the Reading Phrases subtest from the Boston Diagnostic Aphasia Examination (e.g., "The spy fled to Greece").

Comprehension is assessed with various tests and subtests. The Token Test,[104] which assesses propositional language, has the patient manipulate colored tokens in response to the examiner's command (e.g., "Put the red square between the blue circle and the green circle" or "Before picking up the black square, pick up the green square"). Subtests of the Boston Diagnostic Aphasia Examination assess comprehension by testing right–left orientation (e.g., "Show me your right ear") and by requiring the patient to point to pictures representing orally presented words (e.g., "Point to 'dripping' "), to follow complex commands (e.g., "Tap each shoulder twice with two fingers while keeping your eyes shut"), to reply to syntactically more complex ideational material (e.g., "Will a good pair of rubber boots keep water out?"), and to answer "yes" or "no" to questions about stories read to him or her. Bizarre yes-or-no questions asked in a matter-of-fact style (e.g., "Is it true that helicopters in South America eat their young?") can uncover comprehension deficits, especially when followed with a subsequent one that suggests a different answer (e.g., "But how about in Europe?").

Language fluency in tasks can be assessed by listening to the rate, phrase length, ease, and smooth flow of speech (see Chapter 6). Verbal fluency tests, described below, assess the generation of words (e.g., words starting with certain letters, nouns, verbs) or categories.[99,141]

A good test of general word (semantic) knowledge is the Pyramid and Palm Trees Test.[89] Each test item is one target picture or word (pyramid) and two test pictures or words (palm tree and evergreen tree). The patient must determine which of the two test items is most closely associated with the target item. Although this test is mostly a research tool, there are no good alternatives for systematically testing semantic knowledge.

Several subtests from aphasia batteries assess praxis; however, norms are usually absent or minimal, and interpretation is based on pathognomonic signs such as body part substitution (e.g., using a finger to brush the teeth). Diagnostic tests can identify patients with apraxia,[142] although clinical assessment remains the most sensitive and specific tool (see Chapter 7).

Reading and writing are assessed in most aphasia batteries. However, these batteries typically present less difficult items than in achievement tests. For instance, the most complex spelling item on the Boston Diagnostic Aphasia Examination is "conscience." In contrast, achievement tests, such as the Wide Range Achievement Test–3, present increasingly harder items, ending with the most difficult spelling or reading item (e.g., "terpsichorean"). Achievement batteries are usually given to screen for learning disabilities, and aphasia batteries are typically used with the more classic neurological disorders, such as stroke, tumors, or epilepsy.

Writing, both the mechanical aspects in grade school and the creative and expositional aspects in higher education, is the most painfully acquired language function for most people; and individual writing ability varies widely. Therefore, before estimating the writing impairment, it is important to ask the patient with suspected agraphia about writing ability preceding the brain insult. To assess writing, provide unlined paper and begin with the signature, which is the most elementary and overlearned written response. Then, proceed with more complex writing skills by testing the patient's ability to copy and write numbers, letters, words, and sentences on verbal command. Finally, ask the patient to write a paragraph on "an average day in your life" or "how to plan a vacation." Observe the spontaneity, speed, and ease of writing. When the patient has completed this task, check writing for quantity of output, form and size of letters, sentence length, accuracy of spelling, substantive words, grammar, and *paragraphias* (the written equivalent of paraphasias). If mechanical problems of writing are suspected, a typewriter or computer can be used to overcome some apraxic, but not aphasic, disturbances. Writing samples may provide clues to other disorders. In Parkinson's disease, the patient's writing becomes small and tends to run up the paper; and in cerebellar disease, the patient's writing is often enlarged to make it more legible. The Test of Written Language-3[75] is a formal measure of mechanical and thematic writing abilities.

Visuospatial Function

Spatial functions are difficult to quantify and relate to real-world daily activities. The earliest spatial tests, such as the Bender-Gestalt Test[143] and the Graham-Kendall Memory for Designs Test,[144] involved copying tasks, which assess visuoconstructional and planning abilities. These tests are no longer popular among neuropsychologists but are still used by many clinical psychologists to screen for gross evidence of "organicity." More specific and valid tests of spatial abilities are now available. In addition, informal bedside drawing tests (e.g., daisy in a flower pot, bicycle, clock face) assess simple constructional ability and identify hemispatial neglect (see above, under Attention).

The Rey Complex Figure Test[84] is the copying test most commonly used for assessing visuoconstructional abilities. The test is scored for the presence and accuracy of 18 elements within the design, and many neuropsychologists, utilizing a "process" approach, also examine the patient's approach to the test by having him or her use different colored pencils at different stages in the copying process. The copying task is also sensitive to frontal lobe dysfunction, as demonstrated by poor planning and organization, and to left-sided hemispatial neglect, as manifested by the omission or distortion of details on the left side of the figure. In addition, performance may vary according to the side of impairment. Patients with injury to the left hemisphere perform poorly, especially by simplifying the figure and omitting elements; and patients with damage to the right hemisphere tend to distort the perspective or spatial orientation of the figure and may add extraneous details. The Beery-Buktenica Developmental Test of Visual-Motor Integration[106] assesses visual perception and fine motor coordination, necessary for copying and handwriting. In subjects with low scores, further testing may be needed to determine if the problem lies in visual perception or the motor response or both. The copying phase of the Benton Visual Retention Test[96,107] is especially sensitive to hemispatial neglect because most of the designs consist of three figures to a page: two large, complex geometric figures in the center and one small, simple figure in the periphery. All of these drawing tests are confounded by motor function with visuospatial integration because they cannot be properly performed by patients with hemiparesis or peripheral or nonneurological manipulation deficits, which makes their results unreliable.

Several tests are used to assess passive visuospatial perception and integration without a motor component. The Hooper Visual Organization Test[108] consists of a series of line drawings of common objects that have been cut up and randomly presented, rather like a jigsaw puzzle. The patient must mentally assemble the disparate pieces in the "mind's eye" and identify the object. The test is very sensitive to visual synthesis and organization, but performance may be impaired by dysfunction of either the left or the right hemisphere. The Judgment of Line Orientation Test[109] presents two segments of short lines oriented at angles ranging from 0 degrees to 180 degrees, which the patient must match to 10 target lines oriented at the same angles and presented in a sunburst array below the two test items. The test assesses spatial relations and angular displacement and is sensitive to right hemisphere dys-

function, especially of parietal functions. The Benton Facial Recognition Test[110] presents a series of heavily shadowed faces that the patient must match to an array of six faces below. In early trials, only one of the six faces match; and in later trials, three of the six faces match, but they are presented at different angles and different degrees of contrast, brightness, and shadowing compared with the target face. The test assesses facial perception and complex visuospatial integration. The Visual Object and Spatial Perception Battery[111] uses brief, simple tests to identify perceptual problems. The tasks require a minimal motor component but may not reliably assess perception in aphasic patients.

Executive Function

Executive function is a term meant to capture a wide range of abilities that require a cognitively complex synthesis of perceptual and motor systems and is likely dependent on the prefrontal cortex. Typical abilities include concept formation, abstract reasoning, planning, organization, error evaluation, cognitive estimation, cognitive flexibility, and creativity. Executive function is often tested minimally, or not at all, in the typical bedside mental status examination, which may include simple verbal reasoning (e.g., similarities or proverbs). A range of executive functions can be assessed with more complex tasks, and it is for this domain of cognitive abilities that neuropsychological assessment may be the most warranted.

The commonly used Wisconsin Card Sorting Test[112,145] requires the patient to deduce a principle for sorting cards into categories (groups) based on verbal feedback of "right" or "wrong." The stimuli are cards with different shapes, colors, and number of shapes on each card, with four levels of each of these categories, which must be matched to fixed target cards. After the patient deduces the first category (color), the relevant or correct category is changed without the patient's knowledge. The patient must then realize from the verbal feedback that the relevant category has changed, abandon that category, and test new categories. The task requires concept formation and abstraction, maintenance of cognitive set, cognitive flexibility, perseveration, and learning.

Another common test of abstraction and

problem solving is the Category Test from the Halstead-Reitan Battery.[124] The test comprises seven subtests, each requiring the patient to deduce a strategy for categorizing stimuli on a series of cards (20–40 in each category). The sorting principles do not change, as in the Wisconsin Card Sorting Test. The first two subtests have easy categories (Roman numerals, number of stimuli on the card), and the last subtest is a review of the first six subtests. The intervening subtests are much more complex and involve identifying the stimulus that is most different from the other three, the quadrant in Cartesian space of the most different stimulus, and the proportion of dashed to solid lines of a variety of shapes. The Category Test requires abilities similar to those required for the Wisconsin Card Sorting Test but has a stronger learning component and involves the deduction of more complex and abstract categories than the Wisconsin Card Sorting Test.

The Trail Making Test[77,114] requires alternating cognitive set by switching back and forth between a number and letter series. A different type of cognitive flexibility is tapped by the Stroop Test,[115] which requires the patient to rapidly read a list of words printed in black ink (Word Trial), identify the color of printed Xs (Color Trial), and identify the color of words printed in ink of a color discordant to the printed color name (Color–Word Trial) (e.g., the word *RED* printed in green ink must be identified by the patient as "green"). The Stroop Test assesses not only the speed of cognitive processing but also cognitive inhibition and cognitive flexibility by the patient's ability to suppress reading the printed word in the Color–Word Trial.

Verbal fluency is simply the rate of verbal production by the patient, but the term *fluency* is also applied to several verbal production tasks, which are good measures of executive function. One of the most common is word association, in which the patient must generate (orally or, less commonly, in writing) as many words beginning with specific letters as possible in a unit of time. Typically, the patient is given three 1-minute trials with different letters; the letters are usually *CFL* or *FAS*,[100] by which the tests are often called. The Controlled Oral Word Association Test (COWAT)[100] is the most common version of this task. Because of its reliance on verbal productivity, the test is sensitive to frontal lobe, particularly left frontal

lobe, dysfunction.[146] A variation of this task requiring the patient to generate semantic rather than phonemic exemplars (e.g., names of animals, supermarket items, and cities, rather than words beginning with target letters) is more sensitive to temporal lobe than frontal lobe dysfunction.[147] Neurologically healthy persons produce at least 12 words a minute in a phonetic category in 1 minute and at least 10 animal or fruit names in the semantic group. However, the actual number of words generated for these tasks varies by the patient's age and educational status. Nonverbal analogues of the COWAT require the patient to draw random, nonsense geometric figures in a unit of time. These tests of nonverbal fluency, such as the Ruff Figural Fluency Test[116] and the Gotman-Milner Design Fluency Test,[98] are not as commonly utilized as their verbal counterparts but can provide some indication of right frontal lobe integrity.

Sequential motor tasks and tests of motor inhibition, drawn from the theories of Luria,[117] although not generally having norms, can detect premotor and prefrontal dysfunction. The Executive Control Battery[118] utilizes a standardized format for many of Luria's procedures. Typical sequential tasks include rapid sequential finger movements (thumb to digits 2, 3, 4, 5), sequential hand movements (touching the table with the fist, palm, and edge of the hand), and sequential orofacial movements (showing the teeth, protruding the tongue, and placing the tongue between the lower teeth and lower lips). Bimanual tasks, such as alternating between a fist and flared hand, between the two sides of the hands, and tapping rhythmically on the table (e.g., tap twice with the right hand, once with the left hand), are often used. Most of these tasks require repetitive sequences of the given order and are timed, usually for 10 seconds. Response inhibition is tested with Go–No Go tasks. For example, the patient is told "Tap once if I tap twice, tap twice if I tap once" or "If I tap hard, you tap softly; if I tap softly, you tap hard." Although the test score is an important indication of the patient's neuropsychological status, observation and interpretation of the patient's approach to performing the tests provide neuropsychologists with information on the patient's problem-solving and reasoning abilities. For example, planning and organization can be observed when the patient constructs the Rey Complex

Figure Test or the Block Design Test from the WAIS–III. Planning and organization are revealed by clustering strategies used in verbal learning tests, such as the CVLT or the RAVLT (e.g., clumping digits into dyads or triplets on Digit Spans) and generating animal names grouped by family on animal naming or words categorized by phoneme clusters on the COWAT. Although these planning and organization strategies are usually not measured empirically and not scored for deviation from normal (with the exception of the clustering scores on the CVLT), they reveal the workings of executive functions. The Tower of London Test[120] assesses problem solving. Subjects are required to move colored beads on a set of pegs to match a target arrangement. The number of beads and pegs can be varied to increase task complexity. The test is most sensitive in detecting dominant prefrontal dysfunction. The Cognitive Estimation Test[121] asks patients to answer questions that can be answered from general knowledge but for which there are limited strategies available. The original finding that patients with frontal lesions give more bizarre answers than those with posterior or subcortical lesions was questioned in a subsequent investigation.[148]

Several test batteries assess a wider range of executive functions, including the Behavioural Assessment of the Dysexecutive Syndrome[122] and the Frontal Assessment Battery.[123]

Sensory and Motor Function

Tests of sensory and motor function are often included in a neuropsychological evaluation. These tests benefit from a standardized method of administration, which permits comparisons across diagnostic groups and quantification of the degree of deficit. The most common battery for sensory and perceptual problems is the Sensory and Perceptual Examination from the Halstead-Reitan Neuropsychological Test Battery.[124] The first section assesses extinction to double simultaneous stimulation in tactile (left hand, right hand; left face, right hand; left hand, right face), auditory, and visual (superior, midline, inferior aspects) modalities. Visual fields are tested to confrontation in superior and inferior temporal and nasal fields. Graphesthesia (fingertip number writing) and finger agnosia are assessed for

each hand, with four trials on each of the five digits for each test. Stereognosis is tested by presenting small (2 cm) plastic squares, circles, crosses, and triangles to each hand and testing accuracy and response latency. Each portion of the battery generates scores and intermanual differences, which are compared with a large set of normative data. The Boston Parietal Lobe Battery[125] assesses components of Gerstmann's syndrome (see Chapter 6).

Six tests are commonly used to assess motor functioning. The dynamometer, a grip strength meter, is used for quantifying hand strength.[114] The norms for the device are arranged by gender and age and permit intermanual comparisons. The Finger Oscillation Test (also called Finger Tapping Test) presents a telegraph-type key that the patient must rapidly press with the forefinger of each hand separately across multiple 10-second trials.[124] It is sensitive not only to fine motor dexterity but also to fatigue and references age and gender norms. The Grooved Pegboard Test[127] presents a series of holes in a board, with a grooved notch in each hole, arranged in a 5 × 5 matrix, into which the patient must place pegs with a protruding ridge. The test is performed separately for each hand and is sensitive not only to motor speed but also to dexterity because each peg must be placed so that the ridge from the peg matches the groove in the hole. It references age and gender norms. The Purdue Pegboard Test[128] is similar in that the patient places pegs into holes, but the board is larger and requires both gross motor (arm) and fine motor (hand) dexterity. A bimanual trial also permits comparison of unilateral upper extremity performance with bimanual performance. The Tactile Performance Test assesses speed of movement, tactile perception, tactile memory, and problem-solving ability.[114] The Edinburgh Handedness Inventory[129] is a questionnaire that formally assesses hand preference.

Personality, Mood, and Other Psychiatric Traits

Assessment of personality, mood, and psychiatric disorders or traits is usually incorporated into neuropsychological testing through the use of selected instruments (Table 1–10). Depression, anxiety, and psychosis are common behavioral sequelae of neurological disorders

Table 1–10. Selected Instruments for Assessing Psychiatric Symptoms and Quality of Life in Patients with Neurological Diseases

1. Personality
   a. Minnesota Multiphasic Personality Inventory-2 (MMPI-2):[149] most commonly used objective measure of personality functioning
   b. Personality Assessment Inventory (PAI):[150] objective personality instrument that is more brief than MMPI or MCMI
   c. Millon Clinical Multiaxial Inventory–III (MCMI-III):[151,152] questionnaire focusing on personality styles and *Diagnostic and Statistical Manual*, 4th ed. (DSM-IV) diagnoses
   d. Structured Clinical Interview for DSM-IV Axis II Personality Disorders (SCID-II):[153] both self- and clinician-rated versions; developed for general psychiatric, and not neurological, populations; incorporates the DSM-IV system
   e. Rorschach Inkblot Method:[154,155] empirically based scoring and interpretation of Rorschach inkblots
   f. Thematic Apperception Test:[156] projective test based on stories elicited from pictures
2. Affective and other psychiatric symptoms
   a. Hamilton Rating Scale for Depression (HRSD):[157] clinician rating for depression; weighted toward vegetative signs and may be nonspecifically elevated in medically ill populations
   b. Beck Depression Inventory (BDI):[158–160] patient self-rating scale; item content more specific for depression than HRSD
   c. Spielberger State–Trait Anxiety Inventory:[161] self-rating scale, state anxiety (how one feels at a particular moment in time) and trait anxiety (a tendency to perceive certain situations as threatening and to respond to these situations with varying levels of state anxiety)
   d. Hamilton Anxiety Rating Scale (HARS):[162] clinician anxiety rating; weighted toward vegetative signs and may be nonspecifically elevated in medically ill populations
   e. Beck Anxiety Inventory (BAI):[160] patient self-rating scale; item content more specific for depression than HARS; developed to assess anxiety independent of depression; simple to fill out
   f. Millon Behavioral Health Inventory:[151] used to evaluate and screen possible psychosomatic complications or help predict response to illness or treatment, stress-related workers' compensation claims, and potential benefit of rehabilitation programs
   g. Symptom Checklist-90-R (SCL-90-R):[163,164] "Swiss army knife" of Axis I rating scales; covers depression, anxiety, and other symptoms
   h. Brief Psychiatric Rating Scale (BPRS):[165] clinician rating scale covering a range of psychiatric symptoms
   i. Positive and Negative Syndrome Scale (PANSS):[166] clinician rating of psychotic symptoms, designed for use in patients with schizophrenia
3. Neurological disorders
   a. Neurobehavioral Rating Scale:[167] cognitive and behavioral function after traumatic brain injury, also used for other disorders (e.g., dementia)
   b. Mattis Dementia Rating Scale:[51,52] a brief, comprehensive test to measure cognitive status in adults with cortical impairment
   c. Behavior Rating Scale for Dementia:[168] administered by caregivers of demented patients; eight principal domains: depressive features, psychotic features, defective self-regulation, irritability/agitation, vegetative features, apathy, aggression, and affective lability
   d. Neuropsychiatric Inventory (NPI, NPI-Q):[169,170] completed by caregiver, designed to assess behavioral symptoms in patients with dementia, measures symptoms and caregiver distress, available in short or long form
4. Quality of life
   a. Rand 36-Item Short-Form Health Survey (SF-36):[171] widely used generic health-related quality of life measure; 36 items, 12 domains
   b. Sickness Impact Profile:[172] widely used generic health-related quality of life measure; 136 items, 12 domains
   c. Quality of Life in Epilepsy (QOLIE-89, QOLIE-31, QOLIE-10):[173–175] patient-completed rating of quality of life in epilepsy; available in long, medium, or short form
   d. Multiple Sclerosis Quality of Life Inventory:[176] patient-completed rating of quality of life in multiple sclerosis
   e. Parkinson's Disease Questionnaire (PDQ39):[177] patient-completed rating of quality of life in Parkinson's disease
   f. Functional Independence Measure (FIM):[178] evaluates the amount of assistance required by a disabled person to perform basic life activities safely and effectively

(e.g., stroke, head trauma, dementia, Parkinson's disease, epilepsy) that respond readily to psychopharmacological therapies (see Chapter 11). In addition to providing a more comprehensive view of behavioral function, identifying mood disorders and personality traits can result in more accurate interpretation of test findings and symptom reports, as well as suggest therapeutic interventions. For example, memory impairment in depressed patients may partly result from the affective disorder and may improve with antidepressant medication. Similarly, paranoid or neurotic personalities may deny or amplify symptoms, including cognitive and behavioral problems.

Formal personality test batteries can identify the presence and severity of comorbid psychological disorders and the degree of somatization or other neurotic disorders affecting perceived illness. The most common and valid personality inventory is the Minnesota Multiphasic Personality Inventory–2 (MMPI–2).[149] This battery includes three validity scales that assess response sets such as random responding, malingering, faking bad or good, and presenting one's self in a favorable or unfavorable light. It also includes 10 clinical scales originally developed by determining items that best separate normal from 10 diagnostic groups popular at the time. Several of these diagnostic groups are no longer in use (e.g., psychasthenia). Instead, the battery is interpreted by the constellation of profile elevations. There are "cookbooks" derived from numerous large-scale studies identifying the psychopathology associated with patterns of scale elevations, mostly based on the highest two scales. This method of interpretation has withstood the rigor of scientific validation, and the MMPI–2 remains the most valid of personality batteries. The Personality Assessment Inventory[150] provides a briefer systematic assessment of personality than most other scales (e.g., MMPI-2, Millon Clinical Multiaxial Inventory [MCMI]).

Several recent scales focus on the *Diagnostic and Statistical Manual* (DSM) classification system. The MCMI[151,152] is a self-administered questionnaire that assesses DSM-IV personality (Axis I) and psychopathology (Axis II) disorders. It provides scales for 11 personality disorders, three severe personality psychopathologies, seven clinical syndromes, and three severe clinical syndromes. The Structured Clinical Interview for DSM-IV Axis II Personality Disorders (SCID-II)[153] was developed for general psychiatric—not neurological—populations and is available in self-rated and clinician-rated versions.

Projective tests use ambiguous stimuli to elicit responses that reveal underlying personality dynamics. The Rorschach (Inkblot) Test[154,155] is an older technique of personality assessment that once was a common addendum to neuropsychological testing. However, even with more well-controlled studies and validated techniques of interpretation, the Rorschach Test has withstood scientific scrutiny poorly in comparison with the MMPI–2. Additionally, the sensitivity of the test to perceptual disorders from right hemisphere damage has never been adequately addressed. The Thematic Apperception Test[156] is another projective test that elicits stories from pictures. The MMPI-2, MCMI, and SCID-II remain the preferred tools for identifying personality disorders in patients with neurological illnesses.

Mood, anxiety, and psychiatric scales diagnose and determine the severity of affective and other psychiatric disorders. Their growing use in supplementing standard neuropsychological testing reflects the frequency and clinical significance of the target disorders in patients with neurological diseases. For the assessment of depression, the self-reported Beck Depression Inventory[158,160] or the clinician-rated Hamilton Rating Scale for Depression[157] is most often used. The Hamilton scale is weighted toward vegetative signs and may overestimate the frequency and severity of depression in patients with physical disorders. For the assessment of anxiety, the self-reported Spielberger State–Trait Anxiety Inventory[161] is most often used; it provides information on how anxious a patient feels at a particular moment in time (state anxiety) and the tendency to perceive certain situations as stressful (trait anxiety).

More comprehensive batteries for testing mood disturbances and personality styles specific to medical disease, such as the Millon Behavioral Health Inventory,[151] are also commonly used. The Symptom Checklist-90–Revised[163,164] covers a range of Axis I diagnoses, including depression and anxiety. The Brief Psychiatric Rating Scale[165] is another psychiatric inventory casting a broad diagnostic net.

Neurological Disorders

Rating scales for identifying and determining the severity of neurological disorders facilitate clinical research and help to define both their natural history and effective therapy. Many rating scales are available for assessing disease severity, progression, and response to therapy of many neurological disorders.[178,179] Several rating scales focus specifically on neurobehavioral disorders. The Neurobehavioral Rating Scale[167] assesses cognitive and behavioral function after traumatic brain injury but is also used for disorders such as dementia. The Mattis Dementia Rating Scale[52] focuses on cognitive problems in dementia, and the Behavior Rating Scale for Dementia[168] focuses on behavioral problems (i.e., depressive features, psychotic features, defective self-regulation, irritability or agitation, vegetative features, apathy, aggression, and affective lability). The Neuropsychiatric Inventory[169,170] was also developed to assess behavioral symptoms in patients with dementia, measuring symptoms and caregiver distress.

Quality of Life and Quality of Care

Quality of life refers to an individual's well-being and daily functioning. Three principal components comprise health-related quality of life: (1) physical health (e.g., general health; daily functioning; symptoms such as pain, seizures, and medication side effects; strength; ability to ambulate), (2) mental health (e.g., mood, self-esteem, perception of well-being, perceived stigma), and (3) social health (e.g., social activities and relationships). Economic and environmental factors, encompassed by overall quality of life and prominently affected by neuropsychiatric disorders, are not usually included in health-related quality of life.

Quality-of-life issues are most relevant in chronic disorders such as aphasia, epilepsy, and dementia, in which mental and social problems extend far beyond the usual disease symptoms. Quality of life is determined by the patient's perspective, not the physician's. Unfortunately, there is often a poor correlation between the physician's and the patient's assessments of the patient's quality of life. While traditional assessments of a neuropsychiatric disorder and its treatment focus on medical outcomes (e.g., tremor severity, memory score, seizure control,

and adverse medication effects), quality-of-life measures provide essential and complementary information. Quality-of-life measures are increasingly used in clinical trials, nonexperimental outcome studies, cost–utility analyses, and studies of quality of care.[180]

Quality-of-life assessments may be generic or targeted toward a specific disease or disorder. Generic instruments assess a range of functioning and issues of well-being and can evaluate diverse patient populations. Commonly used generic health-related quality-of-life instruments include the RAND 36-item Health Survey,[171] the Sickness Impact Profile,[172] and the McMaster Health Index Questionnaire.[181,182] Generic measurements permit comparisons between patients with different diseases but often lack sensitivity to change or responsiveness to intervention. For example, if a generic instrument does not assess quality-of-life areas relevant to a certain patient group, positive or negative changes in these areas will not be detected when an intervention is made during a longitudinal study. Disease-specific instruments utilize information about the impact of a particular disease on a patient's quality of life. A generic core can be combined with a disease-specific supplement to provide the benefits of both. Neurological disease-specific or combined generic and specific instruments can measure the quality of life for patients with epilepsy, Parkinson's disease, multiple sclerosis, and other disabilities (Table 1–10).

Quality of care is an essential metric for neuropsychiatric practitioners. Measuring quality of care relies on evidence-based assessments of the neurological literature, evaluating the structure, process, and outcomes of care. Outcomes, the impact of care on patients' health, encompass mortality, morbidity, disability, patient functioning, well-being (health-related quality of life), and patient satisfaction with care.[183]

SUMMARY

The cerebral cortex comprises four types in hierarchy of structural complexity: limbic, heteromodal association, unimodal sensory and motor association, and primary sensory and motor. Brain connections are organized into diffuse and specific groups. The diffuse projection systems arise in subcortical nuclei that widely disseminate a specific neurotransmitter throughout the brain. Specific cortical connections permit both serial and parallel processing between cells within a vertical column, in cortical areas involved in a local functional system, and in more extensive cortical and subcortical networks. The brain stem, cerebellum, subcortical nuclei, and cortex have multiple representations of the same functional systems, which are reciprocally connected. Localization of cerebral dysfunction is an integrative process that systematically explores anatomical sites in which a lesion may cause specific behavioral change and synthesizes findings from the patient's medical history and neurological examination with functional neuroanatomy to identify the pathological focus or foci. Patient studies allow us to localize lesions and deficits—not functions—on the cerebral map.

Comprehensive assessment of cognitive and behavioral functions is a necessary component of the neurological examination. At the bedside or in the office, each of the cognitive domains—attention, memory, language, visuospatial skills, and executive function, as well as behavior such as affect, mood, and personality—can easily and thoroughly be assessed within a brief period of time. The components of the mental status examination are separable and individually tested. Coupled with a complete medical history and careful observation of the patient, the mental status examination assesses most functions of the cerebral cortex. Such assessment can potentially reveal focal or diffuse cerebral dysfunction. If further assessment of cognitive or behavioral function is warranted, neuropsychological testing should be performed. Neuropsychological testing is essentially an extension of the bedside mental status examination but is performed in more detail. Its utility in reaching a diagnosis or making therapeutic decisions comes from the normative values for each neuropsychological test derived from a reference group of neurologically healthy persons.

Neurobehavioral assessments of personality, affect, and other psychiatric symptoms often identify clinically significant and treatable problems that complicate neurological disorders. By uncovering mood disorders and personality traits, neuropsychological testing can result in more accurate interpretation of test findings and symptom reports, as well as suggest therapeutic interventions. Quality of life is emerging as a critical concept in the assessment of outcomes for patients with neuropsychiatric disorders.

REFERENCES

1. Meynert T: Der Bau der Grosshirnrinde und seine ortlichen Verschiedenheiten. Vierteljahrsschr Psychiatrie 2:88–113, 1868.
2. Exner S: Untersuchungen uber Localisation der Functionen in der Grosshirnrinde Menschen. W Braumuller, Vienna, 1881.
3. Vogt C and Vogt O: Allgemeine ergebnisse unserer hirnforschung. J Psychol Neurol 25:270–461, 1919.
3a. Brodmann K: Vergleichende Lokalisationslehre der Grosshirnrinde. J.A. Barth, Leipzig, 1909.
4. von Economo C: Zellaufbau der Grobhirnrinde des Menschen. Springer, Berlin, 1927.
5. Mesulam M-M. Principles of Behavioral and Cognitive Neurology. Oxford University Press, New York, 2000.
6. Papez JW: Central reticular path to intralaminar and reticular nuclei of thalamus for activating EEG related to consciousness. Electroencephalogr Clin Neurophysiol 8:117–128, 1956.
7. Zeki S: Localization and globalization in conscious vision. Annu Rev Neurosci 24:57–86, 2001.
8. Kaas JH and Collins CE: The organization of the sensory cortex. Curr Opin Neurobiol 11:498–504, 2001.
9. Picard N and Strick PL: Imaging the premotor areas. Curr Opin Neurobiol 11:663–672, 2001.
9a. Zarow C, Lyness SA, Mortimer JA and Chui HC: Neuronal loss is greater in the locus coeruleus than nucleus basalis and substantia nigra in Alzheimer and Parkinson Disease. Arch Neurol 60:337–341, 2003.
10. Allman J: Evolving Brains. WH Freeman, New York, 1999.
11. Flechsig P: Einige Bemerkungen uber die Untersuchungs methoden der Grosshirnrinde, insbes-ondere des Menschen. Ber Verh sachs Ges Wiss Leipz. Math-Phys Klasse 56:50–104, 177–248, 1904.
12. Holloway RL: The evolution of the primate brain: some aspects of quantitative relations. Brain Res 7:121–172, 1968.
13. Van Hoesen GE, Morecraft RJ, and Semendeferi K: Functional neuroanatomy of the limbic system and prefrontal cortex. In Fogel BS, Schiffer RB, and Rao SM (eds). Neuropsychiatry. Williams & Wilkins, Baltimore, 1996.
14. Bailey P, von Bonin G, McCulloch WS: The Isocortex of the Chimpanzee. University of Illinois Press, Urbana, 1950.
15. Creutzfeldt OD: Cortex Cerebri: Performance, Structural and Functional Organization of the Cortex. Oxford University Press, New York, 1995.
16. Plum F and Van Uitert R: Nonendocrine diseases and disorders of the hypothalamus. In Reichlin S, Baldessarini RJ, and Martin JB (eds). The Hypothalamus. Raven Press, New York, 1978, pp 415–473.
17. Berkovic SF, Andermann F, Melanson D, Ethier R, Feindel W, and Gloor P: Hypothalamic hamartomas and ictal laughter: evolution of a characteristic syndrome and diagnostic value of magnetic resonance imaging. Ann Neurol 23:429–439, 1988.
18. Albert ML, Feldman RG, and Willis AL: The subcortical dementia of progressive supranuclear palsy. J Neurol Neurosurg Psychiatry 37:121–130, 1974.
19. Alexander MP, Naeser MA, and Palumbo C: Correlations of subcortical CT lesion sites and aphasia profiles. Brain 110:961–991, 1987.

20. Bogousslavsky J, Regli F, and Uske A: Thalamic infarcts: clinical syndromes, etiology, and prognosis. Neurology 38:837–848, 1988.
21. Laplane D, Levasseur M, Pillon B, et al.: Obsessive–compulsive and other behavioural changes with bilateral basal ganglia lesions. A neuropsychological, magnetic resonance imaging and positron emission tomography study. Brain 112: 699–725, 1989.
22. Damasio AR, Damasio H, and Chui HC: Neglect following damage to frontal lobe or basal ganglia. Neuropsychologia 18:123–132, 1980.
23. Heilman KM, Bowers D, and Watson RT. Performance on hemispatial pointing task by patients with neglect syndrome. Neurology 33:661–664, 1983.
24. Ferro JM, Kertesz A, and Black SE: Subcortical neglect: quantitation, anatomy, and recovery. Neurology 37:1487–1492, 1987.
25. Squire LR: The neuropsychology of human memory. Annu Rev Neurosci 5:241–273, 1982.
26. Barris RW and Schuman HR: Bilateral anterior cingulate gyrus lesions: syndromes of the anterior cingulate gyri. Neurology 3:44–52, 1953.
27. Ross ED and Stewart RM: Akinetic mutism following hypothalamic damage: successful treatment with dopamine agonists. Neurology 31:1435–1439, 1981.
28. Lashley KS: Brain Mechanisms and Intelligence. University of Chicago Press, Chicago, 1929.
29. Jackson JH: On affections of speech from disease of the brain. Brain 1:304–330, 1878.
30. Walsh FMR. On the role of the pyramidal system in willed movement. Brain 70:329–354, 1947.
31. Mesulam M-M: Large-scale neurocognitive networks and distributed processing in attention, language, and memory. Ann Neurol 28:597–613, 1990.
32. Mesulam M-M: A cortical network for directed attention and unilateral neglect. Ann Neurol 10: 309–325, 1981.
33. Mesulam M-M: Principles of Behavioral Neurology. FA Davis, Philadelphia, 1985.
34. Hodges JR: Cognitive Assessment for Clinicians. Oxford University Press, Oxford, 1994.
35. Strub RL and Black FW: The Mental Status Examination in Neurology, 4th ed. FA Davis, Philadelphia, 2000.
36. Scoville WB and Milner B: Loss of recent memory after bilateral hippocampal lesions. J Neurol Neurosurg Psychiatry 20:11–21, 1957.
37. Levy DE, Knill-Jones RP, and Plum F: The vegetative state and its prognosis following nontraumatic coma. Ann NY Acad Sci 315:293–306, 1978.
38. Jennett B and Teasdale G: Management of Head Injuries. FA Davis, Philadelphia, 1981.
39. Plum F and Posner JB: The Diagnosis of Stupor and Coma. FA Davis, Philadelphia, 1980.
40. Cairns H, Oldfield RC, Pennybacker JB, et al.: Akinetic mutism with epidermoid cyst of the third ventricle. Brain 64:273–290, 1941.
41. Freemon FR: Akinetic mutism and bilateral anterior cerebral artery occlusion. J Neurol Neurosurg Psychiatry 34:693–698, 1971.
42. Kemper TL and Romanul FCA: State resembling akinetic mutism in basilar artery occlusion. Neurology 17:74–80, 1967.
43. Taylor MA: Catatonia: a review of the behavioral neurologic syndrome. Neuropsychiatry Neuropsychol Behav Neurol 3:48–72, 1990.
44. Kahn RL, Goldfarb AI, Pollock M, and Peck A: Brief objective measures for determination of mental status in the aged. Am J Psychiatry 117:326–328, 1960.
45. Pfeiffer E: A short portable mental status questionnaire for the assessment of organic brain deficit in elderly patients. J Am Geriatr Soc 23:433–441, 1975.
46. Folstein MF, Folstein SE, and McHugh PR: Mini-Mental State. A practical method for grading the cognitive state of patients for the clinician. J Psychiatr Res 12:189–198, 1975.
47. Jacobs JW, Bernhard MR, Delgado A, and Strain JJ: Screening for organic mental syndromes in the medically ill. Ann Intern Med 86:40–46, 1977.
48. Fuld PA: Psychological testing in the differential diagnosis of the dementias. In Katzman R, Terry RD, and Bock KL (eds). Alzheimer's Disease: Senile Dementia and Related Disorders. Raven Press, New York, 1978, pp 185–193.
49. Katzman R, Brown T, Fuld P, Peck A, Schechter R, and Schimmel H: Validation of a short Orientation-Memory-Concentration Test of cognitive impairment. Am J Psychiatry 140:734–739, 1983.
50. Kiernan RJ, Mueller J, Langston JW, and Van Dyke C: The Neurobehavioral Cognitive Status Examination: a brief but differentiated approach to cognitive assessment. Ann Intern Med 107:481–485, 1987.
51. Mattis S: Mental status examination for the organic mental syndrome in the elderly patient. In Bellak L and Karasu T. Geriatric Psychiatry; Grune & Stratton (ed.), New York, 1976, pp. 77–101.
52. Gardner R Jr, Oliver-Munoz S, Fisher L, and Empting L: Mattis Dementia Rating Scale: internal reliability study using a diffusely impaired population. J Clin Neuropsychol 3:271–275, 1981.
53. Spreen O and Strauss E: A Compendium of Neuropsychological Tests. Oxford University Press, New York, 1991.
54. Lezak M: Neuropsychological Assessment, 3rd ed. Oxford University Press, New York, 1995.
55. Grant I and Adams KM (eds): Neuropsychological Assessment of Neuropsychiatric Disorders, 2nd ed. Oxford University Press, New York, 1996.
56. Binder LM: Assessment of malingering after mild head trauma with the Portland Digit Recognition Test. J Clin Exp Neuropsychol 15:170–182, 1993.
57. Tombaugh TN: Test of Memory Malingering (TOMM): normative data from cognitively intact and cognitively impaired individuals. Psychol Assess 9:260–268, 1996.
58. Basso MR, Bornstein RA, Roper BL, and McCoy VL: Limited accuracy of premorbid intelligence estimators: a demonstration of regression to the mean. Clin Neuropsychol 14:325–340, 2000.
59. Russell AJ, Munro J, Jones PB, Hayward P, Hemsley DR, and Murray RM: National Adult Reading Test as a measure of premorbid IQ in schizophrenia. Br J Clin Psychol 39:297–305, 2000.
60. Friend KB and Grattan L: Use of the North American Adult Reading Test to estimate premorbid intellectual function in patients with multiple sclerosis. J Clin Exp Neuropsychol 20:846–851, 1998.
61. Snitz BE, Bieliauskas LA, Crossland AR, Basso MR, and Roper B: PPVT-R as an estimate of premorbid intelligence in older adults. Clin Neuropsychol 14: 181–186, 2000.
62. Wechsler D: Wechsler Preschool and Primary Scale of Intelligence–Third Edition (WPPSI-III). Psychological Corporation, San Antonio, TX, 2002.

63. Wechsler D: Wechsler Intelligence Scale for Children, 3rd ed. Psychological Corporation, San Antonio, TX, 1991.
64. Wechsler D: Wechsler Adult Intelligence Scale, 3rd ed. Psychological Corporation, New York, 1997.
65. Wechsler D: WASI, Manual. Psychological Corporation, Orlando, FL, 1999.
66. Raven JC, Court JH, and Raven J: Manual for Raven's Progressive Matrices and Vocabulary Scales. Western Psychological Services, Los Angeles, 1984.
67. Korkman M, Kirk U, and Kemp S. The NEPSY Manual. Psychological Corporation, Toronto, 1998.
68. Kemp S, Kirk U, and Korkman M: Essentials of NEPSY Assessment. John Wiley & Sons, New York, 2001.
69. Randolph C, Tierney MC, Mohr E, and Chase TN: The Repeatable Battery for the Assessment of Neuropsychological Status (RBANS): preliminary clinical validity. J Clin Exp Neuropsychol 20:310–319, 1998.
70. Kaufman AS and Kaufman NL: Kaufman Brief Intelligence Test (K-BIT). American Guidance Service, New York, 1985.
71. Wilkinson GS: Wide Range Achievement Test (WRAT3). Wide Range, Wilmington, DE, 1993.
72. Wechsler Individual Achievement Test–Second Edition (WIAT–II). Psychological Corporation, San Antonio, TX, 2001.
73. Woodcock RW, McGrew KS, and Mather N: Woodcock-Johnson III (WJ III) Tests of Achievement. Riverside, Itasca, IL, 2001.
74. Wiederholt JL and Bryant BR: Gray Oral Reading Test IV (GORT-IV). Pro-Ed, Austin, TX, 2001.
75. Hammill DD and Larsen SC: Test of Written Language–Third Edition (TOWL–3). Psychological Corporation, San Antonio, TX, 1995.
76. Wechsler D: Wechsler Memory Scale–Third Edition (WMS–III). Psychological Corporation, San Antonio, TX, 1997.
77. Army Individual Test Battery. Adjutant General's Office, War Department, Washington DC, 1944.
78. Gronwall D: Paced auditory serial-addition task: a measure of recovery from concussion. Percept Mot Skills 44:367–373, 1977.
79. Milner B: Interhemispheric differences in the localization of psychological processes in man. Br Med Bull 27:272–277, 1971.
80. Smith A: The Symbol Digit Modalities Test: a neuropsychological test for economic screening of learning and other cerebral disorders. Learn Disord 36:83–91, 1968.
81. Rosvold HE, Mirsky AF, Sarason I, Bransome ED, and Beck LH: A continuous performance test of brain damage. J Consult Psychol 20:343–350, 1956.
82. Wilson B, Cockburn J, and Halligan P: Development of a behavioral test of visuospatial neglect. Arch Phys Med Rehabil 68:98–102, 1987.
83. Williams JM: Memory Assessment Scales Manual. Psychological Assessment Resources, Odessa, FL, 1991.
84. Rey A: L'exam psychologique dans les cas d'encéphalopathie traumatique. Arch Psychol 28:286–340, 1941.
85. Osterrieth PA: Le test de copie d'une figure complexe. Arch Psychol 30:206–356, 1944.
86. Benedict RHB: Brief Visuospatial Memory Test–Revised: Professional Manual. Psychological Assessment Resources, Odessa, FL, 1997.
87. Kopelman MD, Wilson BA, and Baddeley AD: The Autobiographical Memory Interview: a new assessment of autobiographical and personal semantic memory in amnesic patients. J Clin Exp Neuropsychol 11:724–744, 1989.
88. Albert MA, Butters N, and Levin JA: Temporal gradients in the retrograde amnesia of patients with alcoholic Korsakoff's disease. Arch Neurol 36:211–216, 1979.
89. Howard D and Patterson K: Pyramid and Palm Trees: A Test of Semantic Access from Pictures and Words. Thames Valley Test Co, Bury St. Edmunds, UK, 1992.
90. Corkin S: Acquisition of motor skill after bilateral medial temporal lobe excision. Neuropsychologia 6:255–265, 1968.
91. Rey A: L'Examen Clinique en Psychologie. Presses Universitaires de France, Paris, 1964.
92. Delis DC, Kramer JH, Kaplan E, and Ober BA: California Verbal Learning Test, Manual. Psychological Corporation, San Antonio, TX, 1987.
93. Glosser G, Goodglass H, and Biber C: Assessing visual memory disorders. J Consult Clin Psychol 1:82–91, 1989.
94. Buschke H and Fuld PA: Evaluating storage, retention, and retrieval in disordered memory and learning. Neurology 24:1019–1025, 1974.
95. Brandt J: The Hopkins Verbal Learning Test. Development of a new memory test with 6 equivalent forms. Clin Neuropsychol 5:125–142, 1991.
96. Benton AL: Abbreviated versions of the Visual Retention Test. J Psychol 80:189–192, 1972.
97. Benton AL: Revised Visual Retention Test, 4th ed. Psychological Corporation, San Antonio, TX, 1974.
98. Jones-Gotman M and Milner B: Design fluency: the invention of nonsense drawings after focal cortical lesions. Neuropsychologia 15:653–674, 1977.
99. Goodglass H, Kaplan E, and Barresi B: Boston Diagnostic Aphasia Examination–Third Edition (BDAE–3). Psychological Corporation, San Antonio, TX, 2000.
100. Benton AL, Hamsher K.deS, and Sivan AB: Multilingual Aphasia Examination, 3rd ed. AJA Associates, Iowa City, 1994.
101. Kertesz A: Western Aphasia Battery, Manual. Psychological Corporation, San Antonio, TX, 1982.
102. Kaplan EF, Goodglass H, and Weintraub S: The Boston Naming Test, 2nd ed. Lea & Febiger, Philadelphia, 1983.
103. Dunn LM and Dunn LA: Peabody Picture Vocabulary Test–III (PPVT-III). American Guidance Service, Circle Pines, MN, 1997.
104. De Renzi E and Vignolo LA: The Token Test: a sensitive test to detect disturbances in aphasics. Brain 85:665–678, 1962.
105. Boller F and Vignolo LA: Latent sensory aphasia in hemisphere-damaged patients. An experimental study with the Token Test. Brain 89:815–830, 1966.
106. Beery KE: The Beery-Buktenica Developmental Test of Visual-Motor Integration, 4th ed. Modern Curriculum Press, Parsippany, NJ, 1997.
107. Sivan AB: Benton Visual Retention Test, 5th ed. Psychological Corporation, San Antonio, TX, 1992.
108. Hooper HE: Hooper Visual Organization Test (VOT). Western Psychological Services, Los Angeles, 1983.
109. Benton AL, Hannay HJ, and Varney NR: Visual perception of line direction in patients with unilateral brain disease. Neurology 25:907–910, 1975.
110. Benton AL and Van Allen MW: Impairment in facial recognition in patients with cerebral disease. Cortex 4:344–358, 1968.

111. Warrington EK and James M. VOSP: the Visual Object and Space Perception Battery. Thames Valley Test Company, Bury St. Edmunds, UK, 1991.
112. Heaton RK, Chelune GJ, Talley JL, et al.: Wisconsin Card Sorting Test Manual: Revised and Expanded. Psychological Assessment Resources, Odessa, FL, 1993.
113. Halstead WC: Brain and Intelligence. University of Chicago Press, Chicago, 1947.
114. Reitan RM and Davison LA: Clinical Neuropsychology: Current Status and Applications. Hemisphere, New York, 1974.
115. Stroop JR: Studies of interference in serial verbal reactions. J Exp Psychol 18:643–662, 1935.
116. Baser CA and Ruff RM: Construct validity of the San Diego Neuropsychological Test Battery. Arch Clin Neuropsychol 2:13–32, 1987.
117. Luria AR: Higher cortical functions in man. Basic Books, New York, 1966.
118. Goldberg E, Podell K, Bilder R, et al.: The Executive Control Battery. Psych Press, Melbourne, 2000.
119. Leimkuhler ME and Mesulam MM: Reversible gono go deficits in a case of frontal lobe tumor. Ann Neurol 18:617–619, 1985.
120. Shallice T: Specific impairments of planning. Philos Trans R Soc Lond B Biol Sci 298:199–209, 1982.
121. Shallice T and Evans ME: The involvement of the frontal lobes in cognitive estimation. Cortex 14:294–303, 1978.
122. Wilson BA, Alderman NN, Burgess PW, Emslie H, and Evans JJ: Behavioural Assessment of the Dysexecutive Syndrome. Thames Valley Test Company, Bury St. Edmunds, UK, 1996.
123. Dubois B, Slachevsky A, Litvan I, and Pillon B: The FAB: a Frontal Assessment Battery at bedside. Neurology 55:1621–1626, 2000.
124. Reitan RM and Wolfson D: The Halstead Reitan Neuropsychological Test Battery: Theory and Clinical Interpretation. Neuropsychology Press, Tucson, AZ, 1993.
125. Goodglass H, Kaplan E, and Barresi B: The Assessment of Aphasia and Related Disorders, 3rd ed. Lippincott Williams & Wilkins, Philadelphia, 2001.
126. Klove H: Clinical neuropsychology. Med Clin North Am 46:1647–1658, 1963.
127. Matthews CG and Kløve H: Adult Neuropsychology Test Battery. University of Wisconsin Medical School, Madison, 1964.
128. Tiffin J: Purdue Pegboard Examiner's Manual. London House, Rosemont, IL, 1968.
129. Oldfield RC: The assessment and analysis of handedness: the Edinburgh inventory. Neuropsychologia 9:97–113, 1971.
130. Bernard LC and Fowler W: Assessing the validity of memory complaints: performance of brain-damaged and normal individuals on Rey's task to detect malingering. J Clin Psychol 46:432–435, 1990.
131. Paul DS, Franzen MD, Cohen SH, and Femouw W: An investigation into the reliability and validity of two tests used in the detection of dissimulation. Int J Clin Neuropsychol 14:1–9, 1992.
132. Wechsler D: Wechsler Adult Intelligence Scale–Revised, Manual. Psychological Corporation, New York, 1981.
133. Heaton RK, Grant I, and Matthews CG: Comprehensive norms for an expanded Halstead-Reitan Battery. Psychological Assessment Resources, Odessa, FL, 1992.
134. Zachary RA: Shipley Institute of Living Scale. Western Psychological Services, Los Angeles, 1986.
135. Thorndike RL, Hagen EP, and Sattler JM (eds): Stanford-Binet Intelligence Scale, 4th ed. Riverside, Chicago, 1986.
136. Jastak S and Wilkinson GS: Wide Range Achievement Test, 3rd ed. Jastak Assessment Systems, Wilmington, DE, 1993.
137. Brown MB, Giandenoto MJ, and Bolen LM: Diagnosing written language disabilities using the Woodcock-Johnson Tests of Educational Achievement–Revised and the Wechsler Individual Achievement Test. Psychol Rep 87:197–204, 2000.
138. Corwin J and Bylsma FW: Translations of excerpts from Andre Rey's Psychological Examination of Traumatic Encephalopathy and P.A. Osterrieth's The Complex Figure Copy Test. Clin Neuropsychol 7:4–9, 1993.
139. Delis D, Kramer J, Kaplan E, and Ober A: CVLT-C California Verbal Learning Test for Children. Psychological Corporation, Toronto, 1994.
140. Dunn LM: Expanded Manual for the Peabody Picture Vocabulary Test. American Guidance Service, Minneapolis, 1970.
141. Baldo JV and Shimamura AP. Letter and category fluency in patients with frontal lobe lesions. Neuropsychology 12:259–267, 1998.
142. van Heugten CM, Dekker J, Deelman BG, Stehmann-Saris FC, and Kinebanian A: A diagnostic test for apraxia in stroke patients: internal consistency and diagnostic value. Clin Neuropsychol 13:182–192, 1999.
143. Bender L: A Visual Motor Gestalt Test and Its Clinical Use. Research Monographs 3. American Orthopsychiatric Association, New York, 1938.
144. Graham FK and Kendall BS: Memory-for-Designs Test: revised general manual. Percept Mot Skills 11:147–188, 1960.
145. Grant DA and Berg EA: Behavioral analysis of degree of reinforcement and ease of shifting to new responses in a Weigl-type card-sorting problem. J Exp Psychol 38:404–411, 1948.
146. Perret E: The left frontal lobe of man and the suppression of habitual responses in verbal categorical behaviour. Neuropsychologia 12:323–330, 1974.
147. Rosser A and Hodges JR: Initial letter and semantic category fluency in Alzheimer's disease, Huntington's disease, and progressive supranuclear palsy. J Neurol Neurosurg Psychiatry 57:1389–1394, 1994.
148. Taylor R and O'Carroll R: Cognitive estimation in neurological disorders. Br J Clin Psychol 34:223–228, 1995.
149. Butcher JN, Dahlstrom WG, Graham JR, et al.: Manual for the Restandardized Minnesota Multiphasic Personality Inventory: MMPI-2. University of Minnesota Press, Minneapolis, 1989.
150. Morey LC: Personality Assessment Inventory: Professional Manual. Psychological Assessment Resources, Odessa, FL, 1991.
151. Millon T, Green CJ, and Meagher RB: Millon Behavioral Health Inventory: Manual. Clinical Assessment Systems, Miami, FL, 1979.
152. Strack S: Essentials of Millon Inventories Assessment. John Wiley & Sons, New York, 1999.
153. First MB, Gibbon M, Spitzer RL, Williams JBW, and Benjamin L: Structured Clinical Interview for DSM-

IV Axis II Personality Disorders (SCID-II). American Psychiatric Publishing, Washington DC, 1997.

154. Rorschach H: Psychodiagnostics: A Diagnostic Test Based on Perception. Lemkau P and Kronenburg B, translators. Huber, Berne, 1942.

155. Exner JE: The Rorschach: A Comprehensive System. John Wiley & Sons, New York, 1993.

156. Murray HA: Thematic Apperception Test. Harvard University Press, Cambridge, MA, 1943.

157. Hamilton M: Development of a rating scale for primary depressive illness. Br J Soc Clin Psychol 6:278–296, 1967.

158. Beck A, Ward CH, Mendelson M, Mock J, and Erlbaugh J: An inventory for measuring depression. Arch Gen Psychiatry 4: 53–63, 1961.

159. Beck AT, Steer RA, and Garbin MG: Psychometric properties of the Beck Depression Interview: twenty five years of evaluation. Clin Psychol Rev 12:77–100, 1988.

160. Beck AT, Steer RA, and Brown GK: Beck Depression Inventory–II, Manual. Psychological Corporation, San Antonio, TX, 1996.

161. Spielberger C, Gorsuch R, and Lushene R: State–Trait Anxiety Inventory Manual. Consulting Psychologists Press, Palo Alto, CA, 1970.

162. Hamilton M: The assessment of anxiety states by rating. Br J Med Psychol 32:50–55, 1959.

163. Derogatis LR, Lipman RS, and Covi L: SCL-90: an outpatient psychiatric rating scale–preliminary report. Psychopharmacol Bull 9:13–28, 1973.

164. Wetzler S and Marlowe DB: The diagnosis and assessment of depression, mania, and psychosis by self-report. J Pers Assess 60:1–31, 1993.

165. Overall JE: The Brief Psychiatric Rating Scale (BPRS): recent developments in ascertainment and scaling. Psychopharmacol Bull 24:97–99, 1988.

166. Kay SR, Fiszbein A, and Opler LA: The positive and negative syndrome scale (PANSS) for schizophrenia. Schizophr Bull 13:261–276, 1987.

167. Levin HS, High WM, Goethe KE, and Sisson RA: The neurobehavioural rating scale: assessment of the behavioural sequelae of head injury by the clinician. J Neurol Neurosurg Psychiatry 50:183–193, 1987.

168. Tariot PN, Mack JL, Patterson MB, et al.: The Behavior Rating Scale for Dementia of the Consortium to Establish a Registry for Alzheimer's Disease. The Behavioral Pathology Committee of the Consortium to Establish a Registry for Alzheimer's Disease. Am J Psychiatry 152:1349–1357, 1995.

169. Cummings JL, Mega M, Gray K, Rosenberg-Thompson S, Carusi DA, and Gornbein J: The Neuropsychiatric Inventory: comprehensive assessment of psychopathology in dementia. Neurology 44:2308–2314, 1994.

170. Kaufer DI, Cummings JL, Ketchel P, et al.: Validation of the NPI-Q, a brief clinical form of the Neuropsychiatric Inventory. J Neuropsychiatry Clin Neurosci 12:233–239, 2000.

171. Hays RD, Sherbourne CD, and Mazel RM: The RAND 36-Item Health Survey 1.0. Health Econ 2:217–227, 1993.

172. Bergner M, Bobbit RA, Carter WB, and Gilson BS: The Sickness Impact Profile: development and final revision of a health status measure. Med Care 19:787–805, 1981.

173. Devinsky O, Vickrey BG, Cramer J, et al.: Development of the quality of life in epilepsy inventory. Epilepsia 36:1089–1104, 1995.

174. Cramer JA, Perrine K, Devinsky O, and Meador K: A brief questionnaire to screen for quality of life in epilepsy: the QOLIE-10. Epilepsia 37:577–582, 1996.

175. Cramer JA, Perrine K, Devinsky O, Bryant-Comstock L, Meador K, and Hermann B: Development and cross-cultural translations of a 31-item quality of life in epilepsy inventory. Epilepsia 39:81–88, 1998.

176. Fischer JS, LaRocca NG, Miller DM, Ritvo PG, Andrews H, and Paty D: Recent developments in the assessment of quality of life in multiple sclerosis (MS). Mult Scler 5:251–259, 1999.

177. Peto V, Jenkinson C, Fitzpatrick R, and Greenhall R: The development and validation of a short measure of functioning and well being for individuals with Parkinson's disease. Qual Life Res 4:241–248, 1995.

178. Keith RA, Granger C, Hamilton BB, and Sherwin FS: The Functional Independence Measure: a new tool for rehabilitation. Adv Clin Rehab 1:6–18, 1987.

179. Herndon RM (ed): Handbook of Neurologic Rating Scales. Demos Vermande, New York, 1997.

180. Gill TM, Feinstein AR. A critical appraisal of the quality of quality of life measurements. JAMA 272:619–626, 1994.

181. Sackett DL, Chambers LW, MacPherson AS, et al.: The development and application of indices of health: general models and a summary of results. Am J Public Health 67:423–428, 1977.

182. Chambers LW, Haight M, Norman G, and MacDonald L: Sensitivity to change and the effect of mode of administration on health status measurement. Med Care 25:470–480, 1987.

183. Ringel SP and Vickrey BG: Measuring quality of care in neurology. Arch Neurol 54:1329–1332, 1997.

APPENDIX A: The Mental Status Examination

Level of Consciousness
- Is the patient awake or alert or somewhere in between? Be as descriptive as possible (e.g., "Responds verbally only to sternal presssure") and avoid terms that carry different meanings for different clinicians (e.g., *lethargic, stuporous, obtunded*)

  Note: Remember that the mental status examination will have localizing value only if the patient is fully alert

Behavioral Status
- Describe the patient's affect (e.g., depressed, euphoric, inappropriate) and other behaviors (e.g., somatic concerns, delusions, hallucinations)
- Describe the patient's insight into his or her illness

Attention

Simple
- Is the patient distractible? Is the patient's attention captured by every random change in his or her environment?

Mental control
- Have patient count backward from 20
- Have patient name the months forward and backward

Sustained
- Have patient indicate whenever you say the letter *A* buried in a 1-minute random list of letters presented to him or her

  Note: Like patients with a decreased level of alertness, a patient with impaired attention will be impaired in other cognitive domains, which will obscure brain–behavior relationships

Speech/Language

Spontaneous speech
- Articulation, volume, latency, prosody

Language

Fluency
- Is the content empty, circumlocutory? Are there frequent word-finding pauses?
- Phonemic paraphasic errors (e.g., *scoon* for *spoon*)
- Semantic paraphasic errors (e.g., *fork* for *spoon*)

Naming
- Confrontation: "What is this?"
- Recognition: "Is this a watch?"

Repetition
- Multisyllabic single words: *Constitutional*
- Phrases: *Methodist Episcopal*
- Sentences: "We all went over there," "Oak trees grow tall"

Comprehension
- Yes/no questions: "Am I wearing glasses?"
- Pointing: "Point to the watch," "Point to the thing that tells time"
- Grammatical: "With the pen touch the glasses"

Reading/writing
- Have patient read words and sentences, including irregular words: *Cough, Yacht*
- Have patient read for comprehension: "Close your eyes"
- Have patient write spontaneously and to dictation

Praxis
- Buccofacial: "Puff your cheeks," "Show me your teeth"
- Limb: "How do you salute?" "How do you wave goodbye?"
- Axial: "Look up," "Stand up and turn around"

  Note: Remember to ask the patient about handedness and whether he or she has always been right-handed

Visuospatial/Perceptual

Neglect
- Line cancellation, line bisection, object drawing
- Extinction to double simultaneous stimulation (also test in tactile and auditory modalities)

Construction
- Copying of geometric designs
- Freehand drawing of objects (e.g., house, flower)
- Clock drawing

Spatial
- Judgment of line orientations; geographic and map orientation

Agnosia
- Visual recognition of common objects (e.g., pen, watch)
- Face recognition, color recognition

(Continued)

Memory

Short-term	• Digit span (normal: forward 7 ± 2, backward 6 ± 2)
	• Pointing span forward and backward
Long-term	• Orientation: ask patient the place and time; if patient does not know his or her own name, then the problem is likely psychiatric
	• Verbal memory: recall of five words (e.g., *cat, apple, table, purple, bank*) after a 1-minute distracted delay; if patient does not recall the words, first give semantic cues (e.g., color) and then multiple choices (e.g., blue, orange, or purple)
	• Visual memory: recall of three geometric figures after a 1-minute distracted delay; if patient does not recall the designs, give him or her a choice
Remote	• Public events, past presidents, autobiographical events
Semantic	• Factual knowledge: "How many days in a year?" "How many ounces in a pound?" "How many feet in a mile?"
	• Category membership judgment: "Which of these items is a vegetable?"

Executive Function

Verbal fluency	• Semantic ("animals") and phonemic ("F")
Response inhibition	• Go–No Go Task: "When I show you two fingers, you show me one finger"; "When I show you one finger, don't show me any fingers"
	• Luria Three-Step Task: side–fist–palm
Problem solving	• Coin Switch Task
	• "How many nickels in $1.35?"
Perseveration	• Drawing loops and alternating patterns
Set shifting	• Oral Trail Making Test (A–1–B–2–C–3 . . .)
Abstractions	• "Why do we pay taxes?"
Judgment	• "What would you do with a stamped envelope found on the ground?"
Similarities	• "Hammer–saw," "apple–banana," "poem–statue"

At the end of the mental status examination, consider these questions:
- Is this level of function likely to impair the patient's ability to function independently in his or her current living situation?
- Is the patient competent to make his or her own decisions?

APPENDIX B: A Brief But Sensitive Mental Status Examination

1. Attention	• Observe patient's attention
	• Count backward from 20
	• Say months of the year backward
2. Language	• Describe patient's spontaneous speech (e.g., dysarthria)
	• Is patient's speech fluent or nonfluent?
	• Name objects
	• Repeat sentences
	• Comprehension of yes/no questions, ability to point to objects
	• Read and write a sentence
	• Test for apraxia: ability to carry out a learned motor command (e.g., "Lick your lips," "Pretend to brush your teeth")
3. Visuospatial	• Bisect lines
	• Copy a geometric design
	• Draw a clock
4. Memory	• Digit span, forward
	• Five-word recall and recognition
	• Recent public events
5. Executive function	• Generate as many animal names as possible in 1 minute
	• Copy alternating patterns
	• Oral Trail Making Test (A–1–B–2–C–3 . . .)

APPENDIX B: *(continued)*

Attention

Observation of patient_____

20 19 18 17 16 15 14 13 12 11 10 9 8 7 6 5 4 3 2 1

Dec Nov Oct Sep Aug Jul Jun May Apr Mar Feb Jan

Language

Speech   *dysarthric /hypophonic /spastic/scanning*

Fluency   *nonfluent/empty/paraphasic/anomic/circumlocutory*

Naming   *high frequency_____ low frequency_____*

Repetition   *normal   abnormal*

Comprehension   *yes/no   pointing   grammatical*

Reading   *normal   abnormal*

Praxis   *buccofacial_____   limb_____*

Memory

	Recall	Cues	Choice	Recall 2	Cues 2	Choice 2
Cat						
Apple						
Table						
Purple						
Bank						

Memory (continued)

Digit span   Forward_____Backward_____

1	7	3	5			4	0	3	2	
9	7	3	1	2		6	9	2	1	8
4	9	6	7	0	6	5	9	4	3	2	6
5	8	2	6	4	1	5	3	9	7	1	5	1	8
9	1	5	7	3	6	0	9	6	0	8	7	2	5	1

Recent events_____

Executive Function

A–1–B–2–C–3–D–4–E–5–F–6–G– 7–H–8–I–9–J–10–K–11–L–12–
M–13 –N–14–0–15–P–16–Q–17–R–18—S–1 9–T–20–U–21–V–22–
W–23–X–24–Y–25–Z–26

"Animals," "F"

WRITE YOUR NAME AND A SENTENCE

_____

COPY THIS FIGURE

PUT THE HANDS ON THIS CLOCK AT "TEN PAST ELEVEN"

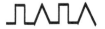

Chapter 2

Functional Neuroimaging of Cognition

Neuroimaging has revolutionized the study of behavioral neurology and cognitive neuroscience. Early studies of brain–behavior relationships relied on a precise neurological examination for hypothesizing the site of brain damage responsible for a given behavioral syndrome. For instance, the association of nonfluent aphasia with right-sided hemiparesis implicated the left hemisphere as the site of language abilities. Clinicopathological correlations were the earliest means of obtaining information about the site of damage causing a specific neurobehavioral syndrome. In 1861, Paul Broca's[1] observations of nonfluent aphasia in the setting of a damaged left inferior frontal gyrus cemented the belief that this brain region was critical for speech output (Fig. 2–1). The introduction of structural brain imaging more than 100 years after Broca's observations, first with computerized tomography and later with magnetic resonance imaging (MRI), paved the way for precise anatomical

localization of the cognitive deficits that develop after brain injury (Fig. 2–1). The anatomical analyses of Broca's aphasia by structural neuroimaging[2–4] determined that damage restricted to the left inferior frontal gyrus causes transient aphasia, with recovery in weeks to months. Damage to deep white matter and insular cortex causes persistent nonfluency. Thus, noninvasive, structural neuroimaging powerfully illuminates the anatomical details of brain injury in living patients. Reliance on the infrequently obtained autopsy is no longer necessary for brain–behavior correlations.

Functional neuroimaging, broadly defined as techniques that measure brain activity, has expanded our ability to study the neural basis of cognitive processes. Measuring regional brain activity in healthy subjects while they perform behavioral tasks links localized brain activity with specific behaviors. For example, these methods detect activation of Broca's area during the performance of a speech-produc-

52

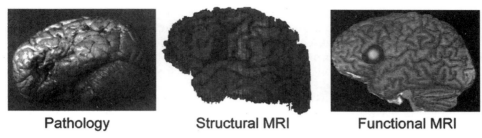

Pathology   Structural MRI   Functional MRI

Figure 2–1. Left panel: The brain of Dr. Paul Broca's patient "Tan," who exhibited nonfluent aphasia after a stroke. Middle panel: MRI scan of patient with Broca's aphasia. Right panel: Functional MRI of the left inferior frontal lobe activated by a speech production task in a healthy subject.

tion task (Fig. 2–1). Functional neuroimaging began with electroencephalography (EEG)[5] and later included magnetoencephalography (MEG).[6] These methods have excellent temporal resolution (i.e., the ability to discriminate neural events occurring on the order of milliseconds), but their spatial resolution is poor as the source of electrical activity, measured over the scalp, cannot be precisely localized. Electrical potentials on the EEG or MEG can be localized only to hemispheric or anterior–posterior differences in the brain. Thus, these methods cannot test hypotheses regarding the precise anatomical location of a brain region serving a given cognitive process.[7] However, EEG or MEG coupled with other functional neuroimaging methods (see below) provides superb complementary information regarding the temporal dynamics of neural events evoked by cognitive processing.[8]

The modern era of functional brain imaging, which brought markedly improved spatial resolution, was introduced in the mid-1970s with the xenon cerebral blood flow technique[9] and was followed in the mid-1980s with positron emission tomography (PET).[10–12] These methods, which measure changes in cerebral blood flow, provide an indirect but highly localized measure of increases in neural activity. However, PET was limited by the need for radioactive tracers to measure cerebral blood flow. In the early 1990s, this problem was surmounted with the introduction of functional MRI (fMRI), which did not require the injection of radioisotopes. Thus, fMRI emerged as an extremely powerful technique for measuring cerebral blood flow and studying the neural basis of cognition.[13] This chapter focuses on the principles underlying fMRI as a tool for exploring brain–behavior relationships.

INFERENCE IN FUNCTIONAL NEUROIMAGING STUDIES OF COGNITIVE PROCESSES

Understanding the link between brain and behavior through a variety of approaches provides tremendous insight into behavioral and cognitive disorders. Because only tentative conclusions can be drawn from studies viewed in isolation, two types of study are needed to provide inferentially sound grounds for the neural basis of cognition. Linking a cognitive process with a specific brain area are *(1)* lesion studies, the examination of deficits caused by specific brain damage in humans or experimental animals, and *(2)* functional neuroimaging studies (e.g., PET or fMRI) of normal, healthy subjects. These dual studies provide complementary but different types of information regarding brain–behavior relationships.

Functional neuroimaging studies support inferences about the association of a particular brain system with a cognitive process. However, these studies cannot prove that the observed activity is necessary for an isolated cognitive process because perfect control over a subject's cognitive processes during a functional neuroimaging experiment is never possible. When a subject performs a task during imaging, it is difficult to demonstrate conclusively that he or she is differentially engaging a single, identified cognitive process. The subject may engage in unwanted cognitive processes that either have no overt, measurable effects or are perfectly confounded with the process of interest. Consequently, the neural activity measured by the functional neuroimaging technique may result from some confounding neural computation that is itself not necessary for executing the cognitive process under study. In other words, functional neuroimaging is an observational, correlative method.[14] The inferences that can be drawn from functional neuroimaging studies apply to all methods of physiological measurement (e.g., EEG, MEG, PET, and fMRI).

The inference of necessity cannot be made without showing that inactivating a brain system disrupts the cognitive process in question. However, unlike precise surgical or neurotoxic lesions in animal models, lesions in patients are often extensive, damaging local neurons and fibers of passage.[15] For example, damage to prominent white matter tracts can cause cognitive deficits similar to those produced by cortical lesions, such as the amnesia resulting from fornix lesions and hippocampal lesions.[16] In addition, connections from region A may support the continued metabolic function of region B, but region A may not be computationally involved in certain processes undertaken by region B. Thus, damage to region A could impair the function of region B via two possible mechanisms: (1) diaschisis[17,18] and (2) retrograde transsynaptic degeneration. Consequently, studies of patients with focal lesions cannot conclusively demonstrate that the neurons within a specific area are themselves critical to the computational support of an impaired cognitive process.

Empirical studies using lesion and electrophysiologic methods demonstrate these issues regarding the types of inference that can be logically drawn from them. In monkeys, single-unit recording reveals neurons in the lateral prefrontal cortex (PFC) that increase their firing during the delay between the presentation of information to be remembered and a few seconds later when that information must be recalled.[19,20] These studies are taken as evidence that the lateral PFC represents a neural correlate of working memory, the cognitive processes supporting the temporary maintenance and manipulation of information (see Chapter 9).[21,22] The necessity of this region for working memory was demonstrated in monkey studies, showing that lesions of the lateral PFC impair performance on working memory tasks but not on tasks that require visual discrimination and saccades without the requirement of temporarily holding information in memory.[23] Delay-specific neurons are also found in the hippocampus,[24,25] a region involved in long-

term memory, as opposed to working, or short-term, memory (see Chapter 8). Hippocampal lesions do not impair performance on most working memory tasks (with short delay periods), which suggests that the hippocampus is involved in maintaining information over short periods of time but is not necessary for this cognitive operation.[26] Observations in humans support this notion. For example, the well-studied patient H.M., with complete bilateral hippocampal damage and the severe inability to learn new information, could nevertheless perform normally on working memory tasks such as Digit Span.[27] The hippocampus may be specifically involved in working memory only when novel information must be remembered.[28]

When the results from lesion and functional neuroimaging studies are combined, a stronger level of inference emerges.[29] As in the example above, in certain instances, a patient with a lesion of a specific brain region shows impairment of a given cognitive process, and when engaged by an intact subject, that cognitive process evokes neural activity in the same brain region. In this instance, the inference that this brain region is computationally necessary for the cognitive process is rendered less vulnerable to the faults associated with each study performed in isolation. Thus, lesion and functional neuroimaging studies are complementary, each providing inferential support that the other lacks.

Other types of inferential failure can occur in the interpretation of functional neuroimaging studies in particular. First, assuming that a particular brain region is activated by a cognitive process (evoked by a particular task), the neural activity in that brain region must depend on engaging that particular cognitive process. For example, a brain region showing greater activation to faces than to other stimuli, such as photographs of cars or buildings, is considered to engage face perception processes. However, this region may also support other cognitive processes.[30] Second, assuming that a particular brain region is activated during the performance of a cognitive task, the cognitive process supported by that region must be engaged by the subject during the task. For example, observing activation of the frontal lobes during a mental rotation task, Cohen et al.[31] proposed that subjects used working memory to recall the identity of the rotated target.

(They derived this assumption from other imaging studies showing activation of the frontal lobes during working memory tasks.) However, in this example, because some other cognitive process supported by the frontal lobes could have activated this region,[32] one cannot be sure that working memory was engaged to activate the frontal lobes. In summary, interpretation of the results of studies attempting to link brain and behavior rests on numerous assumptions. Familiarity with the types of inference that can and cannot be drawn from these studies should be helpful for assessing the validity of the findings of functional neuroimaging studies.

PRINCIPLES OF FUNCTIONAL MAGNETIC RESONANCE IMAGING

Functional MRI is the predominant method for studying cognitive activation. It has several advantages over PET. For instance, in addition to not requiring the injection of a radioisotope, fMRI is noninvasive and has better spatial (on the order of millimeters vs. centimeters) and temporal (on the order of a few seconds vs. tens of seconds) resolution. The temporal and spatial resolutions of fMRI, PET, and other functional neuroimaging methods are shown in Figure 2–2. In selected circumstances, however, PET is superior to fMRI for studying cognition. Currently, fMRI does not clearly image the regions within the orbitofrontal cortex and the anterior or inferior temporal lobe because of the susceptibility to artifact near the interface of the brain and sinuses. Improvements in pulse sequences for acquiring fMRI data should eventually eliminate these artifacts.[33] Electrophysiological recording (e.g., electromyography to measure muscle contraction) during fMRI presents a technical challenge.[34] Functional MRI is exquisitely sensitive to head motion, degrading the images of some subjects, such as agitated patients or normal subjects while talking. However, fMRI scans can be performed

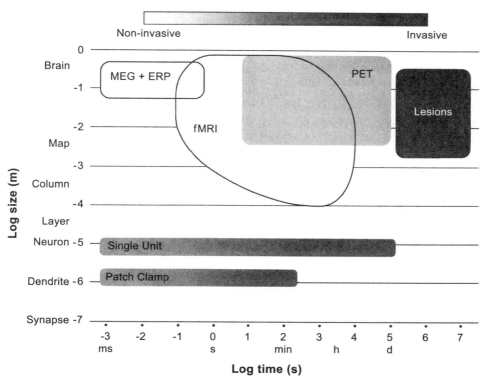

Figure 2–2. Temporal and spatial resolution of different neuroscience methods. fMRI, functional magnetic resonance imaging; PET, position emission tomography; MEG, magnetoencephalography; ERP, event-related potential. (Adapted from Churchland and Sejnowski.[105].)

successfully while the subject makes overt verbal responses.[35] Finally, the pulsing of the fMRI gradient coils is noisy, making the study of auditory processes challenging.[36]

Understanding the proposed physiological basis of the fMRI signal provides a foundation for designing and interpreting fMRI studies of cognition. (For details on the physics of MRI, see the monographs by Horowitz[37] and Buxton[38]) In MRI, hydrogen nuclei in tissue are excited (i.e., put into a higher energy state) by brief exposure to radiofrequency energy. Excitation of the hydrogen protons changes the orientation of their magnetic moments (i.e., changes the direction of the respective magnetic fields of the nuclei in the tissue) away from the main magnetic field of the MRI scanner. After excitation, the magnetic moments take time to reorient with the main magnetic field (i.e., they return to a lower energy state). As they reorient, each nucleus precesses (a wobbling motion similar to a spinning top) about the main magnetic field, releasing radiofrequency energy at a frequency that depends on its precession frequency. The precession frequency of a nucleus depends on the local magnetic field. Deoxyhemoglobin is paramagnetic; it possesses magnetic properties. Because deoxyhemoglobin is paramagnetic, increases in its concentration in a brain region increase the local inhomogeneity in the magnetic field, which decreases the magnetic resonance signal.

Sensitivity for detection of the fMRI signal depends on the blood flow–mediated relation between the concentration of deoxyhemoglobin and neural activity. When a neural event occurs in a brain region, local blood flow subsequently increases[39] and the concentration of deoxygenated hemoglobin in the microvasculature of the activated region paradoxically decreases.[40] This change leads to an increase in the fMRI signal, which is called the *blood oxygenated level-dependent (BOLD) response*.[41,42] In sum, by measuring cerebral blood flow, fMRI indirectly measures neural activity.[43]

The temporal dynamics of neural activity, that is, the time scale on which neural changes occur, are quite rapid, even in frontal or parietal association cortices. For example, neural activity in the lateral intraparietal area of monkeys increases within 100 milliseconds of the visual presentation of a saccade target.[44] In contrast, the fMRI signal gradually increases to its peak magnitude within 4–6 seconds after an experimentally induced brief (<1 second) change in neural activity and then decays back to baseline after several more seconds.[45–47] This slow time course of fMRI signal change in response to such a brief increase in neural activity is informally referred to as the *BOLD fMRI hemodynamic response* or, simply, the *hemodynamic response*. Figure 2–3 shows a hemodynamic response, acquired from the primary sensorimotor cortex of a healthy young subject, during a motor response to a visual stimulus. In contrast, changes in neural activity of primary motor cortex, with simple reaction time tasks, are usually concluded within a few hundred milliseconds after the response cue is presented.[48] Thus, neural dynamics and neurally evoked hemodynamics, as measured with fMRI, are on quite different time scales.

The sluggishness of the hemodynamic response limits the temporal resolution of the fMRI signal to a few seconds as opposed to the millisecond temporal resolution of electrophysiological recordings of neural activity, such as from single-unit recording in monkeys and EEG or MEG in humans. The temporal resolution of fMRI limits the detection of sequential changes in neural activity that occur rapidly with respect to the hemodynamic response. That is, the ability to resolve the changes in the fMRI signal associated with two neural events often requires the separation of those events by a relatively long period of time compared with the width of the hemodynamic response. In general, evoked fMRI responses to discrete neural events separated by at least 4 seconds are well within the range of resolution.[49] However, provided that the stimuli were presented randomly, studies showed significant differential functional responses between two events (e.g., flashing visual stimuli) spaced as closely as 500 milliseconds apart.[50–52] In some tasks, the order of individual trial events cannot be randomized. In working memory tasks, for example, the presentation of the information to be remembered, the delay period, and the period when the subject must recall the information are individual trial events whose order cannot be randomized. In these tasks, short time scales (<4 seconds) cannot be temporally resolved. The temporal resolution issues in fMRI have been extensively reviewed.[53,54]

Paradoxically, brief changes in neural activity can be detected with reasonable statistical

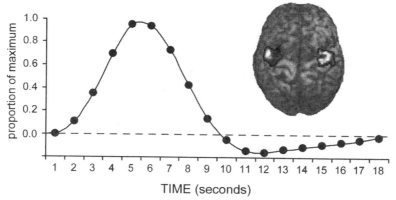

Figure 2–3. A typical hemodynamic response (i.e., functional magnetic resonance imaging [fMRI] signal change in response to a brief increase of neural activity) from the primary sensorimotor cortex. The fMRI signal peaked approximately 5 seconds after the onset of the motor response (at time 0).

power, despite the limited temporal resolution of fMRI (Fig. 2–3). For example, fMRI responses were observed in sensorimotor cortex in association with single finger movements[55] and in visual cortex during very briefly presented (34 milliseconds) visual stimuli.[56] As mentioned, the limitation in temporal resolution is resolving two brief sequential neural events.

In sum, of the functional neuroimaging methods available for human use, fMRI best balances temporal and spatial resolution, making it a powerful method for neuroscience research and, potentially, clinical applications.

ISSUES IN FUNCTIONAL MAGNETIC RESONANCE IMAGING EXPERIMENTAL DESIGN

Blocked Designs

The prototypical fMRI experimental design is a "boxcar," in which two behavioral tasks alternate over the course of a scanning session and the fMRI signal between the two tasks is compared. This is known as a *blocked design.* For example, a given block might present a series of faces for passive perception, which evokes a particular cognitive process, such as face perception. The experimental block alternates with a control block, which is designed to evoke all of the cognitive processes present in the experimental block except for the cog-

nitive process of interest. For example, the control block in an experiment designed to activate a region dedicated to face perception may comprise a series of objects. In this way, the stimuli used in experimental and control tasks have similar visual attributes but differ in the attribute of interest (i.e., faces). The inferential framework of cognitive subtraction[57] attributes differences in neural activity between the two tasks to the specific cognitive process (i.e., face perception) (Fig. 2–4). Originally, the cognitive subtraction method was a major innovation in imaging;[12,57] subtraction was originally conceived by Donders,[58] in the late 1800s for studying the chronometric substrates of cognitive processes.[59] However, the assumptions required for this method may not always hold and could produce erroneous interpretation of functional neuroimaging data.[49]

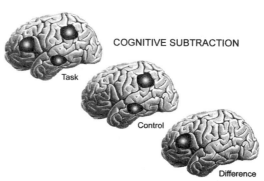

Figure 2–4. Schematic of the principles of cognitive subtraction. fMRI, functional magnetic resonance imaging.

Cognitive subtraction relies on two assumptions: pure insertion and linearity. *Pure insertion* implies that a cognitive process can be added to a preexisting set of cognitive processes without affecting them. This assumption is difficult to prove because one needs an independent measure of the preexisting processes in the absence and presence of the new process.[59] If pure insertion fails as an assumption, a difference in the neuroimaging signal between the two tasks might be observed, not because a specific cognitive process was engaged in one task and not the other but because the added cognitive process and the preexisting cognitive processes interact. For instance, a possible failure of this assumption is illustrated by working memory studies using delayed-response tasks. These tasks (for an example, *see* Jonides et al.[60]) typically present information that the subject must remember (engaging an "encoding" process), followed by a delay period during which the subject must hold the information in memory (engaging a "memory" process) and then by a probe that requires the subject to make a decision based on the stored information (engaging a "retrieval" process). The brain regions engaged by evoking the memory process theoretically are revealed by subtracting the hemodynamic signal measured by PET or fMRI during a block of trials that do not have a delay period (engaging the encoding and retrieval processes) from a block of trials with a delay period (engaging the encoding, memory, and retrieval processes). In this example, if the insertion of a delay period between the encoding and retrieval processes affects these other behavioral processes in the task, the result is failure to meet the assumptions of cognitive subtraction. That is, these "nonmemory" processes may differ in delay trials and no-delay trials.

In functional neuroimaging, the transform between the neural signal and the hemodynamic response (measured by fMRI) must be linear for the cognitive subtractive method to yield valid results. In several studies, linearity did not strictly hold for the BOLD fMRI system.[47,61] In the foregoing example of a delayed-response task, the method fails if the summed transform of neural activity to the hemodynamic signal for the encoding and retrieval processes differs for a delay trial and a no-delay trial. In this example, such artifacts of cognitive subtraction might lead to the inference that a brain region displayed delay-correlated increases in neural activity and, therefore, is a memory region when it is not since the differences might be associated with changes in other cognitive processes. Evidence of such failure exists.[62]

In addition to the limitations of cognitive subtraction, blocked designs do not allow randomization of stimuli order and are constrained to the grouping of trials of the same type with each other in time. The consequent predictability of trial type may confound a blocked experiment. For instance, most early functional neuroimaging studies of the neural substrates of recognition memory presented subjects with blocks of either all old stimuli (i.e., previously presented during an encoding condition) or all new stimuli (i.e., not presented during an encoding condition) together for judgments of recognition.[63,64] This situation highlights the *a priori* undesirability of being constrained to presented blocks of identical trials. The influence of trial order, whether blocked or randomized, on functional neuroimaging data can occur on at least two levels. First, the order of trial presentation can affect the cognitive processes engaged within the trials themselves.[65] Second, blocked or randomized presentation of trials may affect the cognitive processes during the interval between trials. Thus, experiments using blocked designs may be confounded by behaviors resulting from groups of similar trials being presented together, which would not occur with randomized trials. Despite these concerns, blocked designs are most commonly used in fMRI studies.

Event-Related Designs

A newer class of experimental designs, called *event-related fMRI,* attempt to detect changes associated with individual trials, as opposed to the larger unit of time comprising a block of trials.[66] Each individual trial may be composed of one behavioral event, such as the presentation of a single stimulus (e.g., a face or object to be perceived), or several behavioral events (e.g., an item to be remembered, a delay period, and a motor response in a delayed-response task). In the simplest type of event-related fMRI experiment, the temporal separation of behavioral trials allows the hemodynamic response, resulting from the hypothesized brief period of evoked neural activity, to run its course (e.g., 16 seconds). Various analytical approaches allow statistical evaluation of these responses relative to the intertrial interval and to one another. Because the analysis focuses on individual trials, changes in the fMRI signal are attributed to one particular trial type, regardless of presentation order within the experiment. This feature of event-related designs allows for stimulus randomization, thus avoiding the behavioral confounds of blocked trials. Further, it permits separate analysis of functional responses, which are identified only in retrospect (i.e., trials on which the subject made a correct or incorrect response).[67]

In other experiments in which each individual trial is composed of several behavioral events, such as in a delayed-response task, event-related fMRI analysis methods allow the separate determination, at the neural level, of temporally dissociable behavioral components.[49] The design can help to detect and differentiate the fMRI signal evoked by a series of sequential neural events (e.g., presentation of the information to be remembered, the delay period when the subject is remembering the information, or the subsequent retrieval of the remembered information). With event-related analysis of an fMRI study, the PFC consistently displays activity correlating with the delay period,[68] supporting the role of the PFC in temporally maintaining information (*see* Chapter 9). This finding is consistent with single-neuron recording studies in the PFC of monkeys.[19] Figure 2–5 shows memory activity found in monkeys and humans.

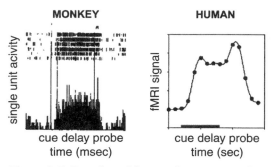

Figure 2–5. Data derived from single-neuron recording in a monkey and functional magnetic resonance imaging scanning in a healthy human during the performance of a spatial working memory task. (Adapted from Funahashi et al.[19] and Zarahn et al.[62])

STATISTICAL ISSUES IN FUNCTIONAL MAGNETIC RESONANCE IMAGING

Many statistical techniques are used for analyzing fMRI data, but no single method has emerged as the ideal or "gold standard." The analysis of any fMRI experiment designed to contradict the null hypothesis (i.e., that there is no difference between experimental conditions) requires inferential statistics. If the difference between two experimental conditions is too large to be reasonably due to chance, then the null hypothesis is rejected in favor of the alternative hypothesis, which typically is the experimenter's hypothesis (e.g., the fusiform gyrus is activated to a greater extent by viewing faces than objects). Unfortunately, since errors can occur in any statistical test, experimenters will never know when an error is committed and can only try to minimize them.[69] Knowledge of several basic statistical issues provides a solid foundation for the correct interpretation of functional neuroimaging studies.

Statistical Errors

Two types of statistical error can occur. A Type I error is committed when the null hypothesis is falsely rejected when it is true; that is, a difference between experimental conditions is found but does not truly exist. This type of error is also called a "false-positive error." In a functional neuroimaging study, a false-positive error would be finding a brain region activated during a cognitive task, when actually it is not. A Type II error is committed when the null hypothesis is accepted when it is false; that is, no difference is found between experimental conditions when a difference does exist. This type of error is also called a "false-negative error." A false-negative error in a functional neuroimaging study would be failing to find a brain region activated during the performance of a cognitive task when actually it is.

TYPE I ERROR

In fMRI experiments, like all experiments, a tolerable probability for Type I error, typically less than 5%, is chosen for adequate control of specificity, that is, control of false-positive rates. Two features of imaging data can cause unacceptable false-positive rates, even with traditional parametric statistical tests. First, there is the problem of multiple comparisons. For the typical resolution of images acquired during fMRI scans, the full extent of the human brain comprises approximately 15,000 voxels (a three-dimensional unit). Thus, with any given statistical comparison of two experimental conditions, there are actually 15,000 statistical comparisons being performed. With such a large number of statistical tests, the probability of finding a false-positive activation, that is, committing a Type I error, somewhere in the brain increases. Several methods exist to deal with this problem. One method, the Bonferroni correction, assumes that each statistical test is independent and calculates the probability of Type I error by dividing the chosen probability ($P = 0.05$) by the number of statistical tests performed. Another method[70] is based on Gaussian field theory and calculates the probability of Type I error when imaging data are spatially smoothed. Some type of correction for multiple comparisons must be adopted to control the false-positive rate.

The second feature of fMRI experiments that might increase the false-positive rate is the "noise" in fMRI data. Data from BOLD fMRI are temporally autocorrelated. Thus, fMRI data collected from human subjects without any experimental task have more noise at some frequencies than at others. The shape of this noise distribution is characterized by a 1/frequency function,[71] with increasing noise at lower frequencies. Traditional parametric and nonparametric statistical tests assume that the noise is not temporally autocorrelated; that is, each observation is independent. Therefore, any statistical test used in fMRI studies must account for the noise structure of fMRI data. If not, the false-positive rates will inflate.[71,72]

TYPE II ERROR

Type II error is rarely considered in functional neuroimaging studies. When a brain map from an fMRI experiment is presented, several areas of activation are typically attributed to some experimental manipulation. The focus of most imaging studies is on brain activation. It is often implicitly assumed that all of the other areas (typically most of the brain) were not activated during the experiment.

Power as a statistical concept refers to the probability of correctly rejecting the null hypothesis.[69] As the power of an fMRI study to detect changes in brain activity increases, the false-negative rate decreases. Unfortunately, power calculations for particular fMRI experiments are rarely performed, although this methodology is evolving.[73] Reports that specific brain areas were not active during an experimental manipulation should provide an estimate of the power required for detection of a change in the region. Experimental design should maximize power. Relatively simple strategies can increase power in an fMRI experiment in certain circumstances, such as increasing the amount of imaging data collected or increasing the number of subjects studied. In addition, behavioral task design can account for the structure of the noise.[74]

Types of Hypothesis Tested by Functional Magnetic Resonance Imaging

Functional neuroimaging experiments test hypotheses regarding the anatomical specificity for cognitive processes (functional specialization), basic mechanisms of cognition (cognitive theory), and direct or indirect interactions among brain regions (functional integration). A powerful approach for the testing of theories on brain–behavior relationships is the analysis of converging data from multiple methods.

FUNCTIONAL SPECIALIZATION

The major focus of fMRI studies is testing theories on functional specialization. The concept of functional specialization is based on the premise that functional modules exist within the brain; that is, areas of the cerebral cortex are specialized for a specific cognitive process. For example, facial recognition is a critical primate function served by a functional module. *Prosopagnosia* is the selective inability to recognize faces (*see* Chapter 5). Patients with prosopagnosia, however, can recognize familiar faces, such as those of relatives, by other means, such as the voice, dress, or body shape. Other types of visual recognition, such as identifying common objects, are normal. Prosopagnosia arises from lesions of the inferomedial temporo-occipital lobe, which are usually due to a posterior cerebral artery infarction. Most early clinical surveys of prosopagnosia concluded that only bilateral lesions caused the disorder,[75] but prosopagnosia also occurs with right hemisphere damage.[76] No lesion studies have precisely localized the area crucial for facial perception. However, they provide strong evidence that a brain area is specialized for processing the face. Functional imaging studies have provided anatomical specificity for such a module.

Kanwisher et al.[77] used fMRI to test healthy young subjects and found that the fusiform gyrus was significantly more active when the subjects viewed faces than when they viewed assorted common objects. The specificity of a "fusiform face area" was further demonstrated by the finding that this area also responded significantly more strongly to passive viewing of faces than to scrambled two-tone faces, front-view photographs of houses, and photographs of human hands. These elegant experiments allowed the investigators to reject alternative functions of the face area, such as visual attention, subordinate-level classification, or general processing of any animate or human forms, demonstrating that this region selectively perceives faces.

COGNITIVE THEORY

An exciting new direction for functional neuroimaging is the testing of theories on the underlying mechanisms of cognition. For example, an fMRI study[78] attempted to answer the question "To what extent does perception depend on attention?" One hypothesis is that unattended stimuli in the environment receive very little processing,[79] but another hypothesis is that the processing load in a relevant task determines the extent to which irrelevant stimuli are processed.[80] These alternative hypotheses were tested by asking normal subjects to perform linguistic tasks of low or high load while ignoring irrelevant visual motion in the periphery of a display. Visual motion was used as the distracting stimulus because it activates a distinct region of the brain (cortical area V5, another functional module in the visual system). Activation of area V5 would indicate that irrelevant visual motion was processed. Although task and irrelevant stimuli were unre-

lated, functional imaging of motion-related activity in V5 showed a reduction in motion processing during the high-processing load condition in the linguistic task. These findings supported the hypothesis that perception of irrelevant environmental information depends on the information-processing load that is currently relevant. Thus, by the finding that perception depends on attention, this functional neuroimaging experiment advanced cognitive theory.

FUNCTIONAL INTEGRATION

Functional neuroimaging experiments can also test hypotheses about interactions between brain regions by focusing on covariances of activation levels between regions.[81,82] These covariances reflect functional connectivity, a concept that was originally developed in reference to temporal interactions among individual neurons.[83] Newer approaches, often using a statistical test called "structural equation modeling," attempt to determine whether covariances among brain regions result from direct or indirect interactions, a concept called "effective connectivity." Using this method, McIntosh et al.[84] found shifting prefrontal and limbic interactions in a working memory task for faces as the retention delay increased (Fig. 2–6). The different interactions between brain regions at short and long delays was interpreted as a functional change. For example, strong corticolimbic interactions were found at short delays, but at longer delays, when the image of the face was more difficult to maintain, strong fronto-cingulate–occipital interactions were

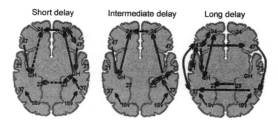

Figure 2–6. Network analysis of functional magnetic resonance imaging (fMRI) data during performance of a working memory task across three different delay periods. Areas of correlated increases in activation (*solid lines*) and areas of correlated decreases in activation (*dotted lines*) are shown. Note the different patterns of interaction among brain regions at short and long delays.[84]

found. The investigators postulated that the former finding was due to maintaining an iconic facial representation and that the latter finding was due to an expanded encoding strategy, resulting in more resilient memory. By characterizing changes in regional activity and the interactions between regions over time, the network analysis in this study added to the original analysis of regional means.

INTEGRATION OF MULTIPLE METHODS

The most powerful approach toward understanding brain–behavior relationships comes from analyzing converging data from multiple methods. This approach has been used in various fMRI studies. The notion that the temporal lobes mediate the retrieval of semantic knowledge arose from studies of patients with focal lesions.[85] These traditional beliefs were challenged by functional neuroimaging studies that consistently showed activation of the left inferior frontal gyrus (IFG) during the retrieval of semantic knowledge. For example, an early cognitive activation PET study revealed IFG activation during a verb-generation task compared with a simple word-repetition task.[12] A subsequent fMRI study[86] offered a fundamentally different interpretation of the apparent conflict between lesion and functional neuroimaging studies of semantic knowledge: left IFG activity is associated with the need to select some relevant feature of semantic knowledge from competing alternatives, not retrieval of semantic knowledge per se. This interpretation was supported by an fMRI experiment in normal subjects in which selection, but not retrieval, demands were varied across three semantic tasks. In a verb-generation task, in a high-selection condition, subjects generated verbs to nouns with many appropriate associated responses without any clearly dominant response (e.g., "wheel"), but in a low-selection condition, nouns with few associated responses or with a clear dominant response (e.g., "scissors") were used. In this way, all tasks required semantic retrieval and differed only in the amount of selection required. The fMRI signal within the left IFG increased as the selection demands increased (see Fig. 2–7). When the degree of semantic processing varied independently of selection demands, there was no

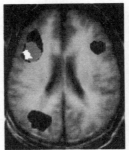
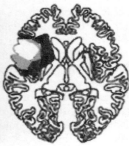

Figure 2–7. Regions of overlap of functional magnetic resonance imaging activity in healthy human subjects (*left panel*) during the performance of three semantic memory tasks, with the convergence of activity within the left inferior frontal gyrus (*white region*). Regions of overlap of lesion location in patients with selection-related deficits on a verb generation task, (*right panel*) with maximal overlap within the left inferior frontal gyrus (white region) (Adapted from Thompson-Schill et al.[86])

difference in left IFG activity, suggesting that selection, not retrieval, of semantic knowledge drives activity in the left IFG.

To determine if left IFG activity was correlated with, but not necessary for, selecting information from semantic memory, fMRI was used to examine the ability of patients with focal frontal lesions to generate verbs.[87] Supporting the earlier claim regarding left IFG function,[86] the overlap of lesions in patients with deficits on this task corresponded to the site of maximum fMRI activation in healthy young subjects during the verb-generation task (Fig. 2–7). In this example, the approach of using converging evidence from lesion and fMRI studies differs in a subtle but important way from the study described earlier that isolated the face-processing module. Patients with left IFG lesions do not present with an identifiable neurobehavioral syndrome reflecting the nature of the processing in this region. Guided by the imaging results from healthy young subjects, the investigators studied patients with left IFG lesions to test a hypothesis regarding the necessity of this region in a specific cognitive process. Coupled with the well-established finding that lesions of the left temporal lobe impair semantic knowledge, these studies further our understanding of the neural network mediating semantic memory (*see* Chapter 8).

CLINICAL APPLICATIONS OF FUNCTIONAL MAGNETIC RESONANCE IMAGING

Methodological Limitations

The clinical applications of fMRI are limited by several potentially problematic methodological issues. One problem is that BOLD fMRI data are unitless. Unlike PET, in which the signal is expressed as a physical quantity (millimeters of blood/100 g of tissue/minute), the BOLD fMRI signal has no absolute interpretation. Consequently, BOLD fMRI experiments generally test for differences in the magnitude of the signal between different conditions within a scanning session, such as in a memory task versus a control task. For example, a difference in the extent of activation between two groups (e.g., Alzheimer's disease patients vs. age-matched control subjects) or a difference in the effect of condition between two behavioral conditions (e.g., memory task vs. control task) can be tested. However, the effect of a single condition (e.g., the memory task) cannot be compared directly between groups of subjects. Advances in MRI perfusion imaging may provide fMRI signals that can be interpreted in concrete physical units,[88] allowing direct comparison between groups of subjects.

Confounding alterations of the BOLD signal by changes in brain physiology or metabolism caused by disease or normal aging may create artifactual results, limiting the clinical application of fMRI. For example, in studies comparing healthy elderly subjects with healthy younger subjects or healthy elderly subjects with stroke patients, a decrease in the fMRI signal in healthy elderly or stroke patients during certain cognitive tasks could be due to altered vascular responses rather than a change in neural activity.[89–91] This is true because fMRI directly measures vascular changes, which are an indirect measure of neural activity. At present, very little is known about the relation of the BOLD fMRI signal and physiological alterations of the vascular system caused by stroke and other neurological diseases as well as normal aging. Histological studies of cerebral microvasculature show considerable age-related variability in the organization of intracerebral arterioles, capillaries, and venules. There are age-related increases in the winding, coiling, and number of "blind ends" in the cerebral vascular microlattice, most notably in the arteriole–venous–capillary bed.[92] More work is needed to clarify the effect of vascular alterations on the BOLD fMRI signal, and new methods are needed to account for these effects before the reliability and validity of clinical fMRI studies are established. Despite these methodological limitations, clinical applications of fMRI have emerged.

Presurgical Planning and Prognosis

INTRACTABLE EPILEPSY

Like the Wada test (for cerebral dominance of language function with intracarotid injection of amobarbital), fMRI provides information on hemispheric lateralization of function. However, the Wada test is expensive and invasive, posing a possible risk to the patient. Replacing this test with the noninvasive fMRI could be extremely advantageous. Language function can be accurately localized with fMRI (for a review, see Binder[93]), as shown in a study of 24 consecutive patients with intractable focal epilepsy who also underwent the Wada test.[94] The correlation between the Wada test and the fMRI lateralization score was 0.96, indicating a very close agreement between the two tests in determining the language-dominant hemisphere. The score was determined by counting the number of voxels activated in each hemisphere by the patients' performance of a language task. A typical language task[94] is a semantic word-categorization task in which subjects hear animal names and must make a semantic decision regarding the animal ("Is it found in the United States and used by people?") versus a nonsemantic task in which subjects hear a sequence of tones and must make a decision about the pitch content of a tone sequence ("Does the sequence contain two high tones?"). In normal right-handed subjects, activation on the semantic task relative to the nonsemantic task is strongly lateralized to the left hemisphere. At present, the types of language task used for both the Wada test and the fMRI vary widely, as does their implementation; more work is needed to standardize the fMRI procedures for widespread clinical use. In addition, the effects of subject movement, medications, and vascular factors (e.g., interhemispheric arterial crossflow) can alter the results.

Functional MRI studies in patients with epilepsy may provide useful prognostic information. The outcome of epilepsy surgery improves with accurate localization of the seizure focus. In contrast to the use of invasive, surgically implanted electrodes, fMRI can accurately localize the seizure focus by detecting the metabolic and hemodynamic changes associated with ictal discharges.[95,96] Unfortunately, this method is useful only in patients who have frequent seizures that are likely to be captured during a short (1 hour) fMRI scanning session. However, new methods, such as EEG-triggered fMRI, may improve its sensitivity and practical use.[97]

Another means of providing prognostic information in patients with epilepsy is based on the premise that asymmetries in interictal blood flow or functional activation might identify diseased brain tissue where seizures may originate. A cognitive task that activates the left medial temporal area in normal subjects activated the left medial temporal lobe in patients with a right-sided seizure focus but not in those with a left-sided focus.[98] Likewise, a cognitive task that activates both medial temporal lobes symmetrically activated the medial temporal lobe asymmetrically, predicting the side of the epileptogenic focus.[99] In this study, the fMRI results were consistent with those of the Wada test, predicting a good outcome of epilepsy surgery.

ARTERIOVENOUS MALFORMATIONS AND BRAIN TUMORS

Functional MRI is potentially useful for presurgical planning in patients with arteriovenous malformations (AVMs) or brain tumors.[100] Identifying functional areas before removal of the AVM or tumor can reduce the risk of a postoperative deficit. Unfortunately, much work is needed before fMRI can safely guide neurosurgical procedures. Unpublished observations from several centers demonstrate that areas activated during the performance of a cognitive task were not necessary for the processes engaged by the task. For example, with a tumor in Broca's area on the left, activation of Broca's area on the right during the performance of a language task does not imply that language will be spared with surgical removal of the tumor. In addition, the absence of activation near the tumor does not indicate that the apparently "silent" area is not necessary for important cognitive processes. The information obtained from clinical studies is complex and warrants further study. So far, no adequate quantitative fMRI data are available to help neurosurgeons tailor their surgical excisions. Such information, however, has provided valuable insight regarding the mechanisms of functional reorganization after brain injury[101] and could potentially direct rehabilitation strategies.

Diagnosis of Neurological Disorders

Functional MRI is a promising diagnostic tool, especially in neurological disorders with normal gross structure on the MRI scan. For instance, fMRI has been used to assess hippocampal function in elderly subjects with normal memory, elderly subjects with isolated memory decline, and patients with probable Alzheimer's disease.[102,103] By anatomically segregating the data into subregions of the hippocampus, investigators observed two distinct patterns of regional dysfunction among the elderly with isolated memory decline; one pattern was similar to that found in elderly subjects with Alzheimer's disease, involving all hippocampal regions, and the other pattern was of dysfunction restricted to only one hippocampal region, the subiculum. These results offer direct evidence of hippocampal dysfunction associated with memory decline in the elderly and suggest that fMRI may assist in the early diagnosis of Alzheimer's disease or other causes of memory decline in aging. Since fMRI is a noninvasive measurement of hippocampal function, it offers significant advantages over PET for developing early diagnostic markers for Alzheimer's disease.[104]

SUMMARY

Functional MRI is an extremely valuable tool for studying brain–behavior relationships. It is the most powerful of functional neuroimaging methods as it is widely available and noninvasive and has superb temporal and spatial resolution. New approaches in fMRI experimental design and data analysis are appearing in the literature at an almost exponential rate, leading to numerous options for testing hypotheses on brain–behavior relationships and developing clinical applications. Combined with information from other methods, such as focal lesion studies, data from fMRI studies provide new insights regarding the organization of the cerebral cortex, as well as the neural mechanisms underlying cognition.

REFERENCES

1. Broca P: Remarques sur le siege de la faculte du langage articule suivies d'une observation d'amphemie (perte de al parole). Bull Mem Soc Anat Paris 6:330–357, 1861.
2. Naeser MA, Palumbo CL, Helm-Estabrooks N et al.: Severe nonfluency in aphasia: role of the medial subcallosal fasciculus plus other white matter pathways in recovery of spontaneous speech. Brain 112:1–38, 1989.
3. Dronkers NF: A new brain region for coordinating speech articulation. Nature 384:159–161, 1996.
4. Alexander MP, Naeser MA, and Palumbo C: Broca's area aphasias: aphasia after lesions including the frontal operculum. Neurology 40:353–362, 1990.
5. Penny WD, Kiebel SJ, Kilner JM, et al.: Event-related brain dynamics. Trends Neurosci 25:387–389, 2002.
6. Michel CM, Thut G, Morand S, et al.: Electric source imaging of human brain functions. Brain Res Brain Res Rev 36:108–118, 2001.
7. Galin D and Ornstein R: Lateral specialization of cognitive mode: an EEG study. Psychophysiology 9:412–418, 1972.
8. Dale AM and Halgren E: Spatiotemporal mapping of brain activity by integration of multiple imaging modalities. Curr Opin Neurobiol 11:202–208, 2001.
9. Ingvar DH and Schwartz MS: Blood flow patterns induced in the dominant hemisphere by speech and reading. Brain 97:273–278, 1974.
10. Frackowiak RS and Friston KJ: Functional neuroanatomy of the human brain: positron emission tomography—a new neuroanatomical technique. J Anat 184:211–225, 1994.
11. Mazziotta JC and Phelps ME: Human sensory stimulation and deprivation: positron emission tomographic results and strategies. Ann Neurol 15:S50–S60, 1984.
12. Petersen SE, Fox PT, Posner MI, et al.: Positron emission tomographic studies of the cortical anatomy of single word processing. Nature 331:585–589, 1988.
13. Menon RS: Imaging function in the working brain with fMRI. Curr Opin Neurobiol 11:630–636, 2001.
14. Sarter M, Bernston G, and Cacioppo J: Brain imaging and cognitive neuroscience: toward strong inference in attributing function to structure. Am Psychol 51:13–21, 1996.
15. Jarrard LE: On the role of the hippocampus in learning and memory in the rat. Behav Neural Biol 60:9–26, 1993.
16. Gaffan D and Gaffan EA: Amnesia in man following transection of the fornix: a review. Brain 114:2611–2618, 1991.
17. Feeney DM and Baron JC: Diaschisis. Stroke 17:817–830, 1986.
18. Price CJ, Warburton EA, Moore CJ, et al.: Dynamic diaschisis: anatomically remote and context-sensitive human brain lesions. J Cogn Neurosci 13:419–429, 2001.
19. Funahashi S, Bruce CJ, and Goldman-Rakic PS: Mnemonic coding of visual space in the monkey's dorsolateral prefrontal cortex. J Neurophysiol 61:331–349, 1989.
20. Fuster JM and Alexander GE: Neuron activity related to short-term memory. Science 173:652–654, 1971.
21. D'Esposito M, Postle BR, and Rypma B: Prefrontal cortical contributions to working memory: evidence from event-related fMRI studies. Exp Brain Res 133:3–11, 2000.
22. Fuster J: The Prefrontal Cortex: Anatomy, Physiology, and Neuropsychology of the Frontal Lobes, 3rd ed. Raven Press, New York, 1997.
23. Funahashi S, Bruce CJ, and Goldman-Rakic PS: Dorsolateral prefrontal lesions and oculomotor delayed-response performance: evidence for mnemonic "scotomas." J Neurosci 13:1479–1497, 1993.
24. Cahusac PM, Miyashita Y, and Rolls ET: Responses of hippocampal formation neurons in the monkey related to delayed spatial response and object-place memory tasks. Behav Brain Res 33:229–240, 1989.
25. Watanabe T and Niki H: Hippocampal unit activity and delayed response in the monkey. Brain Res 325:241–254, 1985.
26. Alvarez P, Zola-Morgan S, and Squire LR: The animal model of human amnesia: long-term memory impaired and short-term memory intact. Proc Natl Acad Sci USA 91:5637–5641, 1994.
27. Corkin S: Lasting consequences of bilateral medial temporal lobectomy: clinical course and experimental findings in H.M. Semin Neurol 4:249–259, 1984.
28. Ranganath C and D'Esposito M: Medial temporal lobe activity associated with active maintenance of novel information. Neuron 31:865–873, 2001.
29. Rushworth MF, Hadland KA, Paus T, et al.: Role of the human medial frontal cortex in task switching: a combined fMRI and TMS study. J Neurophysiol 87:2577–2592, 2002.
30. Druzgal TJ and D'Esposito M: Activity in fusiform face area modulated as a function of working memory load. Brain Res Cogn Brain Res 10:355–364, 2001.
31. Cohen MS, Kosslyn SM, Breiter HC, et al.: Changes in cortical activity during mental rotation: a mapping study using functional MRI. Brain 119:89–100, 1996.
32. D'Esposito M, Ballard D, Aguirre G, et al.: Human prefrontal cortex is not specific for working memory. Neuroimage 8:274–282, 1998.
33. Glover GH and Law CS: Spiral-in/out BOLD fMRI for increased SNR and reduced susceptibility artifacts. Magn Reson Med 46:515–522, 2001.
34. Knuttinen MG, Parrish TB, Weiss C, et al.: Electromyography as a recording system for eyeblink con-

ditioning with functional magnetic resonance imaging. Neuroimage 17:977–987, 2002.

35. Barch DM, Sabb FW, Carter CS, et al.: Overt verbal responding during fMRI scanning: empirical investigations of problems and potential solutions. Neuroimage 10:642–657, 1999.

36. Amaro E Jr, Williams SC, Shergill SS, et al.: Acoustic noise and functional magnetic resonance imaging: current strategies and future prospects. J Magn Reson Imaging 16:497–510, 2002.

37. Horowitz AL: MRI Physics for Radiologists, 3rd ed. Springer-Verlag, New York, 1995.

38. Buxton RB: Introduction to Functional Magnetic Resonance Imaging: Principles and Techniques. Cambridge University Press, Cambridge, 2002.

39. Leniger-Follert E and Hossmann KA: Simultaneous measurements of microflow and evoked potentials in the somatomotor cortex of the cat brain during specific sensory activation. Pflugers Arch 380:85–89, 1979.

40. Malonek D and Grinvald A: Interactions between electrical activity and cortical microcirculation revealed by imaging spectroscopy: implications for functional brain mapping. Science 272:551–554, 1996.

41. Kwong KK, Belliveau JW, Chesler DA, et al.: Dynamic magnetic resonance imaging of human brain activity during primary sensory stimulation. Proc Nat Acad Sci 89:5675–5679, 1992.

42. Ogawa S, Menon RS, Tank DW, et al.: Functional brain mapping by blood oxygenation level-dependent contrast magnetic resonance imaging. A comparison of signal characteristics with a biophysical model. Biophys J 64:803–812, 1993.

43. Heeger DJ and Ress D: What does fMRI tell us about neuronal activity? Nat Rev Neurosci 3:142–151, 2002.

44. Gnadt JW and Andersen RA: Memory related motor planning activity in posterior parietal cortex of macaque. Exp Brain Res 70:216–220, 1988.

45. Bandettini PA, Wong EC, Hinks RS, et al.: Time course of EPI of human brain function during task activation. Magn Reson Med 25:390–397, 1992.

46. Aguirre GK, Zarahn E, and D'Esposito M: The variability of human, BOLD hemodynamic responses. Neuroimage 8:360–369, 1998.

47. Boynton GM, Engel SA, Glover GH, et al.: Linear systems analysis of functional magnetic resonance imaging in human V1. J Neurosci 16:4207–4221, 1996.

48. Georgopoulos AP, Crutcher MD, and Schwartz AB: Cognitive spatial-motor processes. 3. Motor cortical prediction of movement direction during an instructed delay period. Exp Brain Res 75:183–194, 1989.

49. Zarahn E, Aguirre GK, and D'Esposito M: A trial-based experimental design for functional MRI. Neuroimage 6:122–138, 1997.

50. Burock MA, Buckner RL, Woldorff MG, et al.: Randomized event-related experimental designs allow for extremely rapid presentation rates using functional MRI. Neuroreport 9:3735–3739, 1998.

51. Clark VP, Maisog JM, and Haxby JV: fMRI studies of visual perception and recognition using a random stimulus design. Soc Neurosci Abstr 23:301, 1997.

52. Dale AM and Buckner RL: Selective averaging of rapidly presented individual trials using fMRI. Hum Brain Mapping 5:1–12, 1997.

53. Rosen BR, Buckner RL, and Dale AM: Event-related functional MRI: past, present, and future. Proc Natl Acad Sci USA 95:773–780, 1998.

54. D'Esposito M, Zarahn E, and Aguirre GK: Event-related fMRI: implications for cognitive psychology. Psychol Bull 125:155–164, 1999.

55. Kim SG, Richter W, and Ugurbil K: Limitations of temporal resolution in fMRI. Magn Reson Med 37:631–636, 1997.

56. Savoy RL, Bandettini PA, O'Craven KM, et al.: Pushing the temporal resolution of fMRI: studies of very brief stimuli, onset of variability and asynchrony, and stimuli-correlated changes in noise. Proc Soc Magn Reson Med 3:450, 1995.

57. Posner MI, Petersen SE, Fox PT, et al.: Localization of cognitive operations in the human brain. Science 240:1627–1631, 1988.

58. Donders FC: Over de snelheid van psychische processen. Onderzoekingen gedaan in het Physiologisch Laboratorium der Utrechtsche Hoogeschool. Tweede Reeks II:92–120, 1868.

59. Sternberg S: The discovery of processing stages: extensions of Donders' method. Acta Psychol 30:276–315, 1969.

60. Jonides J, Smith EE, Koeppe RA, et al.: Spatial working memory in humans as revealed by PET. Nature 363:623–625, 1993.

61. Vazquez AL and Noll DC: Nonlinear aspects of the BOLD response in functional MRI. Neuroimage 7:108–118, 1998.

62. Zarahn E, Aguirre GK, and D'Esposito M: Temporal isolation of the neural correlates of spatial mnemonic processing with fMRI. Cogn Brain Res 7:255–268, 1999.

63. Kapur S, Craik FIM, Jones C, et al.: Functional role of the prefrontal cortex in retrieval of memories: a PET study. Neuroreport 6:1880–1884, 1995.

64. Rugg MD, Fletcher PC, Frith CD, et al.: Differential activation of the prefrontal cortex in successful and unsuccessful memory retrieval. Brain 119:2073–2083, 1996.

65. Johnson MK, Nolde SF, Mather M, et al.: The similarity of brain activity associated with true and false recognition depends on test format. Psychol Sci 8:250–257, 1997.

66. Postle BR, Zarahn E, and D'Esposito M: Using event-related fMRI to assess delay-period activity during performance of spatial and nonspatial working memory tasks. Brain Res Brain Res Protoc 5:57–66, 2000.

67. Rypma B, Berger JS, and D'Esposito M: The influence of working-memory demand and subject performance on prefrontal cortical activity. J Cogn Neurosci 14:721–731, 2002.

68. Postle BR, Berger JS, Taich AM, et al.: Activity in human frontal cortex associated with spatial working memory and saccadic behavior. J Cogn Neurosci 12:2–14, 2000.

69. Keppel G and Zedeck S: Data Analysis for Research Design. WH Freeman, New York, 1989.

70. Worsley KJ and Friston KJ: Analysis of fMRI time-series revisited—again. Neuroimage 2:173–182, 1995.

71. Zarahn E, Aguirre GK, and D'Esposito M: Empirical analyses of BOLD fMRI statistics. I. Spatially unsmoothed data collected under null-hypothesis conditions. Neuroimage 5:179–197, 1997.

72. Aguirre GK, Zarahn E, and D'Esposito M: Empirical analyses of BOLD fMRI statistics. II. Spatially smoothed data collected under null-hypothesis and

experimental conditions. Neuroimage 5:199–212, 1997.

73. Van Horn JD, Ellmore TM, Esposito G, et al.: Mapping voxel-based statistical power on parametric images. Neuroimage 7:97–107, 1998.

74. Aguirre GK and D'Esposito M: Experimental design for brain fMRI. In Moonen CTW, Bandettini PA (eds). Functional MRI. Springer Verlag, Berlin, 1999, pp 369–380.

75. Damasio A, Damasio H, and Van Hoesen G: Prosopagnosia: anatomic basis and anatomical mechanisms. Neurology 32:331–341, 1982.

76. De Renzi E, Perani D, Carlesimo GA, et al.: Prosopagnosia can be associated with damage confined to the right hemisphere—an MRI and PET study and a review of the literature. Neuropsychologia 32:893–902, 1994.

77. Kanwisher N, McDermott J, and Chun MM: The fusiform face area: a module in human extrastriate cortex specialized for face perception. J Neurosci 17:4302–4311, 1997.

78. Rees G, Frith CD, and Lavie N: Modulating irrelevant motion perception by varying attentional load in an unrelated task. Science 278:1616–1619, 1997.

79. Treisman AM: Strategies and models of selective attention. Psychol Rev 76:282–299, 1969.

80. Lavie N and Tsal Y: Perceptual load as a major determinant of the locus of selection in visual attention. Percept Psychophys 56:183–197, 1994.

81. McIntosh AR: Mapping cognition to the brain through neural interactions. Memory 7:523–548, 1999.

82. Buchel C, Coull JT, and Friston KJ: The predictive value of changes in effective connectivity for human learning. Science 283:1538–1541, 1999.

83. Gerstein GL, Perkel DH, and Subramanian KN: Identification of functionally related neural assemblies. Brain Res 140:43–62, 1978.

84. McIntosh AR, Grady CL, Haxby JV, et al.: Changes in limbic and prefrontal functional interactions in a working memory task for faces. Cereb Cortex 6:571–584, 1996.

85. McCarthy RA and Warrington EK: Disorders of semantic memory. Philos Trans R Soc Lond B Biol Sci 346:89–96, 1994.

86. Thompson-Schill SL, D'Esposito M, Aguirre GK, et al.: Role of left inferior prefrontal cortex in retrieval of semantic knowledge: a reevaluation. Proc Natl Acad Sci USA 94:14792–14797, 1997.

87. Thompson-Schill SL, Swick D, Farah MJ, et al.: Verb generation in patients with focal frontal lesions: a neuropsychological test of neuroimaging findings. Proc Natl Acad Sci USA 95:15855–15860, 1998.

88. Detre JA and Wang J: Technical aspects and utility of fMRI using BOLD and ASL. Clin Neurophysiol 113:621–634, 2002.

89. Pineiro R, Pendlebury S, Johansen-Berg H, et al.: Altered hemodynamic responses in patients after sub-

cortical stroke measured by functional MRI. Stroke 33:103–109, 2002.

90. D'Esposito M, Zarahn E, Aguirre GK, et al.: The effect of normal aging on the coupling of neural activity to the bold hemodynamic response. Neuroimage 10:6–14, 1999.

91. Buckner RL, Snyder AZ, Sanders AL, et al.: Functional brain imaging of young, nondemented, and demented older adults. J Cogn Neurosci 12:24–34, 2000.

92. Fang HCH: Observations on aging characteristics of cerebral blood vessels, macroscopic and microscopic features. In Gerson S, Terry RD (eds). Neurobiology of Aging. Raven Press, New York, 1976, pp. 155–166.

93. Binder JR: Neuroanatomy of language processing studied with functional MRI. Clin Neurosci 4:87–94, 1997.

94. Binder JR, Swanson SJ, Hammeke TA, et al.: Determination of language dominance using functional MRI: a comparison with the Wada test. Neurology 46:978–984, 1996.

95. Richardson MP: Functional imaging in epilepsy. Seizure 11(Suppl A):139–156, 2002.

96. Detre JA, Sirven JI, Alsop DC, et al.: Localization of subclinical ictal activity by functional magnetic resonance imaging: correlation with invasive monitoring. Ann Neurol 38:618–624, 1995.

97. Schomer DL, Bonmassar G, Lazeyras F, et al.: EEG-linked functional magnetic resonance imaging in epilepsy and cognitive neurophysiology. J Clin Neurophysiol 17:43–58, 2000.

98. Bellgowan PS, Binder JR, Swanson SJ, et al.: Side of seizure focus predicts left medial temporal lobe activation during verbal encoding. Neurology 51:479–484, 1998.

99. Detre JA, Maccotta L, King D, et al.: Functional MRI lateralization of memory in temporal lobe epilepsy. Neurology 50:926–932, 1998.

100. Roux FE, Ibarrola D, Tremoulet M, et al.: Methodological and technical issues for integrating functional magnetic resonance imaging data in a neuronavigational system. Neurosurgery 49:1145–1157, 2001.

101. Ances BM and D'Esposito M: Neuroimaging of recovery of function after stroke: implications for rehabilitation. Neurorehabil Neural Repair 14:171–179, 2000.

102. Small SA, Perera GM, DeLaPaz R, et al.: Differential regional dysfunction of the hippocampal formation among elderly with memory decline and Alzheimer's disease. Ann Neurol 45:466–472, 1999.

103. Small SA, Tsai WY, DeLaPaz R, et al.: Imaging hippocampal function across the human life span: is memory decline normal or not? Ann Neurol 51:290–295, 2002.

104. Jagust WJ: Neuroimaging in dementia. Neurol Clin 18:885–902, 2000.

105. Churchland PS and Sejnowski TJ: Perspectives on cognitive neuroscience. Science 242:741–745, 1988.

Chapter 3

The Right Hemisphere, Interhemispheric Communication, and Consciousness

I believe it then to be entirely unphilosophical, and tending to important errors, to speak of the cerebrum as one organ . . . The two hemispheres of the brain are really . . . two distinct and entire organs . . . as fully perfect in all its parts . . . as the two eyes. The corpus callosum, and the other commissures between them, can with no more justice be said to constitute the two hemispheres into one organ than the optic commissure can be called an union of the two eyes into one organ.

Each cerebrum is a distinct and perfect whole capable of independent thought and volition. In the healthy brain one of the two hemispheres is almost always superior in power, and exercises control over the volitions of its fellow. In cases of disease, however, where one cerebrum becomes sufficiently aggravated to defy the control of the other . . . their separate wills struggling against each other, their separate thoughts jumbling together.

A. L. WIGAN, 1844[1]

A powerful bias leads us to view the world as purely dichotomous—good or bad, science or religion, left or right, analytic or holistic, serial or parallel, verbal or nonverbal—but biological and social dichotomies are rarely pure. Likewise, language function and praxis, despite their hemispheric asymmetry, are not exclusively the domain of the left hemisphere. Subtleties of language and fine motor control, paradigms of specialized cerebral hemisphere functions, are ascribed to the right hemisphere. The right hemisphere strongly modulates the speaker's emotional tone, narrative flow, and feedback during verbal communication, as well as the facial expressions and gestures that accompany speech. By focusing on word strings in isolation, the listener can miss the message. Similarly, the neurologist, focusing on symptoms and lesion site, can overestimate, underestimate, or hold false views on the function of damaged cortex.

The two cerebral hemispheres appear as mirror images with redundant cells and circuits, but anatomical differences that emerge during gestation[2] provide a structural basis for hemispheric asymmetry. The left planum temporale (see Fig. 5–11), containing auditory association cortex, is larger in 65% of right-handed persons, averaging one-third larger than on the right side.[3] This increase is largely related to thicker myelin sheaths in the left hemisphere.[4] The left planum temporale is also larger than the right in the human fetus.[5] The cell body and dendrites of pyramidal cells are larger in motor language cortex than in homologous right hemisphere cortex.[6,7] Neuroimaging studies reveal a larger left occipital and right frontal pole in right-handed persons.[8] Anatomical asymmetries occur in the human thalamus[9] and in neurochemical concentrations and receptor sensitivities.[10]

In evolution, human hemispheric specialization likely followed the lead of anthropoid apes for left hemisphere dominance in communication and praxis. Brain asymmetries also exist in early hominids[11] and great apes,[12] including chimpanzees[13] (left planum temporale, a homologue of Wernicke's area). In chimpanzees, referential, intentional gestural communications arise predominantly from the left hemisphere.[14] Hemispheric asymmetry is not novel for either apes or humans. The animal kingdom has many examples of lateralized functions and asymmetrical structures, ranging from the left hemisphere lateralization of bird songs and asymmetrical lobster claws to the production and recognition of calls in monkeys and dolphins.[14]

Language was the first behavior found to have an asymmetrical hemispheric distribution.[15,16] (Dax[16] may have first reported this phenomenon in a presentation to the Congres Meridional de Montpellier in 1836.) Similar findings of an asymmetrical (left-sided) distribution for skilled movements followed.[17] The verbal–nonverbal dichotomy of hemispheric functions persists,[18,19] and the list of lateralized functions grows (Table 3–1). However, the division of brain functions into two hemispheres often excludes negative or contrary evidence[29] and obscures hemispheric similarities. For example, Kimura's studies[19] demonstrating a

right ear (left hemisphere) advantage for verbal stimuli "confirmed" left hemisphere language dominance. However, fewer than half of right-handed subjects consistently show this pattern, and many exhibit the opposite pattern.[59] Similarly, left hemisphere dominance for temporal order judgment was reconceived as "left hemisphere specialization for temporal analysis," ignoring the significant deficits in temporal order judgment produced by right hemisphere lesions.[29] Further, the right hemisphere plays a role in recovery from aphasia caused by left hemisphere damage. The contribution primarily involves receptive language abilities.[60]

In determining lateralized functions, hemispheric specialization is one of several key factors, which also include subject (e.g., sex, age, handedness, strategy), stimulus (e.g., energy, location, complexity), and analytical method (e.g., name, match to sample).[29] For instance, males have stronger lateralization for verbal stimuli, and females have stronger lateralization for nonverbal stimuli.[61] A positive correlation between lesions and symptoms does not imply causation or permit localization (specialization) of function. If so, aphasia after left-sided thalamic lesions would lead to the incorrect conclusion that the left thalamus is specialized for language. Many of the dichotomous functions are relative generalizations, lacking support from controlled studies. Most represent relative degrees of hemispheric specialization that vary by task, individual, and measure.

Right hemisphere–dominant functions include emotions, body schema, visuospatial ability, sensory and motor attention, and certain social behaviors.[58] Dominance for these functions was probably a by-product of left hemisphere specialization. In this model, these skills were initially well developed in both hemispheres but "crowded out" by language and praxis circuitry in the left hemisphere. Simultaneously, more complex and novel aspects of these right hemisphere–dominant functions may have emerged during hominid evolution. The presence of these right hemisphere functions in other primates[57] and the ontogenic dominance of the right hemisphere in infants[62] favor crowding out over new development (emergence) as the primary mechanism. However, the larger right frontal lobes may be a cor-

Table 3–1. **Postulated Dichotomous Relations of the Cerebral Hemispheres***

Behavioral Dimension	Left Hemisphere	Right Hemisphere
Cognitive mode	Expressive,[20] propositional[21]	Perceptual (gnosis)[22]
	Verbal[20–22]	Nonverbal, spatial, performance[23]
	Denotative lexicon	Connotative lexicon[24]
	Detail oriented[25]	Gestalt, holistic- oriented[25–27]
	Probabilistic[28]	Deductive[28] (except statement decoding)
	Serial processing[29]	Synthetic, parallel processing[30]
	Temporal, sequential[29]	Nontemporal, nonsequential
	Logical,[31] abstract,[32] symbolic[22]	Creative[33]
	Propositional[34]	Appositional (i.e., compares percepts, schemas, engrams)[34]
	Concrete[34,35]	Metaphorical,[24] inferential[36]
	Not bound by context[32]	Context-bound[32]
	Categorical data coding[37]	Spatial coordinate coding[37,38]
Perceptual mode	Auditory[20]	Tactile,[39] visual imagery,[20] olfactory[40]
Attentional focus	Right space and body[41]	Left greater than right space and body[41]
	Central,[42] intentional[42]	Peripheral,[43] incidental[43]
Emotionality	Neutral[43]	Affective,[43,44] emotional
Emotional focus	Social emotions (e.g., embarrassment)[45]	Primary emotions (e.g., fear)[45]
Emotional valence	Positive[44,46–48]	Negative[44,46–48]
Knowledge–memory	Factual	Emotional–social,[49,50] autobiographical[42,51,52]
	Verbal[53]	Nonverbal, visuospatial,[23,54,55] topographic[56]
Consciousness	Verbal[57]	Corporeal–emotional[58]

* Many of these dichotomies are speculative, and others are supported by evidence from studies of specific cognitive or behavioral tasks.

relate of emergent, complex social behavior as a dominant function of the right hemisphere.

Commissures functionally link the homologous areas of the hemispheres, providing enormous avenues for them to inhibit, evoke, and synchronize function. Neocortical commissures help to integrate primary perceptual information at early stages of cortical processing. Callosal fibers help to coordinate bimanual tasks and bilateral axial movements, especially during the learning stage. Callosal connections help to mediate sustained attention. Most importantly, perhaps, the corpus callosum allows one hemisphere to deactivate the other and take command over a behavioral function. Lesions of the corpus callosum can disrupt attentional, memory, sensory, motor, and emotional functions. Rarely, callosal lesions isolate two spheres of consciousness, producing the alien hand syndrome.

Consciousness, a subjective state of awareness of something,[63] may be explained by two concepts: modularity of mind[64] and binding of

the modules by synchronizing activity.[65] Disorders of neural synchronicity may underlie certain unexplained aspects of neurological disease. While these concepts help to explain conscious awareness, the existence of two distinct, yet connected cerebral hemispheres poses the following question: Do we possess one consciousness or two? Each hemisphere "sees" a different half of the world, yet our visual and mental world is a seamless whole. The intuitive notions that consciousness is unitary and that most cognition results from an "aware" consciousness may be wrong. Consciousness appears seamless but is woven from distinct modules of awareness (e.g., visual, emotional, and verbal). The nonconscious mind performs most cognitive, perceptual, and motor functions. For example, when running or comprehending speech, we do not consciously monitor the foot's position on landing or discriminate phonemes. For a specific brain function, such as speech production, awareness of the processes underlying the function and awareness of the function itself, that is, self-consciousness regarding speech output, are independent but related functions that utilize overlapping structures. Because automatized or practiced functions extensively utilize subcortical areas,[66] awareness of the underlying processes is often impossible.

THE RIGHT HEMISPHERE

Historically, neurology has focused on left hemisphere functions; the right hemisphere was viewed as "primitive," "silent," or "redundant." Our understanding of right hemisphere functions evolved slowly. The swearing of aphasic patients, often their only means of verbal communication, led John Hughlings Jackson,[22] in 1874, to postulate that "automatic" or "emotional" speech came from the right hemisphere and voluntary expression and conscious awareness of propositional speech from the left hemisphere. Later, in 1880, Jackson[67] reported an association between right temporal lobe seizures and reminiscence (*déjà vu*), as well as dreamy, voluminous mental states. Late nineteenth century clinicians (1879–1885) linked the right hemisphere with madness,[68] emotion,[69] and dissociative and conversion phenomena.[70] Not until Brain's 1941 report on visual disorientation after right hemisphere lesions[71] and Critchley's 1953 monograph on parietal lobe disorders[72] was interest in the right hemisphere rekindled. Current functional–anatomical correlates of right hemisphere dominance are summarized in Table 3–2.

RIGHT HEMISPHERE DOMINANCE OF THE CORPOREAL SELF

The right hemisphere dominates our physical being, that is, our awareness of our corporeal body and its relation to its affective state and to the environment. Right hemisphere injury causes disorders of the corporeal self, impairing perception, constructional and visual skills, body image, and awareness of left-sided sensory and motor deficits, and can also impair the corporeal self's relation to the environment, resulting in disorders of ego boundary, geographic disorientation, and dressing ability.

Perception

The right hemisphere is dominant for many purely perceptual domains (*see* Chapter 5). These include the visuospatial, somesthetic,[73] auditory (melody and tone discrimination and spatial, directional, and temporal auditory processing),[75,77] olfactory,[40] and pain,[87] as well as the domain for comprehending emotional tone in voice and body gestures.[86,89] Evidence supports right hemisphere dominance for apperceptive recognition, or meaningless stimuli, in tactile, auditory, visual, and visuospatial modalities; but the left hemisphere appears dominant for associative recognition, or meaningful stimuli.[117]

Constructional Praxis

Constructional praxis is the capacity to assemble and organize an object from disarticulated pieces. These skills range from constructing a square by drawing four lines to creating a pattern by juxtaposing blocks. *Constructional apraxia,* the inability to spatially group or integrate objects, is most often associated with right parietal lobe disorders.[118] Congenital right hemisphere injuries permanently impair constructional praxis, and patients often produce heaps or disordered clumps when complex grouping procedures are required.[119] Constructional disability has many causes, including impaired strategies and working memory. Thus, right frontal lobe and left frontoparietal lobe lesions can also impair constructional skills.[120,121]

Disorder of dressing ability, the impaired orientation and placement of clothes on one's body, is associated with injury of the right hemisphere, in particular, the right parietal lobe.[71,78,122] The disorder most commonly occurs in patients with Alzheimer's disease. Although the disorder is commonly referred to as "dressing apraxia," patients usually do not have a primary disorder of praxis, such as the inability to button a shirt. Impaired dressing skills can result from factors such as left-sided neglect, impaired body image, and defective visuospatial constructional ability (*see* Chapter

Table 3–2. **Functional–Anatomical Correlation of Right Hemisphere Dominance***

Function	Brain Area
Sensory processing	
Odor perception	Temporal[40]
Tactile orientation	Parietal[73]
Thermal sensation	Anterior insula, orbitofrontal[74]
Auditory: spatial, directional, and temporal processing	Temporal, insula[75–77]
Corporeal self and relation to the environment	
Body image	Parietal[72]
Orientation of body parts to each other	Parietal[71,72]
Orientation of body parts to environment	Parietal[71,72,78]
Topographic orientation	Parietal or temporal[56,79,80]
Topographic memory	Parahippocampal gyrus[38]
Mental rotation	Parietal, temporal[81]
Attention	
Directed spatial attention	Parietal, dorsolateral, prefrontal, or cingulate[41,82]
Sustained mental attention	Dorsolateral prefrontal, anterior cingulate[83]
Sustained intentional movements (i.e., motor attention)	Prefrontal[84,85]
Emotion	
Perception of emotional stimuli (e.g., pain)	Temporal lobe, anterior cingulate[86,87]
Labeling of memories	Amygdala, prefrontal[51,52]
Expressing emotional tone and gesture	Prefrontal[88–90]
Drive-related behavior	
Sexual arousal[90a,90b,90c]	Frontal, temporal
Regulation of food consumption[90d,90e]	Frontal, temporal
Visuoconstructive skills	Parietal, prefrontal[72]
Autonomic	
Stress and sympathetic responsiveness	Temporal, insula, orbitofrontal[91–93]
Intentional movements	
Volitional eye movements	Frontal lobe, premotor[94,95]
Aspects of social behavior	
Eye contact	?Prefrontal[96,97]
Insight	Dorsolateral prefrontal, orbitofrontal, anterior cingulate[98–100]
Self monitoring (e.g., modulating speech discourse)	Prefrontal, orbitofrontal[99,101–103]
Suppress inappropriate behaviors (e.g., impulsive, drive-related behaviors)	Orbitofrontal, prefrontal, basal temporal[99,104,105]
Ego boundary (response-to-next-patient stimulation)	Frontal and parietal greater than temporal[106]
Motivation	Anterior cingulate, prefrontal
Time perception/estimation	Prefrontal, temporal[107–109]
Memory	
Temporal order	Prefrontal, temporal[77,110]
Source information	Prefrontal, temporal[111,112]
Retrieval of episodic (autobiographical) knowledge	Temporal, prefrontal[42,51,52]
Musical	
Appreciation of melody (not timbre)	Temporal, insula[61]
Emotional experience	Temporal[113]
Visual fluency	Prefrontal[114,115]
Constructing novel explanatory scenarios	Prefrontal, parietal[116]

* The lateralization and localization of these functions are relative.

5). Patients' awareness of the left side may be diminished *(sensory neglect),* or they may fail to activate motor programs for dressing *(motor neglect).* In the former instance, they omit dressing or insufficiently dress that side, and in the latter they do not make the hand, arm, and truncal adjustments needed to place the left arm through a shirt or jacket sleeve. Left-sided sensory or motor neglect not only impairs dressing skills but can also hinder shaving, washing, or other grooming activities.

Disorder of dressing ability associated with left-sided neglect (Fig. 3–1) is exemplified by one of our cases:

A 42–year-old attorney awoke one morning, a month after learning he had a right-sided parieto-occipital oligodendroglioma, and was unable to dress himself. He had no difficulty getting out of bed and performing his usual bathroom activities, including showering and shaving. After more than 5 minutes, he was able to put on his underwear but was unable to put on his shirt. He called for his wife to help

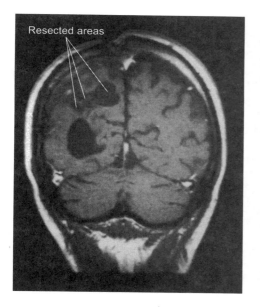
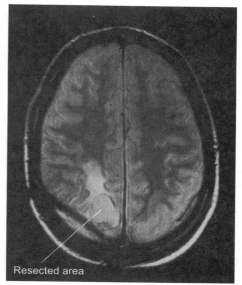
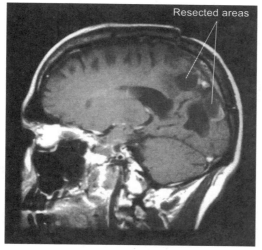

Figure 3–1. Magnetic resonance imaging of a patient with disorder of dressing ability after resection of a parieto-occipital oligodendroglioma.

him, and when she came into the bedroom, his right arm was in the left sleeve and he was attempting to button the shirt. Examination at the hospital later that day showed no abnormalities other than left-sided neglect, demonstrated only with double simultaneous stimulation by a proximal right and distal left tactile stimulus. When attempting to place a shirt on his body, he had difficulty orienting the shirt properly or deciding which arm to place into a sleeve. When the left arm was placed correctly in the left sleeve, he was unable to orient his right arm for placement into the right sleeve.

Nonlinguistic Visuospatial Functions

The right parietal lobe is dominant for nonlinguistic visuospatial functions. Right parietal lobe lesions can impair simple and complex visuospatial, perceptual, and motor tasks.[81,123–128] The visuospatial disorders include difficulty with visual orientation of lines or patterns, orientation of clothing on the body (e.g., top versus bottom, front versus back), geometric block design and assembly, visual maze performance, learning and recall of topographic relations, mental rotation, and drawing complex figures (see Chapter 5).

The two hemispheres make different contributions to drawing and copying (Table 3–3). The right hemisphere mediates visuospatial perception and the overall gestalt of figures, and the left hemisphere is concerned with detail, graphic formulas, and executive motor functions of praxis. Copies of the Rey-Osterreith Complex Figure (Fig. 3–2A) show characteristic patterns after unilateral parietotemporal injury.[128] Patients with right- sided lesions often make spatially disorganized copies that preserve detail (Fig. 3–2B), but those with left-sided lesions may produce simplified copies that lack detail but preserve overall shape and spatial relations (Fig. 3–2C). When a model is provided, the figures of patients with left-sided lesions are improved more than those of patients with right-sided lesions.[129] For example, when copying a rectangle, patients with right-sided lesions may draw four poorly formed squares to duplicate the original rectangle, rather than tracing an outline.

Right parietal lobe lesions disrupt figure copying and immediate recall, and right temporal lobe lesions are strongly correlated with failure on immediate and, particularly, delayed recall. Congenital right hemisphere injury is associated with long- term impairments in drawing skills, especially for creative elements and altering spatial configuration.[130]

Relation of the Self to the Environment

The right hemisphere is essential for spatial and topographic orientation (i.e., perceiving and manipulating the body image in space). Tactile and visceral perception is our earliest awareness of self. Right hemisphere lesions impair tactile attention[39] and the ability to detect the direction of tactile movements.[73] When a patient's arm is moved by an examiner (patient's eyes are closed), those with right-sided, but not left-sided, frontal lesions cannot correctly reproduce the movement.[131] Patients with right temporal and parietal lobe lesions can experience topographic disorientation and

Table 3–3. Effect of Cerebral Lesion Lateralization on Drawing and Copying

Feature	DRAWING AND COPYING	
	Left-Sided Lesion	Right-Sided Lesion
Overall shape	Preserved	Fragmented, disrupted
Orientation	Preserved	Impaired
Spatial relations	Preserved	Disrupted
Three-dimensional figures	Relatively preserved	Impaired
Details	Lacking	Preserved
Motor performance	Slow, effortful (apraxia)	Preserved (temporoparietal), nonfluent (frontal)
Effect of model on copying	Improved	Slightly improved
Neglect	Uncommon, right side	Common, left side

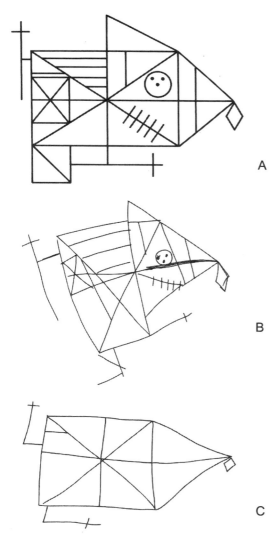

A

B

C

Figure 3–2. Copies of (A) the Rey-Osterreith Complex Figure by a patient with (B) a unilateral right parietotemporal lesion (detail is preserved, overall shape and sense of figure as a whole are lacking) and a patient with (C) a left temporoparietal lesion (overall shape and gestalt are preserved, impoverished detail throughout).

loss of topographic memory (*see* Chapter 5). Topographic disorientation may be related to reduplication for place (*see below, under* Delusional Disorders), which is associated with similar lesions that often extend to frontal regions.

Attention to representational space is a dominant function of the right hemisphere (*see* Chapter 4). Right hemisphere damage can produce unilateral neglect of representational space. For example, a patient with a right pari-

etal lobe lesion omitted details of the left side when asked to imagine the perspectives of familiar surroundings,[94,132] and a large stroke of the right frontal lobe selectively impaired visual imagery for familiar places or objects.[133] Further, the right hemisphere is the more specialized in mediating mental rotation.[81,127]

Body Schema and Disorders of the Corporeal Self

The *body schema,* our awareness of our body and the spatial relations of its parts to each other and to the environment, is formed from prior and current sensory and, in particular, somatosensory information. Within the network that contributes to our sense of physical self, the parietal lobes largely control the body schema, and the right parietal lobe is dominant.[57,104] Right hemisphere lesions can impair the body image, especially on the left side (Table 3–4). Impaired body image also contributes to allesthesia, asomatognosia, and anosognosia.

ALLESTHESIA AND ASOMATOGNOSIA

Allesthesia, the perception of a stimulus at a position remote from the actual stimulus, is usually the result of right parietal lobe lesions. Most often, a left-sided stimulus is incorrectly identified as coming from the right side.[128,134] *Asomatognosia,* the failure to perceive a body part, is also related to right parietal lobe dysfunction.

ANOSOGNOSIA

Patients with acute frontoparietal lobe lesions, almost always involving the right hemisphere, may deny or fail to recognize their own deficit, a symptom called *anosognosia.*[135] Although many patients with anosognosia are unconcerned about their deficit, others may exhibit delusional denial and become paranoid, agitated, and fearful concerning their left side.[72,136] Unilateral neglect and denial of left-sided deficits adversely affect rehabilitation.[137] Patients with left-sided hemiplegia may recognize their deficit but be indifferent to it, a symptom called *anosodiaphoria,* or show unusual reactions.[72,136] These reactions encom-

Table 3-4. Disorders of Body Schema

Disorder	Clinical Feature	Localization	Cause
Hemiasomatognosia			
Conscious type	Patient reports loss of perception of body half or part	Left- or right-sided, ?subcortical	Destructive lesion
Nonconscious type (neglect)	Patient is unaware of body half or part (e.g., may shave only one side of face)	Right parietal, occasionally right frontal, subcortical, or left-sided	Destructive lesion; rarely, seizures
Macrosomatognosia	Perception that a body part is enlarged	Temporal or parietal	Destructive or irritative lesion
Microsomatognosia	Perception that a body part is abnormally small	Temporal or parietal	Destructive or irritative lesion
Autotopagnosia	Inability to name or localize body parts (e.g., finger agnosia)	Left posteroinferior parietal region, occasionally right parietal region homologous	Destructive lesion
Anosognosia for left hemiplegia			
Verbal	Patient is unaware of left-sided hemiparesis and verbally denies paralysis	Right parietal	Destructive lesion
Nonverbal	Patient is unaware of left-sided hemiparesis and exhibits behavioral neglect (i.e., fails to compensate for paralysis)	Right parietal	Destructive lesion
Autoscopy (Doppelgänger)	Perception of seeing one's double	Temporal or parietal, ?right	Destructive or irritative lesion
Out-of-body experience	Perception of one's consciousness leaving the body	Temporal or parietal, ?right	Irritative lesion
Phantom limb phenomenon	Perception of a limb that was amputated or in which sensation was lost (rarely with congenital disorders)	Peripheral nervous system, the thalamus parietal	Amputation, sensory lesion in peripheral or central nervous system; destructive or irritative central nervous system lesion
Asymbolia for pain	Failure to exhibit normal behavioral and subjective reaction to painful stimuli	Insula and anterior cingulate; left greater than right	Destructive lesion

pass various changes in mental attitude toward the paralyzed left extremity and its relation to the self, including lack of emotional insight, excuses for the cause of the dysfunctional limb, claims that the paralyzed limb moves when it does not, attribution of limb ownership to another person, morbid revulsion leading to concealment of the arm from view, personification of the paralyzed limb, or the delusion that the right limb has increased in strength and dexterity.[72] Anosognosia often resolves days or weeks after a stroke.

The inability of the left hemisphere to recognize the deficit—the essence of anosognosia—is remarkable. Two elements must seemingly coexist for anosognosia to occur: the body schema is strongly lateralized in the right hemisphere (i.e., the profound deficit cannot

be "sensed" by the left hemisphere) and, paradoxically, when the left hemisphere is informed that an injury caused a left-sided weakness, this information, supported by sensory data input, cannot overcome the false belief. The inability to understand the explanation despite preservation of language suggests that the body schema module is needed for "corporeal comprehension." The "lying" or "confabulating" by the left hemisphere of patients with anosognosia, who often tell fantastic stories, is consistent with studies in callosotomy patients.[57] The left hemisphere will weave a story to fit the available information (Fig. 3–3), and the right hemisphere is more veridical.

The mechanism underlying anosognosia may be related to the delusional disorders that follow right hemisphere lesions and, possibly, to

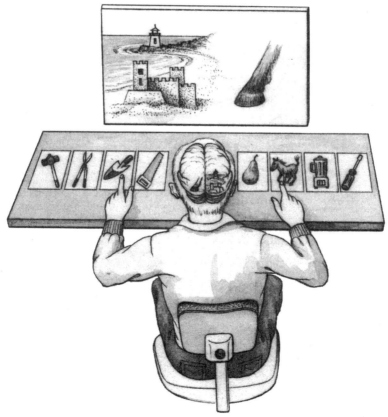

Figure 3–3. Verbal lying: left hemisphere dominance in a patient after corpus callosotomy. A picture of a sand castle is presented to the patient's left visual field (right hemisphere). He has to choose with his left hand (right hemisphere) the item that goes with the scene and correctly chooses the shovel. When asked why he made this choice, his left (language) hemisphere answers ("The shovel is the only tool found in a stable"). The left hemisphere saw the horse's hoof; therefore, he incorporates this into his explanation. (Modified from Gazzaniga.[57])

conversion disorder (see below). Anosognosia may be considered an *organic* delusional disorder, as exemplified by the delusion of body part reduplication, which is associated with right frontoparietal lesions.[138,139] The right hemisphere may detect conceptual errors and help the left hemisphere to recognize ideas and concepts that are wrong, even if they are verbally conceived. In conversion disorder, for example, the left hemisphere may verbally express shock and bewilderment that symptoms are "self-generated," even if through nonconscious processes. This speculation is supported by the predominance of right hemisphere lesions among conversion disorder patients with unilateral cerebral lesions.[140] Further, studies in callosotomy patients suggest that the left hemisphere will "lie," fabricating responses to information presented selectively to the right hemisphere instead of admitting "I don't know." [57] Disrupting the flow of information on corporeal and emotional status from the right to the left hemisphere, by right hemisphere or callosal injury, may contribute to conversion symptoms, with left hemisphere verbal responses similar to those in anosognosia or delusional disorders.

DISORDERS OF APPETITE

The right hemisphere, dominant in emotional control, may be critical in controlling drive-related behaviors, including hunger and possibly others, such as sex, that have strong corporeal features.[90a,90b,90c] Lesions and seizure foci of the right hemisphere are more likely than those of the left hemisphere to produce anorexia.[90d,90e,141] Vomiting during temporal lobe seizures is associated with a right hemisphere focus.[90f,142] Right hemisphere dysfunction or injury may contribute to eating disorders (a paradigm of distorted body image) or changes in eating patterns.

The gourmand syndrome is a benign eating disorder associated with lesions of the right anterior cerebral hemisphere. Regard and Landis[143] studied 36 patients with the gourmand syndrome who had lesions of the right frontal lobe, basal ganglia, or limbic areas. After cerebral injury, the patients became preoccupied with food and often expressed a strong preference for distinct food types and fine eating. They had normal hunger and satiety signals but often craved food. Only 7 of the 36 patients

(19.4%) were mildly obese. Other behaviors associated with "disinhibition" or diminished impulse control after right hemisphere injury include loquaciousness, heightened aggression and drive, and affective lability. The gourmand syndrome may result from impaired impulse control for eating.

Paradoxically, right hemisphere lesions can produce improvement in some psychophysiological conditions. This phenomenon is illustrated by our experience in caring for a young woman with anorexia nervosa and medically refractory partial epilepsy:

After counseling and psychotropic therapy for her eating disorder, the patient gained 10 pounds and underwent a successful left temporal lobectomy. However, she subsequently lost weight despite further psychiatric treatment. One year after the temporal lobectomy and after stopping her antiepileptic medications, she had a tonic-clonic seizure and struck her head on a radiator, resulting in a right-sided subdural hematoma with coma and left-sided hemiparesis. After rehabilitation, her neurological examination results improved to near baseline, although neuroimaging studies revealed right-sided inferofrontal and temporal encephalomalacia. She was no longer anorexic and had insight into her previously abnormal behavior. She observed, "There was something inside me that told me I was fat, not to eat. It was not a voice. A part of myself that was stronger than me. It's gone now."

The resolution of the anorexia may have resulted from destruction of a "dysfunctional body-image module." Right temporal lobectomy led to the resolution of bulimia in one woman (personal observation) and obsessive–compulsive disorder in another.[144]

RIGHT HEMISPHERE DOMINANCE OF THE PSYCHIC SELF

The self is the complete sum of essential qualities constituting an individual person and distinguishing him or her from others. The self is a composite of reflective, verbal, motor, psychic, and corporeal, as well as other, elements. The psychic component consists of emotional and social elements, forming a core of personality. Normal nondominant frontotemporal function helps to maintain the psychic self.[145] Patients with nondominant frontotemporal lobe lesions often lack previously learned self-concepts despite preserved memory and language.

The right hemisphere is dominant for emotion,[88,146–148] but observational, physiological, and neuroimaging studies in patients with unilateral cerebral injury and in normal subjects refute simple left–right theories.[44,149–151] The range of right hemisphere strategies and functions supports the networks that mediate primary emotions: nonverbal functions, synthetic and holistic functions, arousal and attention, recognition of faces and facial expressions, visuospatial functions, and gestalt-pattern recognition.[57,152] Although the emotional range is restricted after massive right hemisphere lesions, emotional function persists. The limbic system is formed by *both* hemispheres and their subcortical structures (*see* Chapter 10). Projections from the cortical limbic areas (anterior cingulate cortex, posterior orbitofrontal cortex, and anterior insula cortex) to the amygdala, hippocampus, hypothalamus, and brain stem regions modulate the arousal state, autonomic and visceral activity, motivation, mood, and movement (*see* Table 10–1).

The valence hypothesis of emotion proposes that negative emotions are lateralized to the right hemisphere and positive emotions to the left hemisphere.[43,45] This was suggested by observations that right hemisphere lesions cause emotional flattening, indifference, euphoria, and mania[43,134] and that left hemisphere lesions, especially of the frontal lobe, more often cause depression and anxiety.[104,153,154] In addition, right-sided intracarotid amobarbital injections may elicit euphoria and mania, but left-sided injections may produce little or negative affective change.[155,156]

Although some studies in normal subjects and patients with focal brain deficits support the valence theory,[45–47,155,157] others do not.[89,158–161] Severe depression can develop after right hemisphere strokes.[154,162] Euphoria can complicate Wernicke's aphasia. Emotional changes during the intracarotid amobarbital test vary, depending on individual factors (e.g., a history of emotional trauma), the test setting, and the presence or absence of brain lesions.[155,163,164]

Hemispheric differences in cognitive processing styles may parallel differences in emotional valence. Cognitive processes predominantly served by right hemisphere systems are specialized for recognizing and reacting to dangerous stimuli, such as attention to peripheral space, arousal, and gestalt perception.[89] Positive emotions may have greater linguistic, communicative, and social components, features that may be best served by left hemisphere processes.[45,165] These mechanistic explanations are limited, and functional neuroimaging studies reveal complex bilateral activation with univalent emotional stimuli.

Hemispheric valence may differ for the expression and experience of emotion,[48,57,89,166,167] although this hypothesis is controversial. For emotional expression, the right hemisphere may mediate negative emotions, and the left hemisphere may mediate positive emotions; for emotional perception, the right hemisphere may mediate both positive and negative emotions. A related approach-and-avoidance model[166,167] stipulates that the right hemisphere mediates avoidance and withdrawal reactions that are reactive and automatic and the left hemisphere mediates approach responses involving sequential or fine motor responses. Thus, the posterior right hemisphere dominates all emotional perception, and the frontal regions are specialized for expressive aspects of negative avoidance and for withdrawal responses versus approach responses.[166,167]

Primary and Secondary Emotions

Darwin's division of emotions into primary (e.g., fear, anger) and secondary, or social (e.g., embarrassment, pride), forms[168] was speculatively extended to hemispheric function. Experiential and noncognitive display behaviors associated with primary emotion may originate mainly in right hemisphere limbic areas, and those associated with social emotion may arise mainly in left hemisphere limbic areas.[45] Right hemisphere emotional responses may be biased negatively because primary emotions are chiefly negative, focusing on survival. In contrast, left hemisphere emotional responses may be biased positively because social display rules encourage affiliative, not antagonistic, behavior. However, the prominent social deficits observed after right frontal lobe injury suggest that social emotions are found in both hemispheres.

Each frontal region probably inhibits contralateral emotional responses.[11,46,163,166,169] Depression after left-sided lesions may result partly from disinhibition. The left hemisphere normally inhibits right hemisphere expression of sadness and anxiety through autonomic, visceral, and experiential responses. Left frontal lobe lesions unleash emotional responses in the right hemisphere, magnifying the normal depressive reaction to a physical disability from a neurological insult. Thus, depression after left frontal lobe damage may partly be a reaction to the disabling neurological deficits,[44] but this mechanism cannot explain abnormal results on the dexamethasone suppression test[170] and the depressive reactions occurring moments after left-sided internal carotid amobarbital infusion.[163] The excessive and socially inappropriate verbalization and behavioral changes observed after right frontal lobe injury are caused, in part, by the lack of inhibition normally imposed on the left frontal lobe by the right frontal lobe.[99] Such patients often display some combination of jocularity, grandiosity, and poor self-monitoring. They fail to "read" social–emotional cues and to consider the consequences of their actions. Right basal temporal and orbitofrontal lobe lesions lead to mania, with elevated mood, impaired impulse control, and heightened arousal.[171]

Emotional Perception

Emotional perception analyzes and categorizes environmental and internal events. Visual and auditory sensory modalities predominate in humans and, along with visceral, autonomic, and skeletomotor signals, such as bladder distention or heart rate, can influence emotional perception. Visceral stimuli, such as chest pressure, and crude modality-specific stimuli, such as a loud noise, buzzing insect, or intense vibration, signal emotionally relevant data to the amygdala directly from the thalamus (see Fig. 10–5). Emotional perception is predominantly nonconscious, but conscious components contribute. Preliminary studies support right hemisphere dominance in detecting emotionally relevant visceral[172] and environmental[173] signals, such as olfaction. When exposed to unpleasant movie scenes, normal subjects and patients with left-sided brain injury divert their gaze from the screen but patients with right hemisphere lesions do not exhibit this avoidance behavior.[158]

A complex sensory stimulus, such as an angry facial expression, reaches limbic areas af-

ter neocortical analysis. The right hemisphere is dominant in understanding emotional facial expression,[151,174] humorous cartoons,[175] cartoons with positive and negative emotions,[176] voice tone,[146] intonation and contextual inference based on nonverbal speech elements,[146,177–179] gesture,[85] and body posture.[87] Frightening films are judged more horrible and cause greater heart rate changes when projected to the right hemisphere.[180]

Modality-specific categorization of emotional stimuli is largely mediated by modality-specific association cortex and interconnected limbic areas. Right inferior occipitotemporal lobe lesions selectively impair imagery for facial emotion.[181] White matter lesions near the forceps major (callosal connections with occipital lobe) can disconnect recognition of emotional facial displays from language cortex. Such patients can recognize similar and different emotional expressions but cannot name or point to displays described by the examiner.[182,183] Bilateral amygdala damage impairs the recognition and recall of emotion in human facial expression.[184]

Emotional Expression

The right hemisphere is dominant in cortical control of emotional expression[91] and arousal.[185] Aphasic patients can affectively color their nonfluent speech, sometimes using expletives,[186] and often become more fluent when relating an emotional message, functions mediated by the right hemisphere.[21,22] Further, patients with agraphia and aphasia are better at writing emotional words than neutral words.[187] The right hemisphere generates the emotional prosody and tone of spoken and written language (see Chapter 6). Right frontal opercular lesions can severely reduce spontaneous gestural behavior,[188] and large lesions of the right frontal lobe, encompassing medial and lateral areas, can dramatically reduce affective behavior in language and gesture.[99]

Studies in patients with unilateral brain injury and normal subjects reveal right hemisphere dominance for expressing facial emotions,[189,190] although facial expression can be reduced by right or left frontal lobe lesions.[191,192] Both hemispheres likely contribute to posed facial expressions, but the right hemisphere dominates spontaneous facial expressions. In portraits, subjects usually show their left cheek more prominently, a bias that becomes exaggerated when they are asked to display emotion and reduced when they have to conceal emotion.[193] Right hemisphere dominance of emotional expression may also extend to sexual interest,[90a,194] orgasm,[90c,195] pain,[196] and reaction to neurological deficits.[136]

Right hemisphere injury, especially involving frontotemporal areas, often produces emotional indifference.[162] Such a patient may learn, for example, that a close family member has died and show little sadness; his or her first question after learning of the death may be inappropriate, as in "What's for lunch?" In contrast, patients with left hemisphere lesions often display exaggerated ("catastrophic") emotional responses.[153]

Emotional Cognition and Memory

Emotional cognition refers to the cerebral processes that interface feeling and thought. It plays the primary role in the analysis, understanding, and meaning of emotional feelings and signals and helps to create social intelligence. The right hemisphere is dominant in emotional cognition,[197] which includes comprehending internal and external emotional signals in light of experience, anticipating the consequences of emotional actions, learned reflexive responses, inhibiting innate tendencies, sending "test" emotional messages to assess responsiveness, and other integrations of emotion with current and planned behaviors. The amygdala primarily provides emotional valence to environmental stimuli and activates emotional responses. Anterior cingulate and posterior orbitofrontal cortices provide motivational and social context for emotional behavior.

The right hemisphere plays a critical role in providing figural or narrative "gestalt" and coherence,[198] inferential reasoning,[199] and inhibiting responses based on initial cognitive analysis.[105] Ramachandran[116] postulated a critical role of the right hemisphere in creating a new model to explain data when anomalies exceed a threshold. In contrast, the left hemisphere typically deals with small, local anomalies or discrepancies by imposing order and maintaining the status quo. This cognitive model may help to account for disorders such as anosognosia.

Right hemisphere neocortical areas may be dominant for retrieval and, possibly, represention of emotional autobiographical memories.[51,52] In normal subjects, these memories are selectively processed by the right temporal lobe and nondominant neocortical and limbic areas.[200] Markowitsch et al.[51,201] described a patient with a traumatic brain injury who was in a coma for 6 weeks. Lesions were bilateral but involved mainly the right prefrontal and anterolateral temporal regions. Following recovery, the patient could encode, consolidate, and retrieve verbal information but had severe retrograde amnesia for autobiographical data. Despite pictorial and verbal cues, for example, the patient could not recall climbing Mount Kilimanjaro. Recall of personal possessions, such as photographs of loved ones, was impaired, but semantic and procedural knowledge was largely preserved. Although he did not recognize his favorite pocketwatch, he recalled the trick of how to open its back. When, with his eyes closed, he smelled the aftershave he had used for 7 years before the trauma, he was unfamiliar with the scent but recalled the name.

Emotional memories form a base for emotional cognition, providing a template upon which new and planned events can be compared and analyzed. Memory relies on emotion to color, classify, and weigh experience, thereby creating a hierarchy for limited storage space. Mnemonic illusions (e.g., *déjà vu*, *jamais vu*) are more frequent with right-sided than left-sided temporal lobe seizures.[202,203] The association of mnemonic illusions with emotional auras, also more frequent with right-sided temporal lobe seizures, supports a dominant role of this area in emotional memories.[204] Species-specific instincts include preprogrammed memories for emotional stimuli, as shown, for example, by baby monkeys' fear of snakes on initial exposure. Genetically determined behavioral tendencies may be specific for species and individuals. The bank of personal emotional memories together with inherited tendencies contribute to personality. A stressful event such as a mugging can exert long-lasting effects on behavior. Through studies with his dogs, Pavlov[205] recognized that strong and extraordinary stimuli (e.g., the great flood in Petrograd) could produce long-lasting psychopathological changes on a neurophysiological (functional or neurotic) basis.

Emotional Experience of Self

Functional imaging and electrophysiological studies reveal a right hemisphere dominance for self-recognition. The ability to recognize one's own face (e.g., in a mirror) is limited to a few species. While face recognition in general selectively activates the fusiform gyrus in humans, self-recognition also activates the ventral prefrontal areas on the right.[205a] A lesion of the right frontal, temporal, or parietal lobe impairs recognition of one's own face, but not the faces of others, in a mirror.[205a] These findings, together with others cited, support the concept of right hemisphere dominance in recognition and processing of "self."

Alexithymia, the diminished ability to identify and describe one's own feelings, is associated with right hemisphere dysfunction.[206,207] Alexithymia occurs in callosotomy patients, who are verbally unable to report on their mood.[208] Psychophysiological studies of normal subjects with high and low alexithymia scores on rating scales support the right hemisphere dysfunction or impaired transfer from right to left hemispheres as models of alexithymia.[207]

Many ictal emotional and experiential phenomena occur more frequently with right than left temporal lobe seizures. Phenomena reported more often with right temporal lobe seizures include depersonalization, fear, grief, crying, theme of death, ecstatic and religious feelings,[204,209,210] and familiarity (*déjà vu*) or unfamiliarity (*jamais vu*).[200,202,203] Right temporal lobe seizures can evoke seeing one's entire life as a series of multisensory mental film clips[202] and feeling "someone being nearby or coming up from behind."[202,211,212] Experiential phenomena with "a current autobiographical element" are more common with right than left temporal lobe seizures.[202]

Survival demands an acute sense of *familiarity,* the relation between past and present experiences with other living beings, inanimate objects, and locales. Humans use extensive visual input to distinguish the familiar from the foreign, as in, faces. The right hemisphere predominantly analyzes stimuli for familiarity and links emotion to familiar stimuli. Impairment of this function produces an altered sense of familiarity and likely contributes to deficits in autobiographical memory, source memory, or false recognition of faces or information,[42,213]

as well as delusional reduplication syndromes associated with right hemisphere lesions.

The higher frequency of *déjà vu* experiences with right than with left temporal lobe seizures or electrical stimulation suggests that the right temporal lobe predominates in generating the emotion of familiarity. Anosognosia, in which the intact left hemisphere fails to perceive the impaired left body as familiar, may partly result from loss of right hemisphere capacity to recognize something as familiar.

Landis and Regard[214] reported a double dissociation in two patients with ischemic infarction of the posterior cerebral artery in opposite hemispheres. The patient with the left-sided lesion had alexia without agraphia and was unable to say what was written but could tell by whom it was written through recognition of the handwriting. In contrast, the patient with the right-sided lesion had prosopagnosia and was able to say what was written but not who had written it, complaining that she had lost the sense of familiarity of handwriting, including her own.

Volition

Volition is strongly modulated by the right hemisphere. Volition, or will, is the conscious process of selecting a mental or physical activity and deciding when to do it. William James,[215] in 1890, wrote that the most voluntary aspect of will "is to ATTEND to a difficult object and hold it fast before the mind." Volition includes both the decision for and the initiation of behavior. Intentional movement is a product of will. Several observations support the dominance of the right hemisphere over intention and motivation. For instance, impairment in raising the contralateral shoulder is greater with strokes in the right hemisphere than in the left hemisphere, regardless of the severity of the hemiparesis.[216] Further, *motor impersistence,* the inability to sustain action, occurs almost exclusively with acute right-sided frontocentral lesions.[181] The mean duration of performance on such motor tasks as "Close your eyes," "Protrude your tongue," "Open your mouth," "Gaze to the right side," and "Say 'aah' " is much shorter in patients with acute right hemisphere injuries than in those with left-sided acute injuries.[84] *Simultanapraxia,* a subset of motor impersistence, is the inability to perform two motor acts simultaneously. It is associated with right hemisphere lesions (Brodmann's areas 6 and 8), often occurring after an infarction of the right middle cerebral artery.[217]

Disorders of the Social Self

Developmental and acquired right hemisphere disorders can impair social awareness and behavior. Affected patients may fail to comprehend emotional and social cues; may not express such social displays as greetings, goodbyes, eye contact, and facial expressions; and may be unable to plan actions in a social context. Developmental impairments in social and emotional processing cause a spectrum of behaviors ranging from a nonverbal learning disorder to Asperger's syndrome, a severe and sustained impairment of social interaction, with restricted and repetitive patterns of behaviors, interests, and activities. A nonverbal learning disorder may result from right hemisphere abnormalities.[50,96,206] Patients with this disorder may have normal to high verbal intelligence and academic success but often are isolated and socially withdrawn, with few close interpersonal relations. They often avoid eye contact and have impoverished gestural and prosodic communication. Many have difficulty in arithmetic and visuospatial skills, which together with the neurological and neuropsychological signs suggests right hemisphere dysfunction.[96] Acquired right hemisphere lesions disrupt social behavior and interpersonal skills, often leading to loss of friends, unemployment, or divorce.[100] Large right frontal lobe lesions encompassing medial and lateral prefrontal areas profoundly reduce the affective range, causing emotional flattening, apathy, and impaired awareness and responsiveness to social context.[99,218] In patients with frontotemporal dementia, socially undesirable behaviors predominate in those with right-sided lesions. Criminal activity, aggression, loss of job, alienation from family or friends, financial recklessness, sexually deviant behavior, and abnormal response to spousal crisis were found in 11 of 12 such patients with right-sided lesions and only 2 of 19 with left-sided lesions.[219] A man with trauma to the right orbitofrontal and prefrontal areas, who exhibited sociopathic behavior and severe aggression, was unable to recognize and autonomically respond to negative emotional expressions and to identify aberrant social behavior[220] (see Chapter 10).

IMPOVERISHED EYE CONTACT

Eye contact is an intimate and powerful form of communication. We learn about the motives and interests of others and reveal our feelings through eye contact and facial expression. Among anthropoid apes, direct, sustained eye contact is a threat.[221] In humans, direct eye contact signals a strong interpersonal context, which can be positive, as in love or trust, or negative, as in anger or threat. Infants who avert their gaze from their parents develop maladaptive relationships, behavioral problems, and developmental delays in later childhood.[222]

The right temporal lobe dominates perception of gaze.[97] Brain injury can disrupt eye contact.[223] In humans, right hemisphere dysfunction impairs both the understanding and the transmission of affective messages delivered through gaze, although complete dissociation of emotions expressed in the eyes from other facial expressions is unusual.[178] Children with a nonverbal learning disorder (with predominantly right hemisphere dysfunction) and adults with right hemisphere lesions often make little eye contact and are unable to derive social cues from eye contact.[50,96] Gaze directed toward another person selectively activates that person's right amygdala.[224] In some brain-injured patients, eye contact triggers intense distress.[225]

NONVERBAL EMOTIONAL COMMUNICATION

The right hemisphere modulates nonverbal, as well as verbal, emotional communication. Although words convey complex concepts, much information is transmitted by nonverbal behaviors. The direction of gaze and facial expression, for example, can contradict a person's words and reveal his or her true feelings. Right hemisphere dominance of nonverbal emotional expression extends to facial movements (emotional expressions produce greater motor activity in the left lower face),[89,190,226] autonomic responses,[227] gestures,[188] and eye contact.[96] Changes in heart rate, respiratory rate, and perspiration are easily measured and form the basis of the polygraph, or lie detector, test.

Most nonverbal behavior is poorly documented in clinical and research neurology. Early on, John Hughlings Jackson[21] recognized that patients with left hemisphere lesions and aphasia can communicate emotions through right hemisphere "nervous arrangements:"

He smiles, laughs, frowns and varies his voice properly. His recurring utterance comes out now in one tone and now in another, according as he is vexed, glad, etc. . . . he may swear when excited, or get out more innocent interjections, simple or compound (acquired parts of emotional language).

Emotional elements and contours of speech are recognized mainly by the right hemisphere.[177,178,228] However, both hemispheres comprehend *propositional prosody*, the rhythm or pitch that confers semantic, lexical, or syntactic meaning, and understand the emotion conveyed by descriptive sentences[88] (see Chapter 6). Right hemisphere lesions impair the comprehension of emotional messages in language[89] and the capacity to determine whether prosodically intoned statements are questions or commands.[178] In contrast, left hemisphere lesions cause *pure word deafness*, a disorder in which patients cannot comprehend speech but can recognize environmental sounds and emotional aspects of speech. After left hemisphere injury, patients comprehend spoken or written emotional words and sentences more readily than neutral words[229] and produce emotional discourse more effectively than neutral discourse,[230] which probably reflects right hemisphere participation. Lesions of the right hemisphere impair verbal communication of nonverbal affective signals[88] and higher-level inferential reasoning, such as interpreting humorous statements and figures of speech.[36,231]

Injury of the right anterior hemisphere impairs emotional speech tone[89,188] and diminishes emotional words in discourse.[186] After a stroke involving the right anterior hemisphere, a woman gave up teaching because she could no longer control the children through the tone of her voice, despite attempts at strongly worded verbal discipline.[232] Such patients often speak in a flat monotone, lacking emotional prosody.

Modulating nonverbal emotional communication is a critical influence of the right hemisphere on social function. Gestural behaviors can communicate linguistic (semiotic or pantomime) and emotional components. However, disorders causing *affective prosody*, the imparting of emotional tone to speech, caused by right hemisphere injury, can also impair spontaneous gesturing and the comprehension of affective gestures.[147] Further, left hemisphere lesions can impair comprehension of symbolic, nonemotional gestures, such as pantomime,[233] but emotional gesturing can increase in patients with aphasia.

SOCIAL LANGUAGE IMPAIRMENTS

The right hemisphere dominates the social aspects of speech.[99,178] Right hemisphere lesions impair social aspects of language comprehension, including nonliteral verbal humor,[234] metaphor,[231] connotative (associative) word meanings,[24] ambiguous word meanings,[235] indirect requests,[36] sarcasm,[236] and affect.[237] Impaired use of personal referents, such as inappropriately using formal rather than informal descriptors, can disturb interpersonal behavior in patients with right hemisphere lesions.[238]

Right frontal lobe lesions can impair the coherent stream and organization of conversation.[198] Patients may produce speech that is excessive, tangential, rambling, and filled with irrelevant personal and vague comments.[36,101] Inferential clues in other people's speech are often missed.[236,239] Right frontal lobe lesions can lead to disinhibited, excessive, and loquacious speech, or *logorrhea*.[101,102,105] Patients fail to recognize nonverbal and verbal cues to end a conversation or stop talking about a topic that upsets another person. They fail to monitor the impact of their comments on listeners, as in this example:

One of us treated a woman with encephalomalacia after resection of a meningioma in the right frontal lobe, who routinely produced a 40–minute monologue despite being informed that office visits were limited to 20 minutes. She could not be interrupted for more than a few seconds. In response to a plea for the examiner to speak, she said "There are a dozen more things I must tell you. By the way, is something wrong with your watch? You keep looking at it."

Right-sided frontotemporal lesions can impair verbal and nonverbal decorum. These patients produce socially embarrassing comments, without cause or insight, that can degrade themselves, family members, or strangers.[98,99] They cannot withhold thoughts or answers. Their humor is coarse, inappropriate, and sometimes accompanied by their own isolated, intense laughter. The opposite social emotion, embarrassment, can result from right frontal lobe activation during a partial seizure.[240]

The right hemisphere's role in modulating the social context of language is reflected in the response of one of our patients:

A 22–year-old man had epilepsy and low self-esteem. During bilateral frontotemporal depth electrode recording, he had a seizure in which ictal activity was restricted to the right temporal lobe but with slowing in the right frontal lobe. During the seizure, he emotionally responded to the nurse's request "Tell me your name" by saying "Have you ever heard anyone called stupid. That's my name. Stupid."

This man later said that an "inner voice," not under his will yet not considered foreign, would comment on his actions as "stupid."

DISORDERS OF EGO BOUNDARY

Among the disorders of ego boundary is the "response-to-next- patient stimulation." It occurs in patients with acute right hemisphere strokes who obey commands such as "Open your mouth," addressed to a patient in the adjacent bed.[106] This response is a defect in distinguishing verbal information directed at others versus self. The left hemisphere comprehends the question and executes the correct response but cannot identify the social context.

Delusional Disorders

Delusions are false, sustained beliefs based on incorrect inferences about the self or the environment that cannot be overturned by refuting evidence, and delusional disorders take many forms (Table 3–5). Content-specific delusions focus on a single theme, such as misidentification of people, places, objects, or sexual issues, as with jealousy or penile retraction, or somatic complaints, as with disease or body part distortion. Delusions most often occur in patients with psychiatric or diffuse neurological disorders, including metabolic disturbances and dementia. Delusions frequently

follow right hemisphere lesions,[241] and focal brain lesions associated with delusional disorders are often found in the right frontal lobe.[242–244] In studies of linguistic interpretation, patients with right hemisphere injuries had difficulty revising an initial interpretation in light of subsequent, contradictory information.[36] Their inability to revise a point of view of a word, sentence, or discourse may partly reflect the same defect that allows other patients with right-sided lesions to become fixed on an idea or belief despite evidence to the contrary.

Patients with right middle cerebral artery infarctions may exhibit delusional jealousy (Othello syndrome), fears of infidelity,[245] or paranoid delusions, as of poisoning.[246] Right hemisphere injury superimposed on generalized brain atrophy may contribute to delusions.[241,246]

Capgras' syndrome, a delusional reduplication, is the delusional belief that familiar people, often family members, are being impersonated by identical doubles.[247] Delusional belief in doubles can also involve the self, as in autoscopy (Doppelgänger),[248] or a persecutor who assumes the appearance of others (de Fregoli's syndrome).[244] Some delusions involve the belief that the physical or mental self is wholly or partly replaced or that others mistake the patient for someone else. Other content-specific reduplicative delusions extend to objects and environmental settings, as in reduplicative paramnesia.[249,250] Capgras' syndrome and related reduplicative delusions may occur in stroke, brain tumor, encephalitis, and other neurological disorders.[241,244] Neurodiagnostic studies in these secondary cases of Capgras' syndrome reveal bilateral or right frontotemporal abnormalities.[244]

Conversion Disorder

Conversion disorder is common, with symptoms suggesting a physical disorder but resulting from psychological factors. Risk factors for conversion disorder include female sex, sexual or physical abuse, other emotional traumas, and minor traumatic brain injury.[251,252] The risk is also increased in patients with neurological disorders.[140] Clinical observations from the late nineteenth century[253,254] to recent times[255–258] show that conversion symptoms more often affects the left side of the body. The

Table 3–5. **Delusional Disorders**

Disorder	Symptom or Belief
Paranoid or persecutory delusions (schizophrenia, severe depression, stimulant toxicity of the central nervous system)	
Referential ideas	People are talking about, insulting, spying on, or harassing one
Theft	One's property or inheritance is being stolen or cheated away
Jealousy	—
Poisoning	
Influence	Outside forces are controlling one's mind or actions
Delusions of illness	
Hypochondriasis: monosymptomatic	Disease of specific organ, or specific disease (parasitosis)
Hypochondriasis: somatization disorder (Briquet's syndrome)	Disease of multiple organ systems simultaneously
Somatic delusions	Bizarre beliefs regarding body image
Delusions of grandeur (confabulation, mania; formerly with neurosyphilis)	
Delusions of love (structural brain lesions, epilepsy)	
de Clerambault's syndrome	Erotomania with the belief that a person, often famous, is in love with one
Phantom lover	—
Jealousy or fears of infidelity	
Delusions of poverty	
Delusion of negation (Cotard's syndrome)	
Negative ideas	Part of the body is missing, the material or conceptual world ceases to exist
Delusions of possession (psychosis, usually; may complicate epilepsy)	
Delusions of reduplication (psychiatric disorders, bifrontal or right hemisphere disorders)	
Reduplicative paramnesia	Reduplication of place
Capgras' syndrome	Reduplication of another person
Double (doppelgänger)	Reduplication of self
de Fregoli's syndrome	A person changes identity by disguise or magic and often torments one
Reduplication or misidentification of objects	Objects are replaced, moved, or altered

left-sided extremities also appear more malleable to hypnotic suggestion.[258a,b] Further, structural or physiological disorders of the right hemisphere may be complicated by conversion symptoms, including seizures, weakness, amnesia, and astasia-abasia.[140,259] Among 60 patients with unilateral cerebral abnormalities, 43 (71%) had right hemisphere structural lesions or physiological dysfunction $(P < 0.02)$.[140] Conversion symptoms also occur in patients with left hemisphere disorders.[260]

The coexistence of neurological and conversion disorders, with neurological impairment typically the preceding event, suggests that brain dysfunction contributes to the development of conversion symptoms. Three patients with partial epilepsy whose seizures evolved into conversion seizures had right frontotemporal seizure foci.[261] The report of a case from this series illustrates how right hemisphere dysfunction may help to uncouple components of self:

A 62-year-old man with a right frontotemporal glioma and partial seizures began having atypical seizures, strongly suggesting conversion symptoms. During video-EEG monitoring, seizures characterized by bizarre, complex, purposeful motor activity were induced and terminated by normal saline injection and suggestion. During a simple partial seizure with an ictal discharge on EEG, he complained of fear, and while talking to a nurse, had a conversion seizure in which he was holding both bedrails and shaking wildly from side to side while still answering the nurse's questions. There were no additional abnormal EEG changes during the attack.
                            Devinsky and Gordon[261]

Presumably, ictal fear superimposed on right hemisphere dysfunction contributed to the elaboration of the patient's conversion symptoms.

Conversion disorder is associated with simultaneous restriction of conscious awareness and aberrant expression of nonconscious will. In contrast with the nonconsciously mediated processes dominating normal cognition,[27] conversion symptoms may result from nonconscious elements of mind that alter sensory, motor, or behavioral function. The production of conversion symptoms (e.g. seizures, paresis) may result from right hemisphere areas that become disinhibited, similar to the willful and independent behaviors of the alien hand syndrome (see Below). Right hemisphere dysfunction can impair conscious awareness of body parts, sensory input, emotional and social cues and neurological deficits (e.g., anosognosia). Failure of the left hemisphere to recognize the "self-generated" symptoms of conversion may be caused by disconnection or destruction of brain areas needed for such recognition. Alternatively, a part of the nonconscious mind that may normally inhibit conscious awareness of emotional content may become may extend inhibition over a wider, pathological field of behavior. Right hemisphere lesions may thus simultaneously impair the capacity to "psychologically handle" painful emotions and erode the awareness of self-features (e.g., anosognosia) and self- generated behaviors (e.g., conversion symptoms) that would otherwise be accessible to consciousness.

THE CEREBRAL COMMISSURES

The corpus callosum is the largest interhemispheric commissure, increasing phylogenetically with associative neocortical volume.

Callosal fibers interconnect homologous association areas of the two hemispheres, but the connections between primary sensorimotor areas are minimal.[262] Two other intercortical connections in humans are the hippocampal commissure, which interconnects the hippocampal and entorhinal areas, and the anterior commissure, which interconnects the olfactory bulbs, amygdalae, and entorhinal and other temporal areas.

The functions of the corpus callosum remain incompletely defined. This massive fiber bundle may be absent at birth (agenesis of the corpus callosum) or severed to control seizures (corpus callosotomy), but intellect and behavior may be near normal.[263–265] The corpus callosum can rapidly inform the hemisphere on one side of what is happening on the other side. However, approximately 40% of callosal fibers are unmyelinated, and these slow-conducting fibers primarily inhibit contralateral activity.[266] Preserved functions after callosotomy may reflect the normal role of the callosum in maintaining hemispheric independence through inhibition.[265] Further, noncallosal routes can support many interhemispheric communications. However, by disrupting the transfer of information and callosum-mediated inhibition, callosal lesions can severely disrupt behavior.

Callosotomy and Functional Impairment

Knowledge of callosal functions and deficits after callosal lesions comes from anatomical studies, animal studies, patients with strokes, and, most importantly, elective division of the corpus callosum for seizure control. In the cognitive laboratory, stimuli can be selectively presented to each hemisphere. For instance, sensory stimuli were presented to one hand of a blindfolded patient, or vision was fixated centrally while a brief stimulus was presented with a tachistoscope. Early studies revealed that the right hemisphere could comprehend single words and simple commands. Later, the Z-lens, a contact lens projecting to the hemiretina, allowed more prolonged visual stimulation of one hemisphere (hemifield) and greater exploration of lateralized functions.[208] Extensive interhemispheric communication, including simple sensory and motor signals,[267] abstract concepts,[208] and inhibitory control signals,[265] persists after neocortical commissurotomy.

Each hemisphere is capable of emotional comprehension and expression, self-awareness, and social judgment.[268] Callosotomy studies support left hemisphere dominance for language, analytical functions, and skilled praxis movements and right hemisphere dominance for visuospatial functions, constructional (manipulative) tasks that rely on spatial concepts, facial recognition, and emotional responsiveness.[31,57,208,265] However, a function is rarely fully lateralized. In most subjects, for example, the right hemisphere can comprehend single words but its language competence varies.

MOTOR FUNCTION

Human evolution has transformed perceptual dominance from the olfactory, gustatory, and tactile modalities to the visual and auditory modalities and motor dominance from an automatized quadruped to a novel bimanual modality, with one hand dominating in dexterity and power. The hand and foot areas of the human primary motor and somatosensory cortices have no callosal connections.[269] The dominance of one side may reflect active inhibition mediated by fibers arising in motor association cortices.

Cats and monkeys trained to perform a task using one hemisphere can transfer the skills to the other hemisphere. After commissurotomy, however, they fail to perform the task in the untrained hemisphere.[270] Similar behavior occurs in patients with callosotomy.[271] In animals, however, the untrained hemisphere gains slight improvements, suggesting that subcortical structures transfer rudimentary data to the unexposed hemisphere.[208]

After callosotomy, patients have difficulty learning new tasks requiring cooperative interaction between the two hands, as in drawing on an Etch-A-Sketch.[272] In contrast, acquired bimanual cooperative tasks, such as playing piano, typing, or bicycling, as well as alternating and parallel movements, are performed normally. Preservation of these functions supports the partial transfer of programs for habituated, complex motor tasks from motor association cortex to primary motor cortex, as well as from cortical to subcortical structures, such as the basal ganglia and cerebellum.

ATTENTION AND MEMORY

Attention becomes unstable and less sustained after callosotomy, contributing to fluctuating neglect and difficulty completing tasks requiring vigilance, such as reading a book.[273] Callosotomy also impairs nonverbal learning and memory.[274] Topographic memory is particularly impaired: patients may forget the location of their wallets and cars and navigate poorly through buildings or streets that should be familiar through repetitive exposure. Verbal memory can be affected as well, leading some patients to abandon reading and watching television or movies because the partly forgotten, fragmented plots are rendered incomprehensible. Working memory may be impaired by callosotomy.[208]

EMOTION

Callosotomy reduces the negative affective range. Patients do not react, or display muted reactions, to unpleasant stimuli or situations.[275] The restricted experience and expressiveness extends from primary emotions such as fear, anger, aggressiveness, or disgust to social emotions such as hatred, bitterness, embarrassment, envy, jealousy, or shame. These patients may relate spousal infidelity or a family member's death in a matter-of-fact manner.[208] Verbal and nonverbal emotional expressions are biased positively. Verbal humor, a left hemisphere function, remains intact. Patients spontaneously create and comprehend jokes. One patient commented "I am a lot smarter than him [her husband]; I have two brains and he has only one."[208]

When emotional stimuli are presented selectively to the right hemisphere, patients react with laughter or surprise but cannot verbally explain their response. For instance, when the right hemisphere of a patient was shown a series of geometric shapes, he was unable to name them. When shown a swastika, he responded differently. Moving in his chair, he said "What was this that you just showed me! . . . A terrible thing, an awful thing."[208]

VOLITION AND ALIEN HAND SYNDROME

Callosotomy occasionally disrupts behavioral expression as an integrated self, resulting in two spheres of independent volition. The most striking example is alien hand syndrome, of which there are two forms: callosal and hemispheric. Alien hand syndrome most commonly results from anterior callosal or medial frontal lesions but may also follow posterior callosal lesions.[276–278] In many patients, including those with anterior cerebral artery strokes, medial frontal and callosal damage coexists.

The callosal form of alien hand syndrome is a dramatic disorder in which one hand "takes on a will of its own" and interferes with the actions of the other hand. The disorder was originally described by Goldstein[279] in 1909. The patient was a 57-year-old woman with right hemisphere and callosal infarctions who experienced intermanual conflict: her left hand opposed her conscious will and the actions of her right hand. Once, when the left hand attempted to choke her, it took all her strength to pull it away from her throat. Isolated callosal lesions, including callosotomy, can produce this syndrome in the hand ipsilateral to the language-dominant hemisphere.[277,278] Later, Akelitis[276] described a case of alien hand syndrome in a woman who had undergone callosotomy:

In tasks requiring bimanual activity, the left hand would frequently perform oppositely to what she desired to do with the right hand. For example, she would be putting on clothes with her right hand and pulling them off with her left, opening a door or drawer with her right hand and simultaneously pushing it shut with the left. These uncontrollable acts made her increasingly irritated and depressed.

In another case of alien hand syndrome following callosotomy, a patient's "left hand (right brain) preferred different foods and even television shows and would interfere with the choices made by the right hand (left hemisphere)."[49,280]

In the callosal form of alien hand syndrome, the right hemisphere acts intentionally outside the awareness of verbal consciousness. The left hemisphere experiences the left hand's "antagonistic" movements as foreign and intrusive and is unable to identify a motivation for the movements or suppress them without force. Among callosotomy patients, alien hand syndrome is uncommon and often transient. Two-stage procedures with initial division of only the anterior two-thirds of the callosum has greatly reduced the frequency of this complication.

The hemispheric form of alien hand syndrome occurs in the hand contralateral to the lesion, regardless of cerebral dominance. In patients with this form of the disorder, infarction of the left anterior cerebral artery (which is approximately three times as likely as the right artery to become infarcted) with medial frontal and anterior callosal injury is the most common cause.[281] When a patient with left frontal lobe stroke and hemispheric alien hand syndrome tried "to write with her left hand, the right hand would reach over and attempt to take the pencil. The left hand would respond by grasping the right hand and trying to restrain it."[282] Medial frontal injury can cause both grasp reflex and utilization behavior (*see* Chapter 9). Together, these factors can cause the hemispheric form of alien hand syndrome. In such cases, the pathological hand does not have a will of its own but demonstrates a reflexive need to grasp and compulsively manipulate objects, as if environmental cues release automated actions, that is, an environmental dependence syndrome.

Callosotomy and Consciousness

The left hemisphere is conscious, dominating verbal behavior, introspection, and behavioral plans. Is the right hemisphere also conscious? Theories of consciousness link the phenomenon to language[283] and a left hemisphere "integrator system" that synthesizes independent brain modules and links the sequence of experiences into a unified consciousness.[57] In this view, the left hemisphere mediates consciousness.

Callosotomy patients rarely experience a "split" in their consciousness, goals, or feelings. The right hemisphere, operating independently and in isolation, shows intelligence. It can perceive, analyze, remember, perform complex reasoning, comprehend and express emotion, demonstrate cultural knowledge, and creatively respond to new environmental situations.[86,268,284–286] The right hemisphere is conscious, dominating awareness of corporeal and emotional self.

Sperry[287] posited two independent spheres of intelligent consciousness after callosotomy, one in each hemisphere; and Sperry et al.[268] reported evidence of right hemisphere intelligence in callosotomy patients. When a patient's right hemisphere was shown a picture of a familiar person, the left hand traced the first letter of the person's name on the right hand, providing the clue needed for a verbal response. In addition, when a patient's own picture was projected to the right hemisphere, the patient responded with emotional reactions such as laughter and self-conscious grins and expressed simple emotional phrases such as "Oh no! Oh God!" The right hemisphere also responded with the socially correct "thumbs up" or "thumbs down" to pictures of famous figures, such as Winston Churchill or Hitler, or attractive strangers. Thus, these experiments, demonstrating that the right hemisphere deliberately cues the left hemisphere and can recognize self, support the notion of a conscious right hemisphere.

CONSCIOUSNESS

The Modular Mind

The hierarchical, serial model of cerebral information processing dominated twentieth century neuroscience. In the visual model of this theory, for example, visual input passes sequentially to the retina, the thalamus, the primary visual areas, the visual association areas, and, finally, the visual recognition areas, creating visual conscious awareness (see Chapter 5). However, cerebral mechanisms of conscious awareness can also be understood through the more recent concept of modularity of mind[64] and the binding of modules through synchronization,[65,288] a nonhierarchical, parallel processing model. Brain function fits a modular model composed of distinct but overlapping and integrated structures and circuits that perform specific, related functions. Modular systems include hard-wired connections and instinct but allow for plasticity and learned behavior. The modules are concerned with traditional components of behavioral neurology, such as perception, memory, motor functions, language, topographic space, emotion, body image, eye–hand coordination, and visuospatial function. Other modules likely reflect critical functions in hominid evolution, such as facial recognition, predicting other people's behavior, and intuitive knowledge of motions and forces.

The visual module, for instance, contains submodules that categorize color, form, movement, and spatial location. Synchronization of activity among these submodules, as well as the primary visual cortex and subcortical visual areas, creates the mental visual image and visual consciousness (*see* Chapter 5). The visual module is linked with the language module. Synchronization of activity between these modules is necessary for reading. Destruction of critical submodules in the visual or language module or of connections between visual and language modules can impair reading. The core process of brain function leading from vision to movement to consciousness is the synchronization of activity in cells involved in a related function.

PARALLEL DISTRIBUTED PROCESSING

Despite the critical role of serial processing, the concept of parallel distributed processing (PDP) may be the dominant mode of information processing in the brain.[64,289] The PDP model, also known as connectivity, postulates large numbers of independent modules and submodules that carry out simple and complex perceptual and cognitive functions. These form various networks that are anatomically and functionally distinct, with different programming rules and modulating influences. When a module is activated, it excites and inhibits many other modules through massive associative connections that rapidly process information until a steady state is reached. Parallel processing is nonconscious, but when a steady state is reached, conscious awareness of information is possible. Consciousness may rely more heavily on the slower serial processing model than on nonconscious PDP processes. Consciousness can access the products of PDP processes but cannot introspectively report on how the information was obtained.

The parceling of cognitive functions into modules and submodules (nodes) is relative, not absolute. Nodes in each module help to coordinate the overall function, but each node is specialized for certain behavioral elements; the nodes are not interchangeable.[290] In the attentional system, for example, the posterior parietal, dorsolateral frontal, and anterior cingulate areas and the frontal eye fields are interconnected nodes that have different but overlapping roles in sensory, motor, cognitive, and motivational aspects of attention. Similarly, patients with lesions of Wernicke's area are deficient in comprehending spoken or written language and decoding individual word meanings. However, they may have mild deficiencies in syntax and articulation, functions more specialized in Broca's node of the language module.

THALAMIC INTEGRATION AND SYNCHRONIZATION

The synchronization of massive parallel connections may unify behavior and create consciousness. The ascending reticular activating system originates in the brain stem and is relayed to the cerebral cortex via intralaminar and other thalamic nuclei, with acetylcholine and glutamate as the main neurotransmitters.[291] Arousal and vigilance are associated with activation in the midbrain reticular activating system and thalamic intralaminar nuclei.[287] Projections of the ascending midbrain reticular formation facilitate oscillatory gamma frequency activity (>30 Hz) and desynchronize lower-frequency activity.[292] The intralaminar thalamic nucleus may synchronize subcortical and cortical activity. A proposed model of thalamocortical circuitry has two resonant loops, one between specific thalamic nuclei and the cortex and the other between nonspecific thalamic nuclei and the cortex[293] (Fig. 3–4). The thalamic reticular nucleus and cortical gamma frequency interneurons synchronize oscillations between both loops. The intralaminar nonspecific nucleus, projecting throughout the neocortex, provides the anatomical connections for diffuse but nearly simultaneous neocortical stimulation.[293] Analogous loops may link the basal ganglia with the cortex, thalamus, and brain stem; the thalamus may be the pacemaker. Similarly, within the cortex, discrete channel-specific synchronous connections underlie the content of consciousness and nonspecific loops temporally unite conscious experience. High-frequency brain activity may have a critical role in attention, perception, and language processing.[294]

Fundamental Features of Consciousness

William James,[295] in 1890, equated consciousness with thought and introduced the popular metaphors "stream of thought" and "stream of consciousness." He named and defined five fundamental features of conscious thought: *(1) subjectivity* ("Every thought tends to be part of a personal consciousness"), *(2) change* ("Within each personal consciousness thought is always changing"), *(3) continuity* ("Within each personal consciousness thought is sensibly continuous"), *(4) content* (it is about something; "It always appears to deal with objects independent of itself"), and *(5) selective attention* ("It is interested in some parts of these objects to the exclusion of others, and welcomes or rejects—*chooses* from among them, in a word—all the while"). We actually ignore most of the things before us. Consciousness mediates our awareness of perceptions, feelings, memories, thoughts, and willful actions. However, those functions are included in the contents of consciousness. To be aware of them is to be conscious.

When James[295] wrote "The universal conscious fact is not 'feelings exist' and 'thoughts exist' but 'I think' and 'I feel'," he recognized that the critical feature of consciousness is reference to the self. We must relate our sensations, thoughts, and emotions to our representation of self for conscious awareness. Neurological and psychiatric disorders can result from the failure to link mental activities to self. Further, nonconscious cognition can monitor the relation of stimuli or thoughts to self, but this process and its contents remain isolated from consciousness.

Consciousness is a subjective state of awareness of something, a sensory percept, an emotional feeling, mental imagery, an abstract thought, inner speech, a memory, a volitional act.[63,296] Consciousness is relatively selective, for its contents at any given moment are limited. Most mental processes and knowledge are nonconscious. As we need information about our personal past (episodic memory) or learned data (semantic memory), we retrieve it from long-term memory and store it in working memory, which is accessible to and coexistent with consciousness. Procedural knowledge may be conscious as we acquire the ability to perform a skill, but once we are proficient at the skill, our knowledge of its steps becomes nonconscious and can only partly be understood. Furthermore, self-awareness of an acquired skill can impair its performance, as in thinking about what letters are being typed.

Cognitive Aspects of Consciousness

CONTENTS AND LEVELS OF CONSCIOUSNESS

Consciousness comprises discrete elements that are more easily examined than the global concept of consciousness. The contents of con-

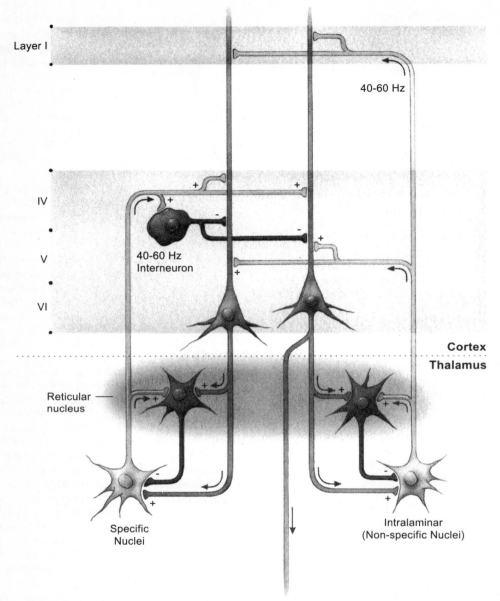

Figure 3–4. Thalamocortical synchronization. The reciprocal thalamocortical neuronal loop function and interactions between the specific and nonspecific thalamic loops. In addition to gating the flow of sensory information to the brain, the thalamus serves as a hub that allows communication and binding (synchronization) between multiple cortical sites using high-frequency (e.g., 40 Hz) activity.

sciousness include attention, internal (interoception) sensations, sensory perception, emotions, mental imagery, inner speech, conceptual thought, remembering, planning, motivation, volition, and self-awareness. Boundaries between conscious and noncon-

scious knowledge and behaviors are discrete or continuous (Fig. 3–5). Some components of nonconscious behavior are purely nonconscious, that is, inaccessible to consciousness. Instinct, the process but not the product of sensory perception, irretrievable memories, and

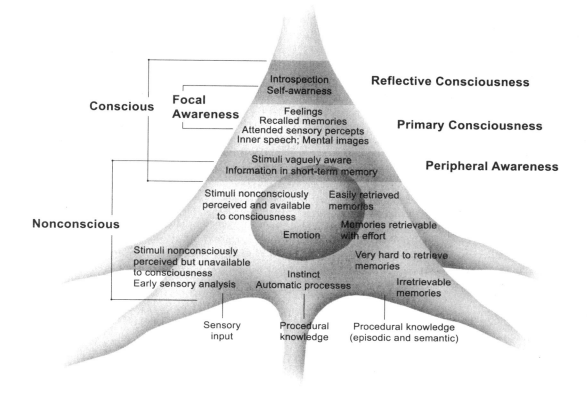

Figure 3–5. Hierarchical levels of nonconscious and conscious mind. Note that more cortical and subcortical resources are devoted to nonconscious cognitive and behavioral functions. Also, although not illustrated, there are strong interconnections between different levels of nonconscious and conscious mind.

much procedural knowledge lie beyond introspection. Complex innate and overlearned behaviors can utilize declarative memories, despite being inaccessible to consciousness.[297]

Preconscious stimuli such as subliminal percepts and implicit memories can influence behavior but remain outside of conscious awareness. Peripheral awareness includes percepts, thoughts, and memories at the fringe of awareness. Directing awareness toward them, with various degrees of attention, persistence, and effort, brings them into consciousness. Primary consciousness is the experience, or awareness, of percepts, feelings, memories, and thoughts. Reflective consciousness is the awareness of one's own primary consciousness, that is, making one's own conscious experience the focus of thought. The capacities to monitor one's own behavior, view a stimulus or scenario from multiple alternative perspectives (as in "seeing things from another person's perspective"), and consciously experience the self as it is integrated over the passage of time are critical elements of human cognition. These capacities may be linked to the emergence of an introspective self and reflective consciousness.

THE COGNITIVE UNCONSCIOUS

Nonconscious states and processes dominate mental life, as in our perception of sensory stimuli, comprehension of spoken and written language, formation of opinions about social acquaintances, selection of a mate, approach to seeking novelty, and coordination of gait. The cognitive unconscious mediates many components of the behavioral sequences that we consider conscious. The cognitive unconscious is most evident in sensory perception, subliminal perception, procedural knowledge, implicit

memory, dreams, hypnosis, and other dissociative states.

SENSORY AND SUBLIMINAL PERCEPTION

In sensory perception, large amounts of sensory information are filtered, processed, and categorized nonconsciously, with only a small fraction selected for conscious awareness. Consciousness has little or no access to raw sensory information or perceptual processes. We cannot introspectively determine how we see or perceive other sensory information.

In subliminal (nonconscious) perception, stimuli lying below the threshold of conscious awareness can affect perceptual, emotional, and cognitive functions. Tachistoscopic presentations of subliminal visual images can reappear in dreams (Poetzel's phenomenon) and influence the detection of a subsequent supraliminal target stimulus.[297,298] The emotional valence of such subliminal stimuli as printed words influences their threshold for detection. Further, simple exposure to subliminal stimuli can afford a nonconscious familiarity that leads subjects to favor one previously viewed, but nonconsciously recognized, stimulus over another.[299]

PROCEDURAL KNOWLEDGE

Procedural knowledge for motor and cognitive skills refers to the mental programs for learned behavior. This knowledge is largely nonconscious. The acquisition of complex motor and cognitive skills requires learning. Procedural knowledge exemplifies how the brain's formatting of processes and information changes as knowledge and skills are acquired. Thus, learned procedures can join the repertoire of sequences that can be automatically activated by appropriate stimuli, such as innate, hardwired behaviors. These are sequences that are stored, retrieved, and, in many cases, executed without conscious awareness.

We learn to read by recognizing both letter sequences and patterns. Once reading is accomplished, letters in common words, as well as syntactic and tense rules, become "invisible to consciousness." A skilled typist, who can type and maintain a conversation, is unaware of the individual letters being typed. Similarly, untrained atheletes first learn athletic skills by repeated conscious attention to the movements and steps, but skilled athletes execute complex motor sequences automatically. Unconscious procedural knowledge becomes automatic, not effortful and controlled,[300] and thereby bypasses the limited capacity of selective attention and working memory. Many of these sequences, as in sports, must be activated faster than consciousness can analyze a situation, use inner language, and react.

Procedural social knowledge is a complex and largely nonconscious behavior. Just as mood influences social decisions, emotional valence of events alters our judgment of them, but often we are unable to describe how we reached our conclusions.[301] Our preference for certain physical features and attraction to some individuals and dislike for others on initial contact incorporate unconscious judgments.[297,302] The most important social decisions we make, such as mate selection, are influenced by factors that cannot be consciously defined. For example, few recognize that mates have a highly significant correlation between interocular distances and digit lengths.[303]

SUMMARY

The left hemisphere dominates verbal behavior, fine motor control, and conscious behavioral planning. Once considered primitive, silent, or redundant, the right hemisphere is now known to dominate the sense of self; an individual's consciousness of being, both corporeally (in relation to external space and to the internal milieu of the body) and psychically; and the relation of that being to the environment. The right hemisphere is critical in primary perception, body schema, emotion, and some social functions.

Functional neuroimaging, studies of focal lesions, and the results of callosotomy show that a function is rarely completely lateralized. Together with subcortical structures, the corpus callosum binds and synchronizes the cerebral hemispheres and behavior. The corpus callosum not only provides an avenue for shared information between the hemispheres but also allows one hemisphere to deactivate the other and take charge of a behavioral function. Callosotomy may reduce the negative affective range and occasionally causes a dramatic interruption in behavior that represents an integrated self, as in alien hand syndrome.

Brain function is modular, with distinct but overlapping and integrated neural structures. Although serial processing is a critical element of sensory, motor, and cognitive behavior, parallel processing appears to dominate cerebral function. Consciousness may result from synchronized activity in multiple cerebral modules. However, nonconscious conditions and activities dominate mental life.

REFERENCES

1. Wigan AL: Duality of the Mind. Longman, Brown, Green, and Longman, London, 1844.
2. Chi JG, Dooling EC, and Gilles FH: Left–right asymmetries of the temporal speech area of the human brain. Arch Neurol 34:346–348, 1977.
3. Geschwind N and Levitsky W: Human brain: left–right asymmetries in temporal speech region. Science 161:186–187, 1968.
4. Anderson B, Southern BD, and Powers RE: Anatomic asymmetries of the posterior superior temporal lobes: a postmortem study. Neuropsychiatry Neuropsychol Behav Neurol 12:247–254, 1999.
5. Wada JA: Pre-language and fundamental asymmetry of the infant brain. Ann NY Acad Sci 299:370–379, 1977.
6. Scheibel AB: A dendritic correlate of human speech. In Geschwind N and Galaburda AM (eds). Cerebral Dominance: The Biological Foundations. Cambridge, MA: Harvard University Press, pp 43–52, 1984.
7. Hayes TL and Lewis DA: Magnopyramidal neurons in the anterior motor speech region: dendritic features and interhemispheric comparisons. Arch Neurol 53:1277–1284, 1996.
8. Weinberger DR, Luchins DJ, Morihisa J, et al.: Asymmetrical volumes of the right and left frontal and occipital regions of the human brain. Ann Neurol 11:97–100, 1982.
9. Eidelberg D and Galaburda AM: Symmetry and asymmetry in the human posterior thalamus. I. Cytoarchitectonic analysis in normal persons. Arch Neurol 39:325–332, 1982.
10. Rodriquez M, Martin L, and Santana C: Ontogenic development of brain asymmetry in dopaminergic neurons. Brain Res Bull 33:163–171, 1994.
11. Holloway RJ and De Lacoste C: Brain endocast asymmetry in pongids and hominids. The paleontology of cerebral hemisphere dominance. Am J Phys Anthropol 58:101–110, 1982.
12. LeMay M, Billig MS, and Geschwind N: Asymmetries of the brains and skulls of nonhuman primates. In Amstrong E and Falk D (eds). Primate Brain Evolution: Methods and Concepts. Plenum, New York, 1982, pp 263–277.
13. Gannon PJ, Holloway RL, Broadfield DC, and Braun AR: Asymmetry of chimpanzee planum temporale: humanlike pattern of Wernicke's brain language area homolog. Science 279:220–222, 1998.
14. Hopkins WD and Leavens DA: Hand use and gestural communication in chimpanzees (*Pan troglodytes*). J Comp Psychol 112:95–99, 1998.
15. Broca P: Perte de la parole, ramollissement chronique et destruction partielle du lobe anterieur gauche du cerveau. Bull Soc Anthropol Paris 2:235–238, 1861.
16. Dax M: Lesion de la moitie gauche de l'encephale coincident avec l'oubli des signes de la pensee (lu a Montpellier en 1836). Gazette Hebdomidaire Med Chir 2:259–260, 1865.
17. Liepmann H: Das Krankheitsbild der Apraxie ("motorischen Asymbolie"). Karger, Berlin, 1900.
18. Milner B: Psychologic defects produced by temporal lobe excision. Res Publ Assoc Res Nerv Ment Dis 36:244–257, 1958.
19. Kimura D: Cerebral dominance and the perception of verbal stimuli. Can J Psychol 15:166–171, 1961.
20. Jackson JH: Notes on the physiology and pathology of the nervous system. In Taylor J (ed). Selected Writings of John Hughlings Jackson, Vol 2. Basic Books, New York, 1958, pp 215–237.
21. Jackson JH: On affections of speech from diseases of the brain. Brain 1:304–330, 1879.
22. Jackson JH: On the nature of the duality of the brain. In Taylor J (ed). Selected Writings of John Hughlings Jackson, Vol 2. Basic Books, New York, 1958, pp 129–145.
23. Corballis PM, Funnell MG, and Gazzaniga MS: Hemispheric asymmetries for simple visual judgements in the split brain. Neuropsychologia 40:401–410, 2002.
24. Brownell HH: Appreciation of metaphoric and connotative word meaning. In Chiarello C (ed). Right Hemisphere Contributions to Lexical Semantics. Springer, Berlin, 1988, pp 19–31.
25. Benson DF and Barton M: Constructional disability. Cortex 19:5–11, 1970.
26. Maurer D, Grand RL, and Mondloch CJ: The many faces of configural processing. Neuropsychologia 1:255–260, 2002.
27. Van Kleeck MH and Kosslyn SM: Gestalt laws of perceptual organization in an embedded figures task: evidence for hemispheric specialization. Neuropsychologia 27:1179–1186, 1989.
28. Parsons LM and Osherson D: New evidence for distinct right and left brain systems for deductive versus probabilistic reasoning. Cereb Cortex 11:954–965, 2001.
29. Efron R: The Decline and Fall of Hemispheric Specialization. Erlbaum Associates, Hillsdale, NJ, 1990.
30. Heinze HJ, Hinrichs H, Scholz M, Burchert W, and Mangun GR: Neural mechanisms of global and local processing. A combined PET and ERP study. J Cogn Neurosci 10:485–498, 1998.
31. Levy-Agresti J and Sperry RW: Differential perceptual capacities in major and minor hemispheres. Proc Natl Acad Sci USA 61:1151, 1968.
32. Deglin VL and Kinsbourne M: Divergent thinking styles of the hemispheres: how syllogisms are solved during transitory hemisphere suppression. Brain Cogn 31:285–307, 1996.
33. Weinstein S and Graves RE: Are creativity and schizotypy products of a right hemisphere bias? Brain Cogn 49:138–151, 2002.
34. Bogen JE: The other side of the brain. II. An appositional mind. Bull LA Neurol Soc 34:135–162, 1969.
35. Jessen F, Heun R, Erb M, et al.: The concreteness

effect: evidence for dual coding and context availability. Brain Lang 74:103–112, 2000.

36. Brownell HH, Potter HH, Birhle AM, and Gardner H: Inference deficits in right brain–damaged patients. Brain Lang 27:310–321, 1986.

37. Trojano L, Grossi D, Linden DE, et al.: Coordinate and categorical judgments in spatial imagery: an fMRI study. Neuropsychologia 40:1666–1674, 2002.

38. Aguirre GK, Detre JA, Alsop DC, and D'Esposito M: The parahippocampus subserves topographical learning in man. Cereb Cortex 6:823–829, 1996.

39. Meador KJ, Loring DW, Lee GP, et al.: Right cerebral specialization for tactile attention as evidenced by intracarotid sodium amytal. Neurology 38:1763–1766, 1988.

40. Savic I, Bookheimer SY, Fried I, and Engel J: Olfactory bedside test: a simple approach to identify temporo- orbitofrontal dysfunction. Arch Neurol 54: 162–168, 1997.

41. Mesulam M-M: Large-scale neurocognitive networks and distributed processing for attention, language, and memory. Ann Neurol 28:597–613, 1990.

42. Tulving E, Kapur S, Craik FIM, Moscovitch M, and Houle S: Hemispheric encoding/retrieval asymmetry in episodic memory: positron emission tomography findings. Proc Natl Acad Sci USA 91:2016–2020, 1994.

43. Bear DM: Hemispheric specialization and the neurology of emotion. Arch Neurol 40:195–202, 1983.

44. Gainotti G: Emotional behavior and hemispheric side of lesion. Cortex 8:41–55, 1972.

45. Ross ED, Homan RW, and Buck R: Differential hemispheric lateralization of primary and social emotions. Neuropsychiatry Neuropsychol Behav Neurol 7:1–19, 1994.

46. Tucker DM: Lateral brain function, emotion, and conceptualization. Psychol Bull 89:19–46, 1981.

47. Davidson RJ and Fox NA: Asymmetrical brain activity discriminates between positive and negative affective stimuli in human infants. Science 218: 1235–1237, 1982.

48. Sackheim HA, Greenberg MS, Weiman AL, et al.: Hemispheric asymmetry in the expression of positive and negative emotions: neurological evidence. Arch Neurol 39:210–218, 1982.

49. Joseph R: The right cerebral hemisphere: emotion, music, visual–spatial skills, body image, dreams, and awareness. J Clin Psychol 44:630–673, 1988.

50. Manoach DS, Sandson TA, and Weintraub S: The developmental social–emotional processing disorder is associated with right hemisphere abnormalities. Neuropsychiatry Neuropsychol Behav Neurol 8:99–105, 1995.

51. Markowitsch HJ, Calabrese P, Liess J, et al.: Retrograde amnesia after traumatic injury of the temporo-frontal cortex. J Neurol Neurosurg Psychiatry 56:988–992, 1993.

52. Markowitsch HJ, Calabrese P, Neufeld H, Gehlen W, and Durwen HF: Retrograde amnesia for world knowledge and preserved memory for autobiographic events. A case report. Cortex 35:243–252, 1999.

53. Weintrob DL, Saling MM, Berkovic SF, Berlangieri SU, and Reutens DC: Verbal memory in left temporal lobe epilepsy: evidence for task-related localization. Ann Neurol 51:442–447, 2002.

54. Lee TM, Yip JT, and Jones-Gotman M: Memory deficits after resection from left or right anterior temporal lobe in humans: a meta-analytic review. Epilepsia 43:283–291, 2002.

55. Jones-Gotman M and Milner B: Right temporal-lobe contribution to image-mediated verbal learning. Neuropsychologia 16:61–71, 1978.

56. Takahashi N, Kawamura M, Shiota J, Kasahata N, and Hirayama K: Pure topographic disorientation due to right retrosplenial lesion. Neurology 49:464–469, 1997.

57. Gazzaniga MS: The split brain revisited. Sci Am 279:50–55, 1998.

58. Devinsky O: Right cerebral hemisphere dominance for a sense of corporeal and emotional self. Epilepsy Behav 1:60–73, 2000.

59. Blumstein S, Goodglass H, and Tartter V: The reliability of ear advantage in dichotic listening. Brain Lang 2:226–236, 1975.

60. Code C: Can the right hemisphere speak? Brain Lang 57:38–59, 1997.

61. Boucher R and Bryden MP: Laterality effects in the processing of melody and timbre. Neuropsychologia 35:1467–1473, 1997.

62. Chiron C, Jambaque I, Nabbout R, et al.: The right brain hemisphere is dominant in human infants. Brain 120:1057–1065, 1997.

63. Farthing GW: The Psychology of Consciousness. Prentice Hall, Englewood Cliffs, NJ, 1992.

64. Fodor JA: Modularity of Mind: An Essay on Faculty Psychology. MIT Press, Cambridge, MA, 1983.

65. Llinas R, Ribary U, Contreras D, and Pedroarena C: The neuronal basis for consciousness. Philos Trans R Soc Lond B Biol Sci 353:1841–1849, 1998.

66. Shadmehr R and Holcomb HH: Neural correlates of motor memory consolidation. Science 227:821–825, 1997.

67. Jackson JH: On right or left-sided spasm at the onset of epileptic paroxysms, and on crude sensation warnings, and elaborate mental states. Brain 3:192–205, 1880.

68. Luys JB: Etudes sur le deboublement des operations cerebrales et sur le role isole de chaque hemisphere dans les phenomenes de la pathologie mentale. Bull Acad Natl Med 8:516–534, 1879.

69. Luys JB: Recherches nouvelles sur les hemiplegies emotives. Encephale 1:378–398, 1881.

70. Myers FWH: Automatic writing. Proc Soc Psychical Res 3:1–63, 1885.

71. Brain R: Visual disorientation with special reference to the lesions of the right hemisphere. Brain 64:244–272, 1941.

72. Critchley M: The Parietal Lobes. Edward Arnold, London, 1953.

73. Carmon A and Benton AL: Tactile perception of direction and number in patients with unilateral cerebral disease. Neurology 19:525–532, 1969.

74. Craig AD, Chen K, Bandy D, and Reiman EM: Thermosensory activation of insular cortex. Nat Neurosci 3:184–190, 2000.

75. Griffiths TD, Rees A, Witton C, Cross PM, Shakir RA, and Green GGR: Spatial and temporal auditory processing deficits following right hemisphere infarction: a psychophysical study. Brain 120:785–794, 1997.

76. Johnsrude IS, Penhune VB, and Zatorre RJ: Func-

tional specificity in the right human auditory cortex for perceiving pitch direction. Brain 123:155–163, 2000.

77. Zatorre RJ. Neural specializations for tonal processing. Ann NY Acad Sci 930:193–210, 2001.

78. Hier DB, Mondlock JR, and Caplan LR: Behavioral abnormalities after right hemisphere stroke. Neurology 33:337–344, 1983.

79. Vighetto A, Aimard G, Confavreux C, and Devic M: Anatomo-clinical study of a case of topographic confabulation [in French]. Cortex 16:501–507, 1980.

80. Fisher CM: Topographic disorientation. Arch Neurol 34:489–495, 1982.

81. Corballis MC: Mental rotation and the right hemisphere. Brain Lang 57:100–121, 1997.

82. Fan J, McCandliss BD, Sommer T, Raz A, and Posner MI: Testing the efficacy and independence of attentional networks. J Cogn Neurosci 1:340–347, 2002.

83. Rueckert L and Grafman J: Sustained attention deficits in patients with right frontal lesions. Neuropsychologia 34:953–963, 1996.

84. Kertesz A, Nicholson I, Cancelliere A, Kassa K, and Black SE: Motor impersistence: a right-hemisphere syndrome. Neurology 35:662–666, 1985.

85. Basso G and Nichelli P: Relations between attentional and intentional neural systems. Percept Mot Skills 81:947–951, 1995.

86. Benowitz LI, Bear DM, Rosenthal R, Mesulam MM, Zaidel E, and Sperry R: Hemispheric specialization in nonverbal communication. Cortex 19:5–11, 1983.

87. Hari R, Portin K, Kettenmann B, Jousmaki V, and Kobal G: Right-hemisphere preponderance of responses to painful CO_2 stimulation of the human nasal mucosa. Pain 72:145–151, 1997.

88. Blonder LX, Bowers D, and Heilman KM: The role of the right hemisphere in emotional communication. Brain 114:1115–1127, 1991.

89. Borod JC, Bloom RL, Brickman AM, Nakhutina L, and Curko EA: Emotional processing deficits in individuals with unilateral brain damage. Appl Neuropsychol 9:23–26, 2002.

90. Wilde MC, Boake C, and Sherer M: Wechsler Adult Intelligence Scale–Revised block design broken configuration errors in nonpenetrating traumatic brain injury. Appl Neuropsychol 7:208–14, 2000.

90a. Arnow BA, Desmond JE, Banner LL, et al: Brain activation and sexual arousal in healthy, heterosexual males. Brain 125:1014–1023, 2002.

90b. Mendez MF, Chow T, Ringman J, Twitchell G, and Hinkin CH: Pedophilia and temporal lobe disturbances. J Neuropsychiatry Clin Neurosci 12:71–76, 2000.

90c. Janszky J, Szucs A, Halasz P, et al: Orgasmic aura originates from the right hemisphere. Neurology 58:302–304, 2002.

90d. Signer S and Benson DF: Three cases of anorexia nervosa associated with temporal lobe epilepsy. Am J Psychiatry 147:235–238, 1990.

90e. Trummer M, Eustacchio S, Unger F, Tillich M, and Flaschka G: Right hemispheric frontal lesions as a cause for anorexia nervosa. Acta Neurochir 144:797–801, 2002.

90f. Kramer RE, Lüders H, Goldstick LP, et al: Ictus emeticus. Neurology 38:1048–1052, 1988.

91. Wittling W: The right hemisphere and the human stress response. Acta Physiol Scand Suppl 640:55–59, 1997.

92. Yoon BW, Morillo CA, Cachetto DF, and Hachinski V: Cerebral hemispheric lateralization in cardiac autonomic control. Arch Neurol 54:741–744, 1997.

93. Hilz MJ, Dutsch M, Perrine K, Nelson PK, Rauhut U, and Devinsky O: Hemispheric influence on autonomic modulation and baroreflex sensitivity. Ann Neurol 49:575–584, 2001.

94. Bisiach E and Luzzatti C: Unilateral neglect of representational space. Cortex 14:129–133, 1978.

95. Hong CC, Gillin JC, Dow BM, et al.: Localized and lateralized cerebral glucose metabolism associated with eye movements during REM sleep and wakefulness: a positron emission tomography (PET) study. Sleep 18:570–580, 1995.

96. Weintraub S and Mesulam MM: Developmental learning disabilities of the right hemisphere. Emotional, interpersonal, and cognitive components. Arch Neurol 40:463–468, 1983.

97. Wicker B, Michel F, Henaff MA, and Decety J: Brain regions involved in the perception of gaze: a PET study. Neuroimage 8:221–227, 1998.

98. Luria AR: The frontal lobes and the regulation of behavior. In Pribram KH and Luria AR (eds). Psychophysiology of the Frontal Lobes. Academic Press, New York, 1973, pp 3–26.

99. Alexander MP, Benson DF, and Stuss DT: Frontal lobes and language. Brain Lang 37:656–691, 1989.

100. Van Lancker D: Rags to riches: our increasing appreciation of cognitive and communicative abilities of the human right cerebral hemisphere. Brain Lang 57:1–11, 1997.

101. Joseph R: Confabulation and delusional denial: frontal lobe and lateralized influences. J Clin Psychol 42:845–860, 1986.

102. Fischer RP, Alexander MP, D'Esposito MD, and Otto R: Neuropsychological and neuroanatomical correlates of confabulation. J Clin Exp Neuropsychol 17:20–28, 1995.

103. Harrington DL, Halland KY, and Knight RT: Cortical networks underlying mechanisms of time perception. J Neurosci 18:1085–1095, 1998.

104. Cummings JL: Neuropsychiatric manifestations of right hemisphere lesions. Brain Lang 57:22–37, 1997.

105. Starkstein SE and Robinson RG: Mechanism of disinhibition after brain lesions. J Nerv Ment Dis 185:108–114, 1997.

106. Bogousslavsky J and Regli F: Response-to-next-patient stimulation: a right hemisphere syndrome. Neurology 38:1225–1227, 1988.

107. Drane DL, Lee GP, Loring DW, and Meador KJ: Time perception following unilateral amobarbital injection in patients with temporal lobe epilepsy. J Clin Exp Neuropsychol 21:385–396, 1999.

108. Brunia CH, de Jong BM, van den Berg-Lenssen MM, and Paans AM: Visual feedback about time estimation is related to a right hemisphere activation measured by PET. Exp Brain Res 130:328–337, 2000.

109. Perbal S, Ehrle N, Samson S, Baulac M, and Pouthas V: Time estimation in patients with right or left medial-temporal lobe resection. Neuroreport 12:939–942, 2001.

110. Milner B, Corsi P, and Leonard G: Frontal-lobe

contribution to recency judgements. Neuropsychologia 29:601–618, 1991.

111. Schacter DL, Harbluk JL, and McLachlan DR: Retrieval without recollection: an experimental analysis of source amnesia. J Verb Learn Verb Behav 23:593–611, 1984.

112. Cansino S, Maquet P, Dolan RJ, and Rugg MD: Brain activity underlying encoding and retrieval of source memory. Cereb Cortex 12:1048–1056, 2002.

113. Jeong J, Joung MK, and Kim SY: Quantification of emotion by nonlinear analysis of the chaotic dynamics of electroencephalograms during perception of 1/f music. Biol Cybern 78:217–225, 1998.

114. Jones-Gotman M and Milner B: Design fluency: the invention of nonsense drawings after focal cortical lesions. Neuropsychologia 15:653–674, 1977.

115. Boone KB, Miller BL, Lee A, Berman N, Sherman D, and Stuss DT: Neuropsychological patterns in right versus left frontotemporal dementia. J Int Neuropsychol Soc 5:616–622, 1999.

116. Ramachandran VS: The evolutionary biology of self-deception, laughter, dreaming and depression: some clues from anosognosia. Med Hypotheses 47:347–362, 1996.

117. Bottini G, Cappa SF, Sterzi R, and Vignolo LA: Intramodal somaesthetic recognition disorders following right and left hemisphere damage. Brain 118:395–399, 1995.

118. Benton A and Tranel D: Visuoperceptual, visuospatial, and visuoconstructive disorders. In Heilman KM and Valenstein E (eds). Clinical Neuropsychology, 3rd ed. Oxford University Press, New York, 1993, pp 165–213.

119. Stiles J and Nass R: Spatial grouping activity in young children with congenital right or left hemisphere brain injury. Brain Cogn 15:201–222, 1991.

120. Borod JC, Carper M, Goodglass H, and Naeser M: Aphasic performance on a battery of constructional, visuo-spatial, and quantitative tasks: factorial structure and CT scan localization. J Clin Neuropsychol 6:189–204, 1984.

121. Platz T and Mauritz KH: Human motor planning, motor programming, and use of new task-relevant information with different apraxic syndromes. Eur J Neurosci 7:1536–1547, 1995.

122. Takayama Y, Sugishita M, Hirose S, and Akiguchi I: Anosodiaphoria for dressing apraxia: contributory factor to dressing apraxia. Clin Neurol Neurosurg 96:254–256, 1994.

123. DeRenzi E, Faglioni P, and Villa P: Topographical amnesia. J Neurol Neurosurg Psychiatry 40:498–505, 1977.

124. Fisher CM: Disorientation for place. Arch Neurol 39:33–36, 1982.

125. Faillenot I, Decety J, and Jeannerod M: Human brain activity related to the perception of spatial features of objects. Neuroimage 10:114–124, 1999.

126. Fink GR, Marshall JC, Shah NJ, et al.: Line bisection judgments implicate right parietal cortex and cerebellum as assessed by fMRI. Neurology 54:1324–1331, 2000.

127. Harris IM, Egan GF, Sonkkila C, et al.: Selective right parietal lobe activation during mental rotation: a parametric PET study. Brain 123:65–73, 2000.

128. Devinsky O: Behavioral Neurology: 100 Maxims. Edward Arnold, London, 1992.

129. Gainotti G, Messerli P, and Tissot R: Quantitative analysis of unilateral spatial neglect in relation to laterality of cerebral lesions. J Neurol Neurosurg Psychiatry 35:545–550, 1972.

130. Stiles J, Trauner D, Engel M, and Nass R: The development of drawing in children with congenital focal brain injury: evidence for limited functional recovery. Neuropsychologia 35:299–312, 1997.

131. Leonard G and Milner B: Contribution of the right frontal lobe to the encoding and recall of kinesthetic distance information. Neuropsychologia 29:47–58, 1991.

132. Meador KJ, Watson RT, Bowers D, and Heilman KM: Hypometria with hemispatial and limb motor neglect. Brain 109:293–305, 1986.

133. Guariglia C, Padovani A, Pantano P, and Pizzamiglio L: Unilateral neglect restricted to visual imagery. Nature 364:235–237, 1993.

134. Meador KJ, Allen ME, Adams RJ, and Loring DW: Allochiria vs allesthesia. Is there a misperception? Arch Neurol 48:546–549, 1991.

135. Babinski J: Contribution a l'etude des troubles mentaux dans l'hemiplegie organique cerebrale (anosognosie). Rev Neurol (Paris) 27:845–847, 1914.

136. Critchley M: Observations on anosodiaphoria. Encephale 5–6:540–546, 1957.

137. Denes G, Semenza C, Stoppa E, and Lis A: Unilateral spatial neglect and recovery from hemiplegia. Brain 105:543–552, 1982.

138. Halligan PW, Marshall JC, and Wade DT: Three arms: a case study of supernumerary phantom limb after right hemisphere stroke. J Neurol Neurosurg Psychiatry 56:159–166, 1993.

139. Hari R, Hanninen R, Makinen T, et al.: Three hands: fragmentation of human bodily awareness. Neurosci Lett 240:131–134, 1998.

140. Devinsky O, Mesad S, and Alper A: Nondominant hemisphere lesions and conversion nonepileptic seizures. J Neuropsychiatry Clin Neurosci 13:367–373, 2001.

141. Griffith JL and Hochberg FH: Anorexia and weight loss in glioma patients. Psychosomatics 29:335–337, 1988.

142. Devinsky O, Frasca J, Pacia SV, et al.: Ictus emeticus: further evidence of nondominant temporal involvement. Neurology 45:1158–1160, 1995.

143. Regard M and Landis T: "Gourmand syndrome": eating passion associated with right anterior lesions. Neurology 48:1185–1190, 1997.

144. Kanner AM, Morris HH, Stagno S, et al.: Remission of an obsessive–compulsive disorder following a right temporal lobectomy. Neuropsychiatry Neuropsychol Behav Neurol 6:126–129, 1993.

145. Miller BL, Seeley WW, Mychack P, et al.: Neuroanatomy of the self: evidence from patients with frontotemporal dementia. Neurology 57:817–821, 2001.

146. Heilman KM, Bowers D, Speedie L, and Coslett B: Comprehension of affective and nonaffective speech. Neurology 34:917–921, 1984.

147. Ross ED: Affective prosody and the aprosodias. In Mesulan MM (ed). Principles of Behavioral and Cognitive Neurology. Oxford University Press, New York, 2000, pp 316–331.

148. Compton RJ, Heller W, Banich MT, Palmieri PA, and Miller GA: Responding to threat: hemispheric

asymmetries and interhemispheric division of input. Neuropsychology 14:254–264, 2000.

149. Etcoff N: Perceptual and conceptual organization of facial emotions. Brain Cogn 3:385–412, 1984.

150. Gainotti G: Lateralization of brain mechanisms underlying automatic and controlled forms of spatial orienting of attention. Neurosci Biobehav Rev 20: 617–622, 1996.

151. Lang PJ, Bradley MM, and Cuthbert BN: Emotion, motivation, and anxiety: brain mechanisms and psychophysiology. Biol Psychiatry 44:1248–1263, 1998.

152. Heilman KM, Schwartz HD, and Watson RT: Hypoarousal in patients with the neglect syndrome and emotional indifference. Neurology 28:229–232, 1978.

153. Goldstein K: Language and Language Disturbances. Grune & Stratton, New York, 1948.

154. Starkstein SE, Robinson RG, and Price TR: Comparison of cortical and subcortical lesions in the production of poststroke mood disorders. Brain 110:1045–1059, 1987.

155. Lee GP, Loring DW, Meador KJ, Flanigin HF, and Brooks BS: Severe behavioral complications following intracarotid sodium amobarbital injection: implications for hemispheric asymmetry of emotion. Neurology 38:1233–1236, 1988.

156. Ahern GL, Herring AM, Tackenberg JN, et al.: Affective self-report during the intracarotid sodium amobarbital test. J Clin Exp Neuropsychol 16:372–376, 1994.

157. Davidson RJ: Cerebral asymmetry, emotion, and affective style. In Davidson RJ and Hugdahl K (eds). Brain Asymmetry. MIT Press, Cambridge, MA, 1995, pp 361–387.

158. Mammucari A, Caltagirone C, Ekman P, et al.: Spontaneous facial expression of emotions in brain-damaged patients. Cortex 24:521–533, 1988.

159. Bradvik B, Dravins C, Holtas S, et al.: Do single right hemisphere infarcts or transient ischemic attacks result in aprosody? Acta Neurol Scand 81:61–70, 1990.

160. Cancelliere AEB and Kertesz A: Lesion localization in acquired deficits of emotional expression and comprehension. Brain Cogn 13:133–147, 1990.

161. Weddel R, Miller R, and Trevarthen C: Voluntary emotional facial expressions in patients with focal cerebral lesions. Neuropsychologia 28:49–60, 1990.

162. Robinson RG, Kubos KL, Starr LB, Rao K, and Price TR: Mood disorders in stroke patients: importance of location of lesion. Brain 107:81–93, 1984.

163. Loring DW, Meador KJ, Lee GP, and King DW: Amobarbital Effects and Lateralized Brain Function: The Wada Test. Springer, New York, 1992.

164. Masia SL, Perrine K, Westbrook L, Alper K, and Devinsky O: Emotional outbursts and post-traumatic stress disorder during intracarotid amobarbital procedure. Neurology 54:1691–1693, 2000.

165. Borod JC, Caron HS, and Koff E: Asymmetry in positive and negative facial expressions: sex differences. Neuropsychologia 19:819–824, 1981.

166. Davidson RJ: Affect, cognition, and hemispheric specialization. In Izard CE, Kagan J, and Zajonc RB (eds). Emotions, Cognition, and Behavior. Cambridge University Press, Cambridge, 1984, pp 320–36.

167. Davidson RJ: The neuropsychology of emotion and affective style. In Lewis M and Haviland JM (eds). Handbook of Emotions. Guilford Press, New York, 1993, pp 143–154.

168. Darwin C: The Expression of Emotions in Animals and Man. John Murray, London, 1872.

169. Damasio AR, Grabowsky TJ, Bechara A, et al.: Subcortical and cortical brain activity during the feeling of self-generated emotions. Nat Neurosci 3:1049–1056, 2000.

170. Finklestein S, Benowitz LI, Baldessarini RJ, et al.: Mood, vegetative disturbance, and dexamethasone suppression test after stroke. Ann Neurol 12:463–468, 1982.

171. Starkstein SE, Mayberg HS, Berthier ML, et al: Mania after brain injury: neuroradiologic and metabolic findings. Ann Neurol 27:652–659, 1990.

172. Hantas MN, Katkin ES, and Reed SD: Cerebral lateralization and heartbeat discrimination. Psychophysiology 21:274–278, 1984.

173. Zatorre RJ and Jones-Gotman M: Human olfactory discrimination after unilateral frontal or temporal lobectomy. Brain 114:71–84, 1991.

174. Anderson AK, Spencer DD, Fulbright RK, and Phelps EA: Contribution of the anteromedial temporal lobes to the evaluation of facial emotion. Neuropsychology 14:526–536, 2000.

175. Gardner H, Ling PK, Flam I, and Silverman J: Comprehension and appreciation of humorous material following brain damage. Brain 98:399–412, 1975.

176. DeKosky S, Heilman KM, Bowers D, and Valenstein E: Recognition and discrimination of emotional faces and pictures. Brain Lang 9:206–214, 1980.

177. Ross ED: The aprosodias: functional-anatomic organization of the affective components of language in the right hemisphere. Arch Neurol 38:561–569, 1981.

178. Weintraub S, Mesulam MM, and Kramer LL: Disturbances in prosody. Arch Neurol 38:742–744, 1981.

179. Wymer JH, Lindman LS, and Booksh RL: A neuropsychological perspective of aprosody: features, function, assessment and treatment. Appl Neuropsychol 9:37–47, 2002.

180. Wittling W and Roschmann R: Emotion-related hemisphere asymmetry: subjective emotional responses to laterally presented films. Cortex 29:431–448, 1993.

181. Bowers D, Blonder LX, Feinberg T, and Heilman KM: Differential impact of right and left hemisphere lesions on facial emotion and object imagery. Brain 114:2593–2609, 1991.

182. Bowers D and Heilman KM: Dissociation between the processing of affective and nonaffective faces: a case study. J Clin Neuropsychol 6:367–379, 1984.

183. Rapcsak SZ, Kaszniak AW, and Rubens AB: Anomia for facial expressions: evidence for a category specific visual-verbal disconnection syndrome. Neuropsychologia 27:1031–1041, 1989.

184. Adolphs R: Neural systems for recognizing emotion. Curr Opin Neurobiol 12:169–177, 2002.

185. Levy J, Heller W, Banich MT, and Burton LA: Are variations among right-handed individuals in perceptual asymmetries caused by characteristic arousal differences between hemispheres? J Exp Psychol Hum Percept Perform 9:329–359, 1983.

186. Bloom R, Borod JC, Ober L, and Gerstman L: Impact of emotional content on discourse production in patients with unilateral brain damage. Brain Lang 42:153–164, 1992.
187. Landis T, Graves R, and Goodglass H: Aphasic reading and writing: possible evidence for right hemisphere participation. Cortex 18:105–112, 1982.
188. Ross ED and Mesulam MM: Dominant language functions of the right hemisphere? Prosody and emotional gesturing. Arch Neurol 36:144–148, 1979.
189. Borod JC, Haywood CS, and Koff E: Neuropsychological aspects of facial asymmetry during emotional expression: a review of the normal adult literature. Neuropsychol Rev 7:41–60, 1997.
190. Sackeim HA, Gur RC, and Savoy MC: Emotions are expressed more intensely on the left side of the face. Science 202:424–435, 1978.
191. Provinciali L and Coccia M: Post-stroke and vascular depression: a critical review. Neurol Sci 22:417–428, 2002.
192. Kolb B and Milner B: Performance of complex arm and facial movements after focal brain lesions. Neuropsychologia 19:491–503, 1981.
193. Nicholls ME, Clode D, Wood SJ, and Wood AG: Laterality of expression in portraiture: putting your best cheek forward. Proc R Soc Lond B Biol Sci 266:1517–1522, 1999.
194. Daniele A, Azzoni A, Bizzi A, et al.: Sexual behavior and hemispheric laterality of the focus in patients with temporal lobe epilepsy. Biol Psychiatry 42:617–624, 1997.
195. Cohen HD, Rosen RC, and Goldstein L: Electroencephalographic laterality changes during human sexual orgasm. Arch Sex Behav 5:189–199, 1976.
196. Hsieh JC, Hannerz J, and Ingver M: Right-lateralised central processing for pain of nitroglycerin-induced cluster headache. Pain 67:59–68, 1996.
197. Nakamura K, Kawashima R, Ito K, et al.: Activation of the right inferior frontal cortex during assessment of facial emotion. J Neurophysiol 82:1610–1614, 1999.
198. Davis GA, O'Neil-Pirozzi TM, and Coon M: Referential cohesion and logical coherence of narration after right hemisphere stroke. Brain Lang 56:183–210, 1997.
199. Winner E, Brownell H, Happe F, Blum A, and Pincus D: Distinguishing lies from jokes: theory of mind deficits and discourse interpretation in right hemisphere brain-damaged patients. Brain Lang 62:89–106, 1998.
200. Fink GR, Markowitsch HJ, Reinkemeier M, et al.: Cerebral representation of one's own past: neural networks involved in autobiographical memory. J Neurosci 16:4275–4282, 1996.
201. Markowitsch HJ, Calabrese P, Haupts M, et al.: Searching for the anatomical basis of retrograde amnesia. J Clin Exp Neuropsychol 15:947–967, 1993.
202. Penfield W and Perot P: The brain's record of auditory and visual experience: a final summary and discussion. Brain 86:595–696, 1963.
203. Weinand ME, Hermann B, Wyler AR, et al.: Long-term subdural strip electrocorticographic monitoring of ictal déjà vu. Epilepsia 35:1054–1059, 1994.
204. Hermann BP, Wyler AR, Blumer D, and Richey ET: Ictal fear: lateralizing significance and implications for understanding the neurobiology of pathological fear states. Neuropsychiatry Neuropsychol Behav Neurol 5:205–210, 1992.
205. Pavlov IP: Conditioned Reflexes. Oxford University Press, London, 1927.
205a. Keenan JP, Wheeler MA, Gallup GG, and Pascual-Leone A: Self-recognition and the right prefrontal cortex. Trends Cogn Sci 4:348–344, 2000.
206. Gross-Tsur V, Shalev RS, Manor O, and Amin N: Developmental right-hemisphere syndrome: clinical spectrum of the nonverbal learning disability. J Learn Disabil 28:80–86, 1995.
207. Jessimer M and Markham R: Alexithymia: a right hemisphere dysfunction specific to recognition of certain facial expressions? Brain Cogn 34:246–258, 1997.
208. Zaidel DW: A view of the world from a split-brain perspective. In Critchley E (ed). The Neurological Boundaries of Reality. Farrand, London, 1994, pp 161–174.
209. Greenberg DB, Hochberg FH, and Murray GB: The theme of death in complex partial seizures. Am J Psychiatry 141:1587–1589, 1984.
210. Luciano D, Devinsky O, and Perrine K: Crying seizures. Neurology 43:2113–2117, 1993.
211. Gloor P, Olivier A, Quesney LF, Andermann F, and Horowitz S: The role of the limbic system in experiential phenomena of temporal lobe epilepsy. Ann Neurol 12:129–144, 1982.
212. Ardila A and Gomez J: Paroxysmal "feeling of somebody being nearby." Epilepsia 29:188–189, 1988.
213. Schacter DL, Curran T, Galluccio L, Milberg WP, and Bates JF: False recognition and the right frontal lobe: a case study. Neuropsychologia 34:793–808, 1996.
214. Landis T and Regard M: The right hemisphere's access to lexical meaning: a function of its release from left-hemisphere control? In Chiarello C (ed). Right Hemisphere Contributions to Lexical Semantics. Springer, Berlin, 1988, pp 33–46.
215. James W: The Principles of Psychology, Vol 2. H. Holt, New York, 1890.
216. Coslett HB and Heilman KM: Hemihypokinesia after right hemisphere stroke. Brain Cogn 9:267–278, 1989.
217. Sakai Y, Nakamura T, Sakurai A, et al. Right frontal areas 6 and 8 are associated with simultanapraxia, a subset of motor impersistence. Neurology 54:522–524, 2000.
218. Stuss DT, Alexander MP, Lieberman A, and Levine H: An extraordinary form of confabulation. Neurology 28:1166–1172, 1978.
219. Mychack P, Kramer JH, Boone KB, and Miller BL: The influence of right frontotemporal dysfunction on social behavior in frontotemporal dementia. Neurology 56(Suppl 4):S11–S15, 2001.
220. Damasio AR, Tranel D, and Damasio H: Individuals with sociopathic behavior caused by frontal damage fail to respond autonomically to social stimuli. Behav Brain Res 41:81–94, 1990.
221. Goodall J: The Chimpanzees of Gombe: Patterns of Behavior. Harvard University Press, Cambridge, MA, 1986.
222. Keller H and Zach U: Developmental consequences of early eye contact behaviour. Acta Paedopsychiatr 56:31–36, 1993.
223. Kleinke CL: Gaze and eye contact: a research review. Psychol Bull 100:78–100, 1986.
224. Kawashima R, Sugiura M, Kato T, et al.: The human amygdala plays an important role in gaze monitoring. A PET study. Brain 122:779–783, 1999.

225. Fleminger S, Murphy L, and Lishman WA: Malignant distress on eye contact after severe head injury. J Neurol Neurosurg Psychiatry 61:114–115, 1996.

226. Borod J, Koff E, Perlman-Lorch J, and Nicholas M: The expression and perception of facial emotions in brain damaged patients. Neuropsychologia 24:169–180, 1986.

227. Wittling W: Psychophysiological correlates of human brain asymmetry: blood pressure changes during lateralized presentations of an emotionally laden film. Neuropsychologia 28:457–470, 1990.

228. Snow D: The emotional basis of linguistic and nonlinguistic intonation: implications for hemispheric specialization. Dev Neuropsychol 17:1–28, 2000.

229. Cicero BA, Borod JC, Santschi C, et al.: Emotional versus nonemotional lexical perception in patients with right and left brain damage. Neuropsychiatry Neuropsychol Behav Neurol 12:255–264, 1999.

230. Bloom RL, Borod JC, Obler LK, and Gerstman LJ: Suppression and facilitation of pragmatic performance: effects of emotional content on discourse following right and left brain damage. J Speech Hear Res 36:1227–1235, 1993.

231. Winner E and Gardner H: The comprehension of metaphor in brain-damaged patients. Brain 100: 717–729, 1977.

232. Ross ED: Right hemisphere syndromes and the neurology of emotion. In Schachter SC and Devinksy O (eds). Behavioral Neurology and the Legacy of Norman Geschwind. Lippincott-Raven, Philadelphia, 1997, pp 183–194.

233. Gainotti G and Lemmo M: Comprehension of symbolic gestures in aphasia. Brain Lang 3:451–460, 1976.

234. Brownell HH, Michel D, Powelson JR, and Gardner H: Surprise but not coherence: sensitivity to verbal humor in right- hemisphere damaged patients. Brain Lang 18:20–27, 1983.

235. Burgess C and Simpson GB: Cerebral hemsispheric mechanisms in the retrieval of ambiguous word meanings. Brain Lang 33:86–103, 1988.

236. Weylman ST, Brownell HH, and Gardner H: "It's what you mean, not what you say." Pragmatic language use in brain-damaged patients. In Plum F (ed). Language, Communication and the Brain. Raven Press, New York, 1988, pp 229–244.

237. Cicone M, Wapner W, and Gardner H: Sensitivity to emotional expressions and situations in organic patients. Cortex 16:145–158, 1980.

238. Brownell H, Pincus D, Blum A, Rehak A, and Winner E: The effects of right-hemisphere brain damage on patients' use of terms of personal reference. Brain Lang 57:60–79, 1997.

239. Foldi NS: Appreciation of pragmatic interpretations of indirect commands: comparison of right and left hemisphere brain- damaged patients. Brain Lang 31:88–108, 1987.

240. Devinsky O, Hafler DA, and Victor J: Embarrassment as the aura of a complex partial seizure. Neurology 32:1284–1285, 1982.

241. Levine DN and Grek A: The anatomic basis of delusions after right cerebral infarction. Neurology 34: 577–582, 1984.

242. Alexander M, Stuss DT, and Benson DF: Capgras' syndrome: a reduplicative phenomenon. Neurology 29:334–339, 1979.

243. Malloy PF and Richardson ED: The frontal lobes and content-specific delusions. J Neuropsychiatry 6:455–466, 1994.

244. Malloy P, Cimino C, and Westlake R: Differential diagnosis of primary and secondary Capgras' delusions. Neuropsychiatry Neuropsychol Behav Neurol 5:83–96, 1992.

245. Richardson ED, Malloy PF, and Grace J: Othello syndrome secondary to right cerebrovascular infarction. J Geriatr Psychiatry Neurol 4:160–165, 1991.

246. Price BH and Mesulam M: Psychiatric manifestations of right hemisphere infarction. J Nerv Ment Dis 173:610–614, 1985.

247. Capgras J and Reboul-Lachaux J: L'illusion des sosies dans un delire systematise chronique. J Bull Soc Clin Med Ment 11:6, 1923.

248. Devinsky O, Feldmann E, Burrowes K, and Bromfield E: Autoscopic phenomena with seizures. Arch Neurol 46:1080–1088, 1989.

249. Pisani A, Marra C, and Silveri MC: Anatomical and psychological mechanism of reduplicative misidentification syndromes. Neurol Sci 21:324–328, 2000.

250. Feinberg TE and Shapiro RM: Misidentification-reduplication and the right hemisphere. Neuropsychiatry Neuropsychol Behav Neurol 2:39–48, 1989.

251. Alper K, Devinsky O, Perrine K, Vazquez B, and Luciano D: Nonepileptic seizures and childhood sexual and physical abuse. Neurology 43:1950–1953, 1993.

252. Westbrook L, Devinsky O, and Geocadin R: Nonepileptic seizures afer head injury. Epilepsia 39: 978–982, 1998.

253. Richer P: Etudes Cliniques sur L'hystero-epilepsie ou Grande Hysterie. Delahaye et Lecrosnier, Paris, 1881.

254. Harrington A: Medicine, Mind, and the Double Brain. Princeton University Press, Princeton, NJ, 1987.

255. Galin D, Diamond R, and Braff D: Lateralization of conversion symptoms: more frequent on the left. Am J Psychiatry 134:578–580, 1977.

256. Stern DB: Handedness and the lateral distribution of conversion reactions. J Nerv Ment Dis 164:122–128, 1977.

257. Axelrod S, Noonan M, and Atanacio B: On the laterality of psychogenic somatic symptoms. J Nerv Ment Dis 168:517–525, 1980.

258. Ley RG: An archival examination of an asymmetry of hysterical conversion symptoms. J Clin Neuropsychol 2:1–9, 1980.

258a. Fleminger JJ, McClure GM, and Dalton R: Lateral responses to suggestion in relation to handedness and the side of psychogenic symptoms. Br J Psychiatry 136:562–566, 1980.

258b. Sackeim HA: Lateral asymmetry in bodily response to hypnotic suggestion. Biol Psychiatry 17:437–447, 1982.

259. Schachter DL, Wang PL, Tulving E, and Freedman M: Functional retrograde amnesia: a quantitative case study. Neuropsychologia 20:523–532, 1982.

260. Krahn LE, Rummans TA, Sharbrough FW, et al.: Pseudoseizures after epilepsy surgery. Psychosomatics 36:487–493, 1995.

261. Devinsky O and Gordon E: Epileptic seizures progressing into nonepileptic conversion seizures. Neurology 51:1293–1296, 1998.

262. Welker WI and Seidenstein S: Somatic sensory representation in the cerebral cortex of the raccoon (Procyon lotor). J Comp Neurol 111:469–501, 1959.

263. Sperry RW: Brain bisection and mechanisms of consciousness. In Eccles JC (ed). Brain and Conscious Experience. Springer, Berlin, 1966, pp 298–308.

264. Lassonde M and Sauerwien C: Neuropsychological outcome of corpus callosotomy in children and adolescents. Neurosurg Sci 41:67–73, 1997.

265. Zaidel E, Clarke JM, and Suyenobu B: Hemispheric independence: a paradigm case for cognitive neurscience. In Scheibel AB and Wechsler AF (eds). Neurobiology of Higher Cognitive Function. Guilford Press, New York, 1990, pp 297–352.

266. Selnes OA: The corpus callosum: some anatomical and functional considerations with special reference to language. Brain Lang 1:111–139, 1974.

267. Clarke S, Maeder P, Meuli R, et al.: Interhemispheric transfer of visual motion information after a posterior callosal lesion: a neuropsychological and fMRI study. Exp Brain Res 132:127–133, 2000.

268. Sperry RW, Zaidel E, and Zaidel D: Self-recognition and social awareness in the disconnected minor hemisphere. Neuropsychologia 17:153–166, 1979.

269. Mesulam MM: Behavioral neuroanatomy. In Mesulam MM (ed). Principles of Behavioral and Cognitve Neurology. Oxford University Press, New York, 2000, pp 80–82.

270. Glickstein M, Arora HA, and Sperry RW: Delayed response performance following optic tract section, unilateral frontal lesion, and commissurotomy. J Comp Physiol Psychol 56:11–18, 1963.

271. Corballis PM, Funnell MG, and Gazzaniga MS: A dissociation between spatial and identity matching in callosotomy patients. Neuroreport 10:2183–2187, 1999.

272. Zaidel D and Sperry RW: Some long-term motor effects of cerebral commissurotomy in man. Neuropsychologia 15:493–504, 1977.

273. Ellenberg L and Sperry RW: Capacity for holding sustained attention following commissurotomy. Cortex 15:421–438, 1979.

274. Zaidel DW: Memory and spatial cognition following commissurotomy. In Boller F and Grafman J (eds). Handbook of Neuropsychology. Elsevier, Amsterdam, 1990.

275. Hoppe KD and Bogen JE: Alexithymia in twelve commissurotimized patients. Psychother Psychosom 28:148–155, 1977.

276. Akelitis AJ: Studies on the corpus callosum. IV. Diagnostic dyspraxia in epileptics following partial and complete section of the corpus callosum. Am J Psychiatry 101:594–599, 1945.

277. Leiguarda R, Starkstein S, and Berthier M: Anterior callosal haemorrhage: partial interhemispheric disconnection syndrome. Brain 112:1019–1037, 1989.

278. Feinberg TE, Schindler RJ, Flanagan NG, and Haber LD: Two alien hand syndromes. Neurology 42:19–24, 1992.

279. Goldstein K: Der makroskopische Hirnbefund in meinem Falle von linksseitiger motorischer Apraxie. Neurol Centralbl 28:898–906, 1909.

280. Joseph R: Dual mental functioning in a '"split-brain" patient. J Clin Psychol 44:770–779, 1988.

281. Feinberg TE: Some interesting perturbations of self in neurology. Semin Neurol 17:129–135, 1997.

282. McNabb AW, Carroll WM, and Mastaglia FL: "Alien hand" and loss of bimanual coordination after dominant anterior cerebral artery territory infarction. J Neurol Neurosurg Psychiatry 51:218–222, 1988.

283. Eccles JC: Conscious experience and memory. Recent Adv Biol Psychiatry 8:235–256, 1965.

284. Zaidel E, Zaidel DW, and Bogen JE: Testing the commissurotomy patient. In Boulton AA, Baker GB, and Hiscock M (eds). Neuromethods. Methods in Human Neuropsychology, Vol 15. Humana Press, Clifton, NJ, 1990, pp 147–201.

285. Sperry R: Some effects of disconnecting the cerebral hemispheres. Science 217:1223–1226, 1982.

286. Gazzaniga MS, Holtzman JD, Deck MD, and Lee BC: MRI assessment of human callosal surgery with neuropsychological correlates. Neurology 35:1763–1766, 1985.

287. Sperry RW: Mental phenomena as causal determinants in brain function. In Globus GG, Maxwell G, and Savodnik I (eds). Consciousness and the Brain: A Scientific and Philosophical Inquiry. Plenum, New York, 1976, pp 163–177.

288. Singer W: Consciousness and the binding problem. Ann NY Acad Sci 929:123–146, 2001.

289. O'Brien G and Opie J: A connectionist theory of phenomenal experience. Behav Brain Sci 22:127–148, 1999.

290. Mesulam M-M: From sensation to cognition. Brain 121:1013–1052, 1998.

291. Steriade M: Arousal: revisiting the reticular activating system. Science 272:225–226, 1996.

292. Munk MHJ, Relfesma PR, Konig P, Engel AK, and Singer W: Role of reticular activation in the modulation of intracortical synchronization. Science 272: 271–274, 1996.

293. Llinas R, Ribary U, Joliot M, and Wang X-Y: Content and context in temporal thalamocortical binding. In Buzaski G, et al. (eds). Temporal Coding in the Brain. Springer, Berlin, 1994, pp 251–272.

294. Pulvermuller F, Birbaumer N, Lutzenberger W, and Mohr B: High-frequency brain activity: its possible role in attention, perception and language processing. Prog Neurobiol 52:427–445, 1997.

295. James W: The Principles of Psychology, Vol 1. H. Holt, New York, 1890.

296. Natsuolas T: Consciousness. Am Psychol 33:906–914, 1978.

297. Kihlstrom JF: The cognitive unconscious. Science 237:1445–1452, 1987.

298. Cheesman J and Merikle PM: Distinguishing conscious from unconscious perceptual processes. Can J Psychol 40:343–367, 1986.

299. Monahan JL, Murphy ST, and Zajonic RB: Subliminal mere exposure: specific, general and diffuse effects. Psychol Sci 11:462–464, 2000.

300. Zeman A: Consciousness. Brain 124:1263–1289, 2001.

301. Zajonc RB: Feeling and thinking: preferences need no inferences. Am Psychol 35:151–175, 1980.

302. Winter L, Uleman JS, and Cunniff C: How automatic are social judgments? J Pers Soc Psychol 49:904–917, 1985.

303. Diamond J: The Third Chimpanzee. Harper Perennial, New York, 1993.

Attention and Attentional Disorders

Everyone knows what attention is. It is the taking possession by the mind, in clear and vivid form, of one out of what seem several simultaneous possible subjects or trains of thought. Focalization, concentration, of consciousness are its essence. It implies withdrawal from some things in order to deal effectively with others.

WILLIAM JAMES (1890)

Attention is a fundamental behavior. It comprises different processes and is integrally involved in diverse cognitive functions. Attention encompasses generalized activation of the cognitive processes of orienting, filtering, and selecting inputs; preparing for action; and maintaining thought on a stimulus, mental activity, or goal. Attention, a vital foundation for higher cognitive functions, maintains a coherent stream of thought. The ability to sustain attention, or vigilance, is necessary for complex behaviors, such as understanding and remembering a story. Therefore, attention must be tested first, before other cognitive functions. An inattentive patient's failure to perform calculations sheds no light on arithmetic skills. Rather, attentional dysfunction is a central feature of syndromes due to diffuse cerebral dysfunction such as delirium, as well as syndromes due to focal cerebral damage such as the neglect syndrome. In addition, attentional dysfunction often accompanies other cognitive impairments in such common neurological

disorders as closed traumatic brain injury and dementia.

FUNCTIONAL ATTENTIONAL NETWORKS

Simplistically, three functional networks underlie attention: a predominantly subcortical diffuse network, which mediates arousal and alerting; a mixed cortical–subcortical network, which mediates orientation to stimuli; and a predominantly cortical network, which mediates selective attention (Fig. 4–1, Table 4–1). Biologically, the three networks communicate and function as a seamless unit. However, dysfunction within one network can impair functions mediated by other networks. For example, impaired arousal and orientation disrupts selective attention. Within each of these three networks, subcortical and cortical areas have different but related functions.[1–3]

Arousal and Alerting Network

The arousal and alerting network, a diffusely distributed attentional system, awakens us from sleep and surveys the internal and external environments for relevant novel or changing stimuli. This "alerting" system includes the ascending reticular activating system, which

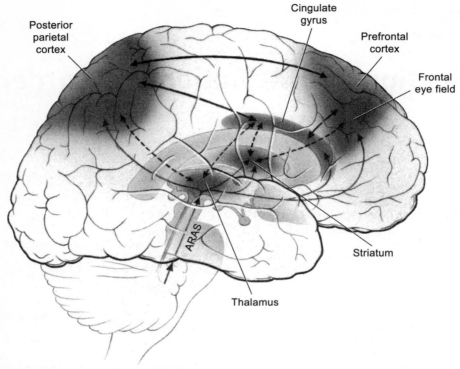

Figure 4–1. Functional anatomical networks of attention. The arousal and alerting network, a predominantly subcortical projection system, includes the reticular structures. The orienting network, a mixed cortical—subcortical system, includes the superior colliculus, pulvinar, and posterior parietal cortex. The selective attentional network, a predominantly cortical system, includes the frontal cortex. The three networks interact with each other and with the cingulate cortex to function as a unit. ARAS, ascending reticular activating system.

arises diffusely from the brain stem and the thalamus (particularly the intralaminar nuclei) and, in turn, influences the limbic system and neocortex. Other ascending projections to the cortex from sites originating in the basal forebrain (releasing acetylcholine), locus ceruleus (releasing norepinephrine), substantia nigra and ventral tegmental area (releasing dopamine), raphe nuclei (releasing serotonin), and hypothalamus (releasing γ-aminobutyric acid and histamine) help to mediate arousal and alerting (Fig. 4–2).[4]

DELIRIUM, A PROTOTYPE

Delirium, also referred to as an acute confusional state or metabolic or toxic encephalopathy, is a protypical example of a disorder affecting the arousal and alerting network. The term *delirium* accurately describes the typical clinical manifestations, while the alternative terms incompletely define the potential causes

of delirium. Delirium is a transient cognitive and behavioral disorder characterized by impairment of attention leading to global cognitive dysfunction, increased sympathetic activity, altered psychomotor activity, disruptions of the sleep–wake cycle, and changes in affect.[5,6] Confusion and clouding of consciousness are the hallmarks of delirium. Delirium may begin acutely or subacutely, symptoms usually fluctuate, and periods of surprising lucidity may be present. The cause is most often diffuse derangement of cerebral function from systemic or intracranial insults but also includes focal brain lesions. The following case report, on one of our patients with delirium, is illustrative:

A 52-year-old man was brought by his wife to the emergency department because he "was not making sense." He had a long history of epilepsy and had had a tonic-clonic seizure during sleep the night before. He appeared tired but normal in the morning and then became confused in the afternoon. He was alert but inattentive. Responses to simple ques-

Table 4–1. **Functional Anatomy of the Attentional Networks**

Network and Anatomical System	Function
Arousal and Alerting Network (Subcortical)	
Ceruleocortical noradrenergic	Arousal, alerting, selective attention
Mesolimbic and mesostriatal dopaminergic	Behavioral activation and motivation, stimulus salience
Basal forebrain cholinergic	Memory and attention
Nonspecific thalamic glutaminergic	Cortical activation, synchronization
Orienting Network (Mixed Cortical–Subcortical)	
Superior colliculus	Detecting novel stimuli, computing target location for attentional shifts, hyperreflexive orienting to ipsilesional field
Pulvinar	Restricts input to selected sensory region, filters irrelevant stimuli, assists in covert orienting, facilitates responses to a cued target
Posterior parietal cortex	Disengages attention from present focus
Selective Attentional Network (Cortical)	
Posterior parietal cortex	Disengages attention from present focus
Right	Greatest effect: mostly disengaging from locations
Left	Least effect: mostly disengaging from objects
Superior parietal lobule	Voluntary shifts of attention
Frontal eye fields	Generates volitional saccades
Premotor cortex	Motor intention
Dorsolateral frontal cortex	Working memory, self-monitoring
Anterior cingulate cortex	Motivation, exploratory behavior, attention to action

tions about time and place were often delayed and varied and usually incorrect. He was distracted by nearby noises and frequently lost his train of thought. When left alone, he would rest quietly but then, suddenly, start shouting for his wife, although she was beside him. On admission, examination revealed impaired comprehension for complex language and verbal discourse. Repetition and naming performance fluctuated. He was unable to do serial seven subtractions and was confused as to right and left on the examiner's body. He had a mild tremor of the outstretched upper extremities. He was found to have an infection (*Clostridium difficile*), which was treated with antibiotics. He was taking valproate for epilepsy, and his blood ammonia concentration was four times the upper limit of normal. Two days after antibiotic therapy and a reduction in the valproate dose, his mental state returned to normal.

Although most common among the elderly, delirium spares no age group. An acute confusional state may be a more common first sign of physical illness in the elderly than fever, pain, or tachycardia.[7] Delirium is found in one-third to one-half of elderly patients admitted to the hospital[8,9] but often remains undetected.[10] Morbidity and mortality are significantly increased in patients with delirium compared to patients with comparable medical illnesses without delirium.[11,12]

The most prominent and consistent feature of delirium is attentional impairment, with distractibility and difficulty in focusing or sustaining attention. Alertness may be reduced or enhanced. Delirious patients often experience visual or auditory hallucinations[5] and often have globally impaired cognition, which affects perception, memory (most prominently, learning new information), abstract thought, and the orderly sequence and organization of behavior. Their speech may be incoherent, with perseverations and circumlocutions, and lacking in content. Language testing reveals dysgraphia, mild word-finding difficulties, and semantic paraphasias.[13]

Delirium commonly impairs psychomotor activity and autonomic function, the sleep–wake cycle, and affect. Dramatic variations in psychomotor activity include displays of motor hyperactivity with agitation, incessant movements, and increased autonomic activity and, in contrast, apathy or abulia. For example, some patients appear "quiet," with mental abnormalities revealed only by questioning (e.g., inco-

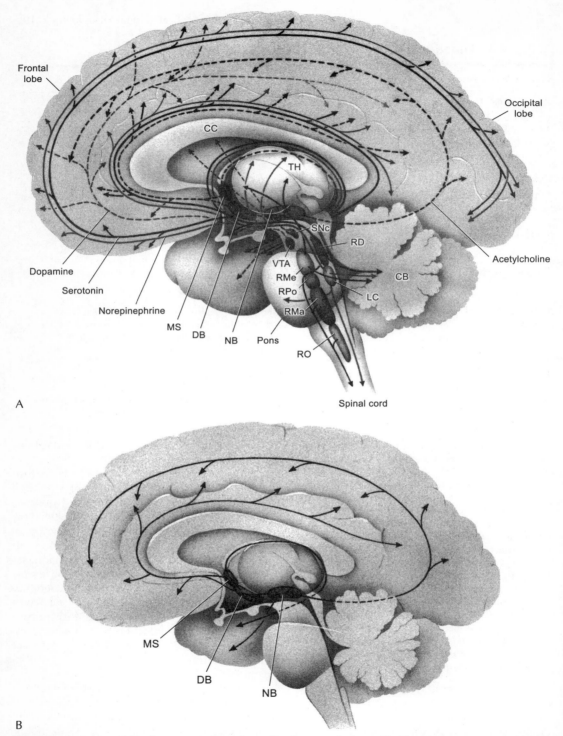

Figure 4–2. *A:* Major diffusely projecting neurochemical pathways in the brain. These neurotransmitters are primarily synthesized in the brain stem and basal forebrain; the thalamus helps to regulate their dispersal. *B:* Acetylcholine mediates attention and arousal in sensory systems.

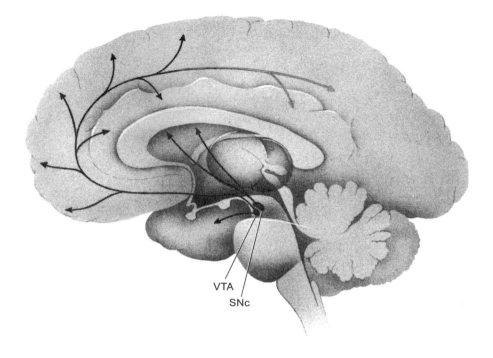

C

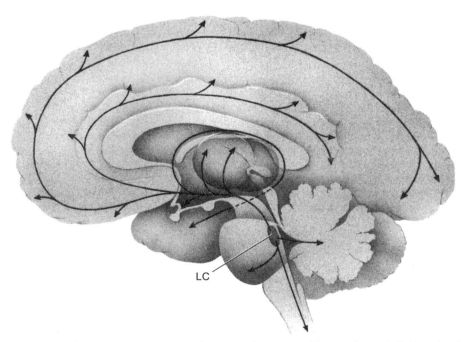

D

Figure 4–2. *Continued. C:* Dopamine sustains psychomotor and motivational focus and arousal. *D:* Norepinephrine helps initiate and sustain arousal and maintains high signal-to-noise ratios in sensory processing areas. CB, cerebellum; CC, corpus callosum; DB, diagonal band (Broca's area); LC, locus ceruleus; MS, medial septum; NB, nucleus basalis; RD, dorsal raphe nuclei; RN, raphe nuclei; SNc, substantia nigra (caudal portion); TH, thalamus; VTA, ventral tegmental area; RME, raphe medianus nuclei; RMA, raphe magnus nuclei; RP, raphe pallidus; RPo, Raphe periolivary; RO, raphe obscuris.

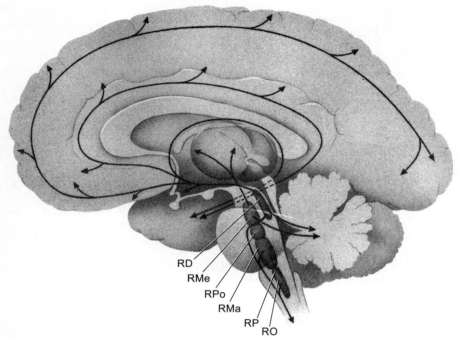

RD
RMe
RPo
RMa
RP
RO

E

Figure 4–2. *Continued. E:* Serotonin modulates affect reduces the impact of incoming information as well as crosstalk between sensory channels. CB, cerebellum; CC, corpus callosum; DB, diagonal band (Broca's area); LC, locus ceruleus; MS, medial septum; NB, nucleus basalis; RD, dorsal raphe nuclei; RN, raphe nuclei; SNc, substantia nigra (caudal portion); TH, thalamus; VTA, ventral tegmental area; RMe, raphe medianus nuclei; RMa, raphe magnus nuclei; RP, raphe pallidus; RPo, Raphe periolivary; RO, raphe obscuris.

herent speech, abnormal associations, or slow, vague thought patterns); and observation of spontaneous behavior may disclose only subtle signs, such as plucking at bedclothes.[14] Daytime somnolence and nocturnal insomnia are often present, and nightmares and vivid dreams during sleep and dreamlike mentation while awake can also occur. Delirium often develops, and is usually worse, at night, leading to "sundowning." The affective state ranges from neutral to profound depression or, less often, euphoria. Fear and anger may be present, usually in response to threatening hallucinations or persecutory delusions, triggering attempts to escape or fight that may endanger the patient and others.

CAUSES OF DELIRIUM

Delirium is often caused by a life-threatening but treatable disorder. Once delirium is recognized, the cause must be identified. Acute or subacute mental changes usually result from underlying cerebral or systemic disorders. A transient cognitive disorder should never be attributed to psychosocial stress alone.[8] Factors

that may predispose to acute confusion or delirium include sleep and sensory deprivation, severe fatigue and stress, age over 60 years, preexisting brain damage (such as in dementia), and addiction to alcohol or other drugs.

The common causes of delirium[5,6] (Table 4–2) include prescription and nonprescription drugs, alcohol intoxication, alcohol withdrawal, intoxication with illicit drugs (e.g., cocaine), cardiopulmonary disorders (a decrease in cerebral blood flow or oxygenation produces transient cognitive disturbances), infections, and metabolic encephalopathies. These last are among the most treatable but potentially devastating causes of delirium. Diffuse central nervous system insults such as traumatic brain injury, radiation, electrical injury, postictal state, and meningeal carcinomatosis can also cause confusional states.

ASSESSMENT OF DELIRIUM

A thorough medical history, physical and neurological examination, and laboratory studies can identify the cause of delirium in almost 90% of cases.[8] Important tests include meas-

Table 4–2. **Causes of Delirium**

Autoimmune disorders
  Serum sickness
  Food allergy
Drugs
  Prescription drugs: anticholinergic agents, sedative-hypnotics, digitalis preparations, cimetidine, opiates, lithium, antiepileptic drugs, salicylates, corticosteroids
  Ethyl and methyl alcohol
  Illicit drugs (e.g., cocaine, phenylcyclidine)
  Abused inhalants: gasoline, glue, nitrous oxide
  Withdrawal from alcohol or sedative-hypnotic drugs
Endocrine disorders
  Hyperinsulinism
  Hypothyroidism, hyperthyroidism
  Hypoparathyroidism, hyperparathyroidism
  Hypopituitarism
  Hypocortisolism, hypercortisolism
Infections
  Systemic: pneumonia, bacteremia, septicemia, hepatitis, bacterial endocarditis, urinary tract infection
  Central nervous system: meningitis, encephalitis, abscess, neurosyphilis
Metabolic disorders
  Hypoxia, severe anemia
  Hypoglycemia
  Hepatic, renal, pancreatic, pulmonary insufficiency
  Disorders of fluid and electrolyte balance
  Dehydration, water intoxication, osmolarity
  Alkalosis, acidosis
  Abnormally elevated or depressed sodium, potassium, calcium, or magnesium
  Porphyria
Neurological disorders
  Epilepsy: ictal and postictal states
  Traumatic brain injury
  Raised intracranial pressure and hydrocephalus
  Intracranial tumors: primary or metastatic
  Transient ischemic attacks and stroke: thrombotic, embolic, vasculitic
  Migraine
Nutritional disorders
  Hypoavitaminosis: nicotinic acid, thiamine, vitamin B_{12}, folate
  Hypervitaminosis: vitamin A or vitamin D intoxication
Poisons
  Industrial toxins: carbon disulfide, organic solvents, methyl chloride, methyl bromide, organophosphate insecticides, heavy metals, carbon monoxide
  Plants and mushrooms
Physical agents
  Heatstroke
  Radiation
  Electrical trauma
Cardiac disorders
  Myocardial infarction
  Congestive heart failure
  Arrhythmias

urement of blood electrolytes, liver and renal function tests, white and red blood cell counts, urinalysis, blood cultures, blood gas measurement, electrocardiogram, chest X-ray, screening for toxic substances, lumbar puncture, electroencephalography (EEG), and computed tomography or magnetic resonance imaging (MRI) of the brain. The EEG is a sensitive indicator of diffuse cerebral function and typically shows bilateral slowing of background activity, which correlates with the degree of cognitive impairment.[15]

Acute confusional states may dominate the clinical presentation in focal strokes or obfuscate other, possibly slight, neurological deficits, leading to the misdiagnosis of toxic or metabolic encephalopathy, postictal states, or psychiatric illness. Delirium can be a prominent manifestation of strokes in the anterior,[16] middle,[17–19] and posterior[20,21] cerebral arteries. These strokes are often misdiagnosed at first, particularly if hemiparesis or other obvious focal deficits do not accompany behavioral changes. The nondominant middle cerebral artery (MCA) is most often involved; delirium occurs in half of patients with this type of stroke.[17,19] Patients frequently display agitation; in some patients, psychosis accompanied by suspiciousness, paranoid delusions, and hallucinations occurs as a presenting[22] or delayed[23] manifestation. Strokes in the right MCA can also cause hemianopia, neglect, visuospatial deficits, and sensorimotor deficits. Fluent aphasia, resulting from dominant posterior temporoparietal lesions, can be mistaken for delirium because it usually begins rapidly and is not associated with focal symptoms such as hemiparesis. Paraphasias and neologisms are much more common with fluent aphasias than with delirium; a prominent comprehension deficit is the hallmark of Wernicke's aphasia (see Chapter 6).

Patients with posterior cerebral artery (PCA) infarction are more likely to experience delirium if the onset is acute and both arteries are involved simultaneously.[24] Unilateral PCA infarcts are more likely to produce confusional states when they affect the dominant hemisphere.[21] The principal manifestations of PCA infarction are visual field loss, hemisensory deficit, and, when the dominant hemisphere is involved, alexia without agraphia; anomia, most severe for colors, can also occur.[25] Other, less common acute symptoms include hemiplegia, transcortical sensory aphasia, memory impairment, release hallucinations in the blind part of the visual fields, visual agnosia, and third nerve palsy. Thalamic pain syndrome and movement disorders, such as cerebellar ataxia, tremor, and choreoatheosis, may develop weeks or months after PCA infarction.[19,21,26]

Anterior cerebral artery infarction can cause a wide range of behavioral changes, including delirium, decreased spontaneity, and socially inappropriate behaviors.[27] Thalamic strokes, too, can produce delirium, as well as personality changes and disorders of language and memory; delirium most often occurs with unilateral anteromedial thalamic lesions.[28,29]

Delirium often develops after surgery. Operative causes include anesthesia (e.g., nitrous oxide narcosis), hypotension, hypoxia, and altered volume status. Postoperative causes are electrolyte and acid-base abnormalities, hypoglycemia, anemia, hypotension, hemorrhage, infection, medications, sleep and sensory deprivation, alcohol withdrawal, and stroke. Physical examination of the patient, scrutiny of the anesthesiologist's operative record, and review of the postoperative medications, as well as blood gas and electrolyte measurements, usually reveal the cause of the delirium.

Dementia is commonly confused with delirium. An important clue to the differential diagnosis is the typical temporal evolution of symptoms: it is insidious in dementia but rapid in delirium. In elderly patients, however, things are not this simple. Indeed, delirium is often superimposed on dementia in the elderly. The insidious onset of cognitive decline may not be appreciated by family or friends, and not until infection or pulmonary disease hastens a sudden deterioration in mental status is the patient brought to medical attention. Further, a patient with known dementia may experience both delirium and depression. The differential diagnosis of delirium and dementia is summarized in Table 4–3.

Orienting Network

The anatomical network for orienting, defined mainly by studies of orientation to visual stimuli, involves the superior colliculus, pulvinar, and posterior parietal cortex.[30–32] Visual orientation involves eye movements that direct peripheral stimuli into foveal view and covert attentional shifts without eye or head movements.[1,32,33]

The superior colliculus mediates reflexive head, eye, and truncal orientation to stimuli (e.g., sudden loud noise) via output in the crossed tectoreticulospinal tract.[34] In the superior colliculus, sensory maps for visual, auditory, and somatosensory systems are aligned with each other and with motor maps,[35,36] al-

Table 4–3. **Differential Diagnosis of Delirium and Dementia**

Feature	Delirium	Dementia
Onset	Rapid, often at night	Insidious
Duration	Hours to weeks	Months to years
Course	Fluctuates over 24 hours, often worse at night	Relatively stable
Awareness	Impaired	
Alertness	Fluctuates	Usually normal
Orientation	Impaired, especially for time	Usually normal
Memory	Impaired for immediate and recent memory, fair fund of knowledge	Impaired or intact
Perception	Visual and auditory illusions common	Impaired for recent memory, variable loss of long-term memory
Sleep–wake cycle	Impaired, normal day–night cycle often reversed	Usually normal
Electroencephalogram	Diffuse slowing	Fragmented sleep
		Normal or diffuse slowing

Source: Modified from Lipowski.[8]

lowing stimuli in one modality to orient attention in other modalities to the relevant spatial area. Input from multisensory neurons in association cortex to the superior colliculus[34] provides higher-level influences on orientational and attentive motor behaviors.

Progressive supranuclear palsy, a degenerative disorder with prominent involvement of the midbrain (including the superior colliculus) and other subcortical regions, impairs volitional eye movements. Patients with this disorder have impaired visual orientation and visually guided behavior.[37] In contrast, patients with lesions of V1 (primary visual cortex) may be hemianopic but often adapt, showing little evidence of their dense field cut. This compensation may be mediated by both retinotectal fibers that project to the superior colliculus and geniculocortical fibers that project to the visual association cortex (see Chapter 5).

The pulvinar helps to filter out irrelevant stimuli from contralateral space[38] and restricts input to an area of interest.[32] Single-neuron recordings reveal activation in response to a visual stimulus that is a target of an impending eye movement or an object of covert attention.[39] The pulvinar connects with the superior colliculus and cortical areas (posterior parietal, inferotemporal, occipital) involved in early visual analysis, preserving topographical relations.[40] Unilateral pulvinar lesions slow a patient's responses to a contralesional cued target, despite having sufficient time for orientation.[1]

The posterior parietal cortex disengages the attentional focus for a contralateral target.[41]

Posterior parietal lesions cause hyperattention to ipsilesional cues, while delaying reflexive saccades and impairing attention to contralesional targets.[32,42]

Selective Attentional Network

Selective (or directed) attention is mediated predominantly by a cortical network that includes the association cortices in the posterior parietal and dorsolateral frontal lobes and the limbic anterior cingulate cortex.[2,43,44] Parietal cortex mediates sensory attentional functions, dorsolateral frontal cortex mediates motor and executive attentional functions, and anterior cingulate mediates motivational aspects of selective attention. This network is distinct from the cognitive processing systems activated passively by exposure to stimuli or execution of automated functions. For example, nonconsciously perceived (i.e., unattended) auditory stimuli activate primary and auditory association cortices. A vast wealth of sensory data are processed without attentional awareness (or consuming attentional capacity). These preattentive processes analyze both elementary and global gestalt features.[41]

Each hemisphere directs the attentional focus to the contralateral body and environment. The cortex of each hemisphere may maintain a spatially organized (e.g., retinotopic) representation of the half-world contralateral to the attentional focus; this representation incorporates current input and memory.[45] Evidence supports right hemisphere dominance for orientation and selective attention,[46,47] with the right parietal lobe being critical for sensory stimuli and the right frontal lobe maintaining motor attention (i.e., intention) and motivation. For instance, acute confusional states occur after an infarct in the right MCA territory;[17] the EEG of the right hemisphere desynchronizes after stimulation of either visual field in healthy subjects;[48] bilateral visual and auditory vigilance tasks performed by healthy subjects predominantly increase glucose metabolism in the right inferior parietal region;[49] and in healthy subjects performing a spatial attention task during positron emission tomography (PET) scanning, the right parietal cortex is activated in response to attention shifts to the left and right visual fields, while the left parietal cortex is activated only for attention shifts to the right visual field.[33] Further, patients with right-sided brain damage neglected stimuli in ipsilateral as well as contralateral hemispace on target cancellation.[50] In another experimental paradigm, patients with left-sided neglect showed significantly more right-sided omissions when left-sided cues were presented than without such cues, suggesting a "general difficulty in deploying attention" as well as a lateralized attentional deficit.[51]

UNILATERAL NEGLECT, A PROTOTYPE

Unilateral neglect is a protypical example of a disorder affecting the selective attentional network. *Unilateral neglect* is the impaired ability to orient toward, perceive, or act on stimuli from one side despite preserved sensorimotor functions. The deficit varies in severity from a minor form, detectable only as a failure to detect left-sided stimuli during simultaneous stimulation to both sides (e.g., extinction), to an inability to perceive all left-sided stimuli, including the side of one's body. Behaviorally, neglect is a more serious disability than primary sensory loss because with sensory loss the patient is aware of the deficit and can compensate. Fortunately, neglect typically improves considerably after the acute insult but can persist. The following describes a case of post-stroke unilateral neglect in one of our patients:

A 62-year-old woman with a history of hypertension and diabetes had the sudden onset of left-sided weakness and was admitted to the hospital. Examination revealed extremely poor attention and marked distractibility. Her speech was hypophonic and monotonous, but there were no obvious paraphasic errors in spontaneous conversation. She had a difficult time staying focused to follow verbal commands. Her head was turned to the right and she did not acknowledge people or objects on the left side. She blinked her eyes in response to threat in her left visual field. Her left arm and leg were markedly hemiplegic. She vehemently denied that there was anything wrong with her and wanted to go home. An MRI scan done 4 days after admission revealed a large right MCA infarct.

One week after her stroke, she appeared depressed but not distractible. Counting backward from 20 or saying the months backward, she would get lost and perform very slowly. Her speech was aprosodic. While reading, she often omitted the first few letters of compound words such as *baseball*, reading only *ball*. Several lines of writing deviated to the right side of the page. She had evidence of significant neglect when bisecting lines and was unable to cross off lines on the left side of the page. She could not close her eyes or stick out her tongue for more than a few seconds despite being told to do so several times. Her copy of a geometric design lacked details on the left side. When asked why she was in the hospital she replied "I had to come here for an operation on my hip; it has been bothering me lately." When asked if she had ever had a stroke, she replied "Not that I am aware of." She was shown her left arm and asked whose it was. She replied "Is it yours?" Even after feeling it with her right hand and tracing it back up to her right shoulder, she denied that it was her arm. On visual field testing, she could sometimes detect finger movement in her left visual field, but she always extinguished left-sided stimuli with double simultaneous stimulation. She also extinguished double simultaneous presentation of tactile stimuli. Her left hemiparesis was maximal in the upper limb.

During the hospital stay, she eventually acknowledged her stroke and her left-sided symptoms. Even several weeks later, however, she still underestimated the extent of her deficit. Her global attention improved markedly, but visuospatial neglect persisted at discharge 5 weeks after the stroke. Despite gaining almost full motor function in her left leg, she left the hospital requiring a wheelchair and home services.

ANATOMY OF UNILATERAL NEGLECT

Unilateral neglect is most common after right inferior parietal lobe injury.[52–54] Unilateral neglect also occurs with lesions of the left parietal lobe or nonparietal areas in the right hemisphere (dorsolateral prefrontal cortex, frontal eye fields, superior temporal gyrus, anterior cingulate cortex, striatum, posterior internal capsule, thalamus [pulvinar], and midbrain).[55-66] Damage to multimodal or heteromodal association cortices causes neglect, which supports the notion that neglect is a high-level attentional deficit rather a deficit in primary sensorimotor processing. Subcortical areas cause neglect when damage interrupts ascending brain stem monoaminergic or cholinergic projections or sensory thalamic relays to the neocortex. Based on clinical observations that neglect can be caused by damage to different cortical or subcortical regions, both Heilman[67] and Mesulam[68] proposed that directed spatial attention is mediated by a large-scale distributed network of brain regions and that different nodes (i.e., specific brain regions) within this network support different aspects of an individual's interaction with the environment.

Right MCA infarction is the most common cause of the neglect syndrome. However, infarction within other arterial territories of the distributed attentional network causes neglect. For example, right PCA infarcts damage the thalamus, and right anterior choroidal artery infarcts damage the posterior limb of the internal capsule, disconnecting sensory input from the left side of the body to the right parietal lobe.[65] Left PCA infarcts also cause delirium.[21] Although unilateral neglect is most commonly caused by stroke, it can present after any structural lesion or even seizures.[69]

CLINICAL FEATURES OF UNILATERAL NEGLECT

The severe form of left-sided unilateral neglect often complicates the acute stage of a right MCA infarction involving the right inferior parietal lobe. The head and eyes are turned toward the right, and patients may fail to bring the eyes left of the midline on command, although leftward eye movements are normal with the doll's eyes maneuver (passive head movements). Therefore, the defect is not oculomotor weakness but failure to direct the gaze toward the left. In addition, visual testing may reveal a dense, left-sided, homonymous visual field loss from interruption of optic radiations projecting to primary visual cortex from the lateral geniculate nucleus. Unilateral left-sided neglect may also affect other sensory modali-

ties. Acutely, patients behave as if the left side of their world no longer exists.

Clinical observations led to the proposal that unilateral neglect results from a deficit in selective or directed spatial attention. Many "attentional" theories of neglect account for the finding that neglect is more commonly associated with right hemisphere lesions. For example, Kinsbourne[70] suggested that left-sided unilateral spatial neglect is due to an innate and powerful bias of the left hemisphere to attend to the contralateral side of space, which is no longer balanced by the damaged right hemisphere. In contrast, Heilman and Watson[71] proposed that the right hemisphere is dominant for arousal and spatial attention. Thus, the right hemisphere directs attention into both fields of space, while the left hemisphere directs attention only into the right side of space. After right hemisphere damage, attention can be directed only into the right side of space, resulting in left-sided neglect. After left hemisphere damage, right-sided neglect would not occur because the intact right hemisphere can direct attention ipsilaterally into the right side of space. Finally, Posner et al.[44] proposed that unilateral spatial neglect is caused by a selective inability to disengage from stimuli present in the ipsilateral space.

Neglect behavior can also manifest as a unilateral deficit of motor program activation, reducing and delaying movements to the contralesional side (i.e., producing "intentional" as opposed to "attentional" neglect). Although parietal cortex is a critical node in the large-scale network supporting perceptual—representational aspects (including attention to stimuli), frontostriatal cortex is essential for exploratory—motor (intentional) aspects.[72-77] In patients with intentional neglect, the initiation and execution of left extremity movements are impaired, a condition that worsens when movements are attempted in the left hemispace. Patients often exhibit hypokinesia, bradykinesia, and hypometria (reduced movement amplitude). Intentional neglect may involve oculomotor as well as appendicular musculature. Attention and intention are closely linked: we direct our attention toward objects in our environment upon which we must act. Thus, even patients with lesions restricted to the parietal cortex can have intentional neglect, but the nature of the deficit may be different from that in patients with lesions restricted to the frontal cortex. For example, parietal lesions may slow the initiation of movements into the left side of space, while frontal lesions may slow the execution of such movements.[78] Intentional neglect may also be caused by impaired motivation for and initiation of action, resulting in diminished exploratory behavior.[79] Most patients with unilateral spatial neglect have deficits in both intentional and attentional aspects of selective attention.

Damage to other cognitive processes lateralized to the right hemisphere causes disorders that accompany left-sided neglect (see Chapter 3). *Motor impersistence,* the inability to maintain a posture, may be present and often occurs after right frontal lobe lesions. Postures such as closing the eyes or sticking out the tongue cannot be maintained, even for a few seconds. When motor impersistence is severe, almost any command from the physician or therapist will not be maintained. *Allesthesia,* the perception of a stimulus at a position remote from the stimulus location, usually occurs with right parietal lobe lesions and may be related to neglect. Most often, a left-sided stimulus is incorrectly identified as coming from the right side. Patients with neglect often exhibit *aprosody,* or the inability to produce the intonation required for adequate speech (see Chapter 6). Patients sound monotonous and cannot inflect their voice to present a question, sound surprised, or sound angry. They may also be unable to understand the inflection in other people's language.[80,81]

Left-sided neglect is often accompanied by personality or affective changes, including combinations of indifference, impaired perception of other peoples' thoughts and emotions, irritability, silliness, and mild euphoria. Mania correlates with extension of the lesion to the basal temporal or orbitofrontal regions on the right.[82] Patients with neglect may deny or fail to recognize their own deficit (e.g., hemiparesis), a symptom termed *anosognosia*[83] (see Chapter 3). Anosognosia is a disorder of body schema, our awareness of our body and of the spatial relations of our body parts to each other and to the environment. In contrast with the severe depression that often complicates left hemisphere strokes and right-sided hemiplegia, patients with acute right frontoparietal strokes may be aware of, but unconcerned about, their left-sided hemiplegia and speak of it as though it were affecting

someone else. However, some patients with anosognosia exhibit delusional denial and may become paranoid, agitated, and fearful concerning their left side.[52,84]

ASSESSMENT OF UNILATERAL NEGLECT

It may be difficult to differentiate homonymous hemianopia from unilateral visual neglect. To distinguish between them, the left hemifield should be tested in a dark room with a small penlight; patients with neglect will detect the left-sided visual stimulus, and those with hemianopia will not. A sensitive test for demonstrating unilateral neglect is the simultaneous presentation of bilateral stimuli.[52] For example, a patient may recognize a tactile stimulus on the left hand but identify the right-sided stimulus only when touched on both hands simultaneously. This can also be tested with visual (e.g., count fingers) or auditory stimuli. However, extinction cannot be tested if the patient has a primary visual, auditory, or somatosensory deficit. Extinction is more pronounced when the bilateral stimuli are identical in the reported attribute.[85]

Visual neglect can also be simply demonstrated by asking the patient to bisect a horizontal line; patients with left-sided visual neglect cut the line off to the right of center. Alternatively, the Cancellation Test may be employed by asking the patient to draw a perpendicular line through a set of randomly oriented lines on a sheet of paper.[86] In this test, patients with left-sided neglect draw only on lines located on the right side of the page.[87] Increasing the number of identifiable targets (e.g., >50) may uncover neglect not found with fewer targets.[88] Neglect behavior is present if, when asked to write prose, patients ignore the left side of the page and start each new line farther toward the right side of the page (Fig. 4–3). When copying simple line drawings (Fig. 4–3), patients with neglect omit details of the left side of the drawing regardless of where they appear on the page.[89,90]

RECOVERY

Rehabilitation clinicians empirically find that patients with right hemisphere infarcts generally have a poorer outcome than patients with

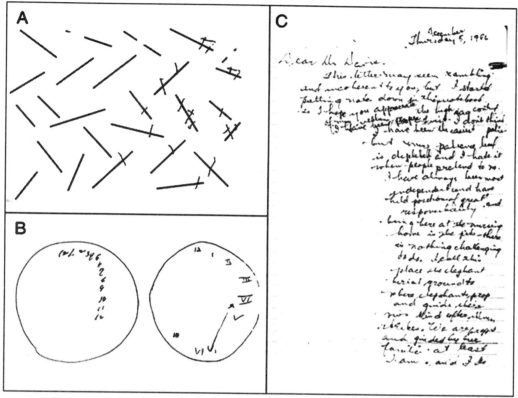

Figure 4–3. Performance of a patient with right parietal lobe stroke and left-sided visual neglect. In each example—the handwriting sample *(A)*, the Cancellation Test *(B)*, and the clock drawing *(C)*,—the left side of the page is ignored.

left hemisphere infarcts. That is, even with comparably sized lesions and sensorimotor deficits, patients with right hemisphere lesions are less likely to leave the rehabilitation hospital walking independently and to live with minimal assistance. Further, neglect acutely following a stroke is associated with longer hospitalizations.[91] Patients with aphasia, even global aphasia, and right hemiparesis often walk independently upon follow-up to the physician's office. In contrast, patients with a right hemisphere lesion and comparable hemiparesis are unable to walk. This appears counterintuitive because the aphasia and apraxia complicating left hemisphere stroke seem to have a more deleterious effect on motor recovery than visual neglect and other behavioral disorders associated with right hemisphere lesions.

This clinical observation was substantiated in a study of patients recovering from left and right hemisphere strokes[92] and has long baffled clinicians. After 6 months, patients with left-sided hemiplegia (right hemisphere strokes) were less independent and less well adjusted socially than patients with right-sided hemiplegia (left hemisphere strokes) and, consequently, had less improvement on performance of activities of daily living. The difference between the patient groups could not be accounted for solely by poorer motor recovery in patients with right hemisphere strokes and left hemiplegia. Neglect seemed to play a major role in deterring recovery after right hemisphere strokes. Outcome was not correlated with anosognosia, impaired intellectual performance, global attentional deficit, or other factors. In another study,[93] the extent of recovery and regaining of functional independence was predicted by the severity of neglect, the presence of anosognosia at 2–3 days, and the patient's age. Anosognosia, rather than neglect per se, may be more important in predicting poor functional recovery.[94]

Lesions outside the right parietal lobe usually cause milder and more transient neglect,[64] but neglect caused by cortical damage extending to underlying white matter tracts, such as the superior longitudinal fasciculus, is longer-lasting.[45,95] Patients with larger right hemisphere lesions and greater premorbid cortical atrophy show the least recovery from neglect.[96] Recovery from neglect depends on the location of damaged tissue as well as the extent and integrity of the undamaged brain tissue. For example, recovery from neglect is accompanied by return of normal metabolic activity in cortical areas within the left and right hemispheres not damaged by the original stroke.[97] Thus, recovery from neglect may be mediated by interactions between hemispheres and interactions within hemispheres. Further supporting this notion is that neglect in monkeys with right hemisphere lesions is more severe if their corpus callosum is transected, which largely interrupts interhemispheric communication.[98]

Prognosis of Neglect

The period of recovery from neglect is similar to that from other neurological deficits caused by stroke. Recovery is greatest over the first 10 days and reaches a plateau by 3 months. Overall, most patients with neglect make a good recovery, and many patients have little or no neglect at 3 months. In a study of 34 patients with left-sided neglect after stroke, only 7 (20%) had significant neglect at 3 months. Neglect recovers much sooner (median 8–9 weeks) than hemianopia (median 32 weeks) or hemiparesis (median 64 weeks).[93] Subtle symptoms of neglect such as extinction (median 19 weeks) and motor impersistence (median 26 weeks) recover more slowly.[61]

Therapeutic Remediation of Neglect

In general, neglect is difficult to treat. Its manifestations are not always obvious. For example, it is a common misconception of family members that patients with neglect cannot see out of the left eye, when actually the patient is unable to attend to objects on the left side of his or her "world," which is being perceived by both eyes. Therefore, family members must be educated about the neglect syndrome. They need to know that in the acute stages, when neglect is severe, it may be necessary to interact with the patient on his or her right, or non-neglected, side. They should understand that a patient with anosognosia is not consciously denying the extent of the illness but suffers from brain damage.

Many strategies seek an effective therapy for neglect.[73] One approach is based on neuropsychological testing. For example, sequential numbering of lines on the Cancellation Test and small financial incentives (e.g., a penny for each target stimulus identified) improve performance, suggesting that strategies to motivate the patient toward visuospatial searching can reduce neglect.[99,100] A modified Cancellation Test requires erasing of all lines. As each line is erased, it no longer competes for attention with the remaining lines. Thus, the patient no longer has to disengage from it before moving on to the next line in contralesional space. Performance is better by patients with left-sided neglect.[101]

Effective therapy for neglect has been developed from experimental programs. In a study of experimental therapy versus standard rehabilitation, Weinberg et al.[102] tested the hypothesis that patients with neglect do not adequately scan their environment. To compensate for impaired visual scanning, patients turned the head to the left to view stimuli in the non-neglected right visual field, a target on the left side of space served as an anchoring point, a high density of stimuli was avoided, and the patient's visual scanning behavior was paced to slow down impulsive tendencies to gaze toward the right side of space. After training sessions of 1 hour a day for 1 month, the experimental therapy group had significantly less visual neglect than the standard rehabilitation group. In a follow-up study, Weinberg et al.[103] trained patients to overcome neglect by improving sensory awareness and spatial organization. Patients were trained in sensory awareness by locating on the back of a mannequin the spot corresponding to the spot on the patient's back touched by the examiner. Patients were trained in spatial organization by estimating the size of rods of various lengths. The experimental therapy group had greater improvement on neglect measures than the group receiving standard rehabilitation.

From the observation that limb movements

on the side contralateral to the lesion improve neglect, Robertson et al.[104] trained patients to place and hold the left arm at the left margin of any activity in which they were engaged. This had the advantage of relying on an ever-present stimulus (i.e., the left arm) for an anchor. The disadvantage was that the patients often had a profound left-sided hemiplegia, making it difficult to use the left arm as an anchor. Viewing the left limb was not necessary for improvement. That is, even when the left arm was placed behind a screen and there were no visual cues, neglect improved.

Fresnel prisms fitted to the inside of a patient's eyeglasses improved visual neglect by shifting a peripheral image in the neglected visual field into the fovea.[105] This treatment improved neglect, but performance on activities of daily living was not improved. In a study of prism adaptation, Rossetti et al.[106] showed that neglect patients wearing prisms displacing visual stimuli to the right improved movements leftward into their neglected field. This effect lasted for at least 2 hours after the prisms were removed, supporting its value in rehabilitation.

Although the results of all of these experimental therapies are encouraging, deficiencies remain. None of the therapies that reduce neglect improves performance on activities of daily living, the primary goal of cognitive rehabilitation. The general attentional deficits that affect patients with right hemisphere damage may limit their ability to learn strategies and utilize them in real-life situations. What is more, the beneficial effects of these therapies do not last long. In a follow-up study of several of the aforementioned neglect therapies,[107] performance on activities of daily living improved, but by 4 months the results were equivalent to those of standard rehabilitation. This finding suggests that these training procedures quickly impart compensatory strategies but leave the final level of performance unaffected.

Other approaches for increasing orientation to the neglected side attempt to alter the neural system subserving attention. Hypothetically, if neglect from a right hemisphere lesion is due to reduced activation of the right superior colliculus, treatments increasing activation of the right (ipsilesional) superior colliculus, a brain region that receives direct visual input from both eyes, would reduce left-sided neglect. This strategy was tested when transient visual stimuli moving in a jerky motion, potent

activators of the superior colliculus, were presented to the neglected (left) visual field of patients with right hemisphere damage.[108] Neglect was substantially reduced, presumably by increased activation of the right superior colliculus. Patients benefitted from this therapy even though they were unaware of the visual stimulation of their neglected visual field. Because this therapy is used automatically and unconsciously, the patient does not have to learn or remember a compensatory strategy.

If unilateral neglect occurs because the left superior colliculus is overactive, driving orientation predominantly to the right, then treatments that reduce activation of the left superior colliculus may also reduce neglect. Theoretically, patching the right eye (i.e., ipsilateral to the cerebral lesion causing neglect) reduces neglect because the left superior colliculus, which gets most of its input from the right eye, is less active.[109] The right superior colliculus might function more effectively because it would no longer be inhibited by the left superior colliculus. This strategy was tested when the right eye was patched in neglect patients, and performance on a line bisection task improved significantly.[110] Neglect was reduced only when the patch was worn. Again, the patient did not have to learn or remember a compensatory strategy. Further, combining monocular patching with dynamic stimulation of the neglected (left) visual field reduced neglect more effectively than either therapy alone.[110] However, none of these therapies improved performance on everyday activities.

Pharmacotherapeutic approaches to neglect are based on the dopaminergic innervation of many structures in the attentional network. Animal experiments show that lesions of ascending dopaminergic pathways lead to neglect-like behavior and that dopaminergic agonists can improve neglect symptoms.[111,112] In two patients, therapy with bromocriptine (a dopaminergic agonist) produced a mild yet statistically significant improvement in neglect. However, when the medication was discontinued, the neglect worsened.[113] Bromocriptine may be more effective than methylphenidate,[114] and dopaminergic agonists may be more effective at improving certain types of behavior,[115] such as perceptual—motor behavior (e.g., pointing to stimuli on a piece of paper) rather than purely perceptual behaviors (e.g., counting stimuli on a piece of paper). In addition to the possibility that dopaminergic agonists may selectively improve certain neglect behaviors, certain behaviors may actually worsen after administration of a dopaminergic agonist. Bromocriptine, for example, caused neglect patients to spend more time exploring the ipsilesional visual field, resulting in increased neglect of the left visual field.[99] Larger, controlled studies are needed to assess the value of pharmacological therapy for neglect.

SUMMARY

Attention, a fundamental behavior, comprises different processes and is integrally involved in diverse cognitive functions. There are at least three distinct functional networks that underlie attention, yet these networks communicate and function as a seamless unit. First, a predominantly subcortical diffuse network mediates arousal and alerting. This network includes the ascending reticular activating system and the thalamus, both of which diffusely influence the limbic system and neocortex. Second, a mixed cortical—subcortical network mediates orientation to stimuli. This network includes the superior colliculus, pulvinar, and posterior parietal cortex. Finally, a predominantly cortical network mediates selective attention. This network is composed of the association areas of the dorsolateral prefrontal cortex and posterior parietal cortex, as well as the anterior cingulate. The interplay of these three functional networks allows us to orient, filter, and select from inputs in the complex world around us, preparing us for action or whatever is necessary to guide our behavior or achieve our goals. Attentional function is impaired by a broad spectrum of diffuse or focal insults to the brain. The clinical manifestations of attentional disorders, such as delirium or spatial neglect, are the direct result of damage to these functional networks in isolation or in combination.

REFERENCES

1. Posner MI: Structures and functions of selective attention. In Boll T and Bryant B (eds). Master Lectures in Clinical Neuropsychology and Brain Function: Research, Management and Practice. American Psychological Association, Washington DC, 1988, pp 171–202.
2. Mesulam MM: Large scale neurocognitive networks and distributed processing for attention, language, and memory. Ann Neurol 28:587–613, 1990.
3. Mesulam M-M: From sensation to cognition. Brain 121:1013–1052, 1998.
4. Saper CB: Diffuse cortical projection systems: anatomical organization and role in clinical function. In Plum, F. (ed.). Handbook of Physiology: Section I. The Nervous System, Vol 5. Higher Functions of the Brain. American Physiological Society, Bethesda, MD, 1986, pp 169–210.
5. Brown TM and Boyle MF: Delirium. BMJ 325:644–647, 2002.
6. Meagher DJ: Delirium: optimizing management. BMJ 322:144–149, 2001.
7. Rabinowitz T: Delirium: an important (but often unrecognized) clinical syndrome. Curr Psychiatry Res 4:202–208, 2002.
8. Lipowski ZJ: Transient cognitive disorders (delirium, acute confusional states) in the elderly. Am J Psychiatry 140:1426–1436, 1983.
9. Trzepacz PT: Delirium: advances in diagnosis, pathophysiology, and treatment. Psychiatr Clin North Am 19:429–448, 1996.
10. Beresin EV: Delirium in the elderly. J Geriatr Psychiatry Neurol 1:127–143, 1988.
11. Cole MG, McCusker J, Dendukuri N, and Han L: Symptoms of delirium among elderly medical inpatients with or without dementia. Br J Neuropsychiatry Clin Neurosci14:167–75, 2002.
12. Elie M, Rousseau F, Cole M, Primeau F, McCusker J, and Bellavance F: Prevalence and detection of delirium in elderly emergency department patients. CMAJ 163:977–981, 2000.
13. Geschwind N and Chedru F: Disorders of higher cortical function in acute confusional states. Cortex 8:395–411, 1972.
14. Treloar AJ and Macdonald AJ: Outcome of delirium. Part 2. Clinical features of reversible cognitive dysfunction—are they the same as accepted definitions of delirium? Int J Geriatr Psychiatry 12:614–618, 1997.
15. Engel GL and Romano J: Delirum, a syndrome of cerebral insufficiency. J Chronic Dis 9:260–277, 1959.
16. Amyes EW and Nielsen JM: Clinicopathologic study of vascular lesions of the anterior cingulate region. Bull Los Angeles Neurol Soc 20:112–130, 1955.
17. Mesulam MM, Waxman SG, Geschwind N, and Sabin TD: Acute confusional states with right middle cerebral artery infarctions. J Neurol Neurosurg Psychiatry 39:84–89, 1976.
18. Caplan LR, Kelly M, Kase CS, Hier DB, et al.: Infarcts in the inferior division of the right middle cerebral artery: mirror image of Wernicke's aphasia. Neurology 36:1015–1020, 1986.
19. Mori E and Yamadori A: Acute confusional state and acute agitated delirium: occurrence after infarction in the right middle cerebral artery territory. Arch Neurol 44:1139–1143, 1987.
20. Ferro JM, Caeiro L, and Verdelho A. Delirium in acute stroke. Curr Opin Neurol 15:51–55, 2002.
21. Devinsky O, Bear D, and Volpe BT: Confusional states following posterior cerebral artery infarction. Arch Neurol 45:160–163, 1988.
22. Price BH and Mesulam M: Psychiatric manifestations of right hemisphere infarctions. J Nerv Ment Dis 173:610–614, 1985.

23. Levine DN and Finkelstein S: Delayed psychosis after right temporoparietal stroke or trauma: relation to epilepsy. Neurology 32:267–273, 1982.

24. Symonds C and MacKenzie I: Bilateral loss of vision from cerebral infarction. Brain 80:415–455, 1957.

25. Nicolai A and Lazzarino LG: Acute confusional states secondary to infarctions in the territory of the posterior cerebral artery in elderly patients. Ital J Neurol Sci 15:91–96, 1994.

26. Fisher CM: Unusual vascular events in the territory of the posterior cerebral artery. Can J Neurol Sci 13:1–7, 1986.

27. Bogousslavsky J and Regli R: Anterior cerebral artery infarction in the Lausanne Stroke Registry. Clinical and etiological patterns. Arch Neurol 47:144–150, 1990.

28. Graff-Radford NR, Eslinger PJ, Damasio AR, and Yamada T: Nonhemorrhagic infarction of the thalamus: behavioral, anatomic, and physiologic correlates. Neurology 34:14–23, 1984.

29. Santamaria J, Blesa R, and Tolosa ES: Confusional syndrome in thalamic stroke. Neurology 34:1618, 1984.

30. Wurtz RH, Goldberg ME, and Robinson DL: Behavioral modulation of visual responses in the monkey: stimulus selection for attention and movement. Prog Psychobiol Physiol Psychol 9:43–83, 1980.

31. Colby CL: The neuroanatomy and neurophysiology of attention. J Child Neurol 6:S90–S110, 1991.

32. Posner MI: Attention in cognitive neuroscience: an overview. In Gazzaniga MS (ed): The Cognitive Neurosciences. MIT Press, Cambridge, MA, 1995, pp 615–624.

33. Corbetta MF, Miezin FM, Shulman GL, and Petersen SE: A PET study of visuospatial attention. J Neurosci 13:1202–1226, 1993.

34. Wallace MT, Meredith MA, and Stein BE: Converging influences from visual, auditory, and somatosensory cortices onto output neurons of the superior colliculus. J Neurophysiol 69:1797–1809, 1993.

35. Sparks DL: Translation of sensory signals into commands for control of saccadic eye movements: role of primate superior colliculus. Physiol Rev 66:116–177, 1986.

36. Stein BE and Meredith MA: The Merging of the Senses. MIT Press, Cambridge, MA, 1993.

37. Rafal RD, Posner MI, Friedman JH, Inhoff AW, and Bernstein C: Orienting of visual attention in progressive supranuclear palsy. Brain 111:267–280, 1988.

38. LaBerge D and Buchsbaum MS: Positron emission tomographic measurements of pulvinar activity during an attentional task. J Neurosci 10:613–619, 1990.

39. Petersen SE, Robinson DL, and Keys W: Pulvinar nuclei of the behaving rhesus monkey: visual responses and their modulation. J Neurophysiol 54:867–886, 1985.

40. LaBerge D: Computational and anatomical models of selective attention in object identification. In Gazzaniga MS (ed). The Cognitive Neurosciences. MIT Press, Cambridge, MA, 1995, pp 649–664.

41. Rafal R and Robertson L: The neurology of visual attention. In Gazzaniga MS (ed). The Cognitive Neurosciences. MIT Press, Cambridge, MA, 1995, pp 625–648.

42. Ro T, Rorden C, Driver J, and Rafal R: Ipsilesional biases in saccades but not perception after lesions of the human inferior parietal lobule. J Cogn Neurosci 2001;13:920–929.

43. Roland PE: Cortical regulation of selective attention in man: a regional cerebral blood flow study. J Neurophysiol 48:1059–1078, 1982.

44. Posner MI, Walker JA, Friedrich FJ, and Rafal RD: Effects of parietal injury on covert orienting of attention. J Neurosci 4:1863–1874, 1984.

45. Gaffan D and Hornak J: Visual neglect in the monkey. Representation and disconnection. Brain 120:1647–1657, 1997.

46. Pardo JV, Pardo P, Janer K, and Raichle ME: The anterior cingulate cortex mediates processing selection in the Stroop attention conflict paradigm. Proc Natl Acad Sci USA 87:256–259, 1990.

47. Posner MI and Petersen SE: The attention system of the human brain. Annu Rev Neurosci 13:25–42, 1990.

48. Heilman KM and Van Den Abell T: Right hemisphere dominance for attention: the mechanism underlying hemispheric asymmetries of inattention (neglect). Neurology 30:327–330, 1980.

49. Reivich M, Gur RC, and Alavi A: Positron emission tomographic studies of sensory stimulation, cognitive processes and anxiety. Hum Neurobiol 2:25–33, 1983.

50. Weintraub S and Mesulam M-M: Right cerebral dominance in spatial attention: further evidence based on ipsilateral neglect. Arch Neurol 44:621–625, 1987.

51. Robertson I: Anomalies in the laterality of omissions in unilateral left visual neglect: implications for an attentional theory of neglect. Neuropsychologia 27:157–165, 1989.

52. Critchley M: The Parietal Lobes. Edward Arnold, London, 1953.

53. Maguire AM and Ogden JA. MRI brain scan analyses and neuropsychological profiles of nine patients with persisting unilateral neglect. Neuropsychologia 40:879–887, 2002.

54. Bjoertomt O, Cowey A, and Walsh V. Spatial neglect in near and far space investigated by repetitive transcranial magnetic stimulation. Brain 125:2012–2022, 2002.

55. Denny-Brown D, Meyers JS, and Horenstein S: The significance of perceptual rivalry resulting from parietal lobe lesion. Brain 74:433–471, 1952.

56. Husain M, Mattingley JB, Rorden C, Kennard C, and Driver J. Distinguishing sensory and motor biases in parietal and frontal neglect. Brain 123:1643–1659, 2000.

57. Ghika-Schmid F and Bogousslavsky J. The acute behavioral syndrome of anterior thalamic infarction: a prospective study of 12 cases. Ann Neurol 48:220–227, 2000.

58. Karnath HO, Himmelbach M, and Rorden C. The subcortical anatomy of human spatial neglect: putamen, caudate nucleus and pulvinar. Brain 125:350–360, 2002.

59. Watson RT, Valenstein E, and Heilman KM: Thalamic neglect: the possible role of the medial thalamus and nucleus reticularis thalami in behaviour. Arch Neurol 38:501–507, 1981.

60. Healton EB, Navarro C, Bressman S, and Brust JCM: Subcortical neglect. Neurology 32:776–778, 1982.

61. Hier DB, Mondlock JR, and Caplan LR: Behavioral abnormalities after right hemisphere stroke. Neurology 33:337–344, 1983.

62. Stein S and Volpe BT: Classical "parietal" neglect syndrome after subcortical right frontal lobe infarction. Neurology 33:797–799, 1983.

63. Ferro JM and Kertesz A: Posterior internal capsule infarction associated with neglect. Arch Neurol 41:422–424, 1984.

64. Viader F, Cambier J, Masson M, and Decroix JP: Subcortical neglect: intentional or attentional? Arch Neurol 42:423–424, 1985.

65. Ferro JM, Kertesz A, and Black SE: Subcortical neglect: quantitation, anatomy, and recovery. Neurology 37:1487–1492, 1987.

66. Karnath HO, Ferber S, and Himmelbach M: Spatial awareness is a function of temporal not parietal lobe. Nature 411:950–953, 2001.

67. Heilman KM: Neglect and related disorders. In Heilman KM and Valenstein E (eds). Clinical Neuropsychology. Oxford University Press, New York, 1979, pp 268–330.

68. Mesulam MM: A cortical network for directed attention and unilateral neglect. Ann Neurol 10:309–325, 1981.

69. Heilman KM and Howell GJ: Seizure-induced neglect. J Neurol Neurosurg Psychiatry 43:1035–1040, 1980.

70. Kinsbourne M: A model for the mechanism for unilateral neglect of space. Trans Am Neurol Assoc 95:143–146, 1970.

71. Heilman KM and Watson RT: Mechanisms underlying the unilateral neglect syndrome. Adv Neurol 18:93–105, 1977.

72. Watson RT, Miller BD, and Heilman KM: Nonsensory neglect. Ann Neurol 3:505–508, 1978.

73. Swan L: Unilateral spatial neglect. Phys Ther 81:1572–1580, 2001.

74. Heilman KM, Bowers D, Coslett HB, Whelan H, and Watson RT: Directional hypokinesia: prolonged reaction times for leftward movements in patients with right hemisphere lesions and neglect. Neurology 35:855–859, 1985.

75. Meador KJ, Watson RT, Bowers D, and Heilman KM: Hypometria with hemispatial and limb motor neglect. Brain 109:293–305, 1986.

76. Nico D: Detecting directional hypokinesia: the epidiascope technique. Neuropsychologia 34:471–474, 1996.

77. Von Giesen HJ, Schlaug G, Steinmetz H, et al.: Cerebral network underlying unilateral motor neglect: evidence from positron emission tomography. J Neurol Sci 125:29–38, 1994.

78. Mattingley JB, Bradshaw JL, and Philips JG: Impairments in movement initiation and execution in unilateral neglect. Brain 115:1849–1974, 1992.

79. Maeshima S, Nakai K, Itakura T, et al.: Exploratory-motor task to evaluate right frontal lobe damage. Brain Inj 11:211–217, 1997.

80. Ross ED: The aprosodias: functional–anatomic organization of the affective components of language in the right hemisphere. Arch Neurol 38:561–569, 1981.

81. Gorelick PB and Ross ED: The aprosodias: further functional:anatomic evidence for the organization of affective language in the right hemisphere. J Neurol Neurosurg Psychiatry 50: 553–560, 1987.

82. Starkstein SE, Mayberg HS, Berthier ML, et al.: Mania after brain injury: neuroradiologic and metabolic findings. Ann Neurol 27:652–659, 1990.

83. Babinski J: Contribution a l'etude des troubles mentaux dans l'hemiplegie organique cerebrale (anosognosie). Rev Neurol 27:845–847, 1914.

84. Bisiach E and Berti A: Dyschiria. An attempt at its systematic explanation. In Jeannerod M (ed). Neurophysiological and Neuropsychological Aspects of Spatial Neglect. Amsterdam, Elsevier, 1987.

85. Baylis G, Rafal R, and Driver J: Extinction and stimulus repetition. J Cogn Neurosci 5:453–466, 1993.

86. Albert ML: A simple test of visual neglect. Neurology 23:658–664, 1973.

87. Schenkenberg T, Bradford DC, and Ajax ET: Line bisection and unilateral visual neglect in patients with neurologic impairment. Neurology 30:509–517, 1980.

88. Chatterjee A, Mennemeier M, and Heilman KM: A stimulus–response relationship in unilateral neglect: the power function. Neuropsychologia 30:1101–1108, 1992.

89. Marshall JC and Halligan PW: Visuospatial neglect: a new copying test to assess perceptual parsing. J Neurol 240:37–40, 1993.

90. Seki K and Ishiai S: Diverse patterns of performance in copying and severity of unilateral spatial neglect. J Neurol 243:1–8, 1996.

91. Kalra L, Perez I, Gupta S, and Wittink M: The influence of neglect on stroke rehabilitation. Stroke 28:1386–1391, 1997.

92. Denes G, Semenza C, Stoppa E, and Lis A: Unilateral spatial neglect and recovery from hemiplegia. Brain 105:543–552, 1982.

93. Stone S, Patel P, Greenwood R, and Halligan P: Measuring visual neglect in acute stroke and predicting its recovery: the visual neglect recovery index. J Neurol Neurosurg Psychiatry 55:431–436, 1992.

94. Pedersen PM, Jorgensen HS, Nakayama H, Raachou HO, and Olsen TS: Hemineglect in acute stroke—incidence and prognostic implications. The Copenhagen Stroke Study. Am J Phys Med Rehabil 76:122–127, 1997.

95. Leibovitch FS, Black SE, Caldwell CB, Ebert PL, Ehlich LE, and Szalai JP: Brain-behavior correlations in hemispatial neglect using CT and SPECT: the Sunnybrook Stroke Study. Neurology 50:901–908, 1998.

96. Levine D, Warach D, Benowitz L, and Calvanio R: Left spatial neglect: effects of lesion size and premorbid brain atrophy on severity and recovery following right cerebral infarction. Neurology 1986:362–366, 1986.

97. Perani D, Vallar G, Paulesi E, Alberoni M, and Fazio F: Left and right hemisphere contributions to recovery from neglect after right hemisphere damage—an [18F]FDG PET study of two cases. Neuropsychologia 40:1278–1281, 1993.

98. Watson RT, Valenstein E, and Heilman KM: The effect of corpus callosum section on unilateral neglect in monkeys. Neurology 34:812–815, 1984.

99. Grujic Z, Mapstone M, Gitelman DR, et al.: Dopaminergic agonists reorient visual exploration away from the neglected hemisphere. Neurology 51:1395–1398, 1998.

100. Ishiai S, Sugishita M, Odajima N, Yaginuma M, Gono S, and Kamaya T: Improvement of unilateral spatial neglect with numbering. Neurology 40:1395–1398, 1990.

101. Mark VW, Kooistra CA, and Heilman KM: Hemispatial neglect affected by nonneglected stimuli. Neurology 38:1207–1211, 1988.

102. Weinberg J, Diller L, Gordon W, et al.: Visual scanning training efffect on reading-related tasks in ac-

quired right brain damage. Arch Phys Med Rehabil 58:479–486, 1977.

103. Weinberg J, Diller L, Gordon W, et al.: Training sensory awareness and spatial organization in people with right brain damage. Arch Phys Med Rehabil 60: 491–496, 1979.

104. Robertson I, North N, and Geggie C: Spatiomotor cueing in unilateral left neglect: three case studies of its therapeutic effects. J Neurol Neurosurg Psychiatry 55:799–805, 1992.

105. Rossi P, Kheyfets S, and Reding M: Fresnel prisms improve visual perception in stroke patients with homonymous hemianopia or unilateral visual neglect. Neurology 40:1597–1599, 1990.

106. Rossetti YGR, Pisella L, Farne A, Li L, Boisson D, and Perenin M: Prism adaptation to a rightward optical deviation rehabilitates left spatial neglect. Nature 395:166–169, 1998.

107. Gordon W, Hibbard M, Egelko S, et al.: Perceptual remediation in patients with right brain damage: a comprehensive program. Arch Phys Med Rehabil 66:353–359, 1985.

108. Butter C, Kirsch N, and Reeves G: The effect of lateralized dynamic stimuli on unilateral spatial neglect following right hemispheric lesions. Restor Neurol Neurosci 2:39–46, 1990.

109. Posner MI and Rafal RD: Cognitive theories of attention and the rehabilitation of attentional deficits. In Meier MJ, Benton A, and Diller L (eds). Neuropsychological Rehabilitation. Guilford, New York, 1987, pp 182–201.

110. Butter C and Kirsch N: Combined and separate effects of eye patching and visual stimulation on unilateral neglect following stroke. Arch Phys Med Rehabil 73:1133–1139, 1992.

111. Apicella P, Legallet E, Nieoullon A, and Trouche E: Neglect of contralateral visual stimuli in monkeys with unilateral striatal dopamine depletion. Behav Brain Res 46:187–195, 1991.

112. Corwin JV, Burcham KJ, and Hix GI: Apomorphine produces an acute dose-dependent therapeutic effect on neglect produced by unilateral destruction of the posterior parietal cortex in rats. Behav Brain Res 79:41–49, 1996.

113. Fleet WS, Valenstein E, Watson RT, and Heilman KM: Dopamine agonist therapy for neglect in humans. Neurology 37:1765–1770, 1987.

114. Hurford P, Stringer AY, and Jan B: Neuropharmacologic treatment of hemineglect: a case report comparing bromocriptine and methylphenidate. Arch Phys Med Rehabil 79:346–349, 1998.

115. Geminiani G, Bottini G, and Sterzi R: Dopaminergic stimulation in unilateral neglect. J Neurol Neurosurg Psychiatry 65:344–347, 1998.

Chapter 5

Perception and Perceptual Disorders

Perception is our primary awareness of the world; it forms our first and strongest cognitive relation with the environment. In deciphering the cognitive mechanisms underlying normal and abnormal perception, we find that the lines between sensation, perception, memory, and thought processes blur. Sensation is the reception, filtering, and early analysis of external and internal stimuli. Perception requires additional filtering and a higher-order analysis of features in which discriminative and pattern-recognition functions are engaged to categorize sensory information.

PERCEPTUAL AWARENESS

Perception of internal and environmental stimuli requires a series of overlapping stages in sensory processing: reception, analysis of basic features, discrimination and comparison of feature patterns within a modality to form a percept, and comparison of a percept with percepts in other sensory modalities and with experiential memories and goals. Selective attention is critical for perception; it modulates the focus of awareness and biases the associative meanings linked with a sensation. The stages of sensory

processing involve relatively distinct cortical areas that form a synaptic hierarchy (serial links): primary sensory, primary unimodal, secondary unimodal, heteromodal, and limbic areas.[1]

All sensory cortices are organized in a similar pattern in which multiple cortical areas have their own somatotopic representations, cytoarchitecture, and thalamic and intracortical connection patterns. Primary sensory areas, with their densely packed small neurons, contain the most detailed representation of sensory input. Primary sensory and motor cortices are the most highly differentiated and distinctively human areas of the cerebral cortex. Primary sensory cortices are critical in reception (together with peripheral receptors and subcortical areas) and feature analysis and early discriminative analysis of sensory information. Primary sensory areas transfer information to unimodal association areas. The latter areas contain cells that respond to broader fields and more complex stimuli than primary areas. In each sensory modality, the different association areas are relatively specialized for analyzing and categorizing different stimulus features, such as color, shape, and motion of visual stimuli. Unimodal sensory areas are involved in more advanced discriminative analysis and in comparing stimuli with previously experienced stimuli in the same sensory modality. Unimodal areas have "primary" and "secondary" components: *primary* (upstream) areas are one synapse away from the primary sensory area; *secondary* (downstream) areas are two or more synapses removed from the primary area.[1] For example, unimodal visual association cortex includes primary components in extrastriate occipital areas and secondary components in inferior temporal and fusiform gyri.

Heteromodal areas receive convergent sensory input from unimodal areas in two or more sensory modalities. These areas are critical in linking different sensory features of the same stimulus, in comparing a percept with previously experienced percepts from other modalities, and in melding percepts into an ongoing behavioral plan and flexibly adapting to these new percepts. Heteromodal areas connect with limbic areas that provide emotional and motivational context to perception. Limbic areas, which have direct connections to hypothalamic centers for regulating internal body states, are on the opposite pole from the primary sensory and motor cortices, which are directed toward interactions with the external environment (see Figure 7-1).

The primary sensory and sensory association cortices are connected through serial and parallel circuits, with feedback fibers from association to primary areas serving an important role in the influence of higher synaptic levels on lower (earlier) levels of sensory function.

Several mechanisms may simultaneously or sequentially impair perception. For instance, visual perception may be adversely affected by diminished acuity, causing difficulty seeing an object clearly; impaired perception of static, but not moving, objects; and inability to distinguish objects by color, brightness, or size or to recognize shape and contour. Perception may also be impaired by cognitive disorders, including the inability to access visual memories or to connect visual memories to other sensations or language, or by psychological disorders, causing suppression of visual data from consciousness, as in conversion disorder.

Assessment of sensory and perceptual functions is laborious, and complete testing is rarely performed at the bedside. The goal is not a label but a detailed description of a patient's abilities. Testing involves progressively more complex stimuli in a given modality, with an attempt to separate impairments in reception,

feature recognition, discrimination (by a matching test), matching of a discriminated stimulus with other previously experienced sensations from the same modality, cross-modal comparisons, and ability to name or imitate (e.g., draw, vocally mimic) the stimulus.

VISUAL PERCEPTION

Human beings are visual animals. During anthropoid evolution, the auditory, tactile, and vestibular senses remained keen, while taste and olfaction waned. Vision is our most highly developed sense, being critical for survival throughout hominid descent. Sensory cortices have evolved not only to analyze and recognize but also to categorize environmental stimuli.[2] Extensive anatomical and physiological studies on the visual cortex provide insights into patterns of brain function, ranging from the vertical organization of cortical columns to multiple unimodal sensory representations related through serial and parallel connections. Sensory perception and movement are often excluded from the "higher" mental functions, but these functions form the foundation for cognition. Sensation and movement, interwoven with cognition, distinguish humans from other primates. An in-depth review of cortical visual areas and systems reflects the importance of vision in perceptual awareness.

Anatomy and Function of Cortical Visual Areas

Visual input from each hemifield passes in the optic tract to the contralateral lateral geniculate nucleus. Some retinal fibers travel directly from the optic tract to brain stem nuclei, forming the afferent limb of the pupillary light reflex (pretectal region) and serving in other visual functions (e.g., detection of motion by the superior colliculus). The small ventral lateral geniculate nucleus is the principal thalamic visual center, linking the retina and visual cortex. It sends projections via the visual radiations to the primary visual, or calcarine, cortex, with a small fraction passing directly to the visual association cortex.

In humans, the visual cortex occupies the occipital lobe, although other brain areas have functions related to visual perception (Table

Table 5–1. Visual Cortical and Related Areas

Visual Area	Location	Function	Comment
Primary visual cortex (V1)	Medial occipital lobe	Initial cortical analysis of visual input	Involved in orientation, selectivity, and binocularity
Visual association cortex[*]	Lateral and medial occipital lobe	Specialized analysis of visual information	Involved in form, motion, color, and depth analysis
V2	Surrounds V1	?Higher-order processing of data than V1	Cells respond to all major visual modalities
V3	Surrounds V2	Motion and depth perception, form analysis at low contrast	—
V4	Lingual and fusiform gyri (temporal lobe)	Size estimation, color perception	—
V5	Lateral junction of temporal, parietal, and occipital lobes	Motion detection	Bilateral lesions cause akinetopsia
V6	?Caudal aspect of superior parietal lobe[†]	Self-motion, 3-D features, target selection in visual searches	—
V8	Ventromedial occipital lobe	Color perception	Bilateral lesions cause achromatopsia
Related areas			
Frontal eye field	Caudal portion of middle frontal gyrus	Volitional eye movements	Saccades directed toward contralateral space
Lateral and basal temporal	Middle and inferior temporal gyri, fusiform, and lingual gyri	Object identification	"What" system
Parietal	Posterior and superior parietal lobes	Object location	"Where" system, directing visual attention

[*]Areas V4, V5, and V6 are located outside the occipital lobe; area V7 is not clearly defined in humans.
[†]As defined in monkeys, not humans.

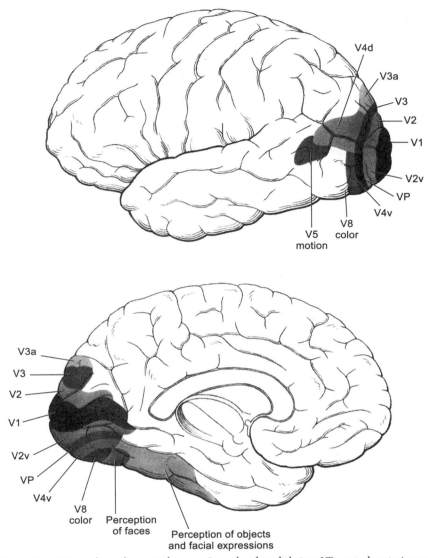

Figure 5–1. Principal visual areas in humans. Lateral and medial view. VP, ventral posterior area.

5–1). The occipital lobe is broadly divided into primary visual cortex (V1) and visual association cortex (V2, V3, V4, V5, V6, and V8; V7 is only preliminarily defined) (Fig. 5–1). Primary visual cortex is called "striate" cortex because a band of white fibers is visible on its surface, and visual association (secondary) cortex is called "extrastriate" cortex. Studies of visual cortex of the monkey provided the first insight into the columnar organization of the cerebral cortex (V1) and visual areas, which are homologous to the human visual cortex (Fig. 5–2).

PRIMARY VISUAL AND VISUAL ASSOCIATION CORTICES

V1 (Brodmann's area [BA] 17) is a 250 million neuron station that processes data from 1.25 million geniculate neurons (Fig. 5–1).[3] The receptive field is the retinal, or visual, field area, which influences the activity of striate cells and defines the cortical unit. Each unit contains simple and complex cells. Simple cells respond to illumination and orientation in a receptive field. Complex cells receive input from simple

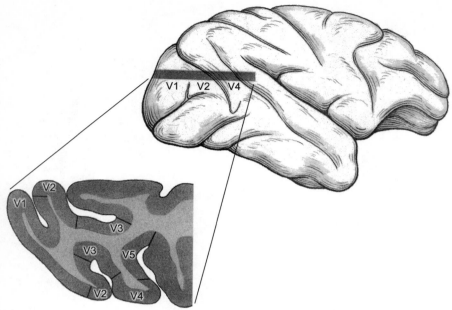

Figure 5–2. Areas on the visual cortex of the macaque monkey (transverse view) homologous to the human visual cortex.

cells, have a larger receptive field than simple cells, and respond to a specifically oriented stimulus (e.g., sharp dark–light contrasts) without regard to visual field location. Hypercomplex cells, found in visual association cortex (BA 18, 19), respond to more specific visual stimuli with input from two or more complex cells. Together with orientation selectivity, a major function of V1 is to combine visual information from the two eyes, resulting in binocular vision. Among the visual areas, V1 and V2 have the most precise retinal maps.

V2 (BA 18) is located adjacent to V1 (Fig. 5–1) and contains cells that respond to all major visual modalities (i.e., orientation, motion, wavelength, and depth). The largest visual association area in the occipital lobe, V2 has intimate connections to V1 and to V3 ipsilaterally and to the contralateral V2 by the corpus callosum. V2 has reciprocal connections with prefrontal, sensory, motor, and auditory areas via long association bundles. Projections from V2 to the frontal regions provide information for voluntary eye movements to coordinate with visual input. Cells in V2 have larger receptive fields and respond to lower spatial frequencies than those in V1. The clinical consequences of selective V2 lesions in humans are unclear. In monkeys, V2 lesions do not impair visual acuity or contrast sensitivity, but monkeys are unable to make complex spatial discriminations.[4]

V3 surrounds V2 along the superior border of the occipital cortex[5] (Fig. 5–1) and responds mainly to spatial orientation, direction, and depth.[6,7] Lesions of V3 may compromise motion and depth perception and form analysis, especially at low contrast levels.

V3a lies superior to V3 in the superior occipital cortex (Fig. 5–1). V3a has a continuous map of the contralateral hemifield, including the upper visual field in the superior occipital cortex.[5] Although in monkeys, V3a is an accessory area to V3 with similar functions and histological characteristics, human V3a appears quite distinct from V3. Although both areas are very sensitive to contrast, human V3a is much more sensitive for motion.[5,8]

The ventral posterior area lies posterior to the ventral portion of V2 in the inferior occipital lobe (Fig. 5–1). The ventral posterior area and V3/V3a form an intermediate hierarchy in the visual system between V1/V2 and higher visual areas.[9] The ventral posterior area may play a role in the early stages of form perception.

Ventral and dorsal components of V4 (Fig. 5–1) have different functional properties, and the nomenclature of the ventral division and its relation to the "color area" is controversial. An area on the lateral aspect of the collateral sulcus on the fusiform gyrus is generally accepted as mediating color perception.[10,11] However, the same area is referred to not only as a part of V4[10,12] but also as V8.[11] We refer to this area as the "color area" and consider it distinct from V4, as discussed later.

The ventral area V4 (V4v) lies in the lingual sulcus and fusiform gyrus (Fig. 5–1). A restricted lesion in V4v impairs hue perception, intermediate form vision, and visual attention in the contralateral superior quadrant.[13] Functional imaging studies in humans support the role of V4v in mediating awareness of object identity[14] and, on the left side, in contributing to visual word processing.[15]

The role of dorsal area V4 (V4d) in humans is less well defined (Fig. 5–1A) but may be critical in size estimation. In humans, mental transformations of size activate the dorsal occipitoparietal areas, including V4d.[16] In monkeys, V4 lesions severely impair the ability to judge the size of objects.[17] In addition, more than 50% of neurons in V1 and V4 of monkeys respond to the distance between the eyes and a visual stimulus.[18] Distance perception may be related to the interaction of two opposing groups of neuronal populations: "nearness" and "farness" cells,[17] which are embedded in all cortical visual areas. Thus, the two-dimensional map of our visual world found in each cortical area appears to have a third dimension encoded by the nearness and farness neurons.

The role of V4 in size estimation, a skill acquired throughout childhood, is relatively unique among cortical visual areas. In the seventeenth century, René Descartes correctly theorized that perception of size for near objects was related to the act of motor fixation (eyes converging), but for far objects, knowledge about the object and its visual context was critical. Children 8 years of age and younger underestimate the size of objects beyond 3 meters. The greater the object's distance, the greater the underestimate. V4 apparently uses visual context for acquiring experience-based spatial perception of object size. For instance, V4 lesions in monkeys do not impair recognition of an object if the object is transformed in size or partly occluded by other stimuli or if information about its contour is reduced. However, when all of these conditions are applied to a visual stimulus, monkeys with V4 lesions fail to recognize objects.[19]

V5 is located on the lateral convexity near the junction of the temporal, parietal, and occipital lobes (Fig. 5–1A).[20,21] V5 responds mainly to motion, detecting binocular disparity, as well as the speed and direction of a moving stimulus.[22,23] Visual data on motion likely reach V5 from the retina via two pathways: a main indirect pathway that passes through V1 and a faster, but smaller, direct pathway.[22,23a] The fast pathway may partly explain the phenomenon of blindsight, in which patients have no awareness of existing visual function (see Cortical Visual Disorders and Defects, below). Bilateral lesions of V5 can cause *akinetopsia,* a defect of movement perception.[23,23a,24] In animals with selective V5 lesions, impaired motion perception wanes with time, indicating that other areas partly compensate.

V6 has not been precisely located in humans; but in monkeys, it lies in the caudal aspect of the superior parietal lobule, with a topographically organized representation of the contralateral visual field. The central field is not magnified relative to the peripheral field. V6 is involved in visual analysis of self-motion and three-dimensional features, selection of targets during visual searching, and control of arm-reaching movements toward nonfoveated targets.[25,26]

V8, the color area, is located in the ventromedial aspect of the occipital lobe and the posterior ventromedial temporal lobe (fusiform gyrus) (Fig. 5–1). (Some investigators consider the color area to be a part of the ventral V4 area, but the controversy surrounds nomenclature, not anatomy.) The prime function of this area is apparently color perception, a role supported by functional imaging studies.[11] Lesions of V8 cause *achromatopsia* (loss of color vision). The color area is close to the area in which lesions cause *prosopagnosia* (impaired facial recognition) (Fig. 5–1B). In both achromatopsia and prosopagnosia, patients are unable to distinguish between items in the same perceptual category.[27] Thus, the ventral occipitotemporal region may mediate recognition of related but different percepts, regardless of whether they are colors or objects. Cells in areas V1–V3 respond to wavelength, but V8 computes *color constancy,* the invariance of object color over changes in luminance.[2,11,17]

HIERARCHICAL, SERIAL MODEL OF VISUAL PROCESSING

The traditional model of brain functioning is serial, or sequential, processing of information. In vision, as input is transferred from the retina to the lateral geniculate nucleus to the primary visual cortex and to the visual association areas, it is processed and more complex features are recognized at each subsequent level. Hierarchical processing of visual input is supported by progressive delays in neuronal response latencies and increasing size of receptive fields from V1 to higher visual association cortices.

The hierarchical model of visual processing conceptualizes visual input traveling down a one-way avenue toward a more complex and integrated visual image. There are, however, robust connections from visual association cortex to primary visual cortex. The forward connections from V1 and V2 are modality-specific, and feedback connections from visual association areas to V1 and V2 are diffuse.[28] For example, the feedback from cortical units in V4 is not limited to cells in V1 and V2, which project to V4, but also includes cells in V1 and V2, which project to V3 and V5.

These feedback fibers may contribute to several functions.[2] The first is access to a detailed visual field map. Although the retinal map of the visual world is reproduced in the specialized visual areas, it is less precise than the one housed in the striate cortex. The benefits of selective recognition, as of motion or color, are balanced by losses in topographic detail. Thus, if an area of visual interest is identified, the feedback fibers access data in V1 and "zoom in" and precisely focus on the area. The second function is linking one visual modality (e.g., motion) with another (e.g., shape) and activating recognition. For example, when a moving structure is recognized by V5, direct and indirect (via V1 and V2) connections to V3 activate the selective cells that recognize the moving structure's shape. The third function is integrating the visual image by providing pathways to join form, color, and motion. These pathways are distinct and complement the integration mediated by direct connections between V3, V4, V5, and V8. The model of multistage integration proposed by Zeki[2] suggests that "each stage of the visual pathways, including area V1, contributes explicitly to perception."

NONHIERARCHICAL, PARALLEL MODEL OF VISUAL PROCESSING

The nonhierarchical, parallel model of visual processing by the brain is a relatively recent concept. Cases supporting this model were reported more than a century ago but rejected because they lacked a theoretical framework. In the late nineteenth century, clinical and neuropathological findings supported the presence of independent, extrastriate areas for color and motion perception.[2] However, neurological authorities of the time emphatically dismissed this evidence as wrong and, in particular, inconsistent with their theories. Henschen, in 1893, correctly localized the "cortical retina" (where the world was "seen") to the striate area but suggested that other cortical areas were visual–psychic (where the world was "understood"; reviewed by Zeki[2]). In 1911, von Monakow,[29] an antilocalizationist and the nemesis of Henschen, argued that visual representation was plastic. With macular sparing as a model, he postulated that the retinal representation in the cortex was mobile or reduplicated and could immediately shift if one area were destroyed. Because there was no fixed retinal representation in the cortex, a local area for motion or color vision was incomprehensible. The concept of separate centers for motion and color vision, with lesions producing an isolated loss of vision for motion (akinetopsia) and color (achromatopsia), vanished from neurology for more than 50 years.

The theoretical structure for acceptance of the late nineteenth century clinical findings was built by more recent anatomical and physiological studies of the visual cortex in monkeys, demonstrating that multiple visual association areas contain independent but different retinal representations.[2,17] Each of these areas is smaller than V1 but contains receptive fields of neurons and cortical columns that are larger than those of V1. Multiple representations of the visual world fit poorly into the hierarchical, serial processing model. These areas are specialized and receive different inputs from V1 and V2. The connections between V3, V4, V5, and V8 strongly support a primarily parallel, not serial, communication network. The concept of parallel visual processing helps to explain feedback, the flow of information from "higher" to "lower" centers, and the nonreplicated role of the lower centers for detailed analysis, synchrony, and awareness (consciousness).

Parallel output is a consistent feature of cortical connectivity. Cortical areas contain functionally distinct cell groups with common properties. The groups have parallel outputs to other cortical and subcortical areas. Each cortical area sends different output signals to different areas, serving as a segregator that undertakes multiple operations. Cortical connections usually exist between areas with similar functions. Thus, portions of V1 and V2 that segregate color input from other inputs have strong connections to V8, the cortical color vision area in the fusiform gyrus. Parallel distributed processing occurs throughout the cortex from primary sensorimotor areas to prefrontal heteromodal association cortex.[30]

Beyond the Occipital Cortex: Parallel Systems

Like a river that forks, visual data flow from the visual association cortex in the occipital lobe to two parallel systems: a dorsal parietal lobe stream for spatial perception and visuomotor performance and a ventral temporal lobe stream for object discrimination and recognition (Fig. 5–3).[31–34] These parallel systems are functionally interwoven.[32,35,36] The inferior parietal and prefrontal cortices integrate the dorsal "where" and ventral "what" visual systems in behavior.[37]

The dorsal visual system connects dorsal occipital cortex with parietal association cortex, which in turn connects with the dorsolateral frontal lobe. Parietal areas attend to peripheral and central visual stimuli, relating visual input to external space and physical self and thus "seeing" the world as a whole. The parietal vi-

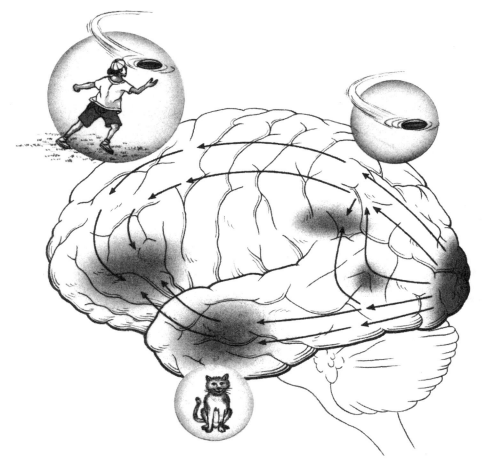

A

Figure 5–3. Major pathways of visual perception. Incoming information is analyzed in specialized sensory association areas; the frontal lobe utilizes input from these areas. *A:* In the "where" system (dorsal), visual information (the Frisbee) is transmitted through V5 (which perceives motion), the parietal lobe (which notes spatial location), and the motor cortex (which coordinates movement). In the "what" system (ventral), visual information (a cat) passes to the temporal lobe where it is recognized in the posterior inferior temporal region. Animals are semantically labeled mainly in the anterior temporal region.

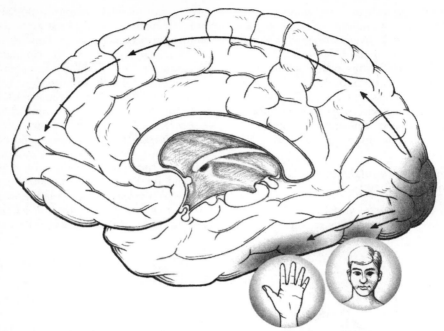

B

Figure 5–3. *Continued. B:* Other objects (e.g., faces and hands) are perceived and identified in different areas of the temporal lobe.

sual area analyzes motion, constructs a representation of visual space, and detects peripheral stimuli. Some cells in parietal visual cortex are gaze-locked, responding only if gaze is directed in a specific direction.[38] In monkeys, lesions of parietal visual areas disrupt sensory and motor aspects of smooth eye movement.[27] Parietal visual areas mediate visually guided ocular and reaching movements. In humans, superior parietal lesions impair coordination of eye and hand movements directed toward visual stimuli and targets. Posterior parietal visual areas are also critical for switching attention from one portion of the visual scene to another.

The inferior lateral temporal cortex includes a posterior area that helps to mediate visual discrimination and an anterior area that contributes to visual recognition and visual memory.[39] In monkeys, the inferior lateral temporal cortex contains cells that mediate facial recognition (most are in the superior temporal sulcus) and visual discrimination and may be the "long-term" storage for visual memories.[40,41] The neuronal receptive field is very large, increasing progressively from V1 to V4 to the inferior lateral temporal cortex. In contrast with the visual cortices described earlier, the infe-

rior lateral temporal cortex contains some neurons with bilateral receptive fields (as opposed to simply callosal connections, as in V2). The inferotemporal visual association cortex contributes to the recognition of color (area V8) and visual patterns, such as faces and birds, as well as the naming of visual stimuli.

Dual Modes of Visual Analysis

In a broader sense, parallel processing can be applied to concepts of "bottom–up" and "top–down" analysis of visual input. The vision system for object discrimination and recognition is largely a bottom–up process, in which tiny parcels of visual input from the retina are processed and constructed into the "object" (Fig. 5–4A). Objects are recognized by populations of cells distributed among one or more visual areas. Object recognition has three distinct stages: visual sensory processing (nonlateralized), perceptual processing (right hemisphere dominance), and semantic processing (left hemisphere dominance).[42] The right hemisphere has a larger responsibility for primary perceptual analysis and the left hemisphere for assigning symbolic language to visual stimuli. Apparently, the right temporal convexity has a larger visual association area, consistent with its role in visuospatial function, and the left temporal convexity has a larger auditory association area, consistent with its role in language comprehension.[43] In contrast to the bottom–up process, top–down processing molds the visual image by influences from other cognitive domains, such as attention, other senses, or emotion (Fig. 5–4B).

NEURONAL SYNCHRONY AND INTEGRATION OF THE VISUAL IMAGE

How is the visual image integrated by the brain? The multiple specialized cortical visual areas "see" different aspects of the world: orientation, depth, form, motion, and color. These areas do not provide convergent input to a "visual integration center" that "sees the whole picture." Instead, they are connected in parallel with each other and reciprocally with V1 and V2. When two specialized visual areas project to a common cortical area, their inputs are largely distinct. Local circuits could integrate

these inputs, but the result would be multiple local circuits in separate areas. Synchronous firing of cells can integrate the visual image.[44]

Synchrony in neuronal populations depends on neuronal groups interconnected by mutually excitatory and inhibitory synaptic connections.[45] Local field potentials resulting from synchronous neuronal firing generate the signals recorded on the electroencephalogram (EEG).[45] Synchronous activity occurs in multiple neurons in the visual cortex,[46] as well as in other areas such as the hippocampus and auditory and motor cortices.[47,48] Stimulation of cells in the retina, lateral geniculate nucleus, and visual cortex produces repetitive oscillatory bursts with frequencies of 30–120 Hz.[49] Further, cells in different visual areas and hemispheres can synchronize their responses to continuous stimuli sharing particular features, such as the same orientation or direction of motion.[50,51] With visual experience, cells become functionally linked with other cells sharing certain properties. As certain cells become synchronously activated over time, they may form repertories or groups and their connections may selectively compete for space on other cells.[52] The stabil-

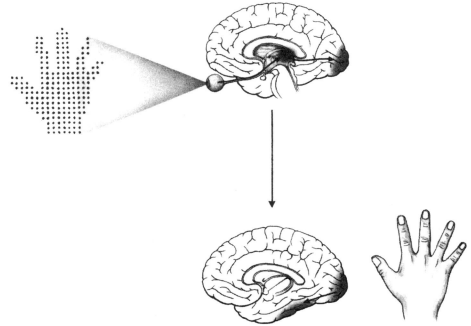

A

Figure 5–4. Dual modes of visual processing. *A:* "Bottom–up" processing. When an object is viewed, individual components (bits of data) are transmitted and processed through the retina, lateral geniculate, and visual cortex to create the visual image.

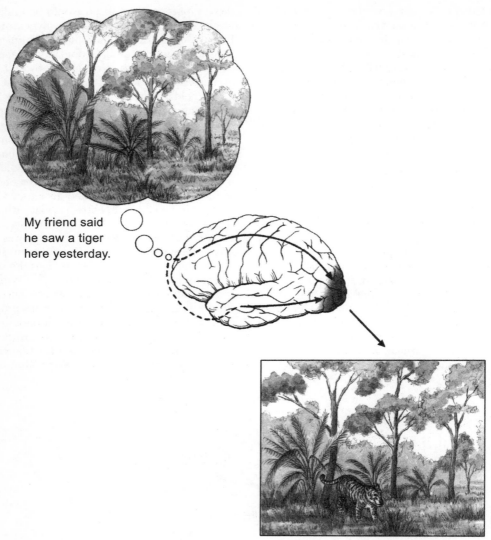

A

Figure 5–4. *Continued. B:* "Top–down" processing. Cognition and affect influence perception. Here, a person who is forewarned of a recent tiger sighting misinterprets ambiguous environmental cues and "sees" a tiger that is not present.

ity of the groups increases if the probability of their firing in synchrony is high.

For synthesis of the visual image, activity in nonspecialized (V1 and V2) and specialized (V3–V8) visual areas must occur in temporal synchrony. Perceptual awareness (consciousness) of visual input may rely on synchronously linked activity in multiple areas. Thus, if a component of visual input such as motion bypasses V1 and V2 and travels via the lateral geniculate nucleus to V5, the specialized area for movement of visual stimuli may detect the motion

but there is no conscious awareness of it.[23a] This phenomenon, which is known as *blindsight,* suggests that the neuronal population for conscious awareness of visual input includes cells in nonspecialized visual areas.

Cortical Visual Disorders and Defects

Cortical visual disorders affect the visual perception of form, face, color, movement, depth, and stereopsis. These disorders range from cortical blindness, in which the perceptual deficit is an absence of all these modalities, to Balint's syndrome and scotoma, in which the perceptual deficits are not as severe or all-encompassing (Table 5–2). *Scotoma* is an area of depressed or defective vision in the visual field, surrounded by an area of less depressed or normal vision. The scotoma is usually negative (a blank, or blind, spot) but may be positive (see Visual Hallucinations, below). Scotoma results from loss of normal sensory input from the optic nerve or striate cortex. Scintillating scotoma (zigzag lines) often occurs in classic migraine but may also result from posterior cerebellar tumors or arteriovenous malformations. Both positive and negative visual phenomena, as well as impaired consciousness and brain stem signs, may be caused by basilar migraine, usually a benign disorder in young women.

CORTICAL BLINDNESS

Blindness is due to bilateral lesions of the visual system at any site, ranging from the eyes to area V1, including the lens, retina, optic nerves and tracts, lateral geniculate nucleus, optic radiations, and striate cortex. Cortical blindness is caused by bilateral lesions of optic radiations or V1. It differs from other forms of blindness in that pupillary light reflexes are preserved by the sparing of fibers from the optic tracts to the midbrain. Patients with cortical blindness have full extraocular movements unless the brain stem is damaged. Optokinetic nystagmus is absent. However, with unilateral vascular lesions of the occipital lobe, it is often preserved toward the side of the hemianopia. Optokinetic nystagmus is typically present in conversion blindness, which, because pupillary light reflexes are preserved in both disorders, helps to distinguish it from cortical blindness. Some patients with conversion disorder can intentionally foveate away from the stimulus and block the nystagmus. Visual imagination and dreaming are usually normal in patients with cortical blindness.[53] Memory impairment, confusion, and simple or complex visual hallucinations are often present.

In cortical blindness, α activity on the EEG is lost but returns with visual recovery. Visual evoked potentials are usually abnormal but not correlated with the severity of visual loss or outcome.[54] Neither the visual evoked potential nor the EEG reliably predicts recovery.[55]

Cortical blindness usually occurs suddenly from a single occlusion of the posterior arterial circulation but may occur gradually or with successive lesions affecting each hemifield.[56,57] Cortical blindness is also caused by cerebral hemorrhage, tumors, cardiopulmonary arrest (especially in children), venous infarcts, cardiac bypass surgery, air and fat embolism, uncal herniation, demyelination, and the Heidenhain variant of Creutzfeldt-Jakob disease.[54] Visual recovery is poor in patients with stroke, age over 40 years, a history of diabetes mellitus or hypertension, or cognitive deficits.[54] Young patients with hypoxic insults and normal visual radiations on neuroimaging studies have the best prognosis.[58] Causes of transient cortical blindness include ischemia, cerebral or coronary arteriography, drugs (e.g., cyclosporin A), migraine, traumatic brain injury, seizures, and myelography.

Patients with cortical blindness are occasionally unaware of their visual loss and will actively deny it. This is known as *visual anosognosia,* or Anton's syndrome.[59] These patients act as if their vision is intact; they walk into walls, bump into furniture, and attempt to walk outside without the precautions a blind person would take. When confronted with their actions and apparent visual impairment, they may confabulate about what they are "seeing" or offer excuses, such as "the lighting stinks" or "these are my bad glasses." In Anton's syndrome, the bilateral lesion often extends beyond area V1 to involve the medial temporal or visual association areas. After weeks or months pass, many patients with visual anosognosia, like patients with anosognosia for hemiplegia, become aware of their deficit.

The mechanisms and precise anatomy of visual anosognosia remain uncertain. Autopsies on patients with permanent visual anosognosia usually reveal posterior cerebral artery infarcts, with lesions of primary visual and visual association cortices, as well as temporal lobe areas, including fusiform, superior temporal, and angular gyri.[60] Although mesial temporal lobe lesions can contribute to memory loss[61] or confusion,[62] neither of these problems accounts for the denial of blindness because either or both may be absent.[63] If primary visual and visual association areas that monitor visual input are destroyed or disconnected from other brain areas, visual awareness may be lost. Consciousness may remain intact, but the patient

Table 5–2. Cortical Visual Disorders and Defects

Disorder*	Visual Field	Principal Perceptual Deficit	Associated Perceptual Deficit	Lesion Site/Cause
Achromatopsia	Normal, contralateral superior quadrantanopia, or bilateral superior defects	No perception of color†	Perception of form usually normal,† perception of face impaired with bilateral defects	Ventral occipital lobe and lingual and fusiform gyrus involving V8 or association white matter, may be unilateral or bilateral, congenital defect in cone pigment cGMP-gated cation channel
Akinetopsia	Normal	No perception of movement	None	V5 bilateral (lateral convexity at junction of temporoparieto-occipital lobes)
Balint's syndrome	Normal or inferior field cut	Perception of depth may be impaired	Simultagnosia, optic ataxia & gaze apraxia	Bilateral occipitoparietal junctions, as in watershed infarcts
Cortical blindness	Absent	No perception of form, face, color, movement, depth, or stereopsis	—	Bilateral V1 or optic radiations
Hemineglect§	Normal or contralateral inferior quadrant defect	None	None	Contralateral hemisphere, R>L; commonly parietal but may be temporal, frontal, or subcortical
Object agnosia	Normal or superior field cut	Perception of form and face impaired or absent	Impaired perception of color	Bilateral infero-occipito-temporal junction, association white matter, or large left inferomedial occipito-temporal; disconnection of VAC to temporolimbic memory area
Prosopagnosia	Normal or superior field cut	No perception of face	Perception of form normal but possible deficit in distinguishing objects in a class	Facial template system: bilateral inferomedial occipitotemporal in VAC or large right inferomedial occipitotemporal
Scotoma	Partial defect, central or peripheral, often circular in general form	Loss of perception, may appear as clouded vision	Zigzag lines or other positive phenomena, possible halo around field defect	V1 and V2, visual pathways (e.g., optic nerve)

*Visual acuity is normal in all disorders, except cortical blindness. Neglect with competing stimuli occurs only in hemineglect and Balint's syndrome. VAC, visual association cortex; cGMP, cyclic guanosine monophosphate; R, right; L, left.
†Vision in peripheral hemifield or quadrant is absent, but foveal vision is usually spared.
‡Perception depends on which field is affected.
§See Chapter 3.

appears to be unaware of the lost function. Verbal consciousness may cause the patient to confabulate from memory and imagination when asked about his vision. Damage to visual consciousness or its connections may provide faulty information to other brain areas.[63] This misinformation may consist of fragmentary visual memories or imagery that prevents consciousness from recognizing the sensory loss and contributes to the confabulations.

BLINDSIGHT

Normal neural function permits conscious awareness of visual input. In other words, we are aware that we can see, and we know what we see. Blindsight is the converse of anosognosia. In blindsight, patients have some visual function but are unaware of it and deny its existence. Patients with blindsight have a visual field defect caused by a lesion of V1.[64] They lack awareness of visual stimuli presented to this area but respond discriminatively.[65,66] Visual acuity is severely impaired in the blind field.[66] Eye movements may be directed toward objects that the patient does not acknowledge seeing.[65,66] Blindsight patients are typically most able to detect a moving stimulus or a flashing stationary stimulus and to localize visual stimuli by eye and hand movements.[64,67] They can usually detect brightness, movement, gross size, and orientation of objects[68] but often cannot perceive such finer visual features as color, shape, or depth.[69] In some cases, blindsight patients can complete figures, summate spatially across the vertical meridian or with the normal hemifield, and detect and discriminate colors.[67,70]

After a tumor in the right occipital area was removed, a patient was unable to name or describe objects in the hemianopic left field.[71] The patient was tested with a forced choice paradigm with a limited number of selections (e.g., point to the target, yes or no, up or down). Forced choice means that the patient must respond to questions, even if it is a guess, but cannot respond "I don't know." Initially, a spotlight was flashed to different parts of the blind field, and the patient was asked to point to where the spotlight was flashed. He responded hesitantly because he was unaware of any stimulus, but his pointing was fairly accurate. He also was able to distinguish horizontal, vertical, and diagonal lines, Xs and Os, and straight from curved lines. In another case, despite having a global cognitive deficit after cardiopulmonary arrest, a girl with cortical blindness was trained to recognize color and form.[72]

Evidence for blindsight is not new. During World War I, Riddoch[73] observed soldiers with occipital cortex injuries who could sometimes see movements in their blind field. Using a conditioning paradigm, Marquis and Hilgard[74] taught monkeys with striate lesions, and apparently blind, to turn and reach toward visual stimuli. In monkeys, fibers project from the lateral geniculate to specialized visual areas in extrastriate cortex, thereby bypassing primary visual cortex.[75] Studies of cortical evoked potentials from the blind field of blindsight patients[76] and transcranial magnetic stimulation studies of V1 and V5[22, 23a] support similar connections in humans. However, blindsight may be mediated by visual input to the pulvinar and superior colliculus. In monkeys, more than 100,000 fibers travel from the ventral geniculate to the midbrain region, and the response properties of these nonstriate pathways parallel capacities of residual vision in blindsight patients.[66] Further, patients who undergo hemispherectomy possess some residual vision.[77] In humans, this subcortical pathway may transmit behaviorally relevant unseen visual events to the amygdala.[78]

Blindsight suggests that the loss of reciprocal connections between nonspecialized (V1 and V2) and specialized (V3–V8) visual areas may be needed for conscious awareness of visual stimuli.[78a] The specialized visual areas may be connected with other cortical areas, but without their link back to V1 and V2, there is no awareness of visual stimuli. If this model is correct and blindsight is not an exclusively subcortical phenomenon, the hierarchical model must be reconsidered. Traditionally, association cortex was considered the vital link between sensory input and consciousness. Consciousness was often considered to reside in the network of parietal or frontal lobe association cortex. However, blindsight challenges these traditional views, suggesting that visual consciousness not only "relies on" but also "inhabits" primary visual as well as visual association cortex.

AKINETOPSIA

Akinetopsia, the inability to perceive motion, results from lesions of V5 (the posterior continuation of the middle temporal gyrus at the lateral occipitotemporal junction).[2,23,79] When some World War I soldiers with gunshot wounds of the striate cortex detected movement in their blind fields, it suggested that movement is represented outside the striate cortex.[73] However, the observation was inconsistent with then-current theory and ignored for more than 60 years.

The inability to see objects move after damage to the extrastriate visual cortex and white matter bilaterally was first reported in 1983.[24] The patient had mild aphasia and acalculia, but her most severe impairment was in motion perception. When she poured tea or coffee into a cup, the "fluid appeared to be frozen, like a glacier." She could not "stop pouring at the right time since she was unable to perceive the movement in the cup (or a pot) when the fluid rose." Crossing the street was another challenge: "When I'm looking at the car first, it seems far away. But then, when I want to cross the road, suddenly the car is very near." When a black cube on a table was moved toward or away from her, she could see changes in postion but not movement in depth. The disorder did not affect her general perception of motion as she could perceive movement of auditory or tactile stimuli. She had lesions of V5 and extending beyond bilaterally.[79] Akinetopsia is rare as bilateral V5 lesions sparing V1 are unusual. Some patients with akinetopsia can perceive global motion and discriminate direction but fail at these tasks when the level of back-

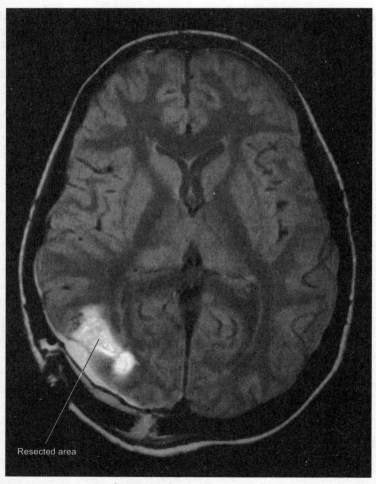

Resected area

Figure 5–5. Magnetic resonance image of a patient's brain with a tumor in V5. Her seizures caused illusions of environmental movement.

ground visual "noise" is moderate,[23] suggesting that visual association cortex extracts salient information from the noise.

We observed a woman with a tumor near V5 (Fig. 5–5) who had seizures characterized by visual illusions of environmental movement. During her seizures, the road appeared to "start waving" and objects appeared to "beat toward and away" from her. In another woman with a lesion in V5, seizures caused sudden illusions of things rapidly moving from side to side. Ictal visual illusions of movement may occur with a seizure focus in V1, V2, or V5 or ictal spread to these areas.

ACHROMATOPSIA

Achromatopsia is an acquired loss of color perception in part or all of the visual field due to lesions of the ventral occipital lobe and the adjacent fusiform (medial occipitotemporal) gyrus, that is, V8, or subjacent white matter.[80,81] Color vision is more than perceiving the wavelength of light. When a colored object such as a red apple is viewed under different sources of illumination (e.g., fluorescent light, daylight, dawn), the perception of shade may change but the color remains constant despite marked changes in the wavelength of light. Hue discrimination and color constancy are critical biological properties of human color perception. If not for these properties, color would no longer be an inherent property of an object, such as an orange, but one that would vary like temperature, as in a "cold" orange and a "hot" orange.[82] Area V8 compares the wavelengths of light reflected by objects to compensate for changes in illumination, thus providing an invariant property: an object's reflectance for light of different wavelengths. Color perception may be a model of how the brain constructs the visual image: extracting the invariant features in stimuli by relating analyzed components to each other.[2]

Achromatopsia is most often the result of a unilateral fusiform lesion involving V8. The signals conveying information about the wavelength of light are normal, but the brain cannot compare wavelengths and construct colors. Achromatopsia usually develops suddenly.[83] Color loss may vary in degree. For some patients, the world may appear washed-out or bleached but color identification is possible. Others may see only drab, "dirty" shades of gray, which may render indistinguishable similar but different-colored objects, such as red and green tomatoes. Visual acuity and the ability to distinguish subtle differences in form and depth are well preserved, and patients have no difficulty reciting the names of colors.[84] Acquired achromatopsia may be transient or permanent. Congenital achromatopsia, an autosomal recessive disorder, is caused by mutations in the gene encoding the α-subunit of the cone photoreceptor cyclic guanosine monophosphate–gated cation channel.[85]

Hemiachromatopsia, loss of color perception in half of the visual field, may exist without other visual defects. Right-sided hemiachromatopsia results from lesions of the left ventral occipital lobe and the occipitotemporal (fusiform and lingual gyri) *cortex*[17,80] and is often accompanied by alexia, visual agnosia, and right-sided superior quadrantanopia if the lesion extends to inferior optic radiations or, less often, to inferior calcarine cortex. Left-sided hemiachromatopsia usually exists as an isolated deficit. Some patients with hemiachromatopsia are unaware of their deficit, which is identified only with specific testing of color perception in each quadrant. Pseudoisochromatic plates (Ishihara or American Optical) are often helpful in diagnosing achromotopsia. The plates contain numbers or geometric designs formed by dots of related hue and varying size juxtaposed against a random background of dots of a different hue. The plates also help to discriminate impaired color vision from optic nerve disease (e.g., retrobulbar neuritis).

Full-field achromatopsia, the loss of color vision in areas of preserved vision, is often associated with prosopagnosia and field defects involving one or both upper quadrants. Achromatopsia may be accompanied by visual object agnosia or alexia. As with prosopagnosia, full-field achromatopsia arises from bilateral lesions of the occipitotemporal areas. The cause is usually an embolic stroke in the posterior cerebral artery bilaterally. After cortical blindness, achromatopsia may develop as vision improves, but color vision often returns early during recovery, especially after hypoxia in infants and children.[57]

The remarkable case of a painter who experienced the development of achromatopsia after a car accident[86] is illustrative:

After 65 years of normal color vision, the artist's world was now seen in black, white, and shades of "dirty" grey. His visual acuity was remarkable ("I can see a worm wriggling a block away"), probably from excessive tonal contrasts. Unfortunately, his tomato juice was black, and his brown dog was dark grey. Following the accident, he developed alexia, which lasted for 5 days, but the achromatopsia was permanent. His intimate relationship with color made his loss devastating, and contributed to an almost suicidal depression. His own color paintings were unfamiliar and meaningless. People looked like "animated grey statues." Flesh was an abhorrent grey that made a look in the mirror or socialization painful, and sexual intercourse impossible. His visual world was wrong, distasteful, and disturbing. It was like living in a world "molded in lead." Eventually, after several years of an anguished adjustment to his loss of color vision, he turned to painting in black and white, and was as productive and successful as he had been when painting in color. He gradually adapted his world to one of black and white, and became a "night person," finding peace in the low illumination.

Because patients with achromatopsia see with their cones and wavelength-sensitive cells in V1, they have access to color and wavelength; however, the color-generating mechanism of V4 and V8 is unusable, and color constancy, that is, what keeps an apple red with different luminance and backgrounds, is lost. Their visual perception of color and wavelength is that of V1, the output of which normally never appears in our awareness; and the sensation is prechromatic, neither colored nor colorless.[86]

COLOR ANOMIA

In spite of preserved color perception, patients with *color anomia* are unable to name colors or point to a color when given its name. Color anomia is usually associated with right-sided homonymous hemianopia and alexia. It is easily tested by asking the patient to name the color of an object to which the examiner points or to point to a color when the examiner names the color. Patients often have greater difficulty in supplying the color name. Color perception, as tested with color-matching tasks, is intact in the preserved left visual field. Unlike patients with achromatopsia, those with color anomia can discriminate hues on testing with pseudoisochromatic plates. The lesion in color anomia is located in the left mesial occipitotemporal region, inferior to the splenium.[87,88] The associated right field cut results from involvement of the optic radiations, striate cortex, or lateral geniculate nucleus.

VISUAL HALLUCINATIONS

Visual hallucinations are caused by destructive and irritative lesions of the visual system. They may be simple or complex. Simple visual hallucinations include spots of light, diffuse color, geometric forms, and positive scotomas (e.g., dark spot, halo of color, area of opacity, or "heat waves" surrounding a black hole), which may persist in the dark or when the eyes are closed. Complex visual hallucinations, such as the image of a face, may occur locally or throughout the visual field and with a clear or clouded sensorium. The major types and causes of visual hallucination are summarized in Table 5–3.

Simple (Unformed) Hallucinations

Photopsia, the appearance of sparks or flashes of light, is the most common simple visual hallucination. Simple visual hallucinations arise from dysfunction in the visual pathways from the eye to the primary visual cortex or, less often, from irritative lesions of the visual association cortex and medial temporal lobe. These types of hallucination have little localizing value but are usually ipsilateral to lesions anterior to the chiasm and contralateral to postchiasmal lesions. Patients with homonymous hemianopia and simple visual hallucinations often incorrectly describe the image as being in the contralateral eye. If a patient is in doubt about which eye is affected, ask him or her to test vision in each eye with the other eye closed. With lesions of the primary visual cortex, visual hallucinations usually arise in areas of visual loss and tend to be continuous and unformed. These hallucinations are often associated with an element of movement, as in weaving patterns, zigzag lines, a shower of sparks, or colored clouds.[89] However, interrupted flashes of light are not typical of hallucinations arising in the primary visual cortex. Unformed visual hallucinations also occur with cerebral lesions outside the primary visual cortex.

COMPLEX (FORMED) HALLUCINATIONS

Complex visual hallucinations usually result from lesions of the temporal, occipital, or parietal visual association area, but may also be caused by lesions throughout the visual system. The images may appear to be moving, multiple, or abnormally large or small; most often,

Table 5–3. **Visual Hallucinations**

Type and Hallucination	Etiology
Simple (unformed)	
Photopsia (light flashes), phosphenes (luminous image), scintillations (zigzag lines), geometric forms, checkerboard patterns, positive scotomas	Sleep or sensory deprivation, febrile states, nutritional deficiencies, drugs (e.g., LSD), alcohol withdrawal, pressure on globe, glaucoma, macular degeneration,° retinal ischemia,° incipient retinal detachment, migraine, release, irritative visual cortex lesion°
Complex (formed)	
People, objects, scenes and landscapes, animals (zoopsia)	Sleep or sensory deprivation, febrile states, nutritional deficiencies, drugs (e.g., LSD), alcohol withdrawal, temporal or parieto-occipital visual association area lesion,° release, irritative temporal lesion,° irritative occipitoparietal lesion

°The most common lesion sites are listed, but lesions in any part of the visual pathway may cause hallucinations. LSD, lysergic acid diethylamide.

they are perceived as being smaller than their real counterparts (*lilliputian hallucinations*). Visual hallucinations caused by seizure discharges typically last less than 3 minutes and are often associated with illusions or hallucinations in other sensory modalities. Complex visual and other experiential unimodal or multimodal hallucinations are more common with nondominant epileptogenic foci and electrical stimuli.[90] Multimodal hallucinations also exist with a systemic illness or the use of hallucinogenic drugs.

Autoscopy

The hallucination or psychic experience of seeing oneself (*autoscopy*) is a complex hallucination manifested in two main forms. The first is seeing one's double. The second is an out-of-body experience, the feeling of leaving one's body and viewing it from another vantage point, usually from above. Autoscopic phenomena may occur in healthy persons, especially with anxiety and fatigue; in patients experiencing near-death phenomena, systemic illness, or migraine; and in those with a temporal or parietal lobe seizure focus.[91]

Charles Bonnet Syndrome

Charles Bonnet syndrome is characterized by formed or unformed hallucinations in blind or partially blind persons. The hallucinations are perceived in the blind portion of the visual field and may be abolished by eye motion or closure of the blind eye. Hallucinations of color, faces, textures, and objects are correlated with cerebral activity in ventral extrastriate visual cortex, both during and between hallucinations.[92] Further, the content of the hallucinations reflects the functional specializations of the region.

Peduncular Hallucinosis

In the rare disorder, peduncular hallucinosis, the visual hallucinations are usually well formed and vivid (e.g., a brightly colored parrot or a dramatic scene with human figures) but may also be unformed. Lesions of the midbrain, diencephalon, or occipitotemporal cortex are usually involved.[93,94] The cause is usually embolic infarction. The pathophysiological mechanism of peduncular hallucinosis is uncertain but likely a release phenomenon, possibly resulting from a sleep abnormality (present in most cases) and related changes in ascending cholinergic or serotonergic activity.[94] Related disorders may be evening hallucinations in elderly subjects with cognitive deficits ("sundowning") and hypnagogic and hypnopompic hallucinations in narcolepsy. In all of these disorders, the mechanisms that activate dreaming during sleep may become pathologically activated during wakefulness.

Dreams

Consisting primarily of colored, formed visual images, dreams are often mixed with other sensory impressions. Although often bizarre, dreams are visually coherent. During dreaming, visual association and limbic cortices are mainly activated and primary visual cortex activity is relatively attenuated.[95]

VISUAL ILLUSIONS

Like visual hallucinations, visual illusions are caused by destructive and irritative lesions of the visual system. In *visual illusions,* the image may be altered in size (micropsia or macropsia), shape (dysmorphopsia or metamorphopsia), position (telopsia), number (polyopia), color, or movement.[96–98] The illusions may be restricted to areas of partial visual loss or may affect the entire visual field. In confused patients, real images may be perceived as familiar and more complex images. In alcohol withdrawal, for example, a patient may "see" a spot on the wall as a spider. Vestibular or oculomotor disorders may cause illusions with altered depth perception, tilting, and changes in shape (e.g., straight edges become curved).

Palinopsia

Visual perseveration (*palinopsia*) is the persistence or recurrence of a visual image after withdrawal of the excitatory stimulus.[99] Palinopsia is illustrated in the words of a patient who shaved repeatedly:[100] "I have shaved one side so that it is beautifully clean to my fingers. I looked back to find that the beard seemed to be still there. Because of that I sometimes shave myself twice, for no earthly reason."

Palinopsia is caused by structural lesions of the parietal and occipital lobes of either the right or left hemisphere, but the right hemisphere is usually involved.[101,102] Palinopsia also occurs in psychiatric disorders (e.g., schizophrenia, depression) and with drug use or abuse (e.g., trazodone, lysergic acid diethylamide [LSD]). When due to a structural lesion, palinopsia is usually a transient phenomenon, occurring during the progressive evolution or resolution of a homonymous visual field defect, and it appears in the area of visual loss. Rarely, palinopsia may persist for years.

The disorder is probably related to the phenomenon of illusory visual spread, in which visual perception extends over a greater area than that which the stimulus would be expected to excite. For example, the subject looks at a clock and sees the area between 6 o'clock and 12 o'clock as being twice as large as the area between 1 o'clock and 6 o'clock.[100] Palinopsia may manifest as an epileptic seizure or release hallucination.[99,102] Psychogenic mechanisms may contribute to palinopsia, for it is said that "things they think about a lot do not go out of vision as quickly, as if they were slow in being switched off."[100]

Visual Synesthesia

An optic percept, visual synesthesia is induced by stimulation of an auditory, tactile, or other sensory modality.[103,104] In response to hearing a specific sound, for instance, a patient may see shapes or colors. Visual synesthesia occurs in both neurologically healthy persons and those with lesions throughout the visual pathways.

Visual Allesthesia

A rare condition, *visual allesthesia* is the transposition of visual images from one homonymous half-field to another. It is usually found with bilateral cerebral lesions but may occur with focal seizures. Auditory and somatic sensations are frequent accompaniments.

VISUAL AGNOSIA

As a general term, *agnosia* refers to the associative disorder in which normal or near-normal perception is preserved but the ability to recognize a stimulus or to know its meaning is lost. A diagnosis of agnosia is critically dependent on establishing preserved perception. Further, it is essential to differentiate agnosia and anomia, when a patient is unable to name an object. In visual agnosia, attention, intelligence, language, and visual sensation are normal but, as in all agnosias, the patient is unable to derive meaning from the preserved primary sensory input.

Visual agnosia is commonly divided into two principal forms: apperceptive and associative. In the first form, higher-order visual perception and, therefore, recognition are impaired; in the second form, perception is largely intact but recognition is selectively impaired.[105] However, some perceptual disorders exist in all visual agnosias.

Apperceptive Visual Agnosia

In *apperceptive visual agnosia*, elementary visual functions, such as acuity, brightness discrimination, depth perception, and color vision, are normal or only mildly disordered (patients may complain of blurred or unclear vision) but recognition is impaired. Patients are unable to recognize, copy, match, or discriminate simple visual stimuli and cannot recognize even simple shapes such as triangles or circles. (Patients with apperceptive visual agnosia may or may not have achromatopsia, but those who do are unable to match stimuli by color.) They may recognize objects by tracing the shape with their fingers or hands, but their tracing and recognition of contours demonstrates a "slavish" dependence on local continuity.[106] They are distracted by irrelevant lines or details and cannot "connect" relevant features. For example, a patient with apperceptive visual agnosia incorrectly read a stimulus with discontinuous lines (Fig. 5–6).[106] The patient's ability to recognize and point to the object may be improved if the object is moving.[105] Patients may display normal object imagery but are unable to relate individual elements to a whole.[107] The inability to "group" and "integrate" object components into a whole may underlie apperceptive visual agnosia.

The lesions in apperceptive visual agnosia are typically diffuse and posterior. The prominence of white matter lesions suggests that disconnection, often of very local intralaminar connections, rather than neuronal loss, causes the visual deficit. Stroke, anoxia, and carbon monoxide or mercury poisoning are common causes of the disorder.[105–107]

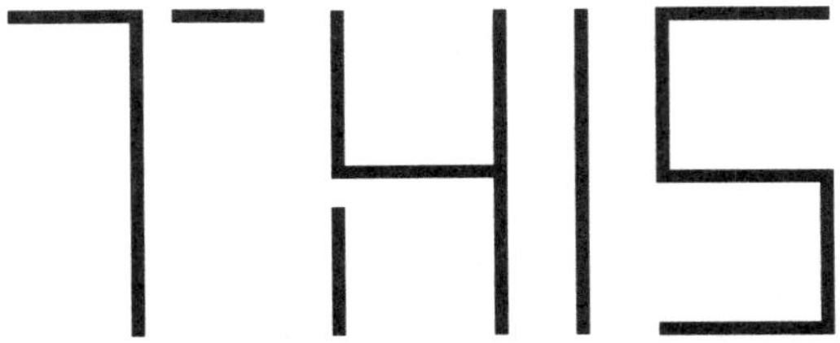

Figure 5–6. A stimulus consistently read as "7415" by a patient with agnosia, who processed only the continuous lines. (From Landis et al.[108] Reprinted with permission of Cambridge University Press.)

Apperceptive visual agnosia is often confused with *simultagnosia,* a disturbance of visual attention in which patients recognize only one element in the visual scene (see Balint's Syndrome, below). In both disorders, despite normal or mildly impaired visual fields, acuity, and color perception, patients may appear blind, often bump into objects in their environment as they maneuver, and make prominent searching movements with their eyes. Careful examination may be required to detect preserved basic visual perception. By definition, patients with simultagnosia can recognize single objects, but those with apperceptive visual agnosia cannot.

Because there is some defect in complex cortical visual processing (downstream from area V1) and often a milder defect in lower-order, more basic cortical visual perceptual functions (closer to area V1, upstream), the traditional apperceptive visual disorder is viewed by some clinicians as "pseudoagnosia."[110,111] They reserve *apperceptive visual agnosia* to describe a small group of patients with right posterior lesions, invariably affecting the posterior inferior parietal lobe, in whom visual recognition is impaired when the perspective is unusual or lighting is uneven. The patients' limited recognition results from misleading clues of color, size, texture, or reflectance.[112]

Associative Visual Agnosia

In visual object agnosia, a form of associative visual agnosia, patients are unable to recognize objects. Patients with visual object agnosia also have prosopagnosia, but those with prosopagnosia do not necessarily have visual object agnosia. The diagnosis depends on establishing normal or near-normal visual perception. Patients must not complain of hazy or otherwise altered vision. The adequacy of visual perception is judged by the patient's description of the visual world. Because aphasia is mild or absent, the patient should be able to describe the visual stimuli in detail (i.e., shape, size, edges and contour, position, and number of stimuli). Many patients with visual agnosia have achromatopsia, as revealed by difficulty describing colors. Copying of a complex figure, matching of similar figures, or matching of an object with a drawing of the object may be used to test normal visual perception. Patients with visual agnosia often use a slow, laborious, line-by-line strategy to make detailed copies of a figure.[113] Even though verbal descriptions, drawing, or matching of visual stimuli may be successfully executed, subtle defects in visual perception may contribute to impaired recognition (Fig. 5–7).[112,114]

Because patients with agnosia often have a misdiagnosis of *anomic aphasia* (inability to name), and vice versa, it is important to use both verbal and nonverbal tests of object recognition. Verbal testing is done first, with patients describing in detail what they see. Patients with associative visual agnosia describe the features and shape of an object but fail to recognize it.

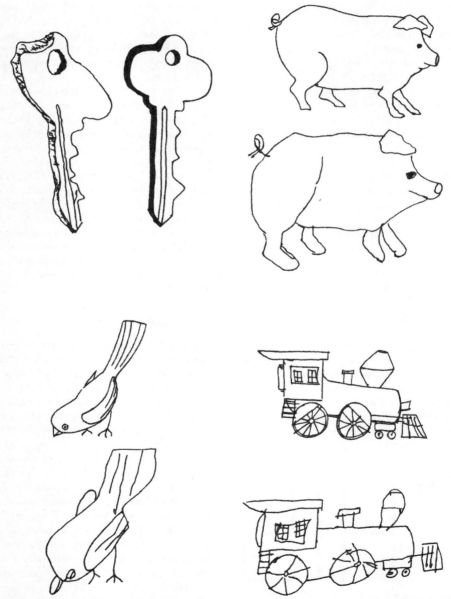

Figure 5–7. A retired physician with associative visual agnosia copied four line drawings. (The original figures are the top ones of each set, except the original key, which is on the right.) He could not identify any of the objects but copied each item well. (From Rubens and Benson,[109] © 1971, American Medical Association.)

When shown a picture of a car, for example, they are unable to state what the object is, what one does with it, or what one puts in it to make it go. In contrast, patients with anomia, when shown the same picture, might say "It's that thing you get in and drive." Patients with anomia know but cannot name the object. Follow verbal testing with nonverbal testing, using such tasks as matching pictures with functionally related objects. Patients with anomia do well on nonverbal tasks (e.g., they easily match pictures of a hammer and a nail), but patients with agnosia fare poorly. The recognition defect in visual agnosia may be incomplete as recognition may range, in order of increasing difficulty, from real (actual) objects to photographs and then to line drawings, reflecting a progressive reduction in visual detail.[114] Common objects, such as a fork or pen, may be more easily recognized than uncommon or complex objects, such as a stethoscope or city skyline. Objects may be recognized through modalities other than vision; for instance, a cat can be recognized by its meow.

Associative visual agnosia is usually the result of bilateral damage to the inferior temporo-occipital junction and subjacent white matter[105] but may also follow unilateral damage to the left or right temporo-occipital region.[115,116] The cause is most often infarction of the posterior cerebral artery bilaterally. Other causes include tumor, hemorrhage, and demyelination.

Associative visual agnosia may result from disconnection of visual association and temporolimbic memory areas[117,118] or destruction of higher-order visual association cortices in the temporo-occipital region.[88,115] The inferior longitudinal fasciculus, which connects the occipital association cortex and medial temporal lobe, is usually destroyed bilaterally in associative visual agnosia, which is consistent with disconnection of visual and memory areas.[88] A bilateral temporo-occipital injury that disconnects visual association and temporolimbic memory areas but does not disrupt the recognition of familiar visual stimuli may cause a visual learning deficit.[119] Visual agnosia may follow selective destruction of temporo-occipital gray matter. Neuronal templates that match a visual stimulus with a visual memory may be stored primarily in ventral visual association cortex.[88,113] Long-term follow-up of a visual agnosia patient suggests that perceptual and mnemonic processes are not independent but have strong interactive relations.[120]

Prosopagnosia

A distinct form of associative visual agnosia, *prosopagnosia* is the inability to recognize familiar faces or to learn and recognize new faces. When the disorder is severe, patients may not recognize their own images in a mirror. When patients with prosopagnosia look at a face, they can identify the nose, eyes, cheeks, and mouth and describe the whole as a face; they have not lost the concept of a face. However, they cannot tell whose face it is. The words of a patient with prosopagnosia[121] illustrate the deficits:

I can see the eyes, nose and mouth quite clearly but they just don't add up. They all seem chalked in, like on a blackboard. I have to tell by the clothes or voice whether it is a man or woman, as the faces are all neutral, a dirty grey colour (he also had achromatopsia). The hair may help a lot, or if there is a moustache . . . All the men appear unshaven . . . I cannot recognize people in photographs, not even myself. At the club I saw someone strange staring at me and asked the steward who it was. You'll laugh at me. I'd been looking at myself in the mirror . . . I later went to London and visited several cinemas and theatres. I couldn't make head or tail of the plots. I never knew who was who . . . I can shut my eyes and can well remember what my wife looked like or the kids.

While the impairment in prosopagnosia generally affects visually triggered memory,[118] it also extends to other classes of visually related stimuli. Thus, the defect is in not only visual identification of relatives and friends but also distinguishing specific types of object in a class, as in discriminating a Cadillac from a Volkswagen (cars), an eagle from an owl (birds), or a pine from an oak (trees). Unlike patients with visual object agnosia, those with prosopagnosia can distinguish the class itself. Some patients can identify facial expression and emotion, sex, and age but cannot identify the face.[122] Unlike patients with prosopagnosia, those with bilateral amygdala lesions can recognize and learn new faces but cannot recognize facial expressions of emotion[118] and are unable to make the social judgment as to whether a face looks approachable and trustworthy.

Prosopagnosia usually develops suddenly, and the patient realizes that a friend's or relative's face appears unfamiliar. Patients identify their spouses by voice, perfume, body shape, or clothes but perceive their faces as foreign. The recognition of familiar individuals by voice and other clues indicates that attention, memory, and intelligence are relatively preserved. In some cases, facial memories are lost as patients cannot visually describe objects from memory, especially faces and animals. Other disorders, including constructional apraxia, left-sided hemianopia, left-sided neglect, or topographic disorientation, may coexist with prosopagnosia. Patients with topographic disorientation are unable to identify correct spatial relations (see Topographic Disorientation, below).

The "facial template system," located in the mesial occipitotemporal visual association cortex (lingual and fusiform gyri), may be the site for storage and recognition of facial memories.[123] Interference with the arrival of visual input at that system, or from its destruction, may cause prosopagnosia. Patients often know that they are viewing a face and can see the details but cannot match the whole image with stored memories. This ability to recognize a "generic" face may result from use of the object recognition system, not the facial template system.

Although patients with prosopagnosia are unable to recognize faces, some may generate a large electrodermal skin conductance response to familiar, but not unfamiliar, faces.[124] The mounting of an autonomic response signifies the nonconscious recognition of familiar facial features, suggesting that an early phase of recognition occurs and influences behavior, even though the data and process are not accessible to consciousness. Studies using correct face–name pairs (larger amplitude of the skin conductance response) and incorrect face–name pairs[125] or eye movement scan paths for familiar versus novel faces[126] support the nonconscious recognition of faces by prosopagnostic patients.

Neocortical neuronal populations in fusiform and lingual gyri selectively respond to different faces, differentiate novel from familiar faces, and are critical for facial recognition and recall.[127,128] The fusiform face area is selective for faces. During functional magnetic resonance imaging (fMRI), for example, the response of the fusiform face area was strongest to stimuli containing human faces,

slightly weaker to human heads, and weakest to whole humans, animal heads, and whole animals.[129] Lesions causing prosopagnosia occupy the bilateral inferomesial visual association cortices (lingual and fusiform gyri) and subjacent white matter (Fig. 5–8), territory similar to that occupied by lesions causing visual object agnosia,[123] but the lesions in prosopagnosia are usually less extensive. Right mesial occipitotemporal lobe lesions rarely produce permanent prosopagnosia.[130] Most patients with unilateral, right-sided lesions and prosopagnosia have transient, mild to moderate deficits. The right hemisphere is superior to the left in recognizing and matching faces, as well as other sensory information that cannot be adequately differentiated with a verbal description.[131] Focal right temporal lobe atrophy may cause isolated, progressive prosopagnosia,[132] which appears to represent the homologue of progressive fluent aphasia resulting from left temporal lobe atrophy.[133,134]

Prosopagnosia usually follows embolic infarction of the posterior cerebral artery distribution. After a right hemisphere infarct, the deficit usually resolves within months. Often, a unilateral stroke in the posterior cerebral artery is followed months or years later by a contralateral infarct that causes prosopagnosia, visual object agnosia, or cortical blindness. Butterfly gliomas traversing the splenium of the corpus callosum to involve the posterior white matter bilaterally may cause prosopagnosia.

BALINT'S SYNDROME

Balint's syndrome is the triad of *simultagnosia*, an inability to perceive the visual field as a whole, with unpredictable perception of only small fragments of the visual field; *gaze apraxia*, an inability to shift the gaze to new stimuli; and *optic ataxia*, impaired target pointing under visual guidance. Caused by bilateral occipitoparietal lesions (Fig. 5–9), Balint's syndrome is a rare but dramatic behavioral disorder.[135] Patients initially appear blind; they are unable visually to detect stimuli approaching them, fail to see a car pass in front of them, bump into walls and furniture, and make wild, inaccurate movements when reaching for things. However, they often describe minute visual details requiring normal visual acuity. Formal visual field testing reveals full fields or inconsistent partial defects. Components of

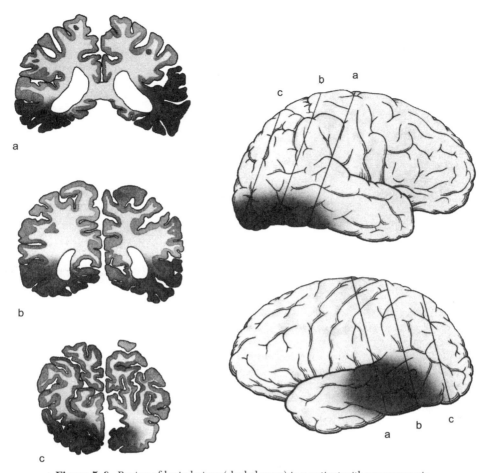

Figure 5–8. Region of brain lesions (shaded areas) in a patient with prosopagnosia.

Balint's syndrome may occur in isolation and probably do more often than reports suggest.

The issue of what can and cannot be seen in Balint's syndrome is explained by simultagnosia, the central feature of the syndrome. Because patients are unable to perceive the visual field as a whole, simultagnosia is sometimes called "piecemeal vision."[136] A patient with simultagnosia may look out the window on a scene of snow, sidewalk, street, trees, bushes, and children but see only a small piece of the picture, such as part of a tree. Suddenly, the patient's gaze may uncontrollably shift to another fragment, such as a child's lower body, and then shift again to a patch of snow. Patients cannot see more than one or two objects at once, but neither object complexity nor size is the major limiting factor for recognition. Rather, the essence of "objecthood" may de-termine what can be identified. Patients who can read letters are able to detect more letters in a sequence when they form a word rather than a nonword.[137] A six-pointed star was presented to a patient with simultagnosia.[138] When the star was a single color, the patient consistently identified it correctly, but when the component triangles were red and blue, he identified only triangles, not a star. Similarly, a patient might fail to recognize an object if "some peculiarity or prominent portion of it at once claimed his attention."[139]

Patients with simultagnosia usually see only with macular vision, which provides good acuity but captures only a tiny fraction of the visual field; and they experience unpredictable jumping of the focus from sector to sector, which does not allow detailed or systematic analysis of a particular region or object. Rapidly

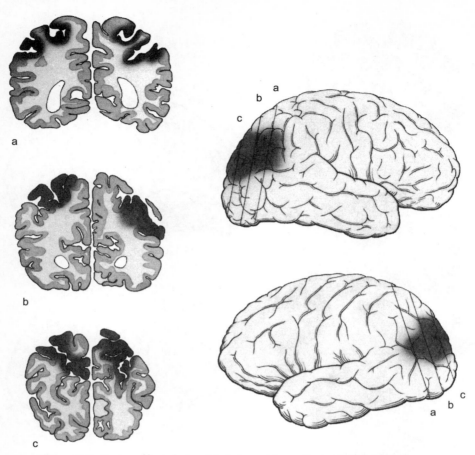

Figure 5–9. Region of brain lesions (shaded areas) in a patient with Balint's syndrome.

or erratically moving targets are much harder for them to see. While watching an auto race on televison, a patient could see a stationary advertisement but never saw the moving cars.[140] A patient with simultagnosia does not respond to threatening visual stimuli directed toward the face,[112,139,141] but responds to auditory stimuli or to his or her own hand thrust suddenly toward his or her face by the examiner.[141] A case of simultagnosia in a patient with Balint's syndrome is vividly described:[142]

When a cigarette was placed between his lips, he could not bring a lighted match into position to light the cigarette. If a pin was placed before his eyes, he recognized it. A tongue depressor was then slowly moved either from the right or from the left. When this was almost touching the pin, he was asked what he saw. He then accurately described the pin but gave no indication that he had seen the tongue depressor . . . two tongue depressors were placed be-

fore him and he acknowledged seeing them. Next he was confronted with a single tongue depressor and then a second depressor was introduced. He continued to see only one, even when the two were very close . . . When the patient was fixing an object and this object was moved, a number of jerky eye movements were observed which soon ceased as though despite the subject's efforts, the original fixation could not be disengaged . . . When addressed by the examiner he would turn his head towards him . . . at this moment, an assistant on the side . . . gesticulated very close to the patient . . . showed no reaction . . . A loud, unexpected noise . . . on the left or right, elicited a blink response but no shift in fixation.

Patients with normal visual acuity and normal ocular motility and scanning may complain that just when they find the target stimulus, it disappears.[126] An impairment in sustained visual attention probably accounts for the disappearance of stationary objects. However, the orientation of attention is preserved.[136] Defects in spatial integration and sustained visual attention most likely underlie simultagnosia. Patients are unable to synthesize the inputs from primary visual and visual association cortices into a unified picture. Thus, simultagnosia is not a true agnosia.

Isolated simultagnosia is caused by lesions of the bilateral superior occipital visual association cortex (BA 18, 19), with sparing of the parietal visuomotor control area.[136] The parietal lobe is critical for disengaging attention.[143] Unilateral parietal lobe injury impairs the disengagement of attention from ipsilateral or contralateral locations and the reengagement of attention at a new stimulus in the contralateral hemifield.[144] Bilateral parietal lobe lesions can severely impair the disengagement process. In such cases, once a visual stimulus is engaged, attention cannot be directed to another visual stimulus. This adhesive attentional disorder prevents patients from seeing more than one object at a time and from volitionally directing gaze to a new visual stimulus. An inability to disengage fixation, although not a central feature of Balint's syndrome, may contribute to both simultagnosia and gaze apraxia, as well as to unilateral neglect.[145]

In gaze apraxia, the second component of Balint's syndrome, patients are unable voluntarily to direct the gaze toward a specific part of the visual field.[140] Gaze wanders aimlessly, and targets are found by chance. Thus, even when patients are told where to look to see an object, they have difficulty directing foveal vision to that spot. Convergence and pursuit movements are usually abnormal. Gaze apraxia, also called *oculomotor apraxia*, is an impairment of visuomotor integration and generation of saccades and not a true apraxia. Normally, when a novel stimulus enters the peripheral vision, a saccadic eye movement brings foveal vision in line with the stimulus. In oculomotor apraxia, however, absent or inaccurate saccades render the subject functionally blind. In isolated oculomotor apraxia, a rare disorder resulting from bilateral posterior parietal lobe lesions,[146] patients can move their eyes on command but the ocular movements are random and aimless. They are unable to follow a moving stimulus.

In optic ataxia, the third element in this syndrome, visually guided reaching movements are impaired. For example, a patient sees the pen she or he wants to pick up, the right hand moves to grasp it, but the pen eludes her or him. In contrast, hand and arm movements under proprioceptive guidance, as in "Close your eyes and touch the tip of your left index finger to the tip of your nose," are performed accurately. Some patients can accurately describe the location and orientation of a visual stimulus but, despite intact motor and proprioceptive functions, are unable to reach for it.[147] Optic ataxia, also called *visuomotor ataxia* or *defective visual localization,* may be limited to the hemifield contralateral to the lesion. Isolated optic ataxia results from lesions of dorsal visual association areas or posterior parietal visuomotor centers or, with more anterior lesions, from disconnection of the projections from visual and visuomotor areas to the frontal lobe.[146,148,149] The critical lesion is centered around the intraparietal sulcus and superior parietal lobe. In monkeys, analogous areas transform retinotopic locations into body-referenced coordinates. Optic ataxia is most likely the result of impaired transformation of retinotopic locations onto a body-referenced frame for motor guidance. A related disorder, *mirror ataxia,* is characterized by the impairment of visually guided reaching through a mirror and is associated with lesions clustered around the postcentral sulcus.[150]

Diagnostic confusion between Balint's syndrome and visual agnosia or alexia is common because patients with Balint's syndrome complain that, although they can see, they cannot recognize what they are seeing and cannot read.[117] It is, therefore, important to use a small visual stimulus when testing patients and to always assess foveal vision. Under these conditions, recognition will occur. Patience is required as it may take time for the fovea to locate the test stimulus. Balint's syndrome may also be mistaken for a visual conversion reaction as some patients may be able to see facial features or other stimuli at a distance but not nearby.[151]

Balint's syndrome arises from disturbance of the dorsal visual system by bilateral parieto-occipital lesions. The cause is most often hypotensive stroke associated with a myocardial infarction with diffuse cerebral atherosclerosis or a cardiac bypass operation. The infarct encompasses the watershed between the territories of the anterior, posterior, and middle cerebral arteries. Multiple emboli, venous infarction (e.g., postpartum), multiple metastases, and butterfly gliomas extending bilaterally across the splenium and posterior corpus callosum may also cause Balint's syndrome.

TOPOGRAPHIC DISORIENTATION

Over the last century, several dozen case reports have presented *topographically disoriented* patients, who appear to have selectively lost their ability to find their way within their environments.[152,153] In 1900, Meyer's[154] experience with three disoriented patients was the first comprehensive study of the disorder. Meyer's first patient, a 49–year-old man, presented with a left-sided homonymous hemianopsia and severe disorientation following a vascular lesion. Despite generally intact intellect, visual perception, and memory, the patient was unable to find his way in his home town or to learn his way around the hospital. He was unable to describe or draw the route between his home and any of the principal public places in his town. In addition, he had great difficulty in recognizing places by their appearance and could deduce their identity only by taking note of small details. Thus, he was able to determine which ward within the hospital was his only by looking for the black beard of his roommate. In contrast, Holmes,[155] in 1919, and Brain,[156] in 1941, described topographically disoriented patients who had impaired immediate spatial perception and were unable to judge the distance and direction of objects. It appears from these and later case reports that topographic disorientation is a heterogeneous disorder, comprising several different types of deficit. A possible taxonomy includes such categories as egocentric disorientation, heading disorientation, landmark agnosia, and anterograde amnesia.[153]

Egocentric Disorientation

Patients with *egocentric disorientation,* classically called topographic disorientation, probably do not have deficits limited to the topographic sphere. These patients have severe deficits in representing the relative location of objects with respect to the self, that is, within the egocentric space. While they can gesture toward visualized objects, this ability is completely lost when their eyes are closed. Performance is impaired on a wide range of visual–spatial tasks, including mental rotation and spatial span tasks.[157] These patients are uniformly impaired in way-finding tasks in both familiar and novel environments. Most remain confined to the hospital or home, willing to venture out only with a companion.[158] Route descriptions are impoverished and inaccurate, and sketch-map production is disordered. In contrast, visual object recognition is relatively intact. Patients with impairments in apprehending egocentric spatial relationships yet possessing intact visual recognition abilities typically have bilateral or right parietal lobe damage. Behavioral neurophysiology studies in animals suggest that posterior parietal cells maintain representations of object position in an egocentric spatial frame.[159]

Heading Disorientation

Patients with *heading disorientation* do not have the dramatic egocentric disorientation and can recognize salient landmarks. Instead, these patients are unable to derive directional information from landmarks they recognize. They have lost their "heading" within their environment. This can be considered a deficit with exocentric (between objects within the environment, including the observer), rather than egocentric, spatial representations. Takahashi et al.[160] described one such patient:

. . . as he was driving his taxi in the same city [in which he had worked for 6 years], he suddenly lost his understanding of the route to his destination. As he could quickly recognize the buildings and landscapes around him, he was able to determine his current location. However, he could not determine in which direction he should proceed. He stopped taking passengers and tried to return to the main office, but didn't know the appropriate direction in which to drive. Using the surrounding buildings, scenery, and road signs he made several mistakes along the way. He remembered, during this time, passing the same places over and over again.

Takahashi et al.[160] suggested that the patient had lost the "sense of direction" that allows recall of positional relationships between the current location and the destination within a space that cannot be entirely surveyed at one time. Although only a few patients have a disorder fitting this description, all have had damage within the right retrosplenial, that is, the posterior cingulate, region. Chen et al.[161] identified in rats a small population of cells within this area that fire only when the rat maintains a certain heading, or orientation, within the environment. These cells, which have been dubbed *head–direction cells,*[162] likely generate their signals from a combination of landmark, vestibular, and idiothetic (self-motion) cues.

Landmark Agnosia

Patients with *landmark agnosia* are unable to use prominent, salient environmental features for the purposes of orientation.[121] Pallis's[121] description of a patient with this disorder is illustrative:

He complained a lot of his inability to recognize places. "In my mind's eye I know exactly where places are, what they look like. I can visualize T . . . square without difficulty, and the streets that come into it . . . I can draw you a plan of the roads from Cardiff to the Rhondda Valley . . . It's when I'm out that the trouble starts. My reason tells me I must be in a certain place and yet I don't recognize it. It all has to be worked out each time . . . For instance, one night, having taken the wrong turning, I was going to call for my drink at the Post Office." He seemed to have difficulty in assimilating new topographical data. "It's not only the places I knew before all this happened that I can't remember. Take me to a new place now, and tomorrow I couldn't get there myself." His topographical memory was good, as could be inferred from his accurate descriptions of paths, roads, the layout of the mine-shafts [the patient was an engineer], and from his excellent performance in drawing maps of places familiar to him before his illness. There was no evidence of neglect or imperception of any part of extra-personal space; localization of objects in space was excellent. He would have difficulty in reconciling the reality about him with the plan in his mind in convincing himself that he was in a given situation. "I have to keep the idea of the route in my head the whole time, and count the turnings, as if I were following instructions that had been memorized." He could at a glance tell terraced council-houses from detached villas, a living room from an office, a country lane from a main road.

Although patients with landmark agnosia are able to provide spatial information regarding a familiar environment, they cannot way-find because of their inability to recognize prominent landmarks. They may also have coexisting neuropsychological deficits such as prosopagnosia, as well as achromatopsia and some degree of a visual field deficit.[163] Patients with landmark agnosia have lesions either bilaterally or of the right medial temporo-occipital region, involving the fusiform and lingual gyrus and sometimes the parahippocampal gyrus.[163] The lesions usually result from a stroke in the right posterior cerebral artery. Convergently, fMRI studies reveal a cortical region within this area of the brain that responds with greater activation to the perception of buildings than to other stimuli, including faces, cars, and general objects.[164,165] This cortical region, through experience, may represent environmental features and visual configurations that have landmark value; that is, they tend to aid spatial navigation.

Anterograde Amnesia

Patients with *anterograde amnesia* tend to have preserved way-finding in environments they have known for at least 6 months before their brain insult but are unable to learn new environments. For example, one patient could draw a very accurate map of his parents' home but could not produce maps of novel environments from memory.[119] Another patient was unable to learn a route within the hospital:[166] "When he had to go from the psychologist's office back to his room, he wandered along the ward, being unable to find his room unless he relied on the sequence of door numbers" and "when asked to draw a floor plan of this simple path, he invariably produced an erroneous drawing, omitting several turns making up the path and misplacing the office in relation to the main landmark (the elevators)." A third patient said she "had to pay attention to verbal cues, such as inscriptions on store windows or street names."[166] Even after 6 days, one patient remained disoriented to the neurology ward where he was staying.[119]

In patients with anterograde amnesia, the lesion is typically in the right basal temporal cortex, centered near the parahippocampal gyrus. Other patients with lesions restricted to the parahippocampus were tested for their way-finding abilities and, relative to control subjects, were impaired on tests of route learning, without any evidence of retrograde topographic disorientation or global memory impairment.[167,168]

ASTEREOPSIS

Stereopsis is depth perception resulting from binocular visual interaction. Separation of the eyes results in the same part of the visual field falling on slightly different portions of the retinas. Binocular visual interaction occurs in area V1. Binocular disparity units in the visual association corte[169] utilize this retinal disparity to generate depth information, permitting accurate localization of objects in visual space. Stereopsis relies on separation of the eyes and overlapping inputs. The benefits of improved localization apparently outweighed the evolutionary cost to primates: restriction of the lateral visual fields. In contrast, animals that are often hunted, such as rabbits or wildebeest, have laterally placed eyes that provide a panoramic view but no stereopsis.

Astereopsis, or *stereoblindness,* is the impairment of binocular depth perception. It occurs as a developmental disorder or is acquired after neurological disease. Studies in humans and monkeys suggest that there is a critical developmental period for stereopsis. Thus, if strabismus is uncorrected for too long, permanent astereopsis and impaired visual acuity may develop. Astereopsis is present from early life in 5%–10% of the general population.[170]

Visual acuity and ocular alignment must be adequate for assessment of stereopsis. Extraocular muscle weakness can be assessed at the bedside with red-glass testing, but formal assessment includes orthoptic techniques (e.g., four-diopter baseout prism). Tests of stereopsis include measurement of stereoacuity (the resolution of a fine binocular disparity) and standard hand-held stereotests that require red–green glasses or polarized glasses.[88,171] In patients with visual complaints or acquired lesions of the visual cortex, especially those with jobs requiring depth perception, such as an architect or airplane pilot, formal assessment of stereopsis is essential.

Astereopsis is commonly acquired from cranial nerve or muscular disorders that weaken extraocular muscles. Diplopia and binocular rivalry occur, but since the binocular visual cortex has developed, diminished vision (amblyopia) does not develop. Ocular realignment with corrective surgery or prism glasses restores stereopsis.

Astereopsis is rarely the result of acquired lesions of the visual cortex. Normally, the left and right visual fields have equal stereoptic functions.[172] Stereoacuity may be reduced by lesions in either the left or right visual cortex.[173] Although the right hemisphere may dominate

stereoptic function,[174] unilateral lesions do not abolish stereopsis. The most severe stereoptic deficits follow lesions of the superior visual cortex bilaterally.[173,174] Bilateral lesions of V5 may impair movement and stereoptic vision.[24]

DISORDERS OF MENTAL IMAGERY

Internal speech and mental imagery are the background of mental life. Mental imagery relies on similar or identical cortical and subcortical systems that are active during perception of environmental stimuli.[175] In neurologically healthy subjects, the use of mental imagery to memorize a word list or answer questions, compared with tasks that rely only on verbal mediation, increases blood flow to the occipital and posterior temporal regions.[176] Similarly, mental motor imagery activates structures similar to those activated with an executed action.[177]

Acquired brain injuries that impair perception generally affect mental imagery to a similar degree. Patients with right parietal lobe lesions and left-sided neglect also fail to mentally image the left portion of figures, objects, and places. Italian patients with visual neglect, who were familiar with the Piazza del Duomo in Milan, were asked to describe the square.[178] From the first observation point, patients omitted landmarks on the left side of the scene. When visualizing the square from the opposite observation point, they omitted the previously described landmarks, which fell on the left rather than the right side of the imaged scene.

Patients with achromatopsia lose the ability to perceive and form mental images in color; they typically are unable to visualize the color of common objects, such as an orange or the sky. However, their verbal memory for colors may be preserved, at least initially, as Sacks[86] wrote of a patient:

From a life-long career as an active and productive painter, "he *knew* the colors of everything, with an extraordinary exactness (he could give not only the names but the number of colors as these were listed in a Pantone chart of hues he had used for many years). He could identify the green of van Gogh's billiard table" . . . For a year or more after the accident, "he *knew* all the colors in his favorite paintings, but could no longer see them, either when he looked or in his mind's eye" . . . As more and more time elapsed without color vision, the painter lost not just his perception of color, but also imagery, even ceasing to dream in color. Finally, he seemed to lose even his memory of color, so that it ceased to be part of his mental knowledge, his mind, and he "no longer *understood* it."

The artist's experience resembled that of a vision researcher who had congenital achromatopsia:[178a]

Although I have acquired a thorough theoretical knowledge of the physics of colours and the physiology of the colour receptor mechanisms, nothing of this can help me to understand the true nature of colours.

The case of achromatopsia in the artist illustrates the complex relationship between perception, mental imagery, memory, and knowledge. Initially, color perception and mental imagery for color were lost but knowledge and memory of color were preserved. How the painter's verbal knowledge and memory of colors slowly waned remains a mystery. Perhaps the color knowledge contained in neuronal networks of the specialized color area was partially represented in verbal and mnemonic form in other cortical areas. However, these areas are needed to keep the "battery of color knowledge charged" via connections to the color area.

Damage to the ventral (temporo-occipital) visual system that recognizes objects ("what" is seen) and to the dorsal (parieto-occipital) visual system that recognizes location ("where" it is seen) may be associated with parallel deficits in imagery, that is, ventral system–visual imagery, dorsal system–spatial imagery.[179] When ventral lesions impair object identification, the result is deficits in describing or drawing objects, animals, or faces; the ability to describe or draw the spatial location of objects or geographic landmarks is preserved. When dorsal lesions impair object location, the result is deficits in describing and drawing the location of objects or geographic landmarks; the ability to describe or draw objects, animals, or faces is preserved. Selective recognition defects parallel imaging defects. Patients with prosopagnosia who have defective recognition of faces but not objects usually are unable to visualize faces.[180]

Although defects in visual recognition and spatial location often correspond to similar defects in imagery, dissociations may occur. Patients with impaired visual recognition may have preserved imagery. Thus, some patients with prosopagnosia can clearly image familiar faces from memory that they cannot visually recognize.[180] The converse also occurs: patients with normal visual function may have impaired mental imagery. Both hemispheres contribute to visual imagery. The left hemisphere may dominate the assembly of mental images from their components and the generation of images for which relative locations are specified.[179] The right hemisphere may be more important in generating images that require spatial mapping relative to a common frame.[181,182] Although a right hemisphere bias exists for mental rotation of visual stimuli,[183] with the right parietal lobe being a critical site, it is unlikely to equal the degree of left hemispheric dominance for language skills, and the contribution of both hemispheres is important.[184,185]

AUDITORY PERCEPTION

Anatomy and Function of Cortical Auditory Areas

The temporal lobes receive and process auditory input and are critical for language and musical comprehension. The primary auditory cortex (Heschl's gyrus, BA 41) is situated on the transverse temporal gyrus, buried in the sylvian fissure (Fig. 5–10). This area receives auditory input from the medial geniculate nucleus. In primates, the primary auditory cortex is organized tonotopically (by sound frequency). Each of the brain's hemispheres receives input from both ears, with some predominance of contralateral input. Because the ascending auditory projections are predominantly bilateral, unilateral lesions of the primary auditory cortex produce minimal hearing loss. Electrical stimulation of Heschl's gyrus evokes unformed auditory hallucinations, such as buzzing and tones.

The auditory association cortex (BA 42) lies lateral to the primary auditory cortex, extends to the convexity of the superior temporal gyrus, and includes the planum temporale (Fig. 5–10). This area receives fibers from primary auditory cortex and is involved in higher-order processing of auditory input.[186] The dorsal surface of the superior temporal gyrus in the sylvian fissure, the planum temporale, is larger in the left hemisphere of right-handed persons

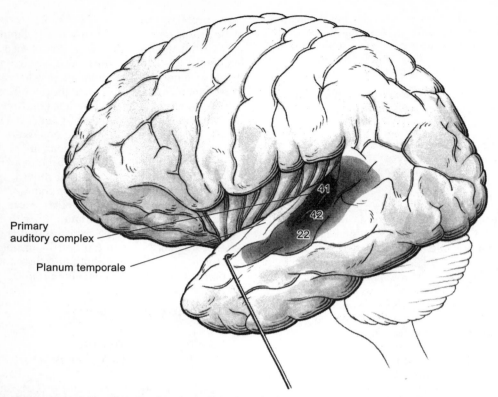

Primary
auditory complex

Planum temporale

41
42
22

Figure 5–10. Map of the principal auditory areas (lateral view). The primary auditory cortex (Brodmann's area [BA] 41) receives input from the medial geniculate nuclei; the auditory association cortex (BA 22, 42) receives input from the primary cortex.

(Fig. 5–11). Electrical stimulation of the auditory association cortex can evoke complex auditory hallucinations, including voices and music.[187] Wernicke's area (BA 22) is higher-order auditory association cortex situated on the posterolateral portion of the left superior temporal gyrus, which functionally extends to the inferior parietal gyri. This area is vital for language comprehension (see Chapter 6). Electrical stimulation of Wernicke's area causes speech arrest and deficits in comprehension, naming, and reading.[188,189] Right and left hemisphere auditory association areas are also involved in music perception.[190–192]

Cortical Auditory Disorders

Cortical auditory disorders result from lesions of the primary auditory or auditory association cortices or their connections. The principal features of these disorders are summarized in Table 5–4.

CORTICAL DEAFNESS

Cortical deafness is a rare disorder in which patients cannot recognize or discriminate sounds. The impairment affects simple and complex sounds ranging from tones to verbal sounds (speech) or familiar nonverbal sounds, such as a dog's barking or a siren.[193] Cortical deafness arises from damage to the primary auditory cortex bilaterally or the auditory radiations from the medial geniculate nucleus. The most common cause is two sequential unilateral strokes.

AUDITORY AGNOSIA

Auditory agnosia is an inability to appreciate the meaning of sounds despite normal perception of pure tones.[194] Nonverbal and verbal forms of auditory agnosia may exist independently or may coexist. Nonverbal auditory agnosia is impaired recognition or understanding of nonlinguistic sounds, such as those produced by a siren, barking dog, or music. This

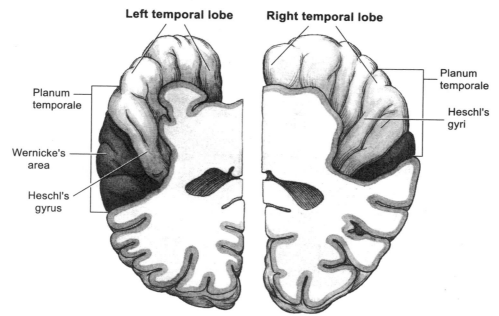

Figure 5–11. Auditory cortex from the upper limit of the sylvian fissure (superior view). The planum temporale (upper surface of the temporal lobe) and Wernicke's area are larger in the left hemisphere.

perceptual–discriminative auditory agnosia is associated with right temporal or parietal lobe lesions[195] or lesions of auditory association cortex bilaterally.[196] Associative–semantic auditory agnosia occurs in patients with posterior left hemisphere lesions and aphasia.[197] These patients make semantic errors in matching sounds and names, as in "bark" and cat. This disorder forms a transition between auditory agnosia and aphasia.

Table 5–4. **Cortical Auditory Disorders**

Disorder	Impairment	Lesion Site
Cortical deafness	Tone sensitivity, recognition and discrimination of sounds	Bilateral AR or PAC
Auditory agnosia		
Nonverbal	Tone sensitivity, recognition of nonverbal sounds; recognition of familiar voices, ?recognition of emotional prosody	Right or bilateral AAC
Verbal°	Tone sensitivity, speech and reading comprehension, ?spontaneous speech (paraphasia),† ?recognition of propositional prosody†	Bilateral AAC or left AR and callosal fibers from right AAC
Sensory amusia	Tone sensitivity, recognition of nonverbal sounds, speech and reading comprehension, spontaneous speech, ?recognition of emotional prosody, recognition of propositional prosody	Right or left AAC
Sensory aprosodia	?Tone sensitivity,† ?recognition of nonverbal sounds,† speech and reading comprehension, spontaneous speech, ?music comprehension,† ?recognition of propositional prosody	Right AAC

°Pure word deafness.
†Hypothesis, not tested clinically.
AAC, auditory association cortex; AR, auditory radiations; PAC, primary auditory cortex.

Paralinguistic aspects of speech, including emotional prosody, are also impaired by right hemisphere lesions. In *phonagnosia,* a paralinguistic auditory disorder in discriminating and recognizing familiar voices after right hemisphere injury,[198] right and left temporoparietal lobe lesions cause different impairments. With left-sided lesions, patients may be unable to distinguish two famous voices (general, declarative knowledge) but may recognize voices with which they are personally familiar (episodic, autobiographical knowledge). Patients with right temporoparietal lobe injuries are impaired at both tasks. Right temporal lobe lesions cause greater impairment of voice discrimination, and right parietal lobe lesions cause greater impairment of voice recognition.[198] Bilateral insular lesions may cause transient mutism and persistent auditory agnosia.[199] Lesions of the right insula may impair auditory processing of speech presented to the left ear.[200]

In verbal auditory agnosia, also called *pure word deafness,* patients are unable to comprehend spoken language despite relatively preserved reading, writing, and nonverbal sound comprehension.[194] Although patients can write spontaneously and copy, they cannot write to dictation. As in Wernicke's aphasia, some patients with pure word deafness experience euphoria or paranoia.[201] Pure word deafness is caused by lesions of Heschl's gyrus in the dominant hemisphere and neighboring white matter fibers that connect the contralateral temporal lobe and the dominant auditory association cortex or by lesions of the primary auditory or auditory association cortices of both hemispheres.[202–204] Pure word deafness is the result of interrupting auditory input to Wernicke's area. Contributing to the speech agnosia is impaired auditory perception and processing and, in some cases, discrimination of prephonemic sound elements, phonemes, or temporal sequencing of phonemes.[205]

Stroke is most often responsible for pure word deafness. Pure word deafness may develop as Wernicke's aphasia resolves. Therefore, patients with this form of aphasia must be reassessed for comprehension of not only spoken language but also written language, which can provide an effective route for communication. Some patients comprehend spoken language more easily when they are spoken to slowly[206] or informed about the topic being discussed.[207] Other patients comprehend paralinguistic aspects of speech, including emotional prosody and visual cues from lip reading.[194]

AMUSIA

The cerebral mechanisms responsible for musical appreciation are incompletely understood, but the auditory association cortex is probably critical for this function. *Amusia,* impaired musical perception or expression, often goes unrecognized because the patient does not consider the problem significant or the physician does not address it. *Instrumental amusia* is the acquired loss of the ability to play a musical instrument not resulting from weakness. *Musical agraphia* is the inability to write music.[208] *Musical alexia* is the inability to read music, and *musical amnesia* is the inability to recall or identify familiar melodies and may be the presenting feature of a posterior cortical dementia syndrome.[209,210]

Expressive (vocal) and receptive (sensory) amusia are common impairments of musical appreciation. *Expressive amusia* is the acquired loss of the ability to sing, whistle, or hum a tune and usually results from right frontotemporal lesions. *Receptive amusia,* the defective perception of music despite normal pure-tone perception, is most often linked with right temporal and insula lesions.[190,211,212] A patient with infarction of the right hemisphere, maximally involving the insula, had impaired musical perception but preserved appreciation of environmental sounds and speech.[190] The patient was unable to analyze a rapid temporal sequence of notes and to perceive sound–source movement.[213] Thus, the insula or adjacent cortex may serve as a sound–motion detector, an area analogous to V5 for visual motion.

Tone discrimination and recall and retention of rhythmic patterns are more greatly impaired by right-sided than by left-sided anterior temporal lobectomy.[214,215] With the simultaneous presentation of different melodies to both ears, the sound of which projects mainly to the contralateral auditory cortex, perception is more accurate from the left ear (right auditory cortex).[216] Expressive and receptive amusia are usually the result of right temporal lobe lesions.[190,217] The exception is professional musicians, who use the left temporal auditory association cortex to analyze rhythm and melody, in which temporal order is important.[216,218] In addition, musicians with perfect pitch appear to have stronger leftward asymmetry of the planum temporale than nonmusicians or musicians without perfect pitch.[219] Volume and appreciation of timbre are probably more dependent on the right temporal auditory cortex in most people,[220] although both hemispheres make significant contributions to musical perception in many. The injection of amobarbital into the right intracarotid artery, producing anesthesia of the right hemisphere, impairs singing and pitch production, with preservation of rhythmic components.

Patients with lesions of the auditory cortex bilaterally may perceive and recognize environmental sounds and speech but have impaired perception of specific voices, tunes, and prosody.[220] This dissociation suggests that distinct classes of auditory material, such as voice, melody, and prosody, share properties. For example, recognizing specific voices and musical instruments depends on timbre, and recognizing tunes depends on pitch. The anatomical systems used for auditory processing of speech and environmental sounds overlap with, but are partly different from, those used for processing music.

Assess receptive amusia by examining the patient's ability to recognize a common melody, such as "Happy Birthday" or "Silent Night" (hummed or whistled by the examiner); to discriminate between a higher and a lower tone (to a hum, whistle, or musical instrument); and to distinguish similar and different rhythmic tap sequences or to repeat the tap pattern made by the examiner on the table top with a finger or pen. Assess expressive amusia by asking the patient to hum or sing a high and a low note and a common song like "Happy Birthday." Test emotional and propositional prosody because they are mediated by similar systems. Interestingly, patients with global aphasia or Broca's aphasia may be able to sing a well-known tune but usually only after someone else initiates the singing. This observation supports the role of the right hemisphere in music.

AUDITORY HALLUCINATIONS AND ILLUSIONS

Auditory hallucinations arise from injury to all portions of the peripheral and central auditory pathways. They may be unformed, as in ring-ing, clicking, buzzing, or humming, or formed, as in voices or music. Both unformed and formed auditory hallucinations occur in deafness, schizophrenia, psychotic depression, salicylate intoxication, cocaine and amphetamine psychoses, alcoholic hallucinosis, delirium, migraine, and simple partial seizures arising in the lateral temporal lobe.[221–224] Electrical stimulation of Heschl's gyrus elicits unformed auditory sensations, often in the contralateral ear.[43] Peripheral lesions cause ipsilateral auditory hallucinations, and cortical lesions cause contralateral or bilateral auditory hallucinations. Complex auditory hallucinations may be produced by stimulation of temporal association or limbic areas.[90,187] Nondominant hemispheric foci often produce musical hallucinations.[90,224,225] Cortical lesions associated with auditory hallucinations are usually located in the posterior superior temporal gyrus, including the primary auditory cortex and the planum temporale.[222] Schizophrenia is the most common cause of prolonged, formed auditory hallucinations in clear consciousness. Typical forms of schizophrenic auditory hallucinations include voices commenting on the patient's actions, voices discussing the patient in the third person, and voices repeating the patient's thoughts. Alcoholic hallucinosis is characterized by the abrupt or gradual onset of auditory (and occasionally transient visual) hallucinations with relatively clear consciousness. These prolonged auditory hallucinations may be persecutory, are often accompanied by paranoid ideation, and occur while the subject is or has recently been abusing alcohol. Recovery usually occurs within hours or days but may take weeks or months.

Simple partial seizures with temporal lobe onset cause both unformed and formed auditory hallucinations.[226] The hallucinations are almost always recognized as unreal, are paroxysmal in onset and cessation, and usually last less than 3 minutes. Migrainous auditory hallucinations typically consist of hissing, rumbling, or growling noises. Both epileptic and migrainous auditory hallucinations are often associated with distortion or partial loss of hearing. Destructive lesions of the auditory end organs, nerves, or brain stem nuclei or pathways may give rise to formed or unformed auditory release hallucinations, which tend to be more prolonged than epileptic hallucinations.

Like auditory hallucinations, auditory illusions arise from all portions of the peripheral and central auditory pathways. Auditory illusions are perceptual distortions of sounds (e.g., muffled, change in volume). These phenomena may occur with all of the same pathological processes associated with auditory hallucinations.

TACTILE PERCEPTION

Anatomy and Function of Cortical Somesthetic Areas

In neonatal life, somesthesis is our primary sensation and defines the boundaries between self and nonself. Later in life, sight or sound is more sensitive than touch in identifying objects. However, touch sensation remains a special human function; it is required for our dexterity. The glabrous skin over the digits and palm is the most sensitive zone in our somatosensory system, the fovea of tactile perception.

The primary somesthetic cortex (SI) is located in the postcentral gyrus, including BA 3a and BA 2 (mirror image representations of inputs from muscle, viscera, and joints), BA 3b and BA 1 (mirror image representations of cutaneous inputs). It receives the massive thalamocortical somatosensory input from ventroposterolateral (VPL, limbs and trunk) and ventroposteromedial (VPM, face) thalamic nuclei and is reciprocally connected with the primary motor and somatosensory association cortices. Lesions of SI impair basic tactile functions, such as light touch, vibration, proprioception, superficial pain, temperature, and two-point discrimination, and some complex tactile functions, such as perception of dimensionality and simple shapes, discriminating weight and texture, recognizing substance, and detecting double simultaneous stimuli.[227] Unlike sensory disorders involving the peripheral nerves, spinal cord, and thalamus, disorders caused by lesions of SI are associated with relatively greater impairment of complex perceptions than basic tactile perceptions.

In addition to SI, somatosensory representations include the somatosensory association cortices (SII, parietal operculum; SIII, inferior parietal cortex; SIV, posterior insula and retroinsular cortex) and the supplementary somatosensory area (SSA). Each somatosensory association cortex contains its own somatotopic

representation of the body. Cortices SII to SIV derive their sensory inputs primarily from SI (some from VPL and VPM) and contralateral SII to SIV. Stimulation of SII evokes contralateral and bilateral paresthesia. Lesions of SII cause transient numbness but peristent tactile agnosia. The dorsomedial SSA is located posterior to the mesial portion of SI. The SSA has larger receptive fields than SI or SII and reciprocally connects to the supplementary, primary, and premotor areas. Stimulation of SSA causes bilateral paresthesia. Lesions of SSA may cause several transient phenomena: apraxia, impaired tactile search strategy and stimulus localization, and relief of thalamic pain syndromes.[227,228] Two parallel streams process somesthetic information: the ventral pathway serves tactile object recognition, tactile learning, and tactile memory and the dorsal pathway integrates sensorimotor, spatial, and possibly temporal components of somesthesis.

Cortical Somatosensory Disorders

TACTILE AGNOSIA

Tactile agnosia, impaired tactile object recognition, is the selective impairment of object recognition by touch despite relatively preserved primary and discriminative somesthetic perception. Tactile agnosia is a unilateral disorder, usually resulting from lesions of the contralateral inferior parietal cortex, affecting mainly the supramarginal gyrus (BA 40) but also the angular gyrus (BA 39).[229–231] Less often, SII lesions are the cause.[231a]

The disorder often goes unnoticed by patients and is rarely assessed in clinical practice. Patients with tactile agnosia often describe specific features of and can draw the palpated object but may confuse it with a physically similar object. Personal experience often facilitates recognition, and patients' tactile perception is better for their own possessions, such as a hairbrush or wallet.[229] Motor search mechanisms, that is, moving the object in the hand while exploring its features, are not deficient in patients with tactile agnosia. Further, hemiparetic patients with lesions of the internal capsule or frontal lobe are unable to move and manipulate the object in their hand, but when the object is moved passively, they rapidly recognize it.[228]

Tactile agnosia is most likely the result of a defect in high-level tactile perception, which provides tactile-specific meaning, that is, learned feature–entity relationships.[230,231] Disconnection of somatosensory association cortices may contribute to tactile agnosia.[232] In monkeys, the posterior insula, which connects SII and mesial temporal structures, is imporant in tactile learning.[233] Disconnecting somatosensory association cortices and mesial temporal memory areas impairs tactile learning but not tactile recognition of familiar objects.

TACTILE ANOMIA

In *tactile anomia*, patients with lesions that disconnect somatosensory association cortices and language areas are unable to name palpated objects. Patients with tactile anomia can identify simple and discriminative tactile features of an object and nonverbally recognize an object by touch, as in matching a palpated object with its picture or showing how it is used. In contrast, patients with tactile agnosia are unable to recognize an object by palpation. Left-sided tactile anomia is a special form of tactile anomia caused by lesions of the caudal body of the corpus callosum.[232] When patients with this disorder palpate an object with their left hand, their right hemisphere somatosensory areas are unable to transfer information to left hemisphere language areas.

IMPAIRED BODY SCHEMA

A body schema is conceptualized from our awareness of our corporeal being, its physical boundaries, spatial layout, and coherence as a structural unit.[234–236] The right hemisphere dominates the body schema (see Chapter 3). Right parietal lesions cause the greatest impairment of body schemas. Knowing the body's orientation in space is critical for interacting with the environment. Somesthesia defines the corporeal limits, but vision is our most critical sense for defining our relation to the environment. To determine corporeal spatial position relative to environmental objects, as in picking apples or avoiding a rock while walking, the brain must transform retinotopic images into body-referenced coordinates. The positions of the eyes, head, trunk, and limbs must be considered when the brain reformats perceived lo-

cations of visual images onto a map based on the body schema as the center. The posterior parietal lobe, including BA 5 and BA 7, performs this transformation in monkeys.[237,238]

PHANTOM LIMB

Phantom limb is a hallucinatory percept of a missing limb. This phenomenon suggests an inborn body schema as it commonly occurs after amputation and is even a feature in some children born without limbs.[234] Corporeal experience strengthens the body schema, as reflected in the correlation between older age at amputation and increased incidence of phantom limb.[239] Phantom limbs are often painful. Phantom sensory phenomena result from lesions of the peripheral nerves, plexus, and spinal cord as well as removal of body parts, such as the eyes, genitalia, women's breasts, and teeth.[240,241] Over time, the phantom limb usually shrinks and "telescopes," with relative preservation of the hand or foot and condensation of the limb. Patients may perceive a hand attached to a proximal stump, probably reflecting the larger cortical representation of the distal limb.

Hallucinations of supernumerary limbs and digits may occur when the deafferentated body parts are still present.[238,240] This disorder most often complicates right hemisphere or bilateral cerebral lesions,[241–244] and is often accompanied by left-sided hemiplegia and, in some cases, delusional reduplication of place or person (Capgras' syndrome). Peripheral and spinal cord lesions may also lead to reduplication of body parts. Hallucinatory reduplication of body parts or the sensation of distorted body shape may occur with partial seizures, migraine, toxic or metabolic encephalopathy, or hallucinogenic drug use.

AUTOTOPAGNOSIA

Autotopagnosia, the inability to locate and identify parts on one's own body, may be considered a disorder of body schema. However, the inability usually extends to parts on another person's body or a model of the human body.[235,245] Some patients who cannot identify parts of the human body can point to parts of animals and objects,[245] but others show a more generalized inability to identify parts of a whole, including objects such as parts of a bicycle. Patients with autotopagnosia usually misidentify body parts by pointing to a body part near the requested one and may make semantic errors, such as saying wrist for ankle. Finger agnosia, a component of Gerstmann's syndrome, is a partial autotopagnosia. In autotopagnosia affecting the identification of proximal body parts, the lesion is usually in the left parietal lobe,[245] but finger agnosia may result from a lesion of the left or right parietal lobe.[246] Diffuse disorders, such as Alzheimer's disease, also cause autotopagnosia.[235]

SOMESTHETIC HALLUCINATIONS

Somesthetic (haptic) hallucinations involve both tactile sensations and internal or corporeal feelings. Corporeal feelings include bone, muscle, ligament, and joint sensations, as well as deep pain to less localizable phenomena, such as fatigue, nausea, hunger, thirst, and sexual pleasure. Somesthetic hallucinations pose a greater diagnostic problem than other sensory hallucinations. Pressure, vibration, and temperature stimuli can be verified by an observer; but pains, aches, itches, tickles, and other sensations, as well as corporeal feelings, cannot be consensually verified.[247]

Visceral hallucinations and illusions may accompany neurological disorders, such as epilepsy and thalamic pain syndrome, and psychiatric disturbances, such as depression, mania, and psychosis. Visceral hallucinations often include poorly localized and sometimes bizarre feelings. One of our patients with a mesial temporal seizure focus said she felt "as if her rib cage was moving and was outside her skin" during a seizure. A patient with a right parietal lobe seizure focus said "my arm burns, as if it were transformed to molten steel, not the skin, the insides. Then it twists as if the bone is about to break; it's excruciatingly painful." A patient with a stroke in the thalamic ventral posterior nuclear complex reported that "the whole left side of my body is like an electrical storm that won't stop. I feel it in my bones, muscles, everywhere. It never lets go."

Tactile hallucinations are common in delirium tremens and intoxication with cocaine, chloral hydrate, or atropine.[248] These drug-induced states may cause formications, a feeling of ants crawling under the skin. Thalamic or parietal lesions may cause unilateral formications.[249,250]

SUMMARY

Perception of internal and environmental stimuli requires a series of overlapping stages in sensory processing: reception, analysis of basic features, discrimination and comparison of feature patterns within a modality to form a percept, and comparison of the percept with percepts in other sensory modalities and with experiential memories and goals. All sensory cortices are organized in a similar pattern: multiple cortical areas with their own somatotopic representations and intracortical connection patterns. The primary sensory areas, analyzing stimulus features and performing early discriminative analysis of sensory information, contain the most detailed representation of sensory input. The unimodal association areas respond to broader fields but more complex stimulus features than the primary areas. In each sensory modality, the different association areas are relatively specialized for analyzing and categorizing the different stimulus features, such as color, shape, and motion of visual stimuli.

Vision, the perceptual system studied most extensively in basic and clinical science, serves as a model for the link between sensation and cognition. Visual data flow from the visual association cortex in the occipital lobe to two parallel systems: a ventral temporal lobe stream for object discrimination and recognition and a dorsal parietal lobe stream for spatial perception and visuomotor performance. Conscious perception results from synchronous binding of activity in primary sensory and sensory association areas with each other and with other cortical areas.

The evolutionary course of primates and humans has led to specialized visual systems, such as facial recognition in the ventral stream. Lesions in the ventral system cause visual agnosia. More restricted lesions in the facial recognition system cause prosopagnosia. Lesions of the dorsal system impair visual attention, coordination of vision with eye and limb movements, and the ability for simultaneously seeing the visual world.

Lesions of the primary auditory cortex and auditory association cortex cause cortical deafness, nonverbal auditory agnosia, and verbal auditory agnosia (pure word deafness). Receptive amusia is most often linked with right temporal and insula lesions. Somesthetic information is processed by two parallel but interactive paths: a ventral pathway serves tactile object recognition, tactile learning, and tactile memory and a dorsal pathway integrates sensorimotor, spatial, and possibly temporal components of somesthesis. Tactile agnosia and disorders of the body schema result from inferior parietal lobe lesions.

REFERENCES

1. Mesulam MM: From sensation to cognition. Brain 121:1013–1052, 1998.
2. Zeki S: A Vision of the Brain. Blackwell, Oxford, 1993.
3. Connolly M and Van Essen D: The representation of the visual field in parvicellular and magnocellular layers of the lateral geniculate nucleus in the macaque monkey. J Comp Neurol 226:544–564, 1984.
4. Merigan WH, Nealey TA, and Maunsell JH: Visual effects of lesions of cortical area V2 in macaques. J Neurosci 13:3180–3191, 1993.
5. Tootell RB, Mendola JD, Hadjikhani NK, et al.: Functional analysis of V3A and related areas in human visual cortex. J Neurosci 17:7060–7078, 1997.
6. Zeki SM: The third visual complex of rhesus monkey prestriate cortex. J Physiol (Lond) 277:245–272, 1978.
7. Poggio GF, Gonzales F, and Drause F: Stereoscopic mechanisms in monkey visual cortex, binocular correlation and disparity selectivity. J Neurosci 8:4531–4550, 1988.
8. Bundo M, Kaneoke Y, Inao S, Yoshida J, Nakamura A, and Kakigi R: Human visual motion areas determined individually by magnetoencephalography and 3D magnetic resonance imaging. Hum Brain Mapp 11:33–45, 2000.
9. Felleman DJ, Burkhalter A, and Van Essen DC: Cortical connections of areas V3 and VP of macaque monkey extrastriate visual cortex. J Comp Neurol 379:21–47, 1997.
10. McKeefry DJ and Zeki S: The position and topography of the human colour centre as revealed by functional magnetic resonance imaging. Brain 120:2229–2242, 1997.
11. Hadjikhani N, Liu AK, Dale AM, Cavanagh P, and Tootell RB: Retinotopy and color sensitivity in human visual cortical area V8. Nat Neurosci 1:235–241, 1998.
12. Bartels A and Zeki S: The architecture of the colour centre in the human visual brain: new results and a review. Eur J Neurosci 12:172–193, 2000.
13. Gallant JL, Shoup RE, and Mazer JA: A human extrastriate area functionally homologous to macaque V4. Neuron 27:227–235, 2000.
14. Bar M and Biederman I: Localizing the cortical region mediating visual awareness of object identity. Proc Natl Acad Sci USA 96:1790–1793, 1999.
15. Tarkiainen A, Helenius P, Hansen PC, Cornelissen PL, and Salmelin R: Dynamics of letter string perception in the human occipitotemporal cortex. Brain 122:2119–2132, 1999.
16. Larsen A, Bundesen C, Kyllingsbaek S, Paulson OB,

17. and Law I: Brain activation during mental transformation of size. J Cogn Neurosci 12:763–774, 2000.
17. Allman JM: Evolving Brains. Scientific American Library, New York, 1999.
18. Dobbins A, Jeo R, Fiser J, and Allman J: Distance modulation of neural activity in the visual cortex. Science 281:552–555, 1998.
19. Schiller P: Effects of lesions in visual cortical area V4 on the recognition of transformed objects. Nature 376:342–344, 1995.
20. Tootell RB, Reppas JB, Dale AM, et al.: Visual motion aftereffect in human cortical area MT/V5 revealed by functional magnetic resonance imaging. Nature 375:139–141, 1995.
21. Dumoulin SO, Bittar RG, Kabani NJ, et al.: A new anatomical landmark for reliable identification of human area V5/MT: a quantitative analysis of sulcal patterning. Cereb Cortex 10:454–463, 2000.
22. Beckers G and Zeki S: The consequences of inactivating areas V1 and V5 on visual motion perception. Brain 118:49–60, 1995.
23. Rizzo M, Nawrot M, and Zihl J: Motion and shape perception in cerebral akinetopsia. Brain 118:1105–1127, 1995.
23a. Schoenfeld MA, Nosselt T, Poggel D, et al.: Analysis of pathways mediating preserved vision after striate cortex lesions. Ann Neurol 52:814–824, 2002.
24. Zihl J, von Cramon D, and Mai N: Selective disturbance of movement vision after bilateral brain damage. Brain 106:313–340, 1983.
25. Sakata H, Taira M, Kusunoki M, et al.: The parietal association cortex in depth perception and visual control of hand action. Trends Neurosci 20:350–357, 1997.
26. Galletti C, Fattori P, Gamberini M, and Kutz DF: The cortical visual area V6: brain location and visual topography. Eur J Neurosci 11:3922–3936, 1999.
27. Desimone R and Ungerleider LG: Neural mechanisms of visual processing in monkeys. In Damasio AR (ed). Handbook of Clinical Neuropsychology. Disorders of Visual Behavior, Vol 2, Sect 4. Elsevier, New York, 1989, pp 267–299.
28. Perkel DJ, Bullier J, and Kennedy H: Topography of the afferent connectivity of area 17 in the macaque monkey: a double-labelling study. J Comp Neurol 253:374–402, 1986.
29. von Monakow C: Localization of brain functions. In con Bonin G (translator). Some Papers on the Cerebral Cortex. CC Thomas, Springfield, IL, 1960.
30. Vanduffel W, Payne BR, Lomber SG, and Orban GA: Functional impact of cerebral connections. Proc Natl Acad Sci USA 94:7617–7620, 1997.
31. Ungerleider LG and Mishkin M: Two cortical visual systems. In Ingle DJ, Goodale MA, and Mansfield RJW (eds). Analysis of Visual Behavior. MIT Press, Cambridge, MA, 1982, pp 549–586.
32. Vaina LM: Functional segregation of color and motion processing in the human visual cortex: clinical evidence. Cereb Cortex 4:555–572, 1994.
33. Corbetta M: Frontoparietal cortical networks for directing attention and the eye to visual locations: identical, independent, or overlapping neural systems? Proc Natl Acad Sci USA 95:831–838, 1998.
34. Humphreys GW: Neural representation of objects in space: a dual coding account. Philos Trans R Soc Lond B Biol Sci 353:1341–1351, 1998.

35. Kraut M, Hart J Jr, Soher BJ, and Gordon B: Object shape processing in the visual system evaluated using functional MRI. Neurology 48:1416–1420, 1997.

36. Schroeder CE, Mehta AD, and Givre SJ: A spatiotemporal profile of visual system activation revealed by current source density analysis in the awake macaque. Cereb Cortex 8:575–592, 1998.

37. Rao SC, Rainer G, and Miller EK: Integration of what and where in the primate prefrontal cortex. Science 276:821–824, 1997.

38. Battaglini PP, Fattori P, Galletti C, and Zeki S: The physiology of area V6 in the awake, behaving monkey. J Physiol (Lond) 423:100P, 1990.

39. Tanaka K, Hikosaka K, Saito H, et al.: Analysis of local and wide-field movements in the superior temporal cortex of the macaque monkey. I. Regional difference in response properties of cells. Soc Neurosci Abstr 13:627, 1987.

40. Mishkin M and Appenzeller T: The anatomy of memory. Sci Am 256:80–89, 1987.

41. Phillips RR, Malamut BL, Machevalier J, and Mishkin M: Dissociation of the effects of inferior temporal and limbic lesions on object discrimination learning with 24–h intertribal intervals. Behav Brain Res 27:99–107, 1988.

42. McCarthy R, Warrington EK: The dissolution of semantics. Nature 343:599, 1990.

43. Penfield W and Jasper H: Epilepsy and the Functional Anatomy of the Human Brain. Little, Brown, Boston, 1954.

44. Usrey WM and Reid RC: Synchronous activity in the visual system. Annu Rev Physiol 61:435–456, 1999.

45. Nunez PL: Neocortical Dynamics and Human EEG Rhythms. Oxford University Press, New York, 1995.

46. Gray CM, Engel AK, Konig P, and Singer W: Synchronization of oscillatory neuronal responses in cat striate cortex: temporal properties. Vis Neurosci 8:337–347, 1992.

47. Faulkner HJ, Traub RD, and Whittington MA: Disruption of synchronous gamma oscillations in the rat hippocampal slice: a common mechanism of anaesthetic drug action. Br J Pharmacol 125:483–492, 1998.

48. Donoghue JP, Sanes JN, Hatsopoulos NG, and Gaal G: Neural discharge and local field potential oscillations in primate motor cortex during voluntary movements. J Neurophysiol 79:159–173, 1998.

49. Castelo-Branco M, Neuenschwander S, and Singer W: Synchronization of visual responses between the cortex, lateral geniculate nucleus, and retina in the anesthetized cat. J Neurosci 18:6395–6410, 1998.

50. Singer W: The formation of cooperative cell assemblies in the visual cortex. J Exp Biol 153:177–179, 1990.

51. Engel AK, Konig P, Kreiter AK, and Singer W: Interhemispheric synchronization of oscillatory neuronal responses in cat visual cortex. Science 252:1177–1179, 1991.

52. Edelman G: Neural Darwinism: The Theory of Neuronal Group Selection. Basic Books, New York, 1987.

53. Chatterjee A and Southwood MH: Cortical blindness and visual imagery. Neurology 45:2189–2195, 1995.

54. Aldrich MS, Alessi AG, Beck RW, and Gilman S: Cortical blindness: etiology, diagnosis, and prognosis. Ann Neurol 21:149–158, 1987.

55. Frank Y and Torres F: Visual evoked potentials in the evaluation of "cortical blindness" in children. Ann Neurol 6:126–129, 1979.

56. Symonds C and Mackenzie I: Bilateral loss of vision from cerebral infarction. Brain 80:415–455, 1957.

57. Bogousslavsky J, Regli F, and Van Melle G: Unilateral occipital infarction: evaluation of the risks of developing bilateral loss of vision. J Neurol Neurosurg Psychiatry 46:78–80, 1983.

58. Lambert SR, Hoyt CS, Jan JE, Barkovich J, and Flodmark O: Visual recovery from hypoxic cortical blindness during childhood: computed tomography and magnetic resonance imaging predictors. Arch Opthalmol 105:1371–1377, 1987.

59. Weinstein EA and Kahn RI: Denial of Illness. CC Thomas, Springfield, IL, 1955.

60. McGlynn SM and Schachter DL: Unawareness of deficits in neuropsychological syndromes. J Clin Exp Neuropsychol 11:143–205, 1989.

61. Benson DF, Marsden CD, and Meadows JC: The amnestic syndrome of posterior cerebral artery occlusion. Acta Neurol Scand 50:133–145, 1974.

62. Devinsky O, Bear D, and Volpe BT: Confusional states following posterior cerebral artery infarction. Arch Neurol 45:160–163, 1988.

63. Heilman KM: Anosognosia: possible neuropsychological mechanisms. In Prigatano GP and Schachter DL (eds): Awareness of Deficit After Brain Injury. Oxford University Press, New York, 1991, pp 53–62.

64. Stoerig P and Cowey A: Blindsight in man and monkey. Brain 120:535–559, 1997.

65. Poppel E, Held R, and Frost D: Residual visual function after brain wounds involving the central visual pathways in man. Nature 243:295–296, 1973.

66. Weisenkrantz L: Blindsight. Oxford University Press, New York, 1986.

67. Marcel AJ: Blindsight and shape perception: deficit of visual consciousness or of visual function? Brain 121:1565–1588, 1998.

68. Weiskrantz L: Neuroanatomy of memory and amnesia: a case for multiple memory systems. Hum Neurobiol 6:93–105, 1987.

69. Perenin MT, Ruel J, and Hecaen H: Residual visual capacities in a case of cortical blindness. Cortex 16:605–612, 1980.

70. Corbetta M, Marzi CA, Tassinari G, and Aglioti S: Effectiveness of different task paradigms in revealing blindsight. Brain 113:603–616, 1990.

71. Weiskrantz L: Some aspects of memory functions and the temporal lobes. Acta Neurol Scand Suppl 109:69–74, 1986.

72. Merrill MK and Kewman DG: Training of color and form identification in cortical blindness: a case study. Arch Phys Med Rehabil 67:479–483, 1986.

73. Riddoch G: Dissociation of visual perception due to occipital injuries, with especial reference to appreciation of movement. Brain 40:15–57, 1917.

74. Marquis DG and Hilgard ER: Conditioned responses to light in monkeys after removal of the occipital lobes. Brain 60:1–12, 1937.

75. Yukie M and Iwai E: Direct projection from the dorsal lateral geniculate nucleus to the prestriate cortex in macaque monkeys. J Comp Neurol 201:81–97, 1981.

76. Celesia GG, Bushnell D, Toleikis SC, and Brigell MG: Cortical blindness and residual vision: is the "second" visual system in humans capable of more than rudimentary visual perception? Neurology 41:862–869, 1991.

77. Faubert J, Diaconu V, Ptito M, and Ptito A: Residual vision in the blind field of hemidecorticated humans predicted by a diffusion scatter model and selective spectral absorption of the human eye. Vis Res 39:149–157, 1999.

78. Morris JS, Ohman A, and Dolan RJ: A subcortical pathway to the right amygdala mediating "unseen" fear. Proc Natl Acad Sci USA 96:1680–1685, 1999.

78a. Fendrich R, Wessinger CM, and Gazzaniga MS: Speculations on the neural basis of islands of blindsight. Prog Brain Res 134:353–366, 2001.

79. Zeki S: Cerebral akinetopsia (visual motion blindness). A review. Brain 114:811–824, 1991.

80. Damasio AR, Yamada T, Damasio H, Corbett J, and McKee J: Central achromatopsia: behavioral, anatomic, and physiologic aspects. Neurology 30:1064–1071, 1980.

81. Beauchamp MS, Haxby JV, Jennings JE, and DeYoe EA: An fMRI version of the Farnsworth-Munsell 100–Hue test reveals multiple color–selective areas in human ventral occipitotemporal cortex. Cereb Cortex 9:257–263, 1999.

82. Hering E: Outlines of a Theory of the Light Sense. Hurvich LM, Jameson D. (translators). Harvard University Press, Cambridge, MA, 1964.

83. Meadows JC: Disturbed perception of colours associated with localized cerebral lesions. Brain 97:615–632, 1974.

84. Bartels A and Zeki S: The architecture of the colour centre in the human visual brain: new results and a review. Eur J Neurosci 12:172–93, 2000.

85. Kohl S, Marx T, Giddings I, Jagle H, Jacobson SG, Apfellstedt-Sylla E, et al.: Total colour blindness is caused by mutations in the gene encoding the alpha-subunit of the cone photoreceptor cGMP-gated cation channel. Nat Genet 19:257–259, 1998.

86. Sacks O: An Anthropologist on Mars. Knopf, New York, 1995.

87. Carlesimo GA, Casadio P, Sabbadini M, and Caltagirone C: Associative visual agnosia resulting from a disconnection between intact visual memory and semantic systems. Cortex 34:563–576, 1998.

88. Damasio AR, Tranel D, and Rizzo M: Disorders of complex visual processing. In Mesulam MM (ed). Principles of Behavioral and Cognitive Neurology. Oxford University Press, New York, 2000, pp 332–372.

89. Russel WR and Whitty CWM: Studies in traumatic epilepsy 3. Visual fits. J Neurol Neurosurg Psychiatry 18:79–96, 1955.

90. Penfield W and Perot P: The brain's record of auditory and visual experience. Brain 86:595–697, 1963.

91. Devinsky O, Feldmann E, Burrowes K, and Bromfield E: Autoscopic phenomena with seizures. Arch Neurol 46:1080–1088, 1988.

92. Ffytche DH, Howard RJ, Brammer MJ, et al.: The anatomy of conscious vision: an fMRI study of visual hallucinations. Nat Neurosci 1:738–742, 1998.

93. Lhermitte J: Syndrome de la calotte du pedoncle cerebral: les troubles psychosensoriels dans les lesions du mesocephale. Rev Neurol 38:1359–1365, 1922.

94. Manford M and Andermann F: Complex visual hallucinations. Clinical and neurobiological insights. Brain 121:1819–1840, 1998.

95. Braun AR, Balkin TJ, Wesensten NJ, et al.: Dissociation pattern in visual cortices and their projections during human rapid eye movement sleep. Science 279:91–95, 1998.

96. Eagleman DM. Visual illusions and neurobiology. Nat Rev Neurosci 2:920–926, 2001.

97. Teuber HI and Bender MB: Alterations in pattern vision following trauma of occipital lobes in man. J Gen Psychol 40:37–57, 1949.

98. Bender MB, Postel DM, and Krieger HP: Disorders in oculomotor function in lesions of the occipital lobe. J Neurol Neurosurg Psychiatry 20:139–l3, 1957.

99. Bender MB, Feldman M, and Sobin AJ: Palinopsia. Brain 91:321–338, 1968.

100. Critchley M: Types of visual perseveration: "paliopsia" and "illusory visual spread." Brain 74:267–299, 1951.

101. Cummings JL, Syndulko K, Goldberg Z, and Treiman DM: Palinopsia reconsidered. Neurology 32:444–447, 1982.

102. Muller T, Buttner T, Kuhn W, et al.: Palinopsia as sensory epileptic phenomenon. Acta Neurol Scand 91:433–436, 1995.

103. Jacobs L, Karpik A, Bozian D, and Gothgen S: Auditory–visual synesthesia: sound-induced photisms. Arch Neurol 38:211–216, 1981.

104. Macaluso E, Frith CD, and Driver J. Crossmodal spatial influences of touch on extrastriate visual areas take current gaze direction into account. Neuron 34:647–658, 2002.

105. De Renzi E: Disorders of visual recognition. Semin Neurol 20:479–485, 2000.

106. Landis T, Graves R, Benson F, and Hebben N: Visual recognition through kinaesthetic mediation. Psychol Med 12:515–531, 1982.

107. Shelton PA, Bowers D, Duara R, and Heilman KM: Apperceptive visual agnosia: a case study. Brain Cogn 25:1–23, 1994.

108. Landis T, Graves R, Benson F, et al.: Visual recognition through kinesthetic mediation. Psychol Med 12:515–531, 1982.

109. Rubens AB and Benson DF: Associative visual agnosia. Arch Neurol 24:310, 1971.

110. Warrington EK: A disconnection analysis of amnesia. Ann N Y Acad Sci 444:72–77, 1985.

111. Warrington EK and James M: Visual object recognition in patients with right-hemisphere lesions: axes or features. Perception 15:355–366, 1986.

112. Farah MJ: Visual Agnosia. MIT Press, Cambridge, MA, 1990.

113. Riddoch MJ and Humphreys GW: A case of integrative visual agnosia. Brain 110:1431–1462, 1987.

114. Levine DN and Calvanio R: Prosopagnosia: a defect in visual configural processing. Brain Cogn 10:149–170, 1989.

115. McCarthy RA and Warrington EK: Visual associative agnosia: a clinico-anatomical study of a single case. J Neurol Neurosurg Psychiatry 49:1233–1240, 1986.

116. Farah MJ: Perception and awareness after brain damage. Curr Opin Neurobiol 4:252–255, 1994.

117. Feinberg TE, Dyckes-Berke D, Miner CR, and Roane D: Knowledge, implicit knowledge and metaknowledge in visual agnosia and pure alexia. Brain 118:789–800, 1995.

118. Damasio AR, Tranel D, and Rizzo M: Disorders of complex visual processing. In Principles of Behavioral and Cognitive Neurology, 2nd ed. Oxford University Press, New York, 2000, pp 332–372.

119. Ross ED: Sensory-specific and fractional disorders of recent memory in man. I. Isolated loss of visual recent memory. Arch Neurol 37:193–200, 1980.

120. Riddoch MJ, Humphreys GW, Gannon T, et al.: Memories are made of this: the effects of time on stored visual knowledge in a case of visual agnosia. Brain 122:537–559, 1999.

121. Pallis CA: Impaired identification for faces and places with agnosia for colours. J Neurol Neurosurg Psychiatry 18:218, 1955.

122. Tranel D, Damasio AR, and Damsio H: Intact recognition of facial expression, gender, and age in patients with impaired recognition of face identity. Neurology 38:690–696, 1988.

123. Dailey MN and Cottrell GW: Prosopagnosia in modular neural network models. Prog Brain Res 121:165–184, 1999.

124. Tranel D and Damasio AR: Knowledge without awareness: an autonomic index of facial recognition by prosopagnosics. Science 228:1453–1454, 1985.

125. Bauer RM and Verfaellie M: Electrodermal discrimination of familiar but not unfamiliar faces in prosopagnosia. Brain Cogn 8:240–252, 1988.

126. Rizzo M and Hurtig R: Looking but not seeing: attention, perception, and eye movements in simultanagnosia. Neurology 37:1642–1648, 1987.

127. Seeck M, Mainwaring N, Ives J, et al.: Differential neural activity in the human temporal lobe evoked by faces of family members and friends. Ann Neurol 34:369–372, 1993.

128. Kim JJ, Andreasen NC, O'Leary DS, et al.: Direct comparison of the neural substrates of recognition memory for words and faces. Brain 122:1069–1083, 1999.

129. Kanwisher N, Stanley D, and Harris A: The fusiform face area is selective for faces not animals. Neuroreport 10:183–187, 1999.

130. Nachson I: On the modularity of face recognition: the riddle of domain specificity. J Clin Exp Neuropsychol 17:256–275, 1995.

131. Gazzaniga MS and Smylie CS: Facial recognition and brain asymmetries: clues to underlying mechanisms. Ann Neurol 13:536–540, 1983.

132. Evans JJ, Heggs AJ, Antoun N, and Hodges JR: Progressive prosopagnosia associated with selective right temporal lobe atrophy. Brain 118:1–13, 1995.

133. Hodges JR: Frontotemporal dementia (Pick's disease): clinical features and assessment. Neurology 56(Suppl 4):S6–S10, 2001.

134. Snowden JS, Neary D, Mann DMA, et al.: Progressive language disorder due to lobar atrophy. Ann Neurol 31:174–183, 1992.

135. Rizzo M and Vecera SP: Psychoanatomical substrates of Balint's syndrome. J Neurol Neurosurg Psychiatry 2002;72:162–178, 2002.

136. Rizzo M and Robin DA: Simultanagnosia: a defect of sustained attention yields insights on visual information processing. Neurology 40:447–455, 1990.

137. Baylis GC, Driver J, Baylis LL, and Rafal RD: Reading of letters and words in a patient with Balint's syndrome. Neuropsychologia 32:1273–1286, 1994.

138. Stasheff SF and Barton JJ: Deficits in cortical visual function. Ophthalmol Clin North Am 14:217–242, 2001.

139. Holmes G and Horrax G: Disturbances of spatial orientation and visual attention, with loss of stereoscopic vision. Arch Neurol Psychiatry 1:385–407, 1919.

140. Girotti F, Milanese C, Casazza M, et al.: Oculomotor disturbance in Balint's syndrome: anatomoclinical findings and the electrooculographic analysis in a case. Cortex 18:603–614, 1982.

141. Holmes G: Disturbances of vision by cerebral lesions. Br J Ophthalmol 2:353–384, 1918.

142. Hecaen H and de Ajuriaguerra J: Balint's syndrome (psychic paralysis of gaze) and its minor forms. Brain 77:373–400, 1954.

143. Fernandez-Duque D and Posner MI: Brain imaging of attentional networks in normal and pathological states. J Clin Exp Neuropsychol 23:74–93, 2001.

144. Steinmetz MA and Constantinidis C: Neurophysiological evidence for a role of posterior parietal cortex in redirecting visual attention. Cereb Cortex 5:448–456, 1995.

145. Morrow LA and Ratcliff G: The disengagement of covert attention and the neglect syndrome. Psychobiology 16:261–269, 1988.

146. Ghika J, Ghika-Schmid F, and Bogousslavsky J: Parietal motor syndrome: a clinical description in 32 patients in the acute phase of pure parietal strokes studied prospectively. Clin Neurol Neurosurg 100:271–282, 1998.

147. Perenin MT and Vighetto A: Optic ataxia: a specific disruption in visuomotor mechanisms. I. Different aspects of the deficit in reaching for objects. Brain 111:643–674, 1988.

148. Battaglia Mayer A, Ferraina S, et al.: Early motor influences on visuomotor transformations for reaching: a positive image of optic ataxia. Exp Brain Res 123:172–189, 1998.

149. Nagaratnam N, Grice D, and Kalouche H: Optic ataxia following unilateral stroke. J Neurol Sci 155:204–207, 1998.

150. Binkofski F, Buccino G, Dohle C, et al.: Mirror agnosia and mirror ataxia constitute different parietal lobe disorders. Ann Neurol 46:51–61, 1999.

151. Juergens SM, Fredrickson PA, and Pfeiffer FE: Balint's syndrome mistaken for visual conversion reaction. Psychosomatics 27:597–599, 1986.

152. Ferrell MJ: Topographical disorientation. Neurocase 2:509–520, 1996.

153. Aguirre GK and D'Esposito M: Topographical disorientation: a synthesis and taxonomy. Brain 122:1613–1628, 1999.

154. Meyer O: Ein-und doppelseitige homonyme Hemianopsie mit Orientierungsstorungen. Mschr Psychiatr Neurol 8:440–456, 1900.

155. Holmes G: Disturbances of spatial orientation and visual attention with loss of stereoscopic vision. Arch Neurol Psychiatry 1:385–407, 1919.

156. Brain R: Visual disorientation with special reference to the lesions of the right hemisphere. Brain 64:244–272, 1941.

157. Alsaadi T, Binder JR, Lazar RM, Doorani T, and

Mohr JP: Pure topographic disorientation: a distinctive syndrome with varied localization. Neurology 5:1864–1866, 2000.

158. Levine DN, Warach J, and Farah M: Two visual systems in mental imagery: dissociation of "what" and "where" in imagery disorders due to bilateral posterior cerebral lesions. Neurology 35:1010–1018, 1985.

159. Andersen RA, Shenoy KV, Snyder LH, Bradley DC, and Crowell JA: The contributions of vestibular signals to the representations of space in the posterior parietal cortex. Ann NY Acad Sci 871:282–292, 1999.

160. Takahashi N, Kawamura M, Shiota J, et al.: Pure topographic disorientation due to right retrosplenial lesion. Neurology 49:464–469, 1997.

161. Chen LL, Lin LH, Green EJ, Barnes CA, and McNaughton BL: Head-direction cells in the rat posterior cortex. I. Anatomical distribution and behavioural modulation. Exp Brain Res 101:8–23, 1994.

162. Taube JB, Goodridge JP, Golob EJ, Dudohenko PA, and Stackman RW: Processing the head direction cell signal: a review and commentary. Brain Res Bull 40:477–484, 1996.

163. Landis T, Cummings JL, Benson DF, and Palmer EP: Loss of topographic familiarity. An environmental agnosia. Arch Neurol 43:132–136, 1986.

164. Aguirre GK, Zarahn E, and D'Esposito M: Neural components of topographical representation. Proc Natl Acad Sci USA 95:839–846, 1998.

165. Haxby JV, Ungerleider LG, Clark VP, Schouter JL, Hoffman EA, and Martin A: The effect of the face inversion on activity in human neural systems for face and object perception. Neuron 22:189–199, 1999.

166. Habib M and Sirigu A: Pure topographical disorientation: a definition and anatomical basis. Cortex 23:73–85, 1987.

167. Maguire EA, Frackowiack RSJ, and Frith CD: Learning to find your way: a role for the human hippocampal region. Proc R Soc Lond B 263:1745–1750, 1996.

168. Bohbot J, Kalina M, Stephankova K, Stephankova N, Petrides M, and Nadel L: Spatial memory deficits in patients with lesions to the right hippocampus and to the right parahippocampal cortex. Neuropsychologia 36:1217–1238, 1998.

169. Hubel DH and Wiesel TN: Stereoscopic vision in macaque monkey. Nature 225:41–42, 1970.

170. Richards W: Stereopsis and stereoblindness. Exp Brain Res 10:380–388, 1970.

171. Rizzo M: Astereopsis. In Damasio AR (ed). Handbook of Clinical Neuropsychology. Disorders of Visual Behavior, Vol 2, Sect 4. Elsevier, New York, 1989, pp 415–427.

172. Julesz B, Breitmeyer B, and Kropfl W: Binocular disparity dependent upper lower hemifield anisotropy and left right hemifield isotropy as revealed by dynamic random dot stereograms. Perception 5:129–141, 1976.

173. Rizzo M and Damasio H: Impairment of stereopsis with focal brain lesions. Ann Neurol 18:147, 1985.

174. Fortin A, Ptito A, Faubert J, and Ptito M: Cortical areas mediating stereopsis in the human brain: a PET study. Neuroreport 13:895–898, 2002.

175. Kosslyn SM, Pascual-Leone A, Felician O, et al.: The role of area 17 in visual imagery: convergent evidence from PET and rTMS. Science 284:167–170, 1999.

176. Goldenberg G: The ability of patients with brain damage to generate mental visual images. Brain 112:305–325, 1989.

177. Jeannerod M and Decety J: Mental motor imagery: a window into the representational stages of action. Curr Opin Neurobiol 5:727–732, 1995.

178. Bisiach E and Luzzatti C: Unilateral neglect of representational space. Cortex 14:713–717, 1978.

178a. Nordby K: Vision in a complete achromat: a personal account. In: Hess RF, Sharpe LT, Nordby K (eds). Night Vision: Basic, Clinical and Applied Aspects. 1990, Cambridge University Press, pp 290–315.

179. Benton A and Tranel D: Visuoperceptive, visuospatial, and visuoconstructive disorders. In Heilman KM and Valenstein E (eds). Clinical Neuropsychology, 3rd ed. Oxford University Press, New York, 1993, pp 165–214.

180. Shuttleworth EC Jr, Syring V, Allen N: Further observations on the nature of prosopagnosia. Brain Cogn 1:307–322, 1982.

181. Farah MJ, Peronnet F, Gonon MA, and Giard MH: Electrophysiological evidence for a shared representational medium for visual images and percepts. J Exp Psychol Gen 117:248–257, 1988.

182. Kosslyn SM: Aspects of a cognitive neuroscience of mental imagery. Science 240:1621–1626, 1988.

183. Hadano K: On block design constructional disability in right and left hemisphere brain-damaged patients. Cortex 20:391–401, 1984.

184. Ratcliff G: Spatial thought, mental rotation and the right cerebral hemisphere. Neuropsychologia 17:49–54, 1979.

185. Corballis MC: Mental rotation and the right hemisphere. Brain Lang 57:100–121, 1997.

186. Read HL, Winer JA, and Schreiner CE: Functional architecture of auditory cortex. Curr Opin Neurobiol. 12:433–440, 2002.

187. Gloor P, Olivier A, Quesney LF, Andermann F, and Horowitz S: The role of the limbic system in experiential phenomena of temporal lobe epilepsy. Ann Neurol 12:129–144, 1982.

188. Lesser RP, Luders H, Morris HH, et al.: Electrical stimulation of Wernicke's area interferes with comprehension. Neurology 36:658–663, 1986.

189. Schwartz TH, Devinsky O, Doyle W, and Perrine K: Function-specific high-probability "nodes" identified in posterior language cortex. Epilepsia 40:575–583, 1999.

190. Griffiths TD, Rees A, Witton C, et al.: Spatial and temporal auditory processing deficits following right hemisphere infarction. A psychophysical study. Brain 120:785–794, 1997.

191. Platel H, Price C, Baron JC, et al.: The structural components of music perception. A functional anatomical study. Brain 120:229–243, 1997.

192. Hugdahl K, Bronnick K, Kyllingsbaek S, et al.: Brain activation during dichotic presentations of consonant–vowel and musical instrument stimuli: a ^{15}O-PET study. Neuropsychologia 37:431–440, 1999.

193. Polster MR and Rose SB: Disorders of auditory processing: evidence for modularity in audition. Cortex 34:47–65, 1998.

194. Bauer RM: Agnosia. In Heilman KM and Valenstein E (eds). Clinical Neuropsychology, 3rd ed. Oxford University Press, New York, 1993, pp 215–278.

195. Fujii T, Fukatsu R, Watabe S, et al.: Auditory sound agnosia without aphasia following a right temporal lobe lesion. Cortex 26:263–268, 1990.

196. Engelien A, Silbersweig D, Stern E, et al.: The functional anatomy of recovery from auditory agnosia. A PET study of sound categorization in a neurological patient and normal controls. Brain 118:1395–1409, 1995.

197. Vignolo LA: Auditory agnosia: a review and report of recent evidence. In Benton AL (ed). Contributions to Clinical Neuropsychology. Chicago, Aldine, 1969, pp 172–208.

198. Van Lancker DR, Kreiman J, and Cummings J: Voice perception deficits: neuroanatomic correlates of phonagnosia. J Clin Exp Neuropsychol 11:665–674, 1989.

199. Habib M, Daquin G, Milander L, Royere ML, Rey M, Lanteri A, Salamon G, and Khalil R: Mutism and auditory agnosia due to bilateral insular damage—role of the insula in human communication. Neuropsychologia 33:327–339, 1995.

200. Fifer RC: Insular stroke causing unilateral auditory processing disorder: case report. J Am Acad Audiol 4:364–369, 1993.

201. Shoumaker RD, Ajax ET, and Schenkenberg T: Pure word deafness (auditory verbal agnosia). Dis Nerv Syst 38:293–299, 1977.

202. Buchman AS, Garron DC, Trost-Cardamone JE, Wichter MD, and Schwartz M: Word deafness: one hundred years later. J Neurol Neurosurg Psychiatry 49:489–499, 1986.

203. Takahashi N, Kawamura M, Shinotou H, Hirayama K, Kaga K, and Shindo M: Pure word deafness due to left hemisphere damage. Cortex 28:295–303, 1992.

204. Klein SK, Kurtzberg D, Brattson A, et al.: Electrophysiologic manifestations of impaired temporal lobe auditory processing in verbal auditory agnosia. Brain Lang 51:383–405, 1995.

205. Coslett HB, Brashear HR, and Heilman KM: Pure word deafness after bilateral primary auditory cortex infarcts. Neurology 34:347–352, 1984.

206. Albert ML and Bear D: Time to understand. A case study of word deafness with reference to the role of time in auditory comprehension. Brain 97:383–394, 1974.

207. Saffran EB, Marin OSM, and Yeni-Komshian GH: An analysis of speech perception in word deafness. Brain Lang 3:255–256, 1976.

208. Benton AL: The amusias. In Critchley M and Henson RA (eds). Music and the Brain. Heinemann, Oxford, 1977, pp 378–397.

209. Brust JCM: Music and language: musical alexia and agraphia. Brain 103:367–392, 1980.

210. Beversdorf DQ and Heilman KM: Progressive ventral posterior cortical degeneration presenting as alexia for music and words. Neurology 50:657–659, 1998.

211. Gates A and Bradshaw JL: The role of the cerebral hemispheres in music. Brain Lang 4:403–431, 1977.

212. McFarland HR and Fortin D: Amusia due to right temporoparietal infarct. Arch Neurol 39:725–727, 1982.

213. Griffiths TD, Bench CJ, and Frackowiak RS: Human cortical areas selectively activated by apparent sound movement. Curr Biol 4:892–895, 1994.

214. Griffiths TD: Central auditory processing disorders. Curr Opin Neurol 15:31–33, 2002.

215. Penhune VB, Zatorre RJ, and Feindel WH: The role of auditory cortex in retention of rhythmic patterns as studied in patients with temporal lobe removals including Heschl's gyrus. Neuropsychologia 37:315–331, 1999.

216. Bever TG and Chiarello RJ: Cerebral dominance in musicians and nonmusicians. Science 185:537–539, 1974.

217. Critchley M and Henson RA: Music and the Brain. Heinemann, London, 1977.

218. Mavlov L: Amusia due to rhythm agnosia in a musician with left hemisphere damage: a nonauditory supramodal defect. Cortex 16:331–338, 1980.

219. Schlaug G, Jancke L, Huang Y, and Steinmetz H: In vivo evidence of structural brain asymmetry in musicians. Science 267:699–701, 1995.

220. Peretz I, Kolinsky R, Tramo M, et al.: Functional dissociations following bilateral lesions of auditory cortex. Brain 117:1283–1301, 1994.

221. Devinsky O, Feldmann E, Bromfield E, Emoto S, and Raubertis R: Structured interview for partial seizures: clinical phenomenology and diagnosis. J Epilepsy 4:107–116, 1991.

222. Ali JA: Musical hallucinations and deafness: a case report and review of the literature. Neuropsychiatry Neuropsychol Behav Neurol 2002;15:66–70.

223. Doune AG and Bourque PR: Musical auditory hallucinosis from *Listeria rhomboencephalitis*. Can J Neurol Sci 24:70–72, 1997.

224. Wieser HG, Hungerbuhler H, Siegel AM, and Buck A: Musicogenic epilepsy: review of the literature and case report with ictal single photon emission computed tomography. Epilepsia 38:200–207, 1997.

225. Berrios GE: Musical hallucinations. A historical and clinical study. Br J Psychiatry 156:188–194, 1990.

226. Devinsky O and Luciano D: Psychic phenomena in partial seizures. Semin Neurol 11:100–109, 1991.

227. Caselli RJ: Tactile agnosia and disorders of tactile perception. In Feinberg TR and Farah MH (eds). Principles of Behavioral Neurology and Neuropsychology. McGraw-Hill, New York, 1996, pp 277–288.

228. Caselli RJ: Ventrolateral and dorsomedial somatosensory association cortex infarctions produce distinct somesthetic syndromes. Neurology 43:762–771, 1993.

229. Reed CL and Caselli RJ: The nature of tactile agnosia. Neuropsychologia 32:527–539, 1994.

230. Platz T: Tactile agnosia. Casuistic evidence and theoretical remarks on modality-specific meaning representations and sensorimotor integration. Brain 119:1565–1574, 1996.

231. Reed CL, Caselli RJ, and Farah MJ: Tactile agnosia. Underlying impairment and implications for normal tactile object recognition. Brain 119:875–888, 1996.

231a. Bohlhalter S, Fretz C, Weder B. Hierarchical versus parallel processing in tactile object recognition: a behavioural-neuroanatomical study of aperceptive tactile agnosia. Brain 125:2537–2548, 2002.

232. Endo K, Miyasaka M, Makishita H, et al.: Tactile

agnosia and tactile aphasia: symptomatological and anatomical differences. Cortex 28:445–469, 1992.

233. Mishkin M: Analogous neural models for tactual and visual learning. Neuropsychologia 17:139–150,1979.

234. Schwoebel J, Coslett HB, Bradt J, Friedman R, and Dileo C: Pain and the body schema: effects of pain severity on mental representations of movement. Neurology 59:775–777, 2002.

235. Berlucchi G and Aglioti S: The body in the brain: neural bases of corporeal awareness. Trends Neurosci 20:560–564, 1997.

236. Sirigu A, Grafman J, Bressler K, and Sunderland T: Multiple representations contribute to body knowledge processing. Brain 114:629–642, 1991.

237. Stein JF: The representation of egocentric space in the posterior parietal cortex. Behav Brain Sci 15:691–700, 1992.

238. Graziano MS, Cooke DF, and Taylor CS: Coding the location of the arm by sight. Science 290:1782–1786, 2000.

239. Poeck K: Phantome nach Amputation und bei angeborenen Gliedma benmangel. Dtsche Med Wochenschr 46:2367–2374, 1969.

240. Frederiks JAM: Phantom limb and phantom limb pain. In Frederiks JAM (ed). Handbook of Neurology, Vol 1. Elsevier, New York, 1985, pp 395–404.

241. Kroner K, Krebs B, Skov J, and Jorgensen HJ: Immediate and long-term phantom breast syndrome after mastectomy: incidence, clinical characteristics and relationship to pre-mastectomy breast pain. Pain 36:327–334, 1989.

242. Halligan PW, Marshall JC, and Wade DT: Three arms: a case study of supernumerary phantom limb after right hemisphere stroke. J Neurol Neurosurg Psychiatry 56:159–166, 1993.

243. Cummings JL: Neuropsychiatric manifestations of right hemisphere lesions. Brain Lang 57:22–37, 1997.

244. Vuilleumier P, Reverdin A, and Landis T: Four legs. Illusory reduplication of the lower limbs after bilateral parietal lobe damage. Arch Neurol 54:1543–1547, 1997.

245. Ogden JA: Autotopagnosia: occurrence in a patient without nominal aphasia and with an intact ability to point to parts of animals and objects. Brain 108:1009–1022, 1985.

246. Gainotti G, Cianchetti C, Tiacci C: The influence of the hemispheric side of lesion on nonverbal tasks of finger localization. Cortex 8:364–377, 1972.

247. Berrios GE: Tactile hallucinations: conceptual and historical aspects. J Neurol Neurosurg Psychiatry 45:285–293, 1982.

248. Perry E, Walker M, Grace J, and Perry J: Acetylcholine in mind: a neurotransmitter correlate of consciousness? Trends Neurosci 22:273–280, 1999.

249. Serra Catafau J, Rubio F, and Peres Serra J: Peduncular hallucinosis associated with posterior thalamic infarction. J Neurol 239:89–90, 1992.

250. Salanova V, Andermann F, Rasmussen T, et al.: Parietal lobe epilepsy. Clinical manifestations and outcome in 82 patients treated surgically between 1929 and 1988. Brain 118:607–627, 1995.

Chapter 6

Language, Aphasia, and Other Speech Disorders

Language, communication through symbols, helps to create and organize the fabric of human consciousness. The acquisition of language is a human instinct, common to all normal individuals exposed to language in childhood. However, the ability to use a visually based language (i.e., reading and writing) rather than a sound-based language (i.e., comprehending speech and speaking) highlights the importance of learning in, as well as the ontogeny of, language acquisition. Written language is a recent part of human history. A common set of principles underlies the grammar (syntax) of diverse languages, which suggests that children innately possess a universal grammar and learn the specific grammar of their native language.

ANATOMICAL AND PHYSIOLOGICAL ASPECTS OF LANGUAGE

Language acquisition involves instinctive, innate systems and learning. Like vision, language development requires exposure at certain critical stages of life.[1] Language acquisition is guaranteed for children up to 6 years of age, steadily compromised between age 6 and puberty, and rare thereafter.[2] After puberty, children who have not acquired a language are known as *feral*. These life stages are also relevant for predicting language recovery after injury to a child's cortical language area. The extensive exposure of infants and young children to speech suggests the importance of learning and more general cognitive systems in language acquisition, including internally representing stimuli, understanding the implications of sequential acts and complex relationships between objects (possibly a by-product of circuitry for primate social structure), sequentially coding data, and making cross-modal associations, such as associating a sound and a visual image.[3]

Cognitive–Linguistic Concepts

Neurological writings on language are dominated by the words *comprehension, speech, prosody,* and *syntax*. Beyond these commonly used terms is an evolving group of cognitive–linguistic concepts. These concepts hold that language is:

1. a code for mapping thoughts (*mentalese*) into signals and signals into thoughts
2. a coordinated system based on phonological, lexical, syntactical, and discourse elements; in other words, a sound-based system of representing and processing words, transforming word order and relation into meaning, and verbal expression
3. information processing, such as *parsing* (mentally grouping words into phrases and sentences) and distinguishing differences in neural coding between written and spoken words
4. lexical categories, such as nouns, verbs, and adjectives, and functional categories, such as determiners, nominal and verbal inflections, and pronouns
5. *discourse,* the temporal organization and flow of narrative speech

These cognitive and linguistic formulations can define both the normal physiological aspects of language and the pathological processes causing aphasia.

Language differs from thought. We use language to communicate with others and as an internal, self-contained process to reflect, understand, explain, and make decisions. The apparent dominance of linguistic thought often obscures the richness of nonverbal thought processes. For example, our understanding of our own and other's feelings, social interactions, mate selection, predicting other people's behavior, justice, and geography are largely nonverbal. Many of humankind's greatest inventions or discoveries, ranging from the wheel to the benzene ring, electrical and magnetic fields, electrical motor, and special relativity, were products of visual thought. Albert Einstein[4] used a thought experiment in which he imagined himself riding parallel to a light beam and looking back at a clock. He viewed the "elements in thought" as "certain signs and more or less clear images which can be 'voluntarily' reproduced and combined. . . . " To him, combinatory play seemed to be "the essential feature in productive thought—before there is any connection with logical construction in words or other kinds of signs which can be communicated with others." In his case, he believed that "the above-mentioned elements are of [the] visual and muscular type. Conventional words or other signs have to be sought laboriously only in a secondary state. . . . "

The identification of the perisylvian areas by Broca,[5] Dax,[6] Wernicke,[7] and others has biased our conceptualization of human language function. Although lesions in Broca's area and Wernicke's area correlate with specific deficits, there are no "language centers." The production and comprehension of human language require an integrated network of diverse cortical areas (Fig. 6–1). To translate a concept into the phonetic–morphological and syntactical structure, or vice versa, discrete regions within the primary and association sensory and motor cortices and higher association areas must be activated. Higher association cortices, separate from the perisylvian language areas, may form a two-directional link between the areas involved in conceptual thought and planning and the areas that implement the understanding and production of language.[8] Recent models postulate critical convergence–divergence sites, called *transmodal areas,* such as Wernicke's area, that transform word forms into meaning; these sites activate images or mediate actions for specific entities in sensorimotor structures. Transmodal areas bind multiple unimodal and other transmodal areas into distributed but integrated multimodal representations.[9]

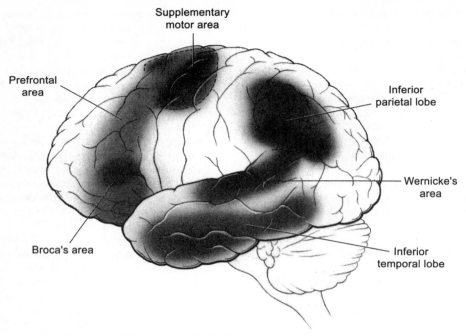

Figure 6–1. Cortical regions involved in language comprehension and production.

Linguistic Components

The four principal components of language are morphemes, lexicon, semantics, and syntax. Other important elements are prosody, pragmatics, and narrative discourse. *Phonology* encompasses the phonetics and phonemics of spoken language. *Phonetics* refers to the sound elements, which may be devoid of meaning. For instance, *dysarthria* is a phonetic disorder affecting articulation. *Phonemics* refers to the meaningful sound elements, the most basic of which is the phoneme (e.g., /p/, /d/). English has approximately 34 phonemes, Spanish has 23, and languages with many dialects, such as Chinese, can have more than 50.

MORPHEMES AND LEXICON

In linguistics, *morphology* is the study of word formation. A *morpheme* is the basic unit of meaning and comprises a word or part of a word. A morpheme can be formed by a single phoneme, such as the personal pronoun *I* or the article *a*, or by multiple phonemes, as in the word *bat* (/b/, /a/, /t/). Lexical morphemes are word roots, such as the word *good*. Grammatical morphemes include modifiers (prefixes

and suffixes that alter the root, as in *goodness*), connectors (e.g., *to, if, and*), and particles. The lexicon comprises all the morphemes in a language.

SEMANTICS

Semantics refers to the meaning of words. Two words that have similar meanings and are often used interchangeably are *synonyms* (e.g., *sad* and *depressed*). Words that have the same sound and often the same spelling but differ in meaning are *homonyms* (e.g., *cord* and *chord*); a word used to designate several different things is also a homonym (e.g., *ball*). Words that sound alike but differ in spelling and meaning are *homophones* (e.g., *aisle* and *isle*).

In the brain, the semantic organization of nouns and verbs can vary. Different categories of nouns and verbs may be closely related to different sources of sensorimotor information within the brain, as shown by the correlation between lesion site and affected category.[10] Some aphasic patients have a selective impairment in reading or writing a word used as a verb but not as a noun.[11] For instance, the difficulty may occur with a word like *crack*, which may be used as a verb, as in "She will crack the eggs to make an omelet," or as a noun, as in "The crack in the wall grew wider over the years."

Semantic fields are formed by hierarchically organized word associations (e.g., animals–mammals–primates–great apes–gorillas). In this sequence, animals and mammals are superordinate to primates, great apes, and gorillas and great apes and gorillas are types of primates. Usually first learned in childhood, superordinate categories are better preserved and more rapidly recovered in patients with aphasia and anomia.

SYNTAX

Syntax refers to the grammatical rules used to construct phrases and sentences. Grammatical connectors such as *and, to,* and *while* link the words in a sentence. The sequence of words conveys meaning, especially in English and other languages where word order communicates intention or action. For example, "The man hit the boy" differs from "The boy hit the man." *Parsing* is the mental spacing between words and the mental grouping of words into phrases and sentences.

PROSODY

Prosody, the intonation of speech, helps to convey the message through variations in the pitch, tone, melody, stress, and rhythm of speech, independent of words (semantics) and organization (grammar). The four components of prosody are described as *dialectical* and *inflectional,* which are intrinsic, as in a rising pitch at the end of a sentence to indicate a question; *attitudinal,* which imparts meaning, as in violent words said in a soft, playful, rising tone or with violent anger; *affective,* which imparts emotional tone; and *nonlinguistic,* inarticulate, such as grunts and moans. Prosody is essential for effective speaking and emotional communication, for example, sarcasm or humor (see Chapter 3).

PRAGMATICS

Pragmatics refers to the functional use of language. Serving practical goals, communication begins simply, as with an infant's crying or a child's pointing to a desired object, and becomes more complex as language develops.

Language can be used to request such things as food or information, give commands, express feelings, and describe events.

NARRATIVE DISCOURSE

The organization of ongoing speech is known as *narrative discourse.* The process includes the topical information, focus of speaker's attention, temporal order of speech elements within and between sentences, sequence of events, digressions and return to main theme, information novelty, and conformity of information for social context, such as the duration of a speech.

HEMISPHERIC HAND AND LANGUAGE DOMINANCE

The origins of anthropoid and human hemispheric hand and language dominance are uncertain. An initial lateralization of circuitry for fine, intentional, sequential manipulation of objects (e.g., throwing a rock, altering material for shelter) may have determined language lateralization, which also requires orchestrated cognitive and motor processes. The development of right-hand dominance for gestural communication may have led to a coupling of left hemisphere language and motor dominance.[12]

Motor dominance is often defined as hand dominance, reflecting the contralateral hemisphere's capacity to acquire skilled motor programs such as fine, distal movements (e.g., writing or using chopsticks). The left hemisphere (right hand) is usually dominant for fine motor control and skilled movements, such as writing and sculpting. The dominant left frontoparietal regions control limb and finger trajectories and coordinate joint motions into a movement plan.[13] Such plans require integrated motor sequences, which may change depending on internal and environmental inputs.[14] Motor dominance extends beyond fine hand (pyramidal) movements. Speech is a bilateral motor activity controlled mainly by the left hemisphere. Emotional prosody and singing are bilateral motor acts with greater right hemisphere control. Skilled truncal (axial) movements, as used in bicycle riding, ice skating, playing basketball, and dancing, require coordinated trunk and proximal limb movements and may be controlled by one hemisphere more than the other. Although pyramidal and axial movements are combined for many complex, learned motor programs, these motor skills also exist independently. Thus, a person may be quite skilled at fine movements, such as playing the piano, but clumsy at sports requiring axial movements, or vice versa. Hemispheric dominance may be different for pyramidal and axial motor skills. For instance, an artist sculpted, engraved, and wrote with his left hand but painted with his right hand.[15] Further, we cared for a 13-year-old boy whose language comprehension, reading and writing skills, and letter production were impaired at the 5-year-old level. Nevertheless, though he was of medium height, he was among the top five scoring basketball players in his age group for the state. Despite impairment of fine motor and language skills, his basketball skills reflected highly developed gross motor skills.

Handedness

Handedness is determined by genetic, developmental, and environmental factors. Right handedness predominates in all human races; 90%–92% of the world's population is right-handed.[16,17] Historically, right handedness has met with greater approval than left handedness. The favorable view of right handedness is reflected in the words *dexterous* and *adroit,* which are derived from Latin *(dexter)* and French *(à droit),* meaning "right" or "the right side." The relatively unfavorable view of left handedness is reflected in the words *sinister* and *gauche,* which are derived from Latin *(sinister)* and Old French *(gauchir),* meaning "left" or "the left side." In some cultures and families, left handedness is treated as an abnormality and children are taught to become right-handed.

Handedness is a heterogeneous trait, ranging from strongly right-handed to ambidextrous to strongly left-handed. A strong family history of left handedness tends to predict ambidexterity.[18] Moreover, left-handed persons tend to be less strongly left-handed, that is, more ambidextrous, than right-handed persons are right-handed.[19] Left-handed individuals may have better mathematical, architectural, spatial, musical, or artistic skills than right-handed individuals[17,20,21] and may more often be homosexual.[22]

Left hemisphere injury in early life may lead to "pathological" left handedness,[23] which may explain why some individuals without a family history of left-handedness are strongly left handed: left hemisphere damage impairs right hand control.[24] Patients with epilepsy, autism, mental retardation, and developmental dyslexia have a high incidence of left handedness. Their left handedness is often pathological but, among other assaults, may reflect fetal exposure to aberrant levels of testosterone or other hormones, which may slow left hemisphere development.[15] Handedness is associated with a complex, interwoven, and variable distribution of hemispheric language functions. In a study of stroke patients, the left hemisphere was dominant for language in 99% of right-handed and approximately 70% of left-handed subjects; but in a functional neuroimaging study of normal subjects, the left hemisphere was dominant in 92.5% of moderately to strongly right-handed men and women.[25] Studies show evidence of sex differences in functional organization of the brain for language. In a phonological processing task, brain activity was lateralized to the left inferior frontal gyrus region in men, but both left and right inferior frontal gyri were activated in women.[26] Right hemisphere lesions in right-handed persons can cause crossed aphasia, but the disorder is rare;[27] and diaschisis, or functional depression of the anatomically normal left hemisphere, may contribute.[28] Clinical and functional neuroimaging studies support the localization of right hemisphere language functions in the rare right-handed person with crossed aphasia.[28]

Left handedness and ambidexterity are associated with greater language capabilities in the right hemisphere. In approximately 30% of left-handed persons, language dominance is in both hemispheres or in the right hemisphere. Non-right-handed subjects tend to have a more bilateral representation of language and visuospatial functions. Among left-handed persons, there is often a dissociation between the hemispheres specialized for handedness, speech, and language comprehension.[25] For example, some have left hemisphere dominance for language comprehension and right hemisphere dominance for skilled manual functions and speech output.[29] Left-handed persons also are more likely to experience stuttering, dyslexia, and language impairments.[30]

Anomalous Dominance

Anomalous dominance refers to a dominance pattern for language and handedness that differs from the standard pattern (language is in the left hemisphere when the right hand is dominant). For example, a person may write with their right hand but throw a frisbee with their left hand and kick a football with their left foot. This irregular pattern is found in approximately one-third of individuals, including those who are left-handed and ambidextrous, which is similar to the percentage of those in whom the planum temporale is not larger on the left side. Anomalous dominance may sometimes result from delayed development of the left hemisphere, which creates a more symmetrical brain.[15] Anomalous dominance is more often identified with standardized test batteries than with self-reports of handedness.[31]

Lateralization of Linguistic Skills

The lateralization of receptive and expressive language skills is a hallmark of the human mind. During hominid evolution, left hemisphere superiority in representing the environment and our inner thoughts symbolically and sequentially may have contributed to its dominance for motor control, language, and logical thought. The left hemsiphere is superior in making temporal order judgments,[32,33] which are critical in language comprehension and production, because speech and other fine motor skills require sequential motor programs.

The lateralization of linguistic skills begins as language develops, around 2 years of age. The right hemisphere acquires language functions if the language areas in the left perisylvian region are damaged before the age of 8–11 years.[34] In most right-handed individuals, the right hemisphere has rudimentary language skills, which, like those in young children, are better for comprehension than speech or writing.[35] Left hemisphere inhibition of the right hemisphere likely contributes to language dominance on the left. Comprehension skills of the right hemisphere may reflect a delay in left hemisphere inhibition, which may be more potent after the age of 2 years, when speech and syntax are learned.[36,37] Furthermore, the right hemisphere may be more involved in acquiring a second language after early childhood.[38]

APHASIA

Aphasia is a disturbance of language formation and comprehension caused by localized brain dysfunction. Structural or physiological disorders in the language network, including its internal and external connections, disrupt the linguistic processing that creates the symbols (words) and structure (grammar) of language from nonverbal thought and produces nonverbal thought from language. The linguistic deficits in aphasia vary, but in most cases there is a primary impairment in decoding and encoding sequential elements of language structure, ranging from the phonemic elements of words to grammatical organization. The exception is *transcortical aphasia,* in which phonemic elements are characteristically preserved and grammar may be intact. Aphasia invariably wreaks havoc on the afflicted person, disrupting communication and the stream of verbal consciousness and, in many cases, compromising social and work roles, decision making, analysis, planning, creativity, and mathematical skills. Aphasia is often complicated by depression and changes in the experience of self.

Aphasia compromises the different forms and stages of language comprehension and formation, creating a rich but confusing variety of clinical profiles. Aphasia impairs the understanding, manipulation, or production of language symbols in three sensory modalities: auditory, as in verbal language; visual, as in written language (based on sounds in Western languages and ideograms in some Asian languages)[39] or in hand and face movements in sign language or Morse code;[40] and tactile, as in Braille reading.[41] Patients with aphasia suffer various combinations of impairments for comprehending, associating, and producing the morphological, lexical, and syntactical features of language. These combinations form the clinical aphasia syndromes, which often overlap and change as the disorder progresses or resolves. In addition to the basic language elements, meaning is conveyed by gesture (nonverbal motor acts, such as eye contact, smiling, thumbs-up sign) and prosody (vocal contours that color language, such as rhythm, melody, intonation, and emotion). These paralinguistic features reveal vital information that can be dissociated from the linguistic message.

Disorders of attention, perception, movement, memory, or thought do not cause aphasia. Attentional impairment from delirium and other causes may impair reception or responsiveness to questions, which can be mistaken as impaired comprehension; it may also disrupt organization of linguistic output with tangential and inappropriate responses, cause errors in word selection, and produce writing errors. The fundamental disorder in delirium is not linguistic processing but global dysfunction of sustained attention and working memory, compromising a spectrum of cognitive functions. In aphasia, impaired cognitive as well as linguistic processing underlies auditory comprehension deficits.[42] A perceptual disorder such as blindness prevents visual language comprehension (reading) but does not impair auditory or tactile language comprehension. Motor disorders may cause mutism, *dysarthria* (imperfect articulation), or *dysphonia* (impairment of the voice) but not aphasia. In adults, memory disorders usually spare language function but may impair retrieval of infrequently used words. In young children, acquisition of the lexicon and grammar requires long-term memory. Thus, primary memory disorders in

children may impair language acquisition, but these are developmental disorders, not childhood aphasia. *Thought disorders* usually refers to psychotic states, in which the coherence, sequencing, and content of mental processes are impaired and often overlaid with paranoia and hallucinations. Patients with dementia, frontal lobe disorders, or severe depression may also have disordered thought or ideation but preserved language.

Any injury to the cerebral hemispheres may result in aphasia, but traumatic brain injury and stroke are the most common antecedents; thrombotic, embolic, and hemorrhagic strokes cause aphasia (Table 6–1). Other causes of aphasia are tumors, degenerative dementias (e.g., Alzheimer's disease, Pick's disease), demyelinating disorders, and infections (e.g., herpes simplex encephalitis, with prominent anomia). When traumatic brain injury causes aphasia, the injury often extends beyond the language areas, causing combinations of memory, behavioral, sensorimotor, and coordination deficits. Aphasia affects approximately 2% of patients after traumatic brain injury of the closed type but is common after open trau-

Table 6–1. Major Arterial Distributions and Aphasic Syndromes in Thrombotic and Embolic Strokes

Arterial Territory	Aphasic Syndrome	Common Associated Findings
Internal carotid	Global aphasia*	Hemiparesis, hemisensory loss, hemianopia
Middle cerebral	Global aphasia	Hemiparesis, hemisensory loss, hemianopia
Middle cerebral branches		
Orbital	None or transient Broca's aphasia	Disinhibited, antisocial behavior
Rolandic	Broca's aphasia, dysarthria	Hemiparesis, possible hemisensory loss, depression
Anterior parietal	Conduction aphasia	Hemisensory loss, face
Posterior parietal	Wernicke's aphasia, TSA	Lower quadrantanopia
Angular	Anomia, Wernicke's aphasia, TSA	Lower quadrantanopia, alexia, agraphia
Posterior temporal	Wernicke's aphasia, TSA	Upper quadrantanopia
Anterior temporal	Mild anomia†	Possible amnesia
Anterior cerebral	TMA	Sensorimotor deficit of the leg
Posterior cerebral	Alexia without agraphia	Hemianopia
Lenticulostriate	Impaired language generation, anomia	Hemiparesis, frontal syndrome features
Thalamoperforant	TSA	Amnesia

*Inadequate collateral circulation can cause global aphasia. TMA, transcortical motor aphasia; TSA, transcortical sensory aphasia.
†Severe anomia is common after inferior infarcts of BA 37.

matic brain injury.[43] The classic aphasia syndromes are less distinct in trauma victims than stroke patients.[44] Recovery from aphasia is more likely after trauma than after stroke or other disorders, due in part to the often younger age of trauma victims and the diffuse versus focal nature of the injury. Aphasia usually results from left hemisphere injury. The asymmetrical distribution of language was recognized early,[5,6] and for more than a century left hemisphere language dominance was repeatedly confirmed by observations in right-handed individuals. Perisylvian and other left hemisphere lesions consistently cause aphasia, but identical right-sided lesions do so in only 0.5%–2% of cases.[45] Left hemisphere language dominance is also true for non-sound-based language, such as American Sign Language. Approximately 70% of left-handed persons have left-sided language dominance, and the remainder have language functions located primarily in the right hemisphere or distributed more or less equally across both hemispheres. Thus, approximately 30% of left-handed individuals are likely to suffer language impairment with a right hemisphere injury.[46] Aphasia is usually milder, and recovery more rapid, in left-handed persons regardless of the side of injury than in right-handed persons with a left-sided insult.[47] However, this clinical maxim is not supported by all studies.[48] Many left-handed patients suffer persistent, severe aphasia.

Diagnosis of Aphasia

Aphasia is usually diagnosed when the language disorder is acquired. Auditory, congenital, and developmental disorders must be excluded. Congenital or developmental disorders usually, but not always, cause language impairment when common brain systems are involved (e.g., memory impairment affects language acquisition in childhood). Language regression may occur in patients with autism and pervasive developmental delay[49] and rarely results from interictal epileptiform activity, as in acquired epileptic aphasia.[50] Developmental language disorders remain imprecisely categorized, their pathogenesis poorly defined, and their differential diagnosis extensive.[51] Because handedness predicts cerebral dominance for speech and language (see Handedness, above), its value for diagnosing and localizing

language disorders cannot be overestimated. Clinically, handedness is determined by asking patients which hand they use for writing. Some persons perform all fine and skilled motor functions with the right hand and foot (e.g., writing, sewing, using a knife, cutting with scissors, throwing and kicking a ball), and others write with their right hand but perform many other skilled tasks with their left hand or foot. Patterns of hemispheric specialization in ambidextrous persons may differ from those of strongly right-handed persons. A family history of left handedness is relevant because a left-handed patient from a large family with no other left-handed members is more likely to be strongly left-handed. A history of conversion from natural left handedness to right handedness is also relevant because the language dominance pattern does not usually join the conversion process. Detailed handedness questionnaires are available.[52]

Tests of language function are the foundation for a diagnosis of aphasia. These functions are fluency, paraphasia, comprehension, repetition, naming, reading, writing, and prosody. It usually is easy to determine the answers to two critical questions about language function: Does the patient speak spontaneously? Is the speech fluent? When entering the room, note whether the patient offers a greeting, returns a greeting, speaks only in response to questions, or gives one- or two-word answers. Some patients conceal major language disorders with yes-and-no answers, so hearing the patient speak in sentences is important. Ask open-ended questions: "Why have you come to the hospital?" "What is your typical weekday like?"

Spontaneity is an important concept in behavioral neurology. The absence of motor and speech spontaneity strongly suggests lesions in the frontal lobe, striatum, or reticular activating system, that is, the upper midbrain or diencephalic reticular formation and its ascending projections. Aspontaneous speech often goes unnoticed because the patient is unaware of the problem and makes no complaints. Broca's aphasia and transcortical motor aphasia are characterized by hesitant, effortful speech, usually only in response to a question.

FLUENCY

Fluent speech flows smoothly without word-finding pauses. Nonfluent speech is slow, with fewer than seven words per phrase present in normal speech. (Technically, some definitions specify fewer than 40 words per minute.) Other deficits may include sparse output, often with the use of single words, effortful speech, dysarthria, dysprosody, and agrammatism. Patients with these deficits often struggle to verbalize; their frustrated grimaces and body posture reveal their awareness of the deficit. Patients with nonfluent aphasias omit grammatical (syntactical) words such as prepositions, articles, and adverbs, and word endings such as plurals and tense. Phrase length is reduced (one or two words/phrase) and composed mainly of substantive words.[53]

Patients with fluent aphasia typically speak effortlessly with normal articulation and prosody. Phrase length, or number of words between pauses, is also normal (three to eight words/phrase). Most patients with fluent aphasia have a normal output (100–150 words/min), but in some the output may be excessive (>200 words/min) or excessively persistent.[54] Fluent aphasia is marked by "empty" speech, containing grammatical words but lacking substantive (lexical) words, as in "Yes, you know, of course, and well yes, as a matter of fact, if you did, yes." Word-finding pauses punctuate the speech of patients with fluent aphasia and are often followed by circumlocutory or nonspecific responses (e.g., "it," "thing"). Patients exhibit paragrammatism with incorrect verb tenses, prefixes, suffixes, inflections, conditional clauses, and prepositional phrases.[55]

Differentiating fluent and nonfluent speech in aphasia is critical in determining whether the lesion is anterior or posterior. Fluency is severely disrupted by some lesions anterior to the rolandic fissure (central sulcus), and most patients with fluent, paraphasic speech have lesions posterior to this landmark.[56,57] Many patients with posterior lesions are acutely nonfluent during the early stages of aphasia. Children with both anterior and posterior lesions usually have nonfluent aphasia, although dysarthria and agrammatism are usually found only with anterior lesions.[58]

Information about articulation, prosody, and paraphasias is revealed by spontaneous speech. Prosody, which also includes a nonaffective (propositional) component, is the chief affective component of speech and introduces subtle shades of meaning or completely changes the impact of a statement[59,60] (see Prosody, below). In a proposed clinical–anatomical correlation of prosody,[59] an anterior right hemisphere lesion (analogue of Broca's area) impairs spontaneous prosody (speech is flat, monotonous, and lacks the emotion and intonation of normal speech), and a posterior right hemisphere lesion (analogue of Wernicke's area) impairs comprehension of prosody; that is, patients are unable to distinguish subtle shades of meaning in the speech of other persons.

PARAPHASIA

Paraphasia, the erroneous substitution of syllables or words, is common in fluent aphasia. *Literal* (phonemic) *paraphasia* is the replacement of letters or syllables in otherwise correct word usages. It means the addition, omission, substitution, or displacement of a phoneme, for example, "John rode my *d*icycle" or "Steve *s*tew the ball." Phonetic errors are the impaired execution of phoneme production and are commonly seen in aphasias produced by anterior lesions. Although they can give rise to "articulatory paraphasias," they are distinct from the linguistic deviations of phonemic paraphasias.[61] *Verbal* (semantic) *paraphasia* is word substitution, often of words related to the intended word, as in "John drove my wheel" and "Steve threw the glove." When anomia is present, superordinate words are often substituted for more specific words. Semantic paraphasias may be composed of morphemes that are inappropriate for the context (e.g., "He was the best on *heavenly* and earth") or may be linguistically incorrect (e.g., "The *clamorific* Martian queen").

COMPREHENSION

Test comprehension after observing spontaneous speech. If the patient constructs well-formulated answers to questions, comprehension is usually normal. It is wrong to assume that comprehension is normal because the patient's speech is verbose and fluent (as in Wernicke's aphasia) or to diagnose a comprehension deficit because the patient cannot verbally respond to a question or command (comprehension in aphasia is often better than tests suggest).[45] A common mistake is asking the patient to perform a learned motor command (e.g., "Show me how you salute"), which also assesses praxis, or a sequence of commands (e.g., "Point to the ceiling, touch your nose, and point to the window"), which also assesses memory and frontal sequencing functions.[62] Another mistake is overestimating language comprehension by providing meaningful nonverbal cues through inflection, tone, or facial expression.

Suspect comprehension deficits if the patient talks but makes little sense, appears confused, or moves from one topic to another without completing a thought. Test comprehension in a mute or aphasic patient by asking the patient to point to body parts, an array of objects placed in front of him or her, or objects in the room. In quadriplegic patients, test comprehension by asking the patient to make eye movements or blinks. In general, asking yes-or-no questions is useful. For example, "Is it true that South American helicopters eat their young?" If the patient says "no," then ask "Do helicopters eat their young in Europe?" If the answer is again "no," ask if that was a silly question or, alternatively, ask "Do two pounds of flour weigh more than one?" and observe the patient for hesitation or uncertainty in the answer. Normally, a person will not ponder long about a nonsense question. Undue hesitation suggests impaired comprehension. The patient has a 50% chance of guessing the correct answer to a yes-or-no question, so ask at least three or four.

REPETITION

Ask a patient with suspected aphasia to repeat words, phrases, and sentences of increasing complexity. With aphasia, the repetition of multisyllabic, difficult-to-articulate phrases ("Methodist Episcopal," "The phantom soared across the foggy heath") and long sentences ("The Tuscan hills are dotted by cypresses and olive trees, whose green shades dance to the sun's music") is challenging. Phrases with multiple relationships ("My mother's brother has had business difficulties with his partners") or complex syntactical words ("There are no ifs, ands, or buts about it") are the most difficult to repeat. If the phrases are repeated correctly, repetition and fluency are normal. Listen carefully for omissions (e.g., plural endings), additions, perseverations, paraphasias, and grammatical errors.

Repetition is usually impaired by lesions of the anterior or posterior perisylvian language areas or their interconnections. Preserved repetition has little localizing value in mild aphasia, but in moderate to severe aphasia, it is indicative of transcortical aphasia with lesions outside the perisylvian language areas. Such patients often have echolalia, echoing phrases or sentences and compulsively completing an incomplete phrase such as "Roses are red, violets are *(blank)*."[63] When repetition is impaired out of proportion to verbal output or language comprehension, conduction aphasia is likely present.

NAMING

Test the patient's ability to name by listening to spontaneous speech for word-finding pauses, circumlocutions, or the use of nonspecific words, such as *it, thing,* and *you know.* (Circumlocution is a circuitous, rambling search for the missing target word or descriptive substitution for objects, such as *hot* for *stove,* or functions, such as *fill my belly* for *eat.*) Test confrontational naming by pointing to objects and asking the patient to name them. Include various categories (e.g., body parts, clothing, appliances, colors) and levels of difficulty (e.g., commonly used words, such as *nose, belt, television, red;* less commonly used words, such as *shin, watch crystal, second hand, tie knot, belt buckle;* and uncommonly used words, such as *watch stem* or *stethoscope*). Patients normally have the least difficulty with superordinate words (e.g., *animal* or *bird* vs. *cardinal*) but may have trouble naming object parts, especially those not commonly used in everyday speech. Avoid cultural bias in selecting items. For example, someone who never wears a necktie may have never heard the word *knot* used in reference to a tie. If the patient fails to name an object pointed to by the examiner but selects the correct word from a short list, comprehension is normal but naming is not. The examiner may assist patients in producing the missing word by phonemic cueing, that is, giving the initial phoneme of the desired word, such as /n/ for *nose,* or by contextual cueing, that is, giving a sentence in which the word is missing, such as "I smell with my *(blank)*." The patient's ability to provide a name in response to a verbal definition or a verbal definition in response to a target word helps to define abstractional thought in word retrieval. Test the patient's ability to name items presented tactilely and auditorily (e.g., touching a key and jangling keys) and to produce not only nouns but also verbs or adjectives to visual confrontation (e.g., *small glass* vs. *large glass*). Finally, testing word retrieval in both spoken and written responses occasionally reveals a dissociation,[64] which may have therapeutic implications.

Naming errors occur with most aphasias and have limited localizing value.[65] However, positron emission tomography (PET) and fMRI studies implicate the left temporal neocortex anterior and inferior to Wernicke's area, the left anterior insula, and the left inferior frontoparietal area in naming different objects (Fig. 6–8).[66,67]

READING

Ask the patient with aphasia to read a few words or sentences aloud. If the patient cannot read aloud but can comprehend written material, test reading comprehension of a menu, newspaper, or magazine with questions that can be answered by nodding the head "yes" or "no." Patients with alexia caused by parietotemporal lesions are unable to recognize words spelled aloud by the examiner, in contrast to those who have occipital alexia (without agraphia), who comprehend well through the auditory route.[68] Alexia resulting from brain damage is usually accompanied by errors in oral reading.

WRITING

Ask the patient to perform a series of writing tasks of increasing difficulty, ranging from his or her signature to writing single words to dictation, and to compose descriptive passages about such subjects as the job, favorite foods, or the weather. When spoken language is aphasic, writing is invariably aphasic. Therefore, the testing of writing is an excellent screen of language function. A patient who can write a short paragraph normally is not aphasic. Disruption of motor or language systems by an acquired brain injury may cause agraphia. Examine written output for mechanics (e.g., large, poorly formed letters in Broca's aphasia), syntax, semantic content, spelling, and spatial distribution.

PROSODY

To test affective (emotional) comprehension, determine the patient's ability to recognize the examiner's emotional tone (e.g., happy, sad, angry, neutral, questioning). (Let patients with nonfluent aphasia select between a set of spoken choices or, ideally, a set of labeled, simple line drawings.) To test affective repetition, ask the patient to repeat the word describing the examiner's mood and determine whether the repetition communicates the correct affect. To test affective expression, ask the patient to produce an emotional tone in a sentence that the examiner states in a neutral manner; the patient is allowed up to three chances to produce the desired effect. Having the patient listen to a tape recording of affective voices or view drawings depicting various affects and identify the affect presented provides a more formal, systematic assessment of prosody.

Localization and Clinical Patterns of Aphasia

Neuropathological and modern neuroimaging techniques show that specific clusters of cerebral signs are consistently associated with damage of a particular brain area. However, the common practice of correlating lesion site and functional deficit to normal function in a specific, circumscribed brain area is incorrect. Language production and functions, such as assembling phonemes into words and words into sentences, involve multiple brain areas organized into a functional network. Most aphasias are easily but imprecisely localized and diagnosed. The clinical findings in an aphasic syndrome vary. Language disorders do not strictly obey anatomical landmarks. However, an examination of language comprehension and production uncovers recognizable and reproducible clinical patterns. The semantic organization of verbs and nouns in the brain differs, with the frontal areas being more critical in verb generation and the temporoparietal areas more critical in noun generation.[10] Analysis of these clinical patterns, along with behavioral and other neurological signs and symptoms, produces fairly accurate localization of the lesion causing the aphasia.

Aphasias are classified as cortical, mixed cortical and subcortical, and subcortical. There are eight forms of cortical aphasia: Broca's aphasia, transcortical motor aphasia, mixed transcortical aphasia, and global aphasia (all marked by nonfluent spontaneous speech), as well as Wernicke's aphasia, conduction aphasia, transcortical sensory aphasia, and anomic aphasia (all marked by fluent speech). Two-thirds of aphasia cases can be classified as one of these cortical forms. Most of the remaining cases are mixed cortical and subcortical aphasias (see Subcortical Aphasia, below). Often, one aphasic disorder evolves, or resolves, into another. For example, global aphasia might change into Broca's aphasia or Broca's aphasia might change into transcortical motor aphasia.

BROCA'S APHASIA

Broca's aphasia, caused by left frontal lobe lesions, is characterized by nonfluent, effortful speech with relatively preserved comprehension. The clinical features of Broca's aphasia are summarized in Table 6–2. The terms *motor aphasia* and *expressive aphasia* are not synonyms for Broca's (anterior) aphasia because speech output (expression) is altered in some way in most aphasic, and many nonaphasic, disorders; avoid this terminology as it fosters confusion.

Patients may be mute at the onset of Broca's aphasia or may produce only single syllables or words; in some cases, a reiterated word or phrase forms a verbal stereotypy. Subsequently, the sparse speech is aspontaneous, slow, effortful, and interrupted by pauses that often overshadow the output. Patients often produce fewer than a dozen words a minute. Speech automaticity is lost as the fluid stream of words disintegrates into individual, strained words. Impaired articulation, with phonetic distortions and impaired melodic intonation and inflection, produces flat and unnatural but usually intelligible speech. Patients automatically produce expletives (e.g., *shit, damn it*) that are correctly articulated, phonemically structured, intonated, and used in appropriate settings (e.g., stubbing one's toe, inability to speak). John Hughlings Jackson,[69] who first recognized this phenomenon in 1878, postulated that the right hemisphere produced this nondeliberate, emotional verbalization. Patients with Broca's aphasia are more articulate and fluent in producing overlearned serial speech, as in counting or reciting the alphabet or months of the year, than in generating spontaneous speech.

Verbal output in Broca's aphasia is called "telegraphic" because patients utter substantive nouns and verbs that carry the meaning of the sentence but omit grammatical connecting words such as prepositions, articles, conjunc-

Table 6–2. **Clinical Features of Broca's Aphasia**

Feature	Observation
Linguistic deficits	Agrammatism: phonemic, morphemic, and syntactic levels
Speech	Aspontaneous, nonfluent, dysarthric, dysprodic, telegraphic, effortful, some phonemic paraphasias
Comprehension, auditory and written	Relatively normal, deficit in complex grammatical structures
Repetition	Impaired
Pointing to named items	Good
Naming	Impaired but improved with cues
Reading	
Aloud	Impaired (similar to speech, see above)
Comprehension	Good, but deficit in complex grammatical structures
Writing	Impaired, poorly formed letters; right-sided hemiparesis often forces writing with left hand
Associated neurological findings	Right-sided hemiparesis; variably, right-sided hemisensory loss
Behavioral findings	Depression, apraxia
Localization of lesion	Left posterior–inferior frontal cortex and underlying white matter
Pathology, typical	Stroke, upper division of left middle cerebral artery; hemorrhage, tumor, trauma

tions, and adverbs. For example, the question "Do you want to go to the store with me?" might come out as "go . . . store . . . me." Nouns are used most often, followed by verbs and adverbs; grammatical connecting words are usually omitted. A hallmark of Broca's aphasia, this telegraphic speech pattern reflects *agrammatism*, the inability to organize written or spoken words into sentences according to grammatical rules, and the misuse of, or failure to use, grammatical words. Grammatical words include the small words that connect sentence components, such as prepositions (e.g., *from, to*), conjunctions (e.g., *and, or, but, if*), and auxiliary verbs that convey tense. When patients with Broca's aphasia act out sentences that can only be understood by syntax, such as "The car is pushed by the truck," their interpretation is correct only half the time.

Repetition is impaired but less severely than spontaneous speech. Thus, although patients with Broca's aphasia can comprehend a sentence such as "The spy fled to Greece," they are unable to repeat it verbatim. Phrases and sentences with many small grammatical words ("There are no ifs, ands, or buts about it") or difficult articulatory sequences ("Methodist Episcopal") are most difficult for these patients to repeat. Sound or syllable substitutions, literal (phonemic) paraphasias, often occur in spontaneous speech and repetition. Patients with Broca's aphasia cannot write normally with either hand, and their writing contains poorly formed and oversized letters. Words are misspelled, letters are omitted, and grammatical errors are numerous.

The "tip-of-the-tongue" phenomenon, in which patients utter the initial letter or syllable of a word but cannot complete the word, is common in Broca's aphasia. Confrontational naming is usually impaired. Difficulties with word finding are often improved by cueing. Both phonetic cues, as in giving the patient the first sound or syllable, and contextual cues, such as "I take my coffee with cream and *(blank),*" are helpful.

Comprehension of auditory and written information is relatively normal in Broca's aphasia. The meaning of nouns and verbs is preserved. When comprehension is impaired, the deficits may be subtle or readily apparent. Subtle deficits may be revealed by testing complex grammatical relationships ("Is it true that my mother's brother's sister is a female?") or reversible passive sentences ("The man had ar-

gued with the shopkeeper"). Comprehension requires the interpretation of lexical and grammatical (syntactical) components of language. The lexical components (nouns, verbs, adjectives) relate the sentence to the physical world, and the grammatical components (word order, articles, and inflection) provide specific meaning. Therefore, "mother's sister's brother" and "mother's brother's sister" are different people and sexes. Damage to cortical areas that sustain lexical processing causes syntactical comprehension deficits.[70,71] Patients with Broca's aphasia have comprehension difficulties with noninflected reversible passive sentences, such as the foregoing, in which the action ("argued") could be attributed to either party ("man" or "shopkeeper"). In contrast, these patients comprehend nonreversible passive or active sentences, such as "The boy kicked the ball."

Sequencing and planning functions are impaired in Broca's aphasia. These patients do fairly well at pointing to a named object but often are unable to point to a series of three objects in sequence. They can order word groups correctly to form a logical sequence of actions but cannot order similar word groups into a syntactically well-formed sentence.[72] Patients with dorsolateral prefrontal lesions perform in an opposite manner.

Extensive left frontal lobe lesions, reaching back to the rolandic fissure and involving the underlying white matter, produce the classic syndrome of Broca's aphasia.[57,73] Persistent, severe nonfluency is associated with white matter lesions in both the rostral portion of the medial subcallosal fasciculus, connecting the cingulate gyrus and the supplementary motor area (SMA) with the caudate, and the areas adjacent to the lateral ventricle body, deep to the sensorimotor cortex for the mouth (Fig. 6–2). The medial subcallosal fasciculus is important for the preparation, initiation, and limbic aspects of speech; the periventricular white matter is critical for motor execution and sensory feedback in spontaneous speech.[57]

Broca's aphasia must be distinguished from Broca's area aphasia (Fig. 6–3), a syndrome of dysarthria and resolving aphasia, and from aphemia, a nonaphasic defect of hypophonia and dysarthria.[73–75] Broca's aphasia is produced by lesions of not only Broca's area (posterior portion of the inferior frontal gyrus, Brodmann's areas [BAs] 44 and 45) but also adjacent frontal areas (BAs 9, 46, 47), under-

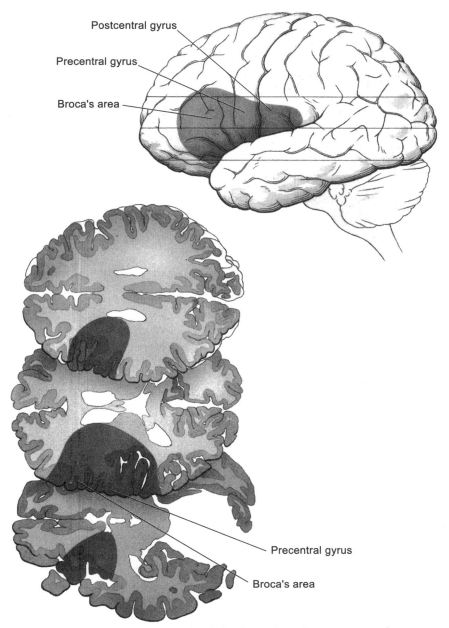

Postcentral gyrus

Precentral gyrus

Broca's area

Precentral gyrus

Broca's area

Figure 6–2. Lesion site associated with the chronic form of severe Broca's aphasia.

lying white matter, and basal ganglia (left head of the caudate and putamen). All of these areas, as well as the sensorimotor areas for face and larynx and the parietal areas (BAs 7, 39, 40) connected with Broca's area, form a network for ordering linguistic elements in time and space, that is, sequencing phonemes into words and words into sentences.[75] In contrast, the lesions in Broca's area aphasia are restricted to Broca's area and spare much of this network. Mutism may be followed by mild aphasia, which in most cases largely resolves[73] despite the selective activation of Broca's area in syntactical tasks.[76]

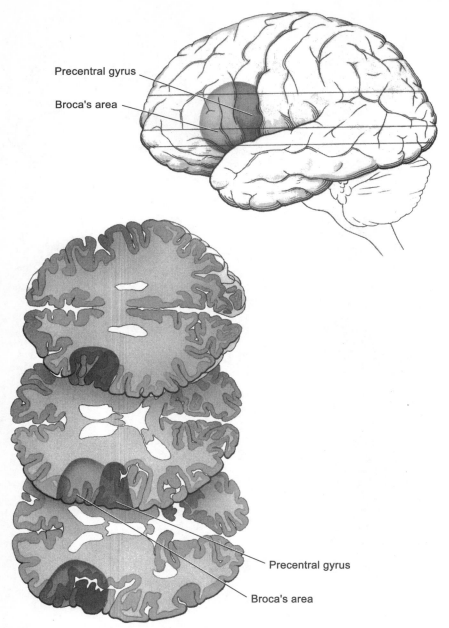

Precentral gyrus

Broca's area

Precentral gyrus

Broca's area

Figure 6–3. Lesion site associated with Broca's area aphasia. Lesions limited to Broca's area cause chronic transcortical motor aphasia. Lesions limited to the precentral gyrus (including primary motor and premotor areas) cause chronic aphemia.

The most common cause of Broca's aphasia is embolic or thrombotic infarction in the distribution of the superior branch of the middle cerebral artery (MCA). Other causes include tumors, traumatic brain injury, infections, and degenerative disorders with isolated aphasia (primary progressive aphasia).[77] In the acute stage of Broca's aphasia resulting from a stroke, right-sided hemiparesis, affecting the face and arm more than the leg, is usually present. When hemiparesis is absent, the aphasia is often transient. Right-sided hemisensory loss is common. Ideomotor apraxia of the left arm and leg (sympathetic apraxia) and orofacial muscles is often present.

Depression occurs in many aphasic patients with small to moderate-sized anterior lesions.[78] Goldstein, in 1948,[79] first described the "catastrophic reaction" to left frontal lobe injuries, in which nonfluent aphasia is associated with profound depression, anxiety, and withdrawal. This affective response is likely mediated by the right hemisphere in response to the profound functional loss. The association between poststroke depression and anterior lesions in the language-dominant hemisphere appears most relevant for patients with typical frontal or occipital asymmetries.[80] After a large stroke, affective symptoms may develop without a lateralized predominance[78] and are common with right-sided[81] lesions.

WERNICKE'S APHASIA

Wernicke's aphasia presents with dramatic linguistic and behavioral features but may be unrecognized when mild or incomplete. The absence of hemiparesis, sensory loss, or other neurological signs and symptoms adds to the risk of underdiagnosis or misdiagnosis, although right superior quadrantanopia or homonymous hemianopia may be present (Table 6–3). Patients with Wernicke's aphasia have fluent speech with normal prosody and inflection, often speak excessively (logorrhea or verborrhea) and effortlessly with paraphasias and neologisms (newly coined words), and have impaired comprehension.[58,75,82] In some cases, patients speak in hesitant, brief phrases, producing a "pseudononfluency." Like patients with Broca's aphasia, those with Wernicke's aphasia are unable to assemble phonemes, repeat sentences, or name things.

Acutely, patients may be mute before the onset of the characteristic fluent speech filled with empty phrases, circumlocutions, and paraphasias. To an English speaker, a foreigner with Wernicke's aphasia, speaking an unfamiliar language, would sound similar to a foreigner with normal speech. As with other anomic patients, patients with Wernicke's aphasia frequently use nonspecific and "filler" words, such as *thing, it, that,* and *you know.* Phonemic and word choice errors may render speech incomprehensible. Paragrammatism refers to several characteristic components of Wernicke's aphasia: abundance of grammatical words (often connectors such as *if, and,* or *but*), underuse of meaningful substantive words (nouns and verbs), errors in selecting grammatical elements, and failure to delimit a sentence with a pause.[45] Paraphasias are common in the spontaneous speech of patients with Wernicke's aphasia, including semantic paraphasias (word substitutions) and phonemic paraphasias (sound substitutions). When several phonemic errors are combined in the same word, unintelligible neologisms, such as *thimplay* for *simple,* are produced. Jargon aphasia refers to fluent, well-articulated, but incomprehensible speech, which is often due to

Table 6–3. **Clinical Features of Wernicke's Aphasia**

Feature	Observation
Linguistic deficits	Phonological discrimination: phonemic and semantic levels
Speech	Fluent, normal prosody and articulation, frequent semantic and phonemic paraphasias
Comprehension, auditory and written	Impaired
Repetition	Impaired
Naming	Impaired, paraphasic errors
Reading aloud	Impaired (similar to speech, see above)
Writing	Well-formed letters but meaningless content
Associated neurological findings	Right superior quadrantanopsia; normal fields or, rarely, hemianopia
Behavioral findings	Unconcern, euphoria, confusion, agitation, irritability, suspiciousness
Pathology, typical	Stroke, lower division of left middle cerebral artery; hemorrhage, tumor, trauma

abundant neologisms.[83] Wernicke's aphasia is less common in children than adults, and children tend to be less fluent but to recover more fully than aphasic adults.[84,85]

Verbal comprehension deficit is the central linguistic component of Wernicke's aphasia but is easily overlooked if not specifically tested. The comprehension deficit may be due to deficits in auditory processing or analysis, fluency of conceptual thinking, or other cognitive processes.[86] Despite impaired comprehension of spoken language, after the acute stage, patients often derive meaning from nonverbal cues such as speech tone, facial expression, and hand and body gestures. Patients may display fatigability of comprehension, initially comprehending several words and then failing to understand additional words of similar difficulty or previously comprehended words. The best test of comprehension in Wernicke's aphasia is a series of nonsense questions asked in a serious, inquisitive manner ("Do two pounds of flour weigh more than one?" "Do helicopters in South America eat their young?"). Patients may have difficulty discriminating phonemes, especially closely related phonemes. Some patients are able to follow commands involving the axial musculature ("Close your eyes," "Stand") but not the extremities ("Flip a coin"). Auditory and reading comprehension are usually impaired to a similar degree; but occasionally one, usually reading comprehension, is relatively spared.[87,88] Test auditory and reading comprehension separately[89] because preservation of one modality may open a rare therapeutic window in which a patient who comprehends written material can learn to communicate with sign language.

Naming and repetition are impaired in Wernicke's aphasia. In both spontaneous speech and confrontation, word finding is severely deficient, and patients may produce bizarre, paraphasic naming errors and perseverate. Comprehension and naming deficits often prevent self-monitoring systems from recognizing the errors. Reading aloud is usually impaired but may be relatively intact with or without some preservation of reading comprehension. Writing is legible but incomprehensible, with the same emptiness, circumlocution, and paraphasic errors that contaminate speech.

Acutely, mood and affect are often prominently altered. Some patients may lack awareness of or concern for the condition and may appear euphoric. Others may act irritable, angry, paranoid, or violent.[90] These behavioral changes may be caused by limbic dysfunction with interrupted neocortical input to preserved medial temporal areas, "emotional comprehension" that something is very wrong, fear and self-referential thoughts because the patients cannot understand what others are saying to them, or disruption of the internal thought that guides behavior.

Wernicke's aphasia may be misdiagnosed as a psychiatric disorder, as illustrated by one of our cases:

A neurological consultation was requested for a 64-year-old man because psychological testing raised the question of "organicity." Family members brought him to the emergency department because of confusion and irritability. The man had no history of a psychiatric disorder and was well until several hours before admission. He was hospitalized on a psychiatric unit for a month, with a diagnosis of atypical psychosis. When the neurologist asked why he was in the hospital, he replied "I don't think that's fair, no, not that thing." He spoke fluently with slightly pressured speech and paraphasias. When asked "Do helicopters in South America eat their young?" he replied "I should hope so." Neuroimaging showed a left posterior, superior temporal lucency consistent with infarction.

The confusion between Wernicke's aphasia and psychiatric illness partly reflects the paucity of neurological signs in the former. The patient's behavior is clearly different and often characterized by family members as "bizarre" or "confused." Fluent aphasia usually can be distinguished from delirium, psychosis, or dementia because the behavioral changes develop suddenly without previous evidence of personality or mood disorders, patients are usually older, and precipitating events, such as the death of a spouse, are absent; most importantly, language examination is diagnostic. The speech patterns in schizophrenia and Wernicke's aphasia are different: responses to open-ended questions are shorter in aphasia, paraphasias are common in aphasia and rare in schizophrenia, and vague responses occur in both disorders but are due to word-finding problems in aphasia and circumstantiality in psychosis; in addition, bizarre and delusional themes are components of psychosis.[90]

Wernicke's area is situated in the posterior third of the left superior temporal gyrus (BA 22), and lesions in this region (Fig. 6–4) and

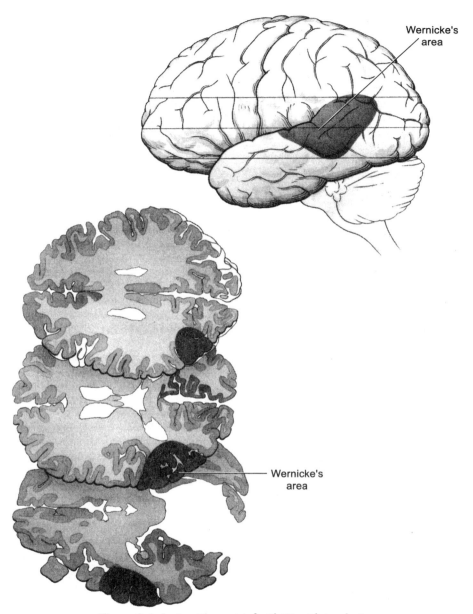

Figure 6–4. Lesion site associated with Wernicke's aphasia.

the adjacent temporal and parietal regions (BA 37, 39, 40) are associated with Wernicke's aphasia.[91] Subcortical lesions in the temporal isthmus interrupt input to Wernicke's area, causing Wernicke's aphasia.[92] Wernicke's area processes speech sounds but is not the site of auditory comprehension or word selection. These processes involve more widespread cortical areas. Speech sounds processed by Wer-

nicke's area are translated into words and then used to evoke conceptual and associative meanings (e.g., *grandmother* is a class of people and a person associated with facial features, emotional valence, and so on). Word selection is accomplished by a network that utilizes Wernicke's area to form an internal auditory representation after the word has been selected.

Lesions confined to Wernicke's area usually

produce persistent aphasia but occasionally cause no language deficits.[91,93] However, when the characteristic features of Wernicke's aphasia are present, lesions are reliably found in the superior posterior temporal region.[94] Involvement of the posteriorly contiguous infrasylvian parietal lobe (supramarginal and angular gyri) is common in these patients and contributes to jargon aphasia and alexia, that is, failure to comprehend written material.[73,94]

The most common cause of Wernicke's aphasia is stroke, usually an embolus to the inferior division of the left MCA. Hemorrhages, especially posterior putaminal hemorrhages extending into the temporal lobe isthmus, also produce Wernicke's aphasia,[95] as do tumors, abscesses, and other lesions involving this area. Epileptic discharges may also produce symptoms of this aphasic syndrome. Partial status epilepticus rarely presents as Wernicke's aphasia.[96]

Patients with Wernicke's aphasia usually recover some auditory comprehension, although the prognosis is less favorable than in Broca's aphasia. Good prognostic features for recovery are mild initial deficit, small lesion, relative sparing of white matter and supramarginal and angular gyri, and, to a lesser degree, relative sparing of the superior and middle temporal gyri.[94,97] Slow presentation of auditory material may improve comprehension.[98] As patients improve, they often acquire insight into the language deficits and become depressed. Paranoia may emerge as a late sequela.

Although theoretically distinct, the rare syndrome of pure word deafness and Wernicke's aphasia often overlap. With pure word deafness, the comprehension deficit is restricted to spoken words.[99] Pure tone hearing is normal. With left-sided lesions, comprehension of nonverbal sounds, such as music, animal vocalizations, and sirens, is preserved. In pure word deafness, spontaneous speech, writing, reading, and naming are intact; only auditory verbal comprehension and repetition are impaired. Mild paraphasic errors in speech or naming indicate the incomplete separation of word deafness and aphasia. In its pure form, word deafness is not an aphasic disorder but a form of auditory agnosia in which input from the primary auditory cortex (Heschl's gyrus) is unable to reach Wernicke's area. In pure word deafness, anatomical lesions conform to this model and are found unilaterally in the left temporal region (isthmus, posterior insula, and superior gyrus) or bilaterally in the subcortical temporal regions.[100,101]

CONDUCTION APHASIA

Conduction aphasia, marked by disproportionate impairment in repeating spoken language, accounts for 5%–10% of all aphasias.[82] The clinical characteristics of conduction aphasia are shown in Table 6–4. As with Wernicke's aphasia, the diagnosis is hampered by a relative paucity of associated neurological changes, although right-sided facial weakness, face and arm somatosensory changes, or a visual field cut may be present. In addition, as in Wernicke's aphasia, the speech patterns in schizophrenia and conduction aphasia are different (see Wernicke's Aphasia, above). In conduction aphasia, spontaneous speech is usually fluent with frequent literal (phonemic) paraphasias, but word-finding pauses may be present. In some cases, hesitations, broken melody (*dysprosody*), and phonemic paraphasias suggest Broca's aphasia. However, preserved grammar and articulation, abundant phonemic paraphasias, and absence of hemiparesis distinguish conduction aphasias with decreased fluency from Broca's aphasia.

Good comprehension of spoken language is a prerequisite for a diagnosis of conduction aphasia. As in Broca's aphasia, comprehension may be entirely normal or impaired only for grammatical components, such as understanding active versus passive sentences or sentences with indirect objects and embedded clauses. However, patients with conduction aphasia have no comprehension difficulties in normal conversation. Moderately impaired comprehension and fluent speech suggest Wernicke's aphasia. In conduction aphasia, unlike Wernicke's aphasia, patients produce fewer words and pause longer between words. These staccato interruptions give rise to a dysprosodic pattern that may cause confusion with a nonfluent aphasia.

Marked impairment of repetition with preserved comprehension is the essence of conduction aphasia. Difficulty in repeating spoken language stands out against a background of fluent, or near fluent, conversational speech. Some patients have difficulty repeating single words; others can repeat simple phrases (e.g., "the boy ran") but not more complex phrases or sentences (e.g., "The spy fled to Greece,"

Table 6–4. **Clinical Features of Conduction Aphasia**

Feature	Observation
Linguistic deficits	Repetition: phonemic level
Speech	Fluent, frequent paraphasias, usually literal; possible hesitation
Comprehension, auditory and written	Normal or mildly impaired
Repetition	Impaired
Pointing to named items	Normal to mildly impaired
Naming	Mild to moderately impaired
Reading aloud	Usually impaired (similar to speech, see above)
Writing	Impaired
Associated neurological findings	Possible right-sided hemisensory loss and hemianopia; uncommonly, right-sided hemiparesis
Behavioral findings	Possible apraxia: buccofacial, bilateral limb
Localization of lesion	Left temporoparietal area
Pathology, typical	Stroke, upper or lower division of left middle cerebral artery or borderzone; tumor

"The phantom soared across the foggy heath"). The phonemic switches in repetition are characterized by simplification, that is, the use of primary, easily produced language sounds, and by alterations in articulatory stress and changes in consonants or, rarely, vowels.[102] Patients with conduction aphasia cannot correctly assemble phonemes or recall auditory sequences, which contributes to the repetition deficit.[75] Conduction aphasia often emerges 1–2 weeks after a stroke. Unlike in Wernicke's aphasia, repetition improves as the patient recovers and may leave only anomia in its wake.

Confrontational naming is usually impaired. Errors may be due to phonemic and, occasionally, verbal paraphasias, as well as anomic word-finding difficulties. The following discourse is from one of our patients with conduction aphasia:

Examiner: Tell me about your illness.
Patient: That fib . . . bibrill . . . bibill . . . bibrill-tatin . . . that funny beating, fast, of my heart. They sway that's it.
Examiner: Atrial fibrillation?
Patient: Yes. That's it. It's done all of this. This sss . . . ssst . . . ssst . . . strake."

Reading aloud is usually abnormal, with paraphasias and hesitation, but reading comprehension is quite good. Significant impairment of reading comprehension suggests that pure conduction aphasia is accompanied by alexia or impaired comprehension, produced,

respectively, by posterior extension of the lesion or involvement of Wernicke's area. Writing is typically impaired, with paraphasias, errors in spelling and word order, and, in some cases, severe inability to express thoughts in writing (agraphia). Buccofacial and limb apraxia may be present.

In 1874, Wernicke[7] postulated that a lesion in the insula would disconnect the anterior (Broca's) and posterior (Wernicke's) language areas, thus causing conduction aphasia, a claim finding modern-day support.[75] Later, Wernicke[103] conceded to von Monakow that a lesion in the arcuate fasciculus is responsible for impaired repetition. However, the arcuate fasciculus need not be involved as lesions in the insula and nearby white matter may cause conduction aphasia.[90,91,104–106] Moreover, repetition may be spared in the presence of arcuate fasciculus lesions.[107] The most common lesion sites, located in the left hemisphere, are in the supramarginal gyrus (BA 40) and subjacent white matter (including the arcuate fasciculus)[3,105] and the insula, primary auditory cortex, and nearby white matter.[83,108,109] (Fig. 6–5). Isolated lesions of the left posterior insula occur in patients with conduction aphasia,[110] impair speech initiation[111] or repetition, damage of the adjacent temporoparietal language cortex or subcortical fibers may be responsible.

Rarely, isolated lesions in the arcuate fasciculus, as found in patients with multiple sclerosis, cause conduction aphasia.[112] Widespread

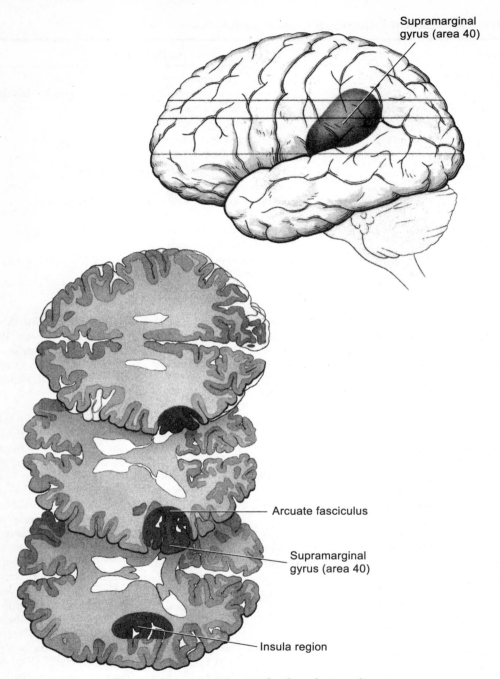

Figure 6–5. Lesion site associated with conduction aphasia.

glucose hypometabolism in temporal and parietal regions, observed on PET, suggests the importance of both cortical and white matter lesions;[113] cortical destruction or disconnection can cause conduction aphasia. Rarely, conduc-

tion aphasia develops when an intact language comprehension area in the right temporal lobe is disconnected from the motor speech areas in the left hemisphere.[114]

Stroke is the most common cause of conduction aphasia, although other structural lesions in these locations are also implicated. Electrical stimulation of the posterior superior temporal gyrus elicits transient conduction aphasia, further supporting the role of cortical, as well as white matter, lesions in conduction aphasia.[106,115]

GLOBAL APHASIA

Moderate to severe impairment of all language functions is known as *global aphasia*. This common syndrome, accounting for roughly a quarter of all aphasias, represents a combination of anterior and posterior aphasic disorders (Table 6–5). Acutely, the patient is mute or limited to groans. Speech is nonfluent, effortful, and sparse. Automatic (nondeliberate) speech with emotional content is often preserved, as in Broca's aphasia. In addition, automated speech sequences, such as counting or reciting the months of the year or the days of the week, are relatively preserved, once they are initiated by the examiner. Patients are often able to hum or sing common melodies and songs (e.g., "Happy Birthday"). Auditory comprehension is usually limited to common nouns, verbs, and phrases (e.g., "Thank you"). Grammatical words and complex grammatical structures are poorly understood. The severe impairment of comprehension prevents testing of praxis (to command but not to imitation) and other higher cognitive functions. Patients with global aphasia are unable to read, write, or name. This syndrome often evolves into Broca's aphasia.

Global aphasia is usually caused by a stroke involving the territory of the entire dominant MCA, resulting from occlusion of the internal carotid artery or the proximal MCA (Table 6–1). Dense right-sided hemiparesis, hemisensory loss, and hemianopia often accompany global aphasia. Patients may be lethargic during the acute stage, and as cerebral edema progresses, some patients lapse into coma after 24–96 hours. A single lesion encompassing the frontal, parietal, and temporal lobes, as well as the insula and basal ganglia, is usually responsible.[104,116,117] Recovery of language and motor function is very poor in patients with single large lesions. Global aphasia caused by dominant frontal lobe lesions extending to the insula and basal ganglia often evolves into severe Broca's aphasia.[75,116,118] Occasionally, patients have discrete, noncontiguous anterior and posterior lesions or large putaminal hemorrhages.[119,120] Global aphasia resulting from lesions in the thalamic region has a poor prognosis.[121] Very rarely, a subcortical stroke with lesions in the putamen, posterior internal capsule, temporal isthmus, and periventricular white matter produces global aphasia.[122] Large tumors in the dominant hemisphere also cause global aphasia, especially when cerebral edema is present.

Global aphasia may occur without hemiparesis but is usually accompanied by right-sided hyperreflexia, Babinski's sign, and upper extremity drift. Lesions involve the language cortex but spare the precentral gyrus and descending pyramidal pathways. This disorder is most often associated with separate lesions in frontal and temporoparietal regions, usually

Table 6–5. **Clinical Features of Global Aphasia**

Feature	Observation
Speech	Mute or nonfluent and telegraphic
Comprehension, auditory and written	Impaired
Repetition	Impaired
Naming	Impaired
Reading aloud	Impaired (similar to speech, see above)
Writing	Impaired
Associated neurological findings	Right-sided hemiparesis,° hemisensory loss, hemianopia
Behavioral findings	Lethargy, decreased attention
Pathology, typical	Stroke, internal carotid artery or proximal middle cerebral artery; hemorrhage, tumor

°Global aphasia without hemiparesis is rare. Unilateral right hemisphere lesions infrequently cause global aphasia because patients with right hemisphere language function usually have incomplete dominance.

encompassing Broca's area and Wernicke's area, respectively.[123] Rarely, a single large lesion anterior to the primary motor cortex but often involving the insula is found in global aphasia without hemiparesis.[120] The comprehension deficit caused by a single anterior lesion may result from secondary dysfunction in temporoparietal language areas that have been disconnected from Broca's area and other association areas, possibly by *diaschisis* (the inhibition of function by an acute lesion of the central nervous system at a site connected with but distant from the injury). Embolic stroke, as well as tumor and hemorrhage, usually causes global aphasia without hemiparesis.[120] Recovery is usually rapid as patients are able to communicate verbally within several weeks and are usually left with anterior aphasia.

TRANSCORTICAL APHASIA

Isolation, not destruction, of the perisylvian language cortex causes transcortical aphasia, which is characterized by preserved repetition. These aphasias are postulated to disconnect, and thereby isolate, speech areas from other cortical regions. In contrast to the classic syndromes, such as Broca's aphasia and Wernicke's aphasia, the speech cortices are spared in extrasylvian aphasia. Transcortical aphasia exists in three forms: the anterior form, called transcortical motor aphasia (TMA); the posterior form, called transcortical sensory aphasia (TSA); and the combined anterior and posterior form, called mixed transcortical aphasia (MTA).

Transcortical Motor Aphasia

The clinical features of TMA (Table 6–6) are similar to those of Broca's aphasia, but TMA is distinguished by preserved repetition. Mutism may occur in the acute stage. Speech and, often, motor activity are characterized by impoverished spontaneity. Verbal output is dysprosodic and nonfluent, with effortful production of short phrases. Speech in TMA resembles that in Broca's aphasia, but grammatical structure is better preserved. For example, telegraphic speech is more common in Broca's aphasia. Patients with TMA often respond to yes-or-no questions in a facile manner. When asked to count to 10, they may have difficulty initiating the sequence; but if the examiner provides the first few numbers, they can often complete the series. In some cases, perseverative and echolalic responses intervene; though aware of the echolalia, the patients are unable to control it.[124] Patients do well at completing open-ended sentences such as "The cow jumped over the *(blank)*."

When repeating, patients with TMA may correct syntactical errors in the original sentence. Comprehension of spoken and written language is intact, except for complex verbal sequences, such as interpreting a series of relations (e.g., "My mother's brother's sister is a woman"). However, lesions extending into the middle frontal gyrus may impair auditory comprehension.[125] Perseverative responses may obscure normal comprehension. Confrontational naming is usually mildly impaired and improved by contextual or phonemic cues but does not distinguish TMA from other aphasias. For example, if the patient cannot generate the word *watch,* providing a cue, such as "This is used to tell time" (contextual cue) or "It starts with *wa*" (phonemic cue), may be helpful. Naming errors may occur when the examiner fails to wait for the patient to respond or the patient exhibits perseveration, responds to a part of the stimulus, or gives a bizarre answer reflecting a loose or random association to the target item (e.g., when shown a picture of a tree, the patient responds "A place for termites"). When asked to generate a word list, patients with TMA often have trouble getting started and maintaining the category.

Writing is impaired in TMA, with poor spelling, absence of grammatical words (telegraphic writing), and, in some cases, oversized and poorly formed letters. Patients have difficulty initiating a writing task on command and may be unable to continue writing unless repeatedly reminded. Reading comprehension is spared, but reading aloud is often clumsy and may resemble spontaneous speech, with dysarthria and repetition of syllables and words.

Hemiparesis–almost always right-sided—affecting the leg and shoulder more than the arm or face is often seen with TMA. Generalized akinesia often improves to right-sided hemiakinesia with perseveration and mild echolalia.[126] Sensory loss is absent or mild and parallels the distribution of motor loss. Apraxia of the left arm and leg is common. Right-sided grasp reflexes (foot and hand) and increased tone (leg and arm) and tendon reflexes, snout reflex, and lack of initiative *(abulia)* may ac-

Table 6–6. **Clinical Features of Transcortical Motor Aphasia**

Feature	Observation	FRONTAL INVOLVEMENT	
		Dorsolateral (Commom)	Mesial (Uncommon)
Linguistic deficits	Initiation, motor automaticity	Impaired sequencing	Impaired motivation
Speech	Nonfluent, effortful	Echolalia	Effortful
Comprehension, auditory and written	Normal or mildly impaired	—	Impaired for complex sequences
Repetition	Normal	—	—
Pointing to named items	Normal	—	—
Naming	Normal to mildly impaired	—	—
Reading aloud	Impaired (similar to speech, see above)	—	—
Writing	Impaired, slow	—	Errors in spelling and word selection, diminished activation
Associated neurological findings	Increased tendon reflexes, Babinski's sign	Hemiparesis only with prominent subcortical involvement	Sensorimotor deficit, right leg and shoulder
Behavioral findings	Diminished motor and verbal spontaneity, features of frontal lobe syndrome	Right-sided motor neglect	Mild abulia, mutism prolonged initially
Pathology, typical	Ischemic stroke, upper division of left MCA or border zone of MCA–ACA or ACA; hemorrhage, tumor, trauma	Left MCA or MCA–ACA border zone	Left ACA

MCA, middle cerebral artery; ACA, anterior cerebral artery.

company TMA but are usually subtle after the acute stage. Extensive or bilateral injury of the frontal lobe usually precludes a diagnosis of TMA because of the prominence of the neurobehavioral syndrome (see Chapter 9).

The lesion in TMA is almost always in the dominant frontal lobe, anterior and superior to Broca's area (Fig. 6–6), and usually involves the dorsolateral prefrontal cortex but occasionally is restricted to the SMA and anterior cingulate cortex.[127–129] In some cases, Broca's area is involved.[118] Destruction of the dominant SMA or its disconnection from Broca's area may be the common pathogenetic mechanism. The SMA and anterior cingulate cortex are important in motivation, including the initiation and maintenance of speech.[124,126] Lesions in the mesial frontal region cause greater leg and

shoulder sensorimotor deficits and more prolonged mutism (2–10 days vs. 1–3 days) than dorsolateral frontal lesions but do not cause echolalia, the forced-completion phenomenon, or impaired comprehension of complex verbal sequences.[130] Prefrontal cortical lesions reduce speech formulation and discourse but do not cause true TMA.[131] TMA rarely follows left-sided thalamic lesions.[132] TMA is caused by hemorrhage, acute internal carotid artery occlusion with infarction in the border zone between the anterior artery and the MCA, thrombotic and embolic infarcts in the anterior cerebral artery distribution, tumors (often following resection), and trauma.[133]

Like other aphasic patients, the majority of patients with TMA improve, but recovery is often incomplete; the greatest changes occur within

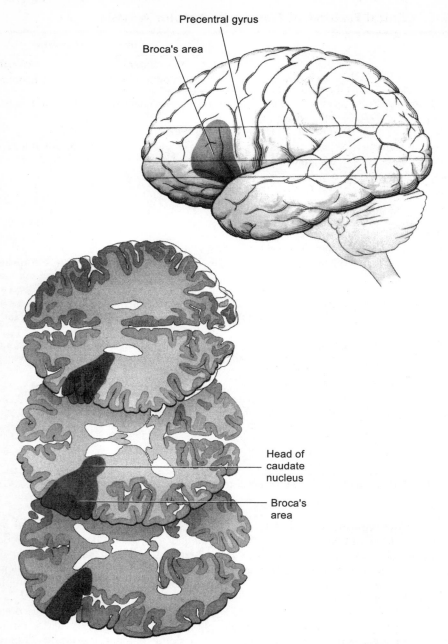

Figure 6–6. Most common lesion site (dorsolateral frontal lobe) associated with transcortical motor aphasia.

the first few weeks after the acute episode. Occasionally, symptoms resolve completely.[130,134]

Transcortical Sensory Aphasia

The clinical features of TSA (Table 6–7) are similar to those of Wernicke's aphasia, except that TSA is distinguished by preserved repetition. Speech is fluent, with neologistic and semantic paraphasias. Some patients with TSA lose the semantic meaning of words and the associative meanings (e.g., visual image or emotional memory) that anchor words to experience. Such patients can repeat the word *dog*

Table 6–7. **Clinical Features of Transcortical Sensory Aphasia**

Feature	Observation
Linguistic deficits	Meaning and relationship of words: semantic level, integration of elements and relations in a sentence
Speech	Fluent, semantic paraphasias, prominent echolalia
Comprehension, auditory and written	Impaired
Repetition	Normal
Pointing to named items	Impaired
Naming	Impaired
Reading aloud	Impaired (similar to speech, see above)
Writing	Impaired
Associated neurological findings	Right superior quadrantanopia or hemianopia, increased tendon reflexes; uncommonly, right-sided hemiparesis
Behavioral findings	Gerstmann's syndrome
Pathology, typical	Stroke, watershed infarcts

and copy a picture of a dog but are unable to link the two. Other patients may have semantic aphasia characterized by the inability to comprehend sentences that include successive subordinate clauses (e.g., *which, that, despite, if*), temporal or spatial combinations that are reversible (e.g., "He did it before she did it," "The cloth is under the table"), comparisons, double negatives, passive verbs (e.g., "The clay was molded by the child"), or relations (e.g., *mother's brother*). Many of these features are also found in Broca's aphasia, but patients with TSA have fluent speech. Some patients cannot integrate the components and relations within a sentence, although individual word meanings may be preserved. In other patients, comprehension of single words is impaired.

The impairments in TSA include auditory and written language comprehension, confrontational naming, pointing to a named object, reading, and writing. Rarely, naming is relatively spared. Echolalia is often a prominent feature of TSA. The examiner's question may be repeated in an automatic, involuntary manner. As with Wernicke's aphasia, TSA may be misdiagnosed as psychosis or delirium.

The most commonly associated neurological sign in TSA is visual field loss, most often a right superior quadrantanopia or right hemianopia. Lesions are posterior, usually in the watershed between the MCA and the posterior cerebral artery (Fig. 6–7) and occasionally in the territory of the MCA in the angular gyrus or at the junction of the parietal, temporal, and occipital lobes (involving the inferior angular gyrus and the upper part of BA 37).[117,135–137] Rarely, lesions involving the left internal capsule and thalamus, left frontal lobe, or right hemisphere may produce TSA.[135,137–139] The prognosis in TSA is variable; the aphasia can evolve into anomic aphasia with recovery of comprehension.

Mixed Transcortical Aphasia

Also called mixed extrasylvian aphasia, MTA is a rare syndrome in which the clinical features (Table 6–8) include the remarkable ability of patients to repeat almost perfectly even though they cannot understand or spontaneously speak fluently. Therefore, in a simplistic way, it is helpful to think of MTA as the opposite of conduction aphasia: in MTA repetition is better than expected, and in conduction aphasia it is worse than expected. The lesion in mixed extrasylvian aphasia spares Broca's area, Wernicke's area, the inferior parietal language (supramarginal gyrus) area, and their white matter interconnections but involves the cortical rim surrounding these perisylvian language areas. All language functions except repetition are impaired.

The speech of patients with MTA is nonfluent and aspontaneous, with impaired naming, comprehension (auditory and written language), and writing. Occasionally, naming is intact.[140] Repetition stands alone as an island of preserved language function. Some patients

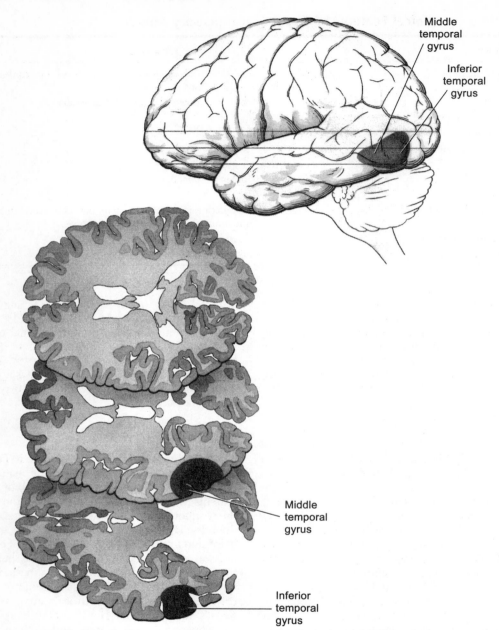

Figure 6–7. Most common lesion site associated with transcortical sensory aphasia.

echolalically repeat everything that is heard, whether spoken or sung. Many patients speak only when spoken to. In milder cases of MTA, comprehension and spontaneous speech are less severely impaired.

The lesion in MTA functionally disconnects language areas from other frontal, parietal, and temporal cognitive association cortices. Lesions often involve primary motor and sensory areas, causing motor, somatosensory, and visual field deficits that may be bilateral. Lesions in the border zone between the anterior artery and the MCA and between the MCA and the posterior artery are the most common cause of

Table 6–8. **Clinical Features of Mixed Transcortical Aphasia**

Feature	Observation
Linguistic deficits	Initiation, relating phonemic elements of word to associated meanings
Speech	Nonfluent, paraphasias, echolalia, normal articulation
Comprehension, auditory and written	Impaired
Repetition	Relatively or fully preserved
Pointing to named items	Impaired
Naming	Impaired
Reading aloud	Impaired (similar to speech, see above)
Writing	Impaired
Associated neurological findings	Commonly, right-sided sensorimotor deficits; increased tendon reflexes, right superior quadrantanopia or hemianopia
Behavioral findings	Abulia
Pathology, typical	Stroke, watershed infarcts

MTA. Rarely, MTA occurs after large strokes in the left anterior cerebral artery with infarction extending posteriorly and medially into the parietal lobe.[141]

Hypoxic–ischemic brain insults from cardiac arrest, shock, hypotension, and carbon monoxide poisoning are the most common causes of severe MTA and produce border zone infarcts bilaterally. High-grade stenosis or occlusion of the left internal carotid artery produces milder MTA. In these cases, hypotension or stenosis of the right internal carotid artery may cause ischemia in the left border zone territory.

ANOMIC APHASIA

Anomic aphasia is characterized by spontaneous, fluent speech interrupted by word-finding pauses and a relatively selective and severe naming impairment. Because anomia is the most ubiquitous finding in the aphasias, the naming impairment must be prominent and other disorders absent or mild for a diagnosis of anomic aphasia. The absence of substantive words (e.g., bookshelf, wristband) and the frequent use of nonspecific nouns and verbs (e.g., thing, this, it) in anomic aphasia produces empty speech. However, in contrast with the empty speech of patients with Wernicke's aphasia, patients with anomic aphasia maintain a more coherent and focused stream of thought. Some patients, when unable to find the correct substantive word, use circumlocution. For example, when trying to find the word

cat, the patient may say You know that thing that likes to, uh, that white stuff and it makes those sounds, you know, meow.

Patients with anomic aphasia do poorly on confrontational naming and word-production tests (e.g., name all the farm animals, name words that begin with the letter *s*). Some patients appear almost unaffected by the disorder as they circumlocute or provide a nonspecific filler without pause. Others are frustrated, impatient, and embarrassed by their disorder.[142] In most of these patients, the meaning of the word that cannot be retrieved is not lost from memory as creative pantomimes and revealing circumlocutions often provide the listener with the meaning. Patients with anomic aphasia have fully or relatively preserved fluency, comprehension, and repetition. Naming (word retrieval) must be distinguished from semantic knowledge (ability to describe verbally an object's functions, features, and so on), perceptual knowledge (object recognition), and praxis (object use).

The following discourse with one of our patients exemplifies anomic aphasia:

Examiner: Can you tell me about what brought you to the hospital?
Patient: My, you know, my well . . . pump thing . . .
Examiner: You're pointing to your heart?
Patient: Yes . . . the doctor did a job on it . . . He . . . he . . . he undid the thing in it . . .
Examiner: Did he perform a bypass?
Patient: Yes, yes . . . a bypass on the . . . uh . . . you know . . . the pump thing.

There are three primary forms of anomic aphasia: word selection anomia, semantic anomia, and disconnection anomia. The key features that distinguish these anomias are knowledge of the desired name, understanding of what the object actually is and how it is used, ability to correctly point to the object when the name is presented, and modality-specific or unilateral (e.g., right visual field only) naming deficits.

Word Selection Anomia

In word selection anomia, the patient knows how to use an object and is able to choose the correct object from a group of objects when given the name but cannot name the object when it is presented in any sensory modality. Patients who cannot retrieve words but can recognize words usually have lesions in the left middle and lateral inferotemporal region and the lateral temporoparietal region. Category-specific anomias challenge our understanding of the cortical organization of language, revealing that separate conceptual categories of entities are mediated by different neural systems. The brain employs different areas, and possibly different strategies, for encoding, understanding, and associatively linking different categories of knowledge. Some patients exhibit selective impairment in naming or recognizing letters, body parts, colors, indoor objects such as furniture,[143] animals,[144] fruits and vegetables,[145] facial emotions,[146] abstract versus concrete entities, and naturally occurring versus manufactured entities.[147,148]

Lesions that cause deficits in naming and understanding specific (unique) and nonspecific categories of certain entities may be distinctly localized. For example, bilateral lesions usually produce deficits in naming living items, and unilateral left hemisphere lesions usually cause deficits in naming nonliving items.[149] Lesions associated with impaired naming of nonunique animals cluster in the inferotemporal region, and lesions impairing conceptual knowledge (recognition) for animals cluster in the mesial occipitotemporal regions. In contrast, lesions correlated with impaired naming and recognition of tools and utensils cluster in the posterior and lateral temporal cortices and the supramarginal gyrus. Thus, the neural systems required to retrieve conceptual information for nonunique animals are partially separate from those used to retrieve words for those

entities. However, these systems largely overlap for tools and utensils.[150] A PET study of naming in normal subjects showed activation of the posterolateral aspect of the left inferotemporal area for tools and utensils and more anteromesial areas for animals,[151] which agrees with the results of lesion studies.

Lesions of the left medial and lateral temporal poles (BA 38), as well as lesions of the middle and inferior temporal gyri (BAs 21, 22), produce selective impairment for specific names (e.g., unique faces, animals, fruits, tools) (Fig. 6–8).[150,152,153] Lesions of the temporal pole impair retrieval of unique names of places, persons, and objects; and more posterior and inferior temporal lesions (BAs 20, 21) impair retrieval for common, nonunique nouns but not for unique entities.[150,154,155] Thus, neural structures mediating word retrieval for unique entities are anterior to those for nonunique entities.[150] The anterior temporal cortices provide access to words that denote physical beings or locations but not verbs, adjectives, or grammatical words that tell us about the features, actions, or relationships of those entities. The ability to name action verbs relies on a separate system located in left inferior motor and premotor regions and dorsolateral prefrontal cortex.[150] Impaired naming of action verbs is usually accompanied by impaired recognition of the actions and poor sentence processing.[156] Patients with fluent paraphasic speech and lesions in parietal or frontotemporal areas may correctly use the noun form but not the verb form when reading and writing the noun and verb forms of a homonym.[11]

Semantic Anomia

The symbolic meaning of words is lost in semantic anomia, which includes not only a naming deficit but also a recognition deficit. Even though the examiner provides the name, the patient is unable to choose the correct object. Semantic anomia often occurs in TSA and Wernicke's aphasia, both posterior aphasias, and forms a continuum with TSA. Lesions in the left posterior temporal (posterior BAs 21, 22) and adjacent inferior parietal areas (inferior BAs 39, 40) result in semantic anomia. Lesions may be confined to the angular gyrus (BA 39) or the posterior middle temporal gyrus (BA 37),[157] but the anatomical localization of semantic anomia is often poorly defined.

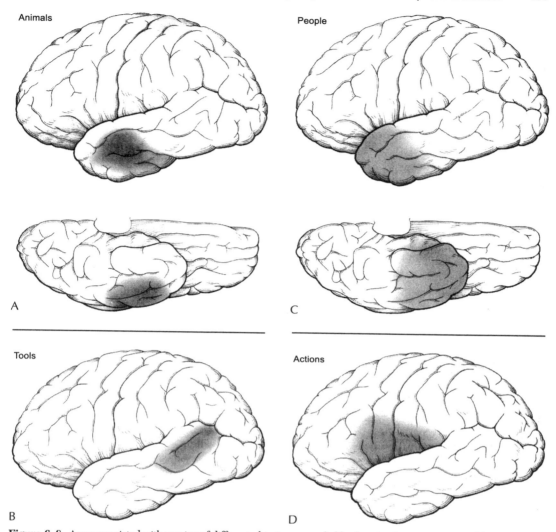

Figure 6–8. Areas associated with naming of different objects, as revealed by functional neuroimaging and lesion studies.

Disconnection Anomia

Lesions that sever connections between sensory and language cortices produce disconnection anomia, of which there are three forms: modality-specific, category-specific, and callosal. In modality-specific anomia, defective naming is limited to one sensory modality. For example, in visual anomia (optic aphasia), patients cannot name objects presented visually but can readily name the same object when touched, heard, or smelled (assuming it has a characteristic shape, sound, or smell). Distinguishing modality-specific anomia and *agnosia* (the inability to recognize objects in a sensory modality despite normal attention, language, and sensory perception) is often difficult. The lesion in modality-specific anomia, usually found in the posterior white matter tracts, disconnects language and sensory association cortices.

Although disconnection may cause category-specific anomia, it is usually caused by damage to specific cortical regions; these are not "centers" that store a permanent memory but dynamic systems containing knowledge for activating word images.[150] For example, patients with selective anomia for facial emotional expression often have lesions in the right inferotemporal area.[146] In humans, the naming of facial emotions activates this area,[158] which if destroyed or disconnected from language areas gives rise to this selective anomia.

Callosal anomia is produced when lesions in the corpus callosum isolate intact sensory areas in the nondominant hemisphere from language areas. Patients who palpate an object in the left hand can accurately assess its size and shape with somatosensory areas in the right hemisphere but cannot transmit that information to language areas. Therefore, they are unable to name the object but can correctly use it or select it from a group of pictures with the nondominant hand.

SUBCORTICAL APHASIA

Human language is viewed as a phylogenetic pinnacle, reflecting the functions of advanced association cortices. However, lesions in subcortical regions cause language dysfunction, but paradoxically, lower vertebrates have the same subcortical structures as humans, albeit in a less developed form. Subcortical aphasia suggests the need for a reexamination of human brain function. Rather than refuting the concept of cortical language areas, the association of subcortical lesions with language dysfunction emphasizes the complex interrelations of cortex and subcortex. Subcortical aphasia may be understood through the extensive cortical projections to the subcortex. The cortex deluges the caudate and thalamus with information, thus endowing these subcortical nuclei with "cognitive" functions via massive input from the neocortex. Projections from cortical language areas to the caudate help to create procedural knowledge for language, that is, automatized learning to comprehend and produce frequently used language components and structures.[75] Evidence that lesions of the thalamus create deficits in highly automatized language supports this role.[159] Projections from cortical language areas to specific thalamic nuclei may be critical for synchronizing activity in the language network.

Subcortical lesions associated with aphasia involve the left head of the caudate, thalamus (anterolateral nucleus), and white matter tracts (subjacent to cortical language areas, arcuate fasciculus, subcallosal connections, other corticocortical connections, and the anterior limb of the internal capsule) (Fig. 6–9).[160–163] Subcortical aphasias are heterogeneous, usually differ from classic cortical aphasic syndromes

and often have a good prognosis. However, any classic aphasic syndrome may be caused by a subcortical lesion.[95] The affect of patients with subcortical aphasia ranges from normal to indifference and unconcern to mild depression but may also include the severe depression often associated with anterior cortical aphasias.[164] Subcortical aphasias usually result from infarction in the territory of the lateral lenticulostriate branches of the MCA, which supply the basal ganglia and internal capsule; infarction in the territory of the thalamoperforant (especially the tuberothalamic) arteries; or hemorrhage.[95,161,162,165]

Striatal–Capsular Aphasia

Lesions involving the head of the caudate and anterior capsule cause language deficits accompanied by hemiparesis.[161,162,166,167] Aphasia arising from left caudate lesions may largely result from adjacent white matter lesions,[92] but the head of the caudate is also involved.[75,161,166,168] The caudate head connects to the auditory cortex and cortical areas involved in emotion, memory, movement, and executive functions.[169] Lesions of the body and tail of the caudate and the putamen do not cause aphasia.[92,161] When lesions of the head of the caudate and the anterior capsule extend to anterior–superior white matter, speech is effortful, slow, and dysarthric but comprehension and grammar are normal.[162] However, executive functions are often impaired.[168] Lesions extending posteriorly involve the auditory radiations and temporal isthmus, causing fluent paraphasic speech with impaired comprehension.[161,162]

Combined lesions of the head of the caudate and the anterior limb of the internal capsule often produce features of anterior and posterior cortical aphasias, with prominent stuttering and stammering.[161,170] The generative language problem impairs verbal fluency and sentence production, increases the latency between verbal utterances, and causes perseveration.[168] Occasionally, speech content is bizarre despite preserved fluency, which is similar to the effects of prefrontal injury. Caudate–capsular lesions are responsible for the right-sided hemiparesis, dysarthria, and dysprosody that usually accompany the aphasia. Acutely, speech is nonfluent and contaminated with semantic and phonemic paraphasias. Comprehension and reading may or may not

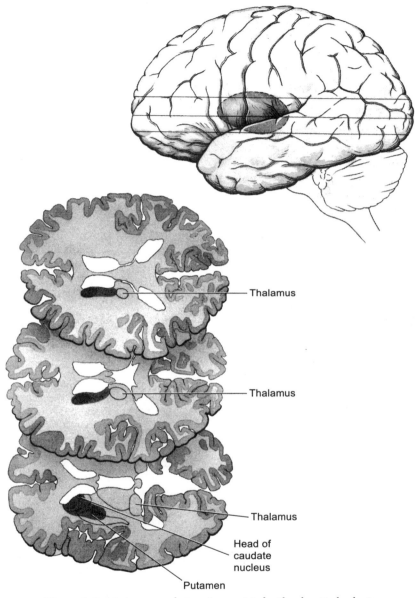

Figure 6–9. Most common lesion site associated with subcortical aphasia.

be affected,[171] but even if moderately impaired, they usually improve rapidly and almost completely.

Rarely, combined lesions of the putamen, posterior internal capsule, temporal isthmus, and periventricular white matter caused by subcortical stroke produce global aphasia. Cortical hypoperfusion of the perisylvian language areas, including Broca's and Wernicke's areas, presumably due to undercutting of the white matter, appears to be the mechanism for subcortical global aphasia.[122]

Small, discrete lesions of the anterior limb of the internal capsule, the adjacent corona radiata, or the head of the caudate cause pure dysarthria (dysarthria without limb weakness).[172] Lacunar infarction is the most common cause. Aphasia is not present, and the dysarthria usually resolves within 2–4 weeks. Isolated lesions of the left putamen result in hypophonia and spasmodic dysphonia.[95,173]

Subcortical lesions of the basal ganglia and thalamus in the right hemisphere produce dysprosody.[59,174] However, clinical, neuroradiological, and pathological information on dysprosody with isolated subcortical lesions is scarce.[175]

Thalamic Aphasia

Thalamic aphasia is characterized by fluctuations in language performance, low speech volume, fading or "withering" of language, and preserved repetition. In contrast to caudate–capsular aphasias, thalamic aphasia is associated with deficits in other cognitive domains. Left-sided lesions involving some combination of the anterolateral, ventral anterior, ventral lateral, and dorsomedial nuclei cause thalamic aphasia.[159,163,165,176] However, aphasia also occurs in left-handed persons after thalamic stroke in the right hemisphere, paralleling the association between right-sided cortical lesions and aphasia in left-handed persons. Thalamic stroke in the right hemisphere of right-handed patients causes left-sided neglect but not aphasia. Causes of thalamic aphasia include infarction, hemorrhage, brain tumor, and stereotactic surgery.[165,177,178]

Acutely, patients are often mute, with right-sided weakness and sensory loss, especially after cerebral hemorrhage. Hypophonia and fluctuating levels of consciousness and language function are common during the acute stage of thalamic aphasia. Patients may alternate between an alert state with fairly normal speech and lethargy with dysarthria, paraphasia, perseveration, and progressive loss of speech volume.[132,160,179] The aphasia closely resembles TSA because repetition is well preserved and not contaminated by paraphasias like those observed in spontaneous speech. Speech is fluent, or nearly so; and comprehension, naming, and reading are often mildly impaired. The language disorder and loss of voice volume often become more evident as the patient's spontaneous speech fatigues, or withers. Thalamic aphasia often resolves or markedly improves over time.[179]

The enormous cortical input to the thalamus likely "programs" specific thalamic nuclei to assist the cortex in executing language functions, but the mechanism by which thalamic lesions in the left hemisphere cause language impairment is uncertain. Secondary effects on other subcortical or cortical areas from cerebral edema and pressure likely contribute to the aphasia, especially with severe hemorrhage. However, lesions restricted to the left thalamus produce language dysfunction. Electrical stimulation of the ventral lateral nucleus and pulvinar produces naming errors, supporting a thalamic role in language.[180] In addition, these thalamic areas are connected with frontal and parietotemporal language areas. Evidence from PET and cerebral blood flow studies in patients with subcortical aphasia suggests that secondary effects on cortical function cause language dysfunction.[181,182] Vascular occlusion or diaschisis may result in cortical hypoperfusion. Thalamic aphasia may partly result from damage to the network linking frontal lobe areas subserving working memory and thalamic gating of attention by the pulvinar and lateral posterior nuclei, thus disrupting lexical–semantic functions which are dependent on these systems.[171]

Other Aphasias and Language Disorders

CHILDHOOD APHASIA

Acquired brain lesions impair language in children, but the aphasias differ from their adult counterparts. Hemispheric asymmetry for language evolves during childhood. Until the age of 10–12 years,[34,85] and to a lesser degree into adolescence and adulthood,[183] aphasia produced by a left hemisphere lesion is compensated for by the right hemisphere or recruitment of regions adjacent to the damaged perisylvian language region. Even in childhood, however, language recovery after dominant hemisphere damage is often incomplete, and language deficits and learning difficulties are common sequelae.[84,85] Compensation by the right hemisphere declines with age, as does overall recovery from aphasia. Usually, the younger the child when aphasia is acquired, the more rapid and complete the recovery.

Initial mutism in aphasia is more common in children than adults.[45] Aphasia in young children is often, though not invariably, nonfluent regardless of the lesion site.[84,85,184] This age-dependent effect is less prominent in adolescents. The speech of children with acquired aphasia is typically effortful, slow, sparse, and hypophonic; and a persistent deficit in syntax is common. Lesions impairing acquired language skills can also impair language development.

APHASIA IN ILLITERATES

The ability to read is a relatively recent human development, realized for no more than 3000 years in humankind's history of more than 125,000 years. Many people remain illiterate. Left hemisphere lesions predominate in aphasic illiterates, as they do in aphasic literates.[185] Illiterates, however, have a greater bihemispheric language representation, possibly because, when language is studied, mastering written codes for language potentiates hemispheric specialization.[186,187] Aphasia may be less severe and recovery more complete in illiterates than literates.[185]

APHASIA IN POLYGLOTS

Acquisition of a native language, as well as subsequent languages, is a function of the left hemisphere.[188] However, the right hemisphere has a greater role in the late acquisition of language in bilingual or multilingual patients, with increased age at the time of additional language aquisition corresponding to greater right hemisphere involvement.[38,189] The cerebral organization of language in polyglots, individuals fluent in more than one language, varies with the age at aquisition. Additional languages acquired during the early stage of language acquisition are usually represented in common frontal cortical areas. Within the temporal lobe language-sensitive region (Wernicke's area), additional languages acquired in adulthood are represented within the same areas; but within the frontal lobe language-sensitive region (Broca's area), the later languages may or may not be spatially separated from the native language.[188,190]

Polyglots with aphasia may have complex patterns of language impairment and recovery. The aphasia may selectively affect one language, but usually all languages are affected. Furthermore, the aphasic features (e.g., nonfluency, poor repetition) are usually very similar in the different languages.

Recovery of language may be better in the language in which thinking and mental calculations are routinely carried out[191] or the one used in the environment in which the patient is recovering.[192] Usually, some recovery occurs in all learned langauges, although it is often uneven and may be selective.[191,193] Differential language recovery of aphasia in polyglots may be modified by the site of the lesion, which, in addition, may affect the recovery of writing when the languages utilize different graphic forms (e.g., Arabic vs. Indo-European vs. Chinese).[194,195]

EPILEPSY AND LANGUAGE DYSFUNCTION

Seizures, either spontaneous or induced, disrupt language functions. Neither of these forms of aberrant cortical activation mimics normal physiological function, so the implications for normal function remain tentative. Cortical stimulation typically is applied over adjacent electrodes (2.3–4.0 mm in diameter; electrodes 1 cm apart, center-to-center) on the convexity. Most cortical areas, buried in the sulci, are not stimulated. Instead of activating selective neuronal groups and their network connections, the electrical stimulus delivers a local surface "blast" of cortical stimulation. This provides a view through a "frosted window" into the language functions of an area, primarily by inactivation. The area is likely rendered inactive by sustained depolarization, activation of inhibitory systems, or disruption of the synchronization process needed for complex functions.

Speech arrest is induced by stimulation of the classic language areas, such as Broca's area, the angular gyrus, and Wernicke's area, as well as the SMA of the dominant hemisphere. However, in the motor and sensory areas, particularly the primary areas, cortical stimulation evokes positive phenomena. Electrical stimulation does not evoke language, although stimulation of the SMA may evoke nonverbal vocalization. Stimulation also causes selective disruption of naming, reading, repetition, comprehension, and fluency.[115,196] Pooled data from a large cohort in a study of stimulation of the posterior language cortex showed that the sites are organized not randomly but as several noncontiguous nodes devoted to different aspects of language processing (Fig. 6–10).[196] In addition, early age at seizure onset[197] and lower

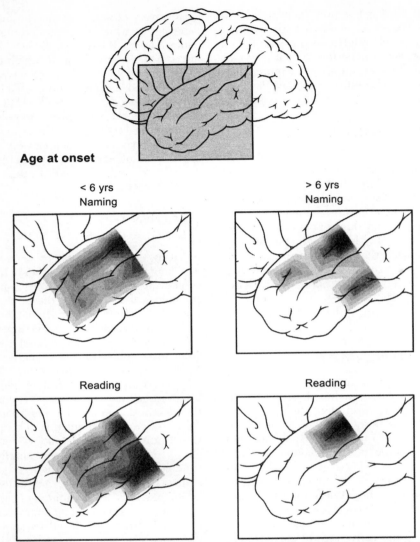

Age at onset

Figure 6–10. Areas of the temporal lobe involved in naming and reading, as revealed by cortical stimulation in patients with epilepsy. Earlier age at seizure onset (<6 years) *(A)* and lower verbal IQ (<90) *(B)* were associated with wider areas of involvement.

IQ[198] are associated with more widely distributed language areas, possibly reflecting physiological dysfunction at sites originally programmed for specific language functions.

Seizures arising from the temporal, frontal, or parietal lobe of the dominant hemisphere often cause ictal and postictal aphasia,[199–201] as well as verbal auditory agnosia, agraphia, alexia, and apraxia.[202,203] Distinguishing language dysfunction from confusion or impaired consciousness during or after seizures can be very difficult. With isolated speech arrest, the patient should be able to reply to a nonverbal command (e.g., mimic a simple motor act) and maintain eye contact during the seizure. Localizing a seizure focus on the basis of clinical symptoms is more uncertain than localizing destructive lesions based on language deficits as ictal and postictal symptoms may reflect ictal spread and associated cognitive deficits. Ictal

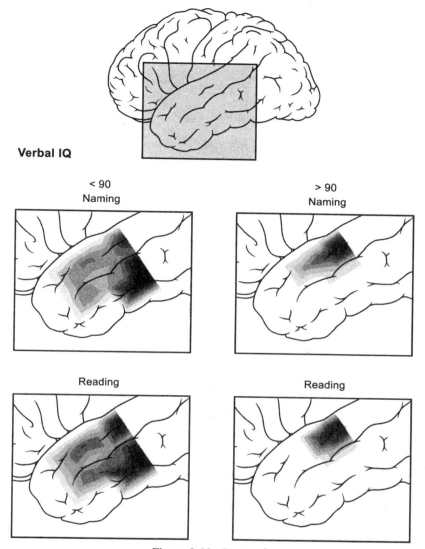

Verbal IQ

Figure 6–10. *Continued.*

aphasias rarely correspond to the classic aphasia syndromes that follow stroke. Rather, they are characterized by more rapidly changing symptoms, often admixed with impairments of attention, memory, and self-awareness. Seizures arising from Broca's area are more likely to cause speech arrest than nonfluent speech, and those caused by a lesion in Wernicke's area are infrequently associated with the fluent paraphasic speech typical of Wernicke's

aphasia. One of our patients with a seizure arising from the vicinity of Wernicke's area provided an insightful account of the event:

A 35-year-old man had a traumatic brain injury at age 20 years, with skull fracture on the right side and loss of consciousness. Subsequent MRI revealed a small area of encephalomalacia in the left posterior portion of the superior temporal gyrus. At age 30, he began to experience episodes of language impairment in which he was unable to speak or un-

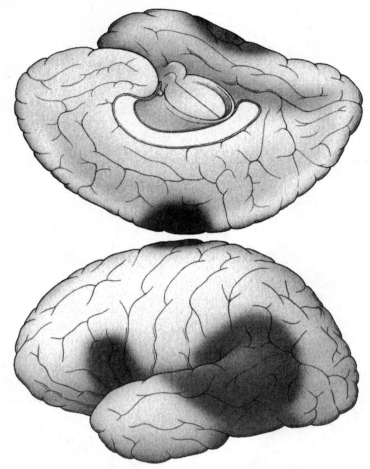

C

Figure 6–10. *Continued. C:* Areas from which electrical stimulation disrupts speech, naming, reading, or writing.

derstand spoken language, although he was able to "think" and recall the events around him in detail, "with a heightened awareness of things going on." During one of these attacks, he was reading, and suddenly everything on the page "didn't make sense. I tried to read, but I couldn't say the words or sound them out in my head, although they all looked familiar. Then I tried to read individual letters, and was unable to do this as well. When I tried to force the words out, gobbledygook came out of my mouth. Finally, after a few minutes, I could read individual letters and then, shortly afterward, I could read again, although infrequently used words caused me to hesitate for a moment."

Ictal speech, with fluent sentences, is most often observed during seizures originating in the nondominant temporal lobe. Such patients often speak as if in a dream, or their speech forms a fragmented continuation of prior conversation or commentary on prior activities. Their responses to questions are usually delayed and lack normal content. In response to open-ended questions, for example, the narrative discourse is sparse. Patients may produce disinhibited speech, containing inappropriate content, including curses and insults. During seizures arising from either the left or the right hemisphere, patients may speak only in brief, often repetitive phrases, such as "Oh boy, oh boy" or "Don't do it, don't do it."

Postictal symptoms usually reflect the functions of the hemisphere and the localized region of seizure onset. However, postictal language dysfunction provides limited information about the location of the focus since differentiation from postictal confusion is difficult. Impaired comprehension, with fluent but incomprehensible speech, as well as anomia, occurs with either a left or a right temporal lobe seizure focus. In complex partial seizures, the delay in spontaneous verbal output, reading, and repetition to command is greater when the focus is in the left temporal lobe.[199,200] Patients with a left-sided temporal lobe focus often cannot correctly read a test phrase until more than 60 seconds after a seizure. Postictal global aphasia, nonfluent speech, or paraphasic errors strongly suggest a seizure focus in the dominant hemisphere.

EPILEPTIFORM ACTIVITY-INDUCED LANGUAGE IMPAIRMENT

The role of interictal epileptiform discharges in impaired linguistic and other cognitive functions remains unclear. Brief or subtle seizures impair cognition.[204] The short-lived ictal discharges usually have the greatest effect on areas from which they originate; when the discharges are generalized, patients have a momentary lapse of awareness. A few studies have reported transient cognitive deficits associated with interictal epileptiform discharges.[204,205] An electroencephalogram (EEG) recorded from the scalp or with invasive electrodes often reveals very frequent interictal epileptiform discharges in the hippocampus and other areas, causing impaired cognitive function. A structural abnormality such as cell loss, persistent electrophysiological dysfunction (as reflected by loss of normal background activity), or intermittent epileptiform discharges may contribute to cognitive impairment. Remarkably, in the common childhood epilepsy syndrome of benign epilepsy with centrotemporal spikes, very frequent epileptiform discharges, especially during sleep, usually have no adverse effect on cognitive function. However, some patients with this syndrome develop language and other learning disorders,[206,206a] which raises the question of whether abundant epileptiform discharges contribute to cognitive impairment in susceptible patients.

Landau-Kleffner syndrome, acquired epileptic aphasia, is characterized by two central symptoms: acquired aphasia and frequent epileptiform discharges predominating over posterior language areas of the dominant hemisphere, especially during sleep, when the discharges are often generalized. Most patients with Landau-Kleffner syndrome have secondary symptoms of occasional seizures and delayed social and behavioral development, including reduced eye contact, impaired attention, and motor hyperactivity. The syndrome, which often begins before 6–8 years of age, shows a male predominance. Auditory verbal (and often nonverbal) agnosia may lead to a mistaken diagnosis of deafness, autism, or attention-deficit disorder. Regression of verbal expression may be the presenting symptom. Antiepileptic drugs usually provide rapid seizure control but are ineffective for treating the language and behavioral symptoms. Steroids may bring about dramatic, but often treatment-dependent, improvement. Multiple subpial transections over spiking areas of language cortex may lead to improvement in linguistic function.[207,208] Magnetoencephalography helps to identify targets, often buried in the sylvian fissure, for intracortical transection.[209] The long-term prognosis for behavioral and language development varies but may be more favorable than commonly thought.[210]

The clinical challenge is to identify true cases of Landau-Kleffner syndrome. Epileptiform activity is associated with language and behavioral regression in two other encephalopathies: autistic epileptiform regression and disintegrative epileptiform regression. These disorders and Landau-Kleffner syndrome have overlapping features, causing diagnostic confusion.[207,211] In addition, continuous spike-and-wave discharges during slow-wave sleep (i.e., electrical status epilepticus during sleep) coexist with Landau-Kleffner syndrome, creating nosological controversies.[212,213] Unfortunately, the diagnostic criteria and therapeutic strategies for these devastating regressive disorders are uncertain, leading to both under- and overdiagnosis and consequent therapeutic errors.

LANGUAGE-INDUCED SEIZURES

Seizures induced by language are characterized by ictal discharges and such clinical symptoms as jerking of the jaw or upper limb triggered by reading or other language functions. Language-induced seizures usually result from partial seizures in the dominant hemisphere but may occur in primary generalized epilepsies, such as absence and juvenile myoclonic epilepsy.[214,215] Reading epilepsy is the most common form of language-induced seizures and usually presents as a partial epilepsy syndrome with autosomal dominant inheritance or from a structural lesion.[216] In its genetic forms, reading epilepsy usually occurs between the ages of 11 and 22 years.[217] Partial seizures induced by reading are associated with epileptiform discharges on the EEG and are maximal over the left posterior temporal and parietal regions and, less often, the frontal regions. In addition to jaw and proximal upper limb jerks, some patients have brief lapses of awareness, alexia, or other nonmotor symptoms. Jerks are often induced by writing or other nonreading linguistic activities, which suggests that the epilepsy is a language-induced disorder rather than a specific reading-induced disorder. In patients with primary generalized epilepsy, thinking and decision making, as well as other cognitive and linguistic activities, especially those that require use of the hands, may induce myoclonus.[216]

Therapy for Aphasia

Speech therapy helps some patients with aphasia, but controversy over its efficacy endures.[218] Most studies support the role of speech therapy in aphasia for nonprogressive disorders such as traumatic brain injury, stroke, and meningioma resection,[219–222] but formal speech therapy may be of no greater benefit than therapy by trained volunteers or no therapy.[223,224] In addition, pharmacological therapy for aphasia has not proved beneficial.

Spontaneous recovery of language function occurs with nonprogressive disorders and is more likely with traumatic brain injury than cerebrovascular disease, reflecting the lesion site and the patient's age.[134] Among the various types of aphasia, acute Broca's aphasia and conduction aphasia are the most likely to improve. Anomic aphasia is often a common end stage for other acute aphasic syndromes, and regardless of the cause or duration of the anomia, phonological and semantic therapies

are of no definite benefit,[225] although reports of positive responses exist.[226]

Long-term follow-up shows that the prognosis is poor for patients with global aphasia, intermediate for patients with Broca's or Wernicke's aphasia, and good for patients with conduction, anomic, or transcortical aphasia.[134] The factors influencing spontaneous improvement and response to speech therapy are summarized in Table 6–9. Functional neuroimaging studies support the role of regions in both the right and left hemispheres in recovery from aphasia.[227]

SPEECH THERAPY

Initially, a speech pathologist or neuropsychologist assesses the patient's language skills and neurobehavioral functions, including attention, memory, praxis, and visuospatial function. Commonly used language inventories include the Boston Diagnostic Aphasia Examination,[228] The Western Battery of Aphasia,[229] Iowa's Neurosensory Center Examination,[230] and The Porch Index of Communicative Ability.[231] The Communication Abilities in Daily Living Test[232] and The Functional Communication Profile[233] are used to assess functional status. Speech therapy may be deferred because of acute medical problems (e.g., myocardial infarction, sepsis), depressed level of consciousness, delirium, dementia, or severe global aphasia. Delaying speech therapy, even as long as 12 weeks, does not appear to compromise ultimate improvement.[222]

Treatment is individualized, which includes identifying the patient's strengths and weaknesses, and first concentrates on relatively preserved language functions so that the patient feels positive about his or her performance. The speech therapist is a supportive counselor to the patient and family. Emotional support is critical, and community stroke and traumatic brain injury support groups are often available. The American Heart Association, The Easter Seal Foundation, the local United Way, and speech pathologists can provide information on community resources. If formal speech therapy is not possible, trained volunteers may be engaged.[223] The volunteers, supervised by speech pathologists, may help to improve the patient's motivation and communication skills.

Speech therapy is successfully provided in the home, residential facility, outpatient clinic, or

Table 6–9. **Prognostic Factors in Aphasia**

| Prognostic Factor | PROGNOSIS | |
	Good	Poor
Age at onset	Young	Old
Handedness	Left	Right
Premorbid status		
Intelligence	High	Low
Creativity	High	Low
Vocabulary	High	Low
Family support	Strong	Weak
Socioeconomic status	High	Low
Education	High	Low
Lesion		
Type	Nonprogressive	Progressive
Size	Small	Large
Location	Frontal, adjacent to language cortex	Temporoparietal language areas
Clinical findings	Normal perception, mood, attentive, normal praxis, normal comprehension	Perceptual deficit, depressed, inattentive, neglect, apraxia, comprehension deficit

hospital. For patients with multiple physical, language, and behavioral problems, therapy in an inpatient rehabilitation center may be more effective. An integrated, multidisciplinary approach involving a neurologist, speech pathologist, occupational and physical therapists, psychologist, social worker, and family members is ideal. Treatment of depression, anxiety, or other psychiatric disorders is critical.

Speech therapy varies with speech pathologists and for different aphasias.[225] Some common forms of speech therapy are shown in Table 6–10. Melodic intonation therapy, relying on the preserved ability of aphasic patients to produce musical tones, is best given in short, frequent sessions for 3–6 weeks.[219,241] This therapy is most effective for patients with Broca's aphasia and variants of nonfluent aphasia and ineffective for those with fluent aphasia. Factors predicting beneficial effects from melodic intonation therapy are unilateral brain injury, relatively preserved auditory comprehension, nonfluent speech with impaired articulation and initiation, poor repetition (even for single words), and a motivated patient with good auditory span.

In general, speech therapy is conducted for 30–60 minutes daily for 1–3 months. If possible, enlist family members or friends to conduct additional homework sessions on language skills.

In addition, they can help the patient to maintain a positive frame of mind and offer encouragement and emotional support during therapy. Maintaining motivation and avoiding depression are essential for the success of aphasia therapy.

Computer-assisted devices can be used by selected patients for augmentative communication, an artificial but effective means of imparting information. Analysis of the lesion site can predict the patient's potential capacity to use the device.[242]

PHARMACOLOGICAL THERAPY

There is no proven medical therapy for aphasia. Anecdotal reports indicate that speech fluency, language content, and nonverbal cognitive skills improve with amphetamines[243] and bromocriptine.[244,245] However, double-blind, placebo-controlled crossover studies show no significant benefits of bromocriptine (15–60 mg daily) on specific skills or the overall severity of aphasia.[246]

AGRAPHIA

In the history of *Homo sapiens*, writing is a very recent development. Although it was developed only in the past 5500 years and was widely

Table 6–10. **Speech Therapies**

Therapy Type	Method	Aphasic Group
Amerind: American Indian Sign Language[234]	Nonverbal system uses hand signs to communicate language	Broca's aphasia, transcortical motor aphasia
Cognitive psychology[226,235]	Analyze language deficit as disordered information processing, target impaired language architecture (see Chapter 11)	All types of aphasia
Communication boards	Uses pointing toward letters, words, or pictures	Broca's aphasia, transcortical motor aphasia
Language comprehension training[236]	Reteaches meaning with use of verbal and nonverbal materials	Wernicke's aphasia, transcortical sensory aphasia, global aphasia
Melodic intonation[237]	Imbeds short phrases in a simple melody; later, the melodic aspect is withdrawn	Broca's aphasia, transcortical motor aphasia
Stimulation approach[238]	Use of a facilitating stimulus to elicit a response in an automatic way, then, by withdrawing the stimulus, in a more voluntary way	All types of aphasia
Syntax stimulation[239]	Combines delayed repetition and story elicitation to facilitate sentence production with correct syntax	Broca's aphasia, transcortical motor aphasia
Visual action therapy[240]	Facilitates gestural communication	Global aphasia
Word retrieval therapy[225]	Provides cues to word meaning (semantic form) and to word sounds (phonological form)	All anomic aphasias

acquired by the general population only in the past few hundred years, writing is a crucial skill in modern societies. Writing can be considered both a language function and a sophisticated form of praxis (see Chapter 7). *Agraphia*, the loss or impairment of writing ability, is caused by acquired brain disease, involving, in particular, the parietal lobe in the dominant hemisphere. The dominant parietal lobe is critical for integrating the body schema for hand and fingers with somatosensory, motor, and spatial information (see Gerstmann's Syndrome, below) and likely mediates motor equivalence (accomplishing the same goal with different effectors and different goals with the same effector) in handwriting so that movements are scale- and plane-invariant. Thus, letter forms are relatively unchanged whether one writes on paper, on a blackboard, or in the sand using the foot.[247] Assessment of writing is particularly important in aphasic patients because it reveals functional severity, helps to localize the lesion, and may identify a relatively preserved avenue for communication.

Agraphia is broadly classified as aphasic and nonaphasic, although components of both forms are often present (Table 6–11). Common non-aphasic causes of writing impairment include pyramidal and extrapyramidal motor disorders, cerebellar lesions, apraxia, sensory and sensorimotor integration disorders, visuospatial disorders, and lower motor neuron lesions, as well as toxic and metabolic insults associated with confusional states.[248,249] In acute confusional states, writing errors usually consist of repeated letters and sloppy mechanics of penmanship. *Musical agraphia*, loss of the ability to write musical symbols and fluently compose such symbols, may or may not parallel aphasic deficits. In addition to agraphia for words, aphasic professional musicians may have musical agraphia and alexia, affecting both pitch and rhythm.[250]

Aphasic Agraphia

Aphasia is almost always accompanied by agraphia as both are the result of impaired lan-

Table 6–11. **Clinical Features of Aphasic and Nonaphasic Agraphia**

Agraphia Form	Clinical Features	Clinical Features	Lesion Localization (Dominant Hemisphere)
Aphasic			
Nonfluent	Writing effortful and sparse, short phrase length, letters large and poorly formed, more nouns than grammatical words	Broca's and transcortical motor aphasia	Frontal lobe
Fluent	Normal sentence length, calligraphy normal, more grammatical words than nouns	Wernicke's, anomic, and transcortical sensory aphasias	Parietotemporal lobes
Phonological	Inability to write unpronounceable nonwords	Disruption of phoneme-to-grapheme conversion system	Supramarginal gyrus or subjacent insula
Lexical	Inability to retrieve and motorically conceptualize whole words	Impaired writing of familiar but atypical words (irregular or ambiguous words)	Angular gyrus
Alexia with agraphia	Nonfluent aphasic agraphia	Anomic aphasia, Gerstmann's syndrome, posterior cortical atrophy	Angular gyrus
Left-hand agraphia	Inability to write with left hand to verbal command	Copies with left hand, Broca's aphasia, sympathetic apraxia	Anterior corpus callosum
Pure agraphia	Inability to write without language disorder, ideomotor apraxia or visuoconstructive deficit	—	Superior parietal lobule (BA 7); less often, posterior frontal or temporal lobe, or subcortical
Nonaphasic			
Extrapyramidal and pyramidal, cerebellar, and visuomotor disorders	—	—	Variable
Confusional states	Repeated letters, sloppy mechanics	Impaired attention	Diffuse

guage functions. Aphasic agraphia is loosely divided, functionally and anatomically, into two forms analogous to those found in aphasia: a nonfluent, anterior form, associated with frontal lobe lesions, and a fluent, posterior form, associated with parietotemporal lobe lesions (Fig. 6–11).[58] Patients with nonfluent agraphia have difficulty initiating writing, and their output is effortful and slow, with large, awkward, and poorly formed letters. Their writing contains such characteristic features as short phrase length, spelling errors, and a lack of grammatical words such as *if, and, or, but,*

and *to.*[251] In contrast, patients with fluent agraphia write with ease; their calligraphy and sentence length are normal, and their output contains an abundance of grammatical words. However, their writing lacks substantive words, such as *basketball* or *computer,* and is contaminated by paragraphias.

Aphasic agraphia is separated into phonological and lexical forms. In *phonological agraphia,* the patient is unable to write pronounceable nonwords owing to disruption of the phoneme-to-grapheme conversion system, which correlates sounds with letters. For ex-

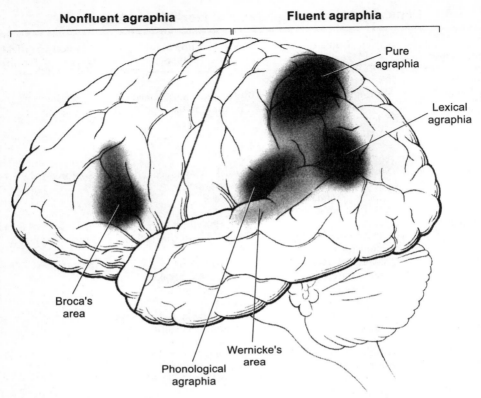

Figure 6–11. Lesion sites associated with different types of agraphia.

ample, when a patient with phonological agraphia hears the sound *ba* (a phoneme), he or she is unable to write the letters *ba* (a grapheme). In *lexical agraphia,* patients are unable to retrieve and motorically conceptualize whole words, and their writing of familiar but atypical words is impaired. The impairment lies within the lexical system, which is important for writing words with irregular or ambiguous spelling. For example, these patients may have difficulty with the irregular words *kerchief* and *circuit* because they contain unusual spelling that prevents simple phoneme-to-grapheme conversion. Additionally, patients may stumble over such ambiguous words as *cotton* and *city,* which require lexical interpretation because they contain sounds that correspond to multiple graphemes. The difference in functional impairment between these two agraphias may be related to the different lesion sites. Patients with lexical agraphia usually have lesions of the angular gyrus, and those with phonological agraphia usually have lesions of the supramarginal gyrus or subjacent insula.[252]

Another form of aphasic agraphia is agraphia with alexia, or acquired illiteracy. It results from lesions of the dominant inferior parietal lobe (angular gyrus) and is often accompanied by anomic aphasia and components of Gerstmann's syndrome, that is, agraphia, acalculia, right–left disorientation, and finger agnosia. Agraphia associated with alexia is typically fluent. It may be found in patients with posterior cortical atrophy.

Aphasic agraphia restricted to the left hand occurs in patients who have language dominance in the left hemisphere and lesions of the anterior corpus callosum.[253] On verbal command, these patients cannot write with the left hand because they are unable to transfer language information from the dominant to the nondominant hemisphere.[3] However, they can copy well with the left hand. Agraphia of the left hand commonly occurs in patients with Broca's aphasia (sympathetic apraxia), whose inability to perform with the left hand on verbal command extends beyond agraphia to encompass all learned motor actions, because language and praxis areas are disconnected from motor association areas in the right hemisphere. In addition, patients with Broca's aphasia often have an aphasic component that contributes to their agraphia.

Pure (isolated, "apraxic") *agraphia* is defined as impaired writing without language disorders, limb (ideomotor) apraxia, or visuoconstructive deficits.[254] Patients with pure agraphia are unable to write letters correctly, but they do not make spelling, reading, or other linguistic errors. This uncommon condition is usually associated with dominant superior parietal lesions (superior to the supramarginal and angular gyri, BA 7).[254,255] However, lesions of the left posterior frontal[256,257] or temporal[258] regions, the caudate or internal capsule,[259] and the thalamus[260] can also cause pure agraphia. Seizures arising from the left superior parietal region produce ictal agraphia.[261]

Nonaphasic Agraphia

Weakness and disorders of movement, visuospatial function, and conversion symptoms produce nonaphasic agraphia. It is not associated with spelling or language errors or with the absence of substantive or grammatical words. In paretic agraphia, the lesion may be located in the muscle, neuromuscular junction, peripheral nerve, peripheral nerve plexus, peripheral nerve root, anterior horn cell, or upper motor neuron. *Micrographia*, or small writing, occurs in two forms: consistently small writing, caused by corticospinal lesions, and progressively smaller writing, caused by parkinsonism.[262] Parkinsonism is also associated with decreased initiative to write, slow writing, crowding of letters, and difficulty maintaining a straight line. Dopaminergic therapy improves micrographia and other writing problems in patients with parkinsonism.

Left-sided thalamo-mesencephalic infarcts cause right-handed micrographia.[263] In hyperkinetic movement disorders, such as tremor, chorea, tics, and dystonia, the intrusion of disordered movements disrupts writing.[251] Writer's cramp, a focal dystonia, usually appears between 20 and 50 years of age and is often associated with abnormal posture and tone in the affected arm.[264] Visuospatial dysfunction also impairs writing. Patients with lesions of the right parietal lobe frequently have left-sided neglect, causing displacement of their writing toward the right side of the page and disruption of the normal spacing and arrangements of letters and sentences. Cerebellar lesions also cause spatial dysgraphia.[249,265] Among patients with conversion disorders, isolated agraphia is rare, but paralysis of the dominant hand commonly causes agraphia.

Hypergraphia, a tendency toward extensive and, in some cases, compulsive writing, may be found in patients with schizophrenia, mania, and, interictally, partial epilepsy.[266,267] Automatic writing, often associated with perseverative and utilization behavior, occurs with bilateral prefrontal injury.[268]

GERSTMANN'S SYNDROME

In the mid-1900s, Gerstmann[269,270] first described the tetrad of agraphia, acalculia, finger agnosia, and right–left disorientation associated with lesions of the left angular gyrus and its transition to the second occipital convolution. Gerstmann suggested that all four deficits are caused by a primary disorder of the body's schema for the hands and fingers, although a primary spatial disorder impairing mental manipulation of images[271] or defective horizontal mapping[272] was later posited. Knowing whether a single mechanism underlies all four deficits in this syndrome would be of great interest, but the question remains unanswered. Developmental Gerstmann's syndrome has been reported in children with or without dyslexia,[273] who may have the classic tetrad plus constructional apraxia or only isolated components of it.

Just as the primary and association somatosensory areas have a disproportionately large representation for the hand, the association posteroinferior parietal cortex has a special relationship to the hand. Ontogenetically, children use their hands and fingers extensively in counting, exploring the world, naming objects as they point toward them, and learning to perform complex motor tasks (praxis). The human is a visual animal who also relies on fine movements and coordination. Cross-modal associations between visual and tactile sensations and motor programs are a hard-wired capacity of the association parietal cortex. The inferior parietal region lies at the junction of the ventral visual stream, which mediates recognition, and the dorsal visual stream, which mediates visuomotor function and peripheral vision.[274]

Recent functional neuroimaging studies have better defined the roles of parietal and extraparietal areas in computational skills. Number-processing tasks activate a circuit comprising bilateral intraparietal, prefrontal, and anterior cingulate components. Task demands modulate the extension and lateralization of this circuit. With multiplication, for example, the inferior parietal regions as well as the fusiform and lingual gyri are activated more on the left than on the right.[275,276] The intraparietal and prefrontal activation is more prominent in the right hemisphere during a comparison task and in the left hemisphere during a multiplication task and is intensely bilateral during a subtraction task.[276] Thus, partially distinct cerebral circuits with the parietal pathway underlie distinct arithmetic operations.

Mathematical intuition relies on the interplay between linguistic and visuospatial representations.[4,277] Exact arithmetic, as in computing an exact sum, is acquired in a language-specific format, transfers poorly to a different language or to novel facts, and recruits networks involved in word-association processes. In contrast, approximate arithmetic, as in computing an approximate sum, is language-independent, relies on a sense of numerical magnitudes, and recruits bilateral areas of the parietal lobes involved in visuospatial processing. Mathematical intuition may emerge from the interplay of these brain systems.

Agraphia and Acalculia

Agraphia is fully covered in a foregoing section (see Agraphia). *Acalculia* is an acquired loss of arithmetic skills. Primary acalculia, the form found in Gerstmann's syndrome, is a pure arithmetic disorder and is not due to language, writing, or spatial disorders. Patients are unable to calculate mentally or with pen and paper. In addition to making reading errors and errors in interpreting signs, such as the plus and the multiplication signs, patients cannot perform simple functions like addition, borrowing, and carrying numbers.[278] Patients with acalculia may correctly answer memorized arithmetic knowledge (multiplication and some addition and subtraction) despite the loss of

conceptual knowledge for calculations.[279] A diagnosis of primary acalculia is valid only in patients who have knowledge of basic arithmetic skills. In addition, the diagnosis cannot be reliably based on errors on the Serial Sevens Subtraction Test because more than half of normal adults make at least one error on this test.[280] Many of our "normal" patients quickly get "100 minus 7 equals 93" but then hesitate with "93 minus 7," and finally answer, incorrectly, "84." In humans, a specific neural substrate, located in the left and right intraparietal areas, is associated with a knowledge of numbers and their relations, that is, a number sense.[281] Acalculia may also be associated with left-sided hemispheric lesions that cause aphasia[282] (although language and calculations can be dissociated[283]) and right-sided hemispheric lesions that cause constructional apraxia, visuospatial disorders, and unilateral neglect.[243,284,285]

Different lesion sites may be associated with different deficits in arithmetic knowledge. Two patients with Gerstmann's syndrome had severe deficits in calculation skills with different lesion sites: a left-sided subcortical lesion and a right-sided inferior parietal lesion.[286] Both could read Arabic numerals and write them to dictation. The patient with the subcortical lesion was selectively deficient at rote verbal knowledge, including arithmetic tables. However, semantic knowledge of numerical quantities was intact. In contrast, the patient with the inferior parietal lesion had a category-specific impairment of quantitative numerical knowledge, which was particularly salient in subtraction and number bisection tasks. The patient's knowledge of rote arithmetic facts was preserved. Proton magnetic resonance spectroscopy in a child with developmental dyscalculia and dysgraphia revealed a focal defect in the left temporoparietal region near the angular gyrus.[287] These cases suggest that a left-sided subcortical network contributes to the storage and retrieval of rote verbal arithmetic facts and that a bilateral inferior parietal network is dedicated to the mental manipulation of numerical quantities.

Finger Agnosia

In Gerstmann's syndrome, damage to the cerebral cortex causes *finger agnosia*, the inability to recognize, identify, differentiate, name, select, indicate, and orient the individual fingers of either one's own hands or another person's hands.[288] Finger agnosia is often a partial defect, with the patient identifying fingers inconsistently. For example, a patient may correctly recognize his or her thumb and little finger but cannot identify his or her index, middle, or ring finger or any of the examiner's fingers. A comprehension deficit and loss of visual or somatosensory input may interfere with finger recognition and must be excluded. Because children first count with their fingers, it may be that the association of finger agnosia and acalculia is a vestige of cognitive development. Finger agnosia is a partial autotopagnosia (see Chapter 3, Table 3–4). Toe agnosia is also present in some cases of Gerstmann's syndrome, suggesting a more generalized digit agnosia.[289]

Mirror agnosia, which is often associated with lesions of the right angular and superior temporal gyri,[290,291] may be related to finger agnosia. Patients with *mirror agnosia* reach toward a virtual object in the mirror and cannot change their behavior even after the object is presented in real visual space. Patients with right-sided inferior parietal injury may have difficulty integrating the body schema for fingers with visuospatial data.

Right–Left Disorientation

Right–left disorientation is the inability to name or point to the right and left sides of objects, including body parts of the self or the examiner. For the diagnosis of right–left disorientation, first exclude a comprehension disorder. With both disorders, it is difficult for patients to follow crossed commands, such as "Touch your left thumb to your right ear." Tests of right–left disorientation and finger agnosia are often combined, as in "Show me your left little finger," but distinguishing these disorders by such commands is difficult because they often occur independently. Right–left disorientation is rare with right hemisphere lesions.[269,292]

A True Syndrome?

Controversy has surrounded the specificity and even the existence of Gerstmann's syn-

drome.[293-296] Skeptics have argued that the degree of intercorrelation among the four components is low, making the existence of a syndrome dubious. However, Geschwind and Strub[295] offer a persuasive counterargument:

It is of no importance whether the intercorrelation is low or whether it is no higher than the correlation of any component with their deficits. Depending on the frequency of acoustic neuromas in the population studied, the correlation of nystagmus with deafness would be higher than, lower than, or equal to the correlation of nystagmus with a Horner's syndrome or a left vagus nerve paralysis. The intercorrelations of components with each other or their correlations with other deficits are thus irrelevant. What is relevant is the predictive ability of the entire complex of components. The predictive value of the Gerstmann syndrome is simply stated: When all four components are present, it predicts with a high degree of accuracy the presence of a left parietal lesion.

Additional clinical observations leave little doubt that the positive correlation of the clinical tetrad with left-sided posterior inferior parietal lesions is valid, assuming that a confusional state and increased intracranial pressure are excluded.[297] Reproduction of the four features with electrical stimulation of the left inferior parietal cortex provides additional support.[298]

NONAPHASIC (NONLINGUISTIC) SPEECH DISORDERS

Nonaphasic speech disorders, like aphasic disorders, cause acquired impairments in understanding spoken or written language. Disorders of auditory or visual sensation and perception, or of their connections to the language cortex, impair the quality of information reaching the language areas. These sensory–perceptual disorders are not aphasia because the language cortex is not directly involved. Syndromes produced by disconnection of sensory input from language areas, such as pure word deafness (see Wernicke's Aphasia, above) and alexia without agraphia (Fig. 6–12), are language disorders, not true aphasias.

Speech requires the coordinated functions of the pyramidal and extrapyramidal motor systems, the cerebellum, lower motor neurons, the neuromuscular junction, and muscles. Le-

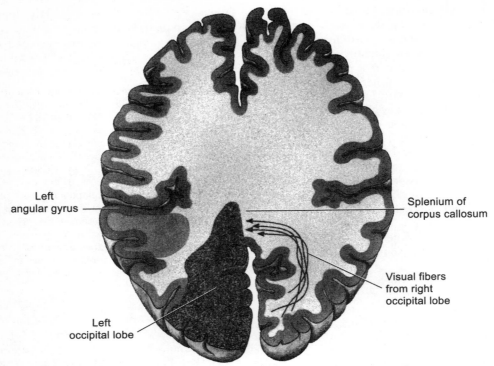

Left
angular gyrus

Splenium of
corpus callosum

Visual fibers
from right
occipital lobe

Left
occipital lobe

Figure 6–12. Lesion site associated with alexia without agraphia. Left posterior cerebral artery infarction of the occipital lobe and splenium of the corpus callosum spares the angular gyrus, but visual input cannot reach it.

sions at these neural levels impair the spontaneity, fluency, articulation, volume, resonance, phonation, and prosody of speech. In addition to transient mutism and persistent dysarthria, right-sided cerebellar lesions can cause agrammatic speech, possibly by interfering with the temporal sequencing of language.[299,300] Structural lesions of the larynx, oropharynx, soft palate, tongue, and lips also affect speech. In contrast with aphasia, these motor speech disorders are not associated with language errors; the patient can, for example, use written language normally.

Dysphonia and Spastic Dysphonia

Speech impairment from laryngeal disorders is called *dysphonia;* if speech is entirely absent, the term is *aphonia.* Dysphonia is distinguished from aphasia by preserved comprehension, fluency, and use of written language. Although dysphonic speech may be mistakenly considered dysfluent, patients are able to produce a grammatical sentence with normal phrase length. Spastic (spasmodic) dysphonia, which usually begins in adulthood, is a gradually progressive focal dystonia of the laryngeal speech musculature. Simultaneous contraction of all speech muscles produces loud, strained, and dysfluent speech, which has been likened to the speech of a person who is being strangled. Although unable to speak in a soft and rhythmic manner, patients typically are able to sing, shout, whisper, and swallow. This dissociation of actions involving the same muscles suggests to some a psychogenic cause. However, like blepharospasm and writer's cramp, spastic dysphonia is an extrapyramidal disorder, and relaxation techniques and psychotherapy are not helpful. Injection of botulinum toxin into a vocal cord (i.e., thyroarytenoid muscle) or thyroplasty (surgically medializing the membranous portion of the vocal fold) may be of benefit.[301]

Dysarthria

Dysarthria refers to abnormal articulation in its strictest sense and to any nonlinguistic speech disorder in its broadest domain. Common in anterior nonfluent aphasia (e.g., Broca's aphasia) and rare in posterior fluent aphasia (e.g., Wernicke's aphasia), dysarthria often occurs without aphasia. According to the qualitative features and neuroanatomical systems involved, dysarthria is classified into four types: paretic, spastic, ataxic, and extrapyramidal.

PARETIC DYSARTHRIA

Weakness of articulatory muscles, usually the vocal cord adductors, causes *paretic dysarthria*, or flaccid speech. Weakness of other muscles, including the laryngeal and pharyngeal, orbicularis oris, masseter, and pterygoid muscles, and of the diaphragm and tongue also impairs oral communication.[302] The lesion may be in the lower motor neurons, as in progressive bulbar palsy, idiopathic polyneuritis, and recurrent laryngeal nerve palsy; the neuromuscular junction, as in myasthenia; or the muscles, as in myositis. The voice is typically soft or barely audible, low-pitched, and nasal. Patients with laryngeal weakness have difficulty with prolonged phonation of vowel sounds, such as *ee*. Weakness of the soft palate, usually from bilateral vagus nerve lesions or myasthenia gravis, also impairs articulation, marked by a nasal voice, especially when the head is tilted forward. Weakness of the tongue, from hypoglossal palsy and myopathies, causes lisping, or muffled speech, and weakness of the lip musculature, from facial palsy, disturbs articulation. Asking the patient to imitate the sounds *ga ga* (soft palate), *ta ta* (tongue), *ba ba* (lips), and *ee* (larynx) helps to distinguish the affected muscles. For example, a patient who cannot repeat the sounds *ga ga* or *ee* most likely has weakness of the soft palate and larynx.

SPASTIC DYSARTHRIA

Upper motor neuron (corticobulbar) lesions, usually multiple, bilateral small lacunar infarcts, cause *spastic* (hypertonic, pseudobulbar) *dysarthria*. Spastic speech is slow, strained, thick, and monopitched; articulation is imprecise, especially of consonants, and volume may be explosive. Jaw jerk is usually increased, and the tongue is unable to make rapid, alternating movements.

Aphemia is spastic dysarthria caused by a cortical lesion, typically from a stroke, involving the frontal motor and premotor cortex (prerolandic gyrus and pars opercularis) and the underlying white matter, sparing Broca's area (Fig. 6–3).[74] As the acute deficits of right-sided hemiparesis and muteness resolve over time, speech recovers, more or less usefully, but at first is slow, hypophonic, and difficult to understand. Broca's aphasia may be present transiently. Patients with aphemia have normal, nonaphasic writing and naming. Aphemia may coexist with orobuccolingual apraxia and is rarely the sole feature of a primary progressive disorder.[303]

ATAXIC DYSARTHRIA

Lesions of the cerebellum or its connections cause *ataxic* (cerebellar) *dysarthria*, or ataxic speech. Slurred speech is dysarticulated into jerky, irregular components. Speech rhythm, volume, and pitch are variable and may be explosive because of poorly regulated expiration. Staccato sentences in a sing-song, monotonous meter, lacking the normal stress on syllables and words, mark "scanning" cerebellar speech. A voice tremor, along with essential tremor in some cases, may further disrupt the phonatory rhythm. Scanning speech is rarely due to a pure cerebellar lesion; cerebellar, pyramidal, and extrapyramidal lesions are usually present.[304] Patients with cerebellar degeneration or multiple sclerosis often have ataxic dysarthria. Rarely, patients with right-sided cerebellar lesions have agrammatic speech with mild dysfluency or anomia, which may be confused with Broca's aphasia, but other aspects of their language are normal.[299,305]

EXTRAPYRAMIDAL DYSARTHRIA

Extrapyramidal dysarthria, or dystonic and hypokinetic speech, takes many forms. Patients with caudate–putamen infarcts have slow, dysarthric speech with or without hemiplegia.[162,170] Parkinsonism is associated with hypokinetic dysarthria, which is characterized by slow, monotonous speech with decreased pitch and variable loudness, low volume, inappropriate silences, and imprecise consonants.[302] Some parkinsonian patients have a more rapid but festinating speech pattern. Patients with Huntington's chorea may have erratic breathing with explosive speech and, in severe cases, only unintelligible utterances.[306] Choreic dysarthria is caused by involuntary respiratory, tongue, and facial movements, resulting in hesitant speech that is irregular in speed, loudness, and articulation.

Nonaphasic Anomia

Nonaphasic naming errors arise from lesions in areas outside the language cortex, including anterior or posterior and cortical or subcortical regions and dominant or nondominant hemispheres. Isolated, nonaphasic anomia, like most aphasic anomia, is of limited localizing value but, as with headache, is often one of the earliest signs of a brain disorder, such as a primary or metastatic tumor.

Misnaming occurs in a variety of nonaphasic disorders.[307,308] Diffuse central nervous system insults, especially those occurring suddenly, as in traumatic brain injury, subarachnoid hemorrhage, sudden increase in intracranial pressure, or systemic illness, may cause nonaphasic anomia. The humorous "frontal" response in the frontal lobe syndrome with deliberate facetiousness (classic witzelsucht) may appear to be anomia. For example, if the examiner asks "What is my profession?" the patient may respond "Someone who asks a lot of questions."[308] In addition, the frontal response superficially resembles the descriptive responses of patients with anomia. In trying to name an apple tree, for instance, the patient may say "That thing the good red fruit grows on." Perseverative errors are often mistaken for naming errors, and responses of patients with conversion disorder or malingering may resemble anomia. As the result of deficits in language, memory, or other functions, anomia is common in dementia.

Foreign Accent Syndrome

An uncommon disorder, foreign accent syndrome is the result of an acquired brain injury, causing the patient's speech to resemble a generic foreign accent. The syndrome is distinct from aphasia, apraxia, and dysarthria but may occur in association with them[309] or in isolation.[310–312] Altered prosody and anomalies of vowel and consonant production (e.g., vowel tensing or lengthening), mediated by the language-dominant hemisphere, appear critical in

producing the foreign accent syndrome. In pure foreign accent syndrome, small lesions (<3 cm) are found in the primary motor cortex (BA 4), association motor cortex (BAs 6, 44), subfrontal white matter, and striatum. Lesions of the middle portion of the primary motor area may produce foreign accent syndrome, impairing prosody, and lesions of the inferior portion may produce aphemia, impairing articulation. The disorder rarely complicates psychotic disorders without lesions on magnetic resonance imaging.[313]

Functional Voice Disorders

Functional (psychogenic) disorders of the voice occur in patients with prominent complaints of impaired phonation despite normal mucosa, full vocal cord movement, and complete closure on phonation.[314] Excessive voice use does not appear to play a role. Increased tension in the laryngeal muscles during speech and psychogenic factors are important. Functional voice impairment is 10 times as common as functional loss of voice.[314]

Stuttering

Although stuttering is usually a developmental disorder of childhood, it may begin after brain injury in adulthood. Acquired stuttering usually occurs acutely and is characterized by involuntary repetitions, prolongations, and blocks not restricted to initial syllables or substantive words; for instance, grammatical words such as *and* and *if* are affected.[315] In most cases of stuttering with aphasia, usually Broca's aphasia, the lesion is in the left hemisphere, although the site varies and rarely involves nondominant and subcortical locations.[82,316,317] Acquired stuttering is often transient but may persist if the lesions are bilateral.[135] Antiepileptic drugs may improve acquired stuttering from stroke. Other causes of acquired stuttering are Parkinson's disease, progressive supranuclear palsy, neurosyphilis, and the multi-infarct state.

Palilalia

Palilalia is involuntary repetition of words, phrases, and, less often, syllables. Usually, speech rate increases and volume decreases with the repetition. Idiopathic parkinsonism, progressive supranuclear palsy, and other diseases with bilateral upper brain stem or basal ganglia lesions, as in pseudobulbar palsy, account for most cases of this uncommon disorder.[318] Trazodone may be helpful in treating palilalia.[319] Postencephalitic parkinsonism was once the most common cause of this disorder. Rarely, palilalia occurs with seizures originating in the left parasagittal region.[320]

Echolalia

Echolalia is the parrot-like repetition of words and phrases that are heard. Echolalia can complicate TMA or MTA.[124] Patients with MTA have no comprehension of what is said but merely repeat what they hear. Echolalia also occurs with autism, schizophrenia, Alzheimer's disease, Tourette's syndrome, and rarely seizures.[320] Echolalia and palilalia may coexist.

Mutism

Mutism, the inability or refusal to speak, occurs in both nonaphasic and aphasic disorders. It has an extensive differential diagnosis (Table 6-12). Patients with Broca's aphasia or global aphasia may be unable initially to speak or may not even attempt to speak. Right-sided facial weakness, or hemiparesis, usually accompanies both types of aphasia; and right-sided hemisensory loss and hemianopia are also found in global aphasia. As mute aphasic patients recover, aspontaneous and nonfluent speech emerges. Aphasic patients with mutism make linguistic writing errors, which distinguishes them from patients with the more common nonaphasic mutism caused by other neurological or functional disorders. These errors include word substitutions, or *paralexias,* such as *pair* instead of *chair;* telegraphic writing, in which connecting grammatical words are deleted, as in "I store rice" for "I want to go to the store to buy rice;" and nonsensical fluent writing, as in "The only thing that I wish well you must know that the other thing yes that thing of course." Patients with pseudobulbar palsy, especially with lesions of limbic–brain stem motor pathways, may be unable to speak.[321]

Table 6–12. **Disorders and Conditions Associated with Mutism**

Aphasic syndromes
  Global aphasia
  Broca's aphasia
Aphemia (pure word mutism)
Supplementary motor area lesions
Pseudobulbar palsy
Abulia
Akinetic mutism
Locked-in syndrome
Chronic vegetative state
Cerebellar lesions
Lower motor neuron lesions
  Idiopathic polyneuritis
  Bulbar poliomyelitis
Laryngeal disorders
Psychiatric and psychogenic disorders

ABULIA AND AKINETIC MUTISM

Abulia and akinetic mutism arise from lesions in different areas of the brain (see Chapter 7). Mutism may be caused by *abulia,* a generalized slowing and decrease in mental and motor activity and speech. Patients with abulia may intermittently fail to respond to questions or commands for minutes at a time, and their responses are slow and apathetic. In akinetic mutism, the most intense form of abulia, the patient appears to be awake but spontaneous motor and verbal responses are absent. Dopaminergic agonists improve akinetic mutism caused by lesions that interrupt dopaminergic input to the cortex[322] but not that caused by diffuse cortical lesions.[323]

MUTENESS FROM SUPPLEMENTARY MOTOR AREA LESIONS

Severe muteness caused by lesions of the SMA in either hemisphere is usually transient, often lasting only days; but with injury of the SMA in the dominant hemisphere, the muteness may last several weeks. The impaired spontaneous speech and repetition caused by SMA damage in the dominant hemisphere usually subsides, but impaired writing may persist.[128] The response to selective SMA ablation is a three-stage process.[324] The first, acute stage is marked by global akinesia, more prominent contralaterally, with speech arrest; the second, subacute stage consists of reduced spontaneous motor activity contralaterally, facial weakness for emotional expression, and reduced spontaneous speech; and the third, chronic stage is marked by slowed rapid alternating hand movements with normal speech. Electrical stimulation during corticography and spontaneous focal seizure discharges from this area cause speech arrest and an "urge to move" and interfere with the organization of future elements in complex movements.[325,326]

MUTENESS FROM BILATERAL CEREBELLAR LESIONS

Acute damage to hemispheric and deep dentate nuclei from bilateral cerebellar lesions causes temporary speech loss.[327] The cognitive impairments mimic the personality changes and deficits in executive function caused by frontal lobe lesions (see Chapter 7);[306] cranial nerve signs may be absent. Muteness lasts less than 3 months, but patients are usually severely dysarthric during recovery.

MUTENESS FROM LOWER MOTOR NEURON LESIONS

Lower motor neuron lesions involving the vagus nerve bilaterally paralyze the laryngeal speech muscles. In addition, the muscles that contribute to speech production, such as the soft palate and tongue, may be weak. Idiopathic polyneuritis is the most common cause of muteness in patients with lower motor neuron deficits. Viral neuronitis usually produces idiopathic vocal cord paralysis.

LOCKED-IN SYNDROME AND CHRONIC VEGETATIVE STATE

The de-efferentation of central motor fibers supplying facial and body musculature produces locked-in syndrome.[328] The ventral pons or, occasionally, the ventral midbrain is the site of the lesion. Pathological processes include infarction, hemorrhage, central pontine myelinolysis, tumor, and encephalitis.[329] Patients are fully alert and conscious but can communicate only by blinking or moving the eyes. The EEG reveals normal or mildly slowed background activity. Ask mute patients to blink or move the eyes on command; otherwise, the diagnosis of locked-in syndrome may be missed.

Patients in the chronic vegetative state emerge from coma and resume relatively normal sleep–wake cycles; the eyes open during "wakefulness," but intellectual activity is minimal or absent. The absence of a clear-cut high-level response to verbal stimuli distinguishes these patients from those with locked-in syndrome. The chronic vegetative state usually follows severe, diffuse brain insults, such as hypoxia, ischemia, hypoglycemia, and head trauma. The EEG usually shows background slowing with decreased voltage. The prognosis for a meaningful recovery is dismal.

LARYNGITIS AND LARYNGEAL DISORDERS

Viral and, less often, bacterial laryngitis causes hoarseness and may produce acute muteness. Tumors and other laryngeal disorders produce a more insidious loss of the voice. Consider laryngeal disorders in all patients with speech disorders who can write normally; examine the vocal cords and obtain imaging studies when indicated. Primary laryngeal disorders causing mutism or dysarthria are occasionally misdiagnosed as aphemia.

PSYCHIATRIC AND PSYCHOGENIC DISORDERS

Mutism is commonly associated with psychiatric disorders.[314] Catatonic depression, schizophrenia, and other psychogenic illnesses may mimic structural brain diseases or laryngeal disorders. Elective mutism is a disorder in which a child refuses to talk in specific social situations, such as school, but comprehends spoken language and speaks in other settings.[330] Predisposing factors in elective mutism are social isolation, parental overprotection (usually the mother), parental shyness and withdrawal (usually the father), language and speech disorders, mental retardation, and immigration before the age of 3 years.[331,332]

SUMMARY

Language is a code for mapping thoughts into signals and signals into thoughts, with a sound-based system used to represent and process words, transform word order and re-lation into meaning, and temporally organize the flow of narrative speech. A network of perisylvian areas in the language-dominant hemisphere implements the understanding (Wernicke's area, angular gyrus) and production (Broca's area) of language. These areas connect with each other and with other association cortices in a bidirectional link between areas involved in conceptual thought and planning and language. Paralinguistic meaning is conveyed by gesture and prosody, for example, emotional tone in speech, which is mediated primarily by the nondominant hemisphere. Aphasia is a disorder of language formation and comprehension caused by structural or physiological disruptions in the language network.

Aphasia must be distinguished from a variety of nonaphasic (nonlinguistic) disorders that impair language comprehension (e.g., hearing deficit) or speech (e.g., motor disorders). Aphasia causes various combinations of impairments for comprehending, associating, and producing the components of language. The resulting aphasia syndromes overlap and change as the disorder progresses or resolves. The aphasias can be separated by spontaneous speech into nonfluent (Broca's aphasia, transcortical motor aphasia, mixed transcortical aphasia, and global aphasia) and fluent (Wernicke's aphasia, conduction aphasia, transcortical sensory aphasia, and anomic aphasia) forms. These eight aphasia syndromes compose the majority of the aphasias, although mixed forms and language disorders resulting from subcortical lesions also occur. The diagnosis of aphasia depends on the assessment of spontaneous speech and specific testing for speech initiation and fluency, comprehension, repetition, naming, paraphasias, reading, writing, and prosody.

Aphasia disrupts communication and the stream of verbal consciousness, often with devastating effects on social and work roles, decision making, creativity, and mathematical skills. Depression is a common comorbid disorder. Therapy for aphasia is of limited efficacy. Acute Broca's aphasia and conduction aphasia are the most likely to improve with speech therapy. Although no known medication improves aphasia, some nonaphasic (nonlinguistic) speech disorders respond to pharmacological therapy (see Chapter 11).

REFERENCES

1. Lewis MB, Gerhand S, and Ellis HD: Re-evaluating age-of-acquisition effects. Are they simply cumulative-frequency effects? Cognition 78:189–205, 2001.
2. Pinker S: The Language Instinct. W Morrow, New York, 1994.
3. Geschwind N: Disconnexion syndromes in animals and man. Brain 88:237–294, 585–644, 1965.
4. Einstein A: Ideas and Opinions. Crown, New York, 1954, pp 25–26.
5. Broca P: Perte de la parole, ramollissement chronique et destruction partielle du lobe anterieur gauche du cerveau. Bull Soc Anthropol Paris 2:235–238, 1861.
6. Dax M: Lesion de la moitie gauche de l'encephale coincident avec l'oubli des signes de la pensee. Gazette Hebdomidaire Med Chir 2:259–260, 1865.
7. Wernicke C: Der Aphasische Symptomenkomplex. Cohn & Wigert, Breslau, Poland, 1874.
8. Papafragou A, Massey C, and Gleitman L: Shake, rattle, 'n' roll: the representation of motion in language and cognition. Cognition 84:189–219, 2002.
9. Mesulam M: From sensation to cognition. Brain 121:1013–1052, 1998.
10. Gainotti G: What the locus of brain lesion tells us about the nature of the cognitive defect underlying category-specific disorders: a review. Cortex 36:539–559, 2000.
11. Lu LH, Crosson B, Nadeau SE, et al.: Category-specific naming deficits for objects and actions: semantic attribute and grammatical role hypotheses. Neuropsychologia 40:1608–1621, 2002.
12. Kimura D: The origin of human communication. In Robson J (ed). Origin and Evolution of the Universe: Evidence for Design? McGill-Queens Press, Montreal, 1987, pp 227–246.
13. Poizner H, Merians AS, Clark MA, Macauley B, Rothi LJ, and Heilman KM: Left hemispheric specialization for learned, skilled, and purposeful action. Neuropsychology 12:163–182, 1998.
14. Rushworth MF, Nixon PD, Renowden S, Wade DT, and Passingham RE: The left parietal cortex and motor attention. Neuropsychologia 35:1261–1273, 1997.
15. Geschwind N and Galaburda AM: Cerebral lateralization: biological mechanisms, associations, and pathology: a hypothesis and a program for research. Arch Neurol 42:428–459, 521–552, 634–654, 1985.
16. Coren S and Porac C: Fifty centuries of right-handedness: the historical record. Science 198:631–632, 1977.
17. McManuse C: Right Hand, Left Hand. Harvard University Press, Cambridge, MA, 2002, pp 202–230.
18. Hecaen H and de Ajuriaguerra J: Left-Handedness: Manual Superiority and Cerebral Dominance. Grune and Stratton, New York, 1964.
19. Szaflarski JP, Binder JR, Possing ET, McKiernan KA, Ward BD, and Hammeke TA: Language lateralization in left-handed and ambidextrous people: fMRI data. Neurology 59:238–244, 2002.
20. Peterson JM and Lansky LM: Left-handedness among architects: partial replication and some new data. Percept Mot Skills 45:1216–1218, 1977.

21. Hassler M and Gupta D: Functional brain organization, handedness, and immune vulnerability in musicians and non-musicians. Neuropsychologia 31: 655–660, 1993.

22. Lalumiere ML, Blanchard R, and Zucker KJ: Sexual orientation and handedness in men and women: a meta-analysis. Psychol Bull 126:575–592, 2000.

23. Dellatolas G, Luciani S, Castresana A, et al.: Pathological left-handedness. Left handedness correlatives in adult epileptics. Brain 116:1565–1574, 1993.

24. O'Callaghan MJ, Burn YR, Mohay HA, Rogers Y, and Tudehope DI: The prevalence and origins of left hand preference in high risk infants, and its implications for intellectual, motor and behavioural performance at four and six years. Cortex 29:617–627, 1993.

25. Knecht S, Deppe M, Drager B, et al.: Language lateralization in healthy right-handers. Brain 123: 74–81, 2000.

26. Shaywitz BA, Shaywitz SE, Pugh KR, et al.: Sex differences in the functional organization of the brain for language. Nature 373:607–609, 1995.

27. Alexander MP and Annett M: Crossed aphasia and related anomalies of cerebral organization: case reports and a genetic hypothesis. Brain Lang 55:213–239, 1996.

28. Bakar M, Kirshner HS, and Wertz RT: Crossed aphasia. Functional brain imaging with PET or SPECT. Arch Neurol 53:1026–1032, 1996.

29. Baynes K, Eliassen JC, Lutsep HL, and Gazzaniga MS: Modular organization of cognitive systems masked by interhemispheric integration. Science 280:902–905, 1998.

30. Hynd GW, Semrud-Clikeman M, Lorys AR, Novey ES, and Eliopulos D: Brain morphology in developmental dyslexia and attention deficit disorder/hyperactivity. Arch Neurol 47:919–926, 1990.

31. Schachter SC: Handedness measurement and correlation with brain structure. In Schachter, SC and Devinsky O (eds). Behavioral Neurology and the Legacy of Norman Geschwind. Lippincott-Raven, Philadelphia, 1997, pp 257–270.

32. Newman MA and Albino RC: Hemisphere differences and judgment of simultaneity of brief light flashes. Percept Mot Skills 49:943–956, 1979.

33. Damasceno BP: Time perception as a complex functional system: neuropsychological approach. Int J Neurosci 85:237–262, 1996.

34. Hertz-Pannier L, Chiron C, Jambaque I, et al.: Late plasticity for language in a child's non-dominant hemisphere: a pre-and post-surgery fMRI study. Brain 125:361–362, 2002.

35. Ansaldo AI, Arguin M, and Roch Lecours A: The contribution of the right cerebral hemisphere to the recovery from aphasia: a single longitudinal case study. Brain Lang 82:206–222, 2002.

36. Regard M, Cook ND, Wieser HG, and Landis T: The dynamics of cerebral dominance during unilateral limbic seizures. Brain 117:91–104, 1994.

37. Zaidel DW: A view of the world from a split-brain perspective. In Critchley E (ed). The Neurological Boundaries of Reality. Farrand, London, 1994, pp 161–174.

38. Wuillemin D, Richardson B, and Lynch J: Right hemisphere involvement in processing later-learned languages in multilinguals. Brain Lang 46:620–636, 1994.

39. Sugishita M, Otomo K, Kabe S, and Yunoki K: A critical appraisal of neuropsychological correlates of Japanese ideogram (*kanji*) and phonogram (*kana*) reading. Brain 115:1563–1585, 1992.

40. Hickok G, Kirk K, and Bellugi U: Hemispheric organization of local- and global-level visuospatial processes in deaf signers and its relation to sign language aphasia. Brain Lang 65:276–286, 1998.

41. Birchmeier AK: Aphasic dyslexia of Braille in a congenitally blind man. Neuropsychologia 23:177–193, 1985.

42. Erickson RJ, Goldinger SD, and LaPointe LL: Auditory vigilance in aphasiac individuals: detecting nonlinguistic stimuli with full or divided attention. Brain Cogn 30:244–253, 1996.

43. Heilman KM, Safran A, and Geschwind N: Closed head trauma and aphasia. J Neurol Neurosurg Psychiatry 34:265–269, 1971.

44. Sarno MT: The nature of verbal impairment after closed head injury. J Nerv Ment Dis 168:685–692, 1980.

45. Benson DF and Ardila A: Aphasia: A Clinical Perspective. Oxford University Press, New York, 1996, p 33.

46. Karbe H, Herholz K, Kessler J, et al.: Recovery of language after brain damage. Adv Neurol 73:347–358, 1997.

47. Brown JW and Hecaen H: Lateralization and language representation. Neurology 26:183–189, 1976.

48. Pedersen PM, Jorgensen HS, Nakayama H, et al.: Aphasia in acute stroke: incidence, determinants, and recovery. Ann Neurol 38:659–666, 1995.

49. Tuchman RF and Rapin I: Regression in pervasive developmental disorders: seizures and epileptiform electroencephalographic correlates. Pediatrics 99: 560–566, 1997.

50. Kolski H and Otsubo H: The Landau-Kleffner syndrome. Adv Exp Med Biol 497:195–208, 2002.

51. Paul R and Marans WD: Assessing speech, language and communication. Child Adolesc Psychiatr Clin N Am 8:297–322, 1999.

52. Oldfield RC: The assessment and analysis of handedness: the Edinburgh inventory. Neuropsychologia 9:97–113, 1971.

53. Goodglass H, Quadfasel F, and Timberlake W: Phrase length and the type and severity of aphasia. Cortex 1:133–153, 1964.

54. Howes D and Geschwind N: Quantitative studies of aphasic language. In Rioch D and Weinstein EA (eds). Disorders of Communication. Proceedings of the Association for Research in Nervous and Mental Disease, Vol 42. Williams & Wilkins, Baltimore, 1964, pp 229–244.

55. Lecours AR, Lhermitte F, and Bryans B: Aphasiology. Bailliere-Tindall, London, 1983.

56. Dick F, Bates E, Wulfeck B, Utman JA, Dronkers N, and Gernsbacher MA: Language deficits, localization, and grammar. Psychol Rev 108:759–788, 2001.

57. Naeser MA, Palumbo CL, Helm-Estabrooks N, Stiassny-Eder D, and Albert ML: Severe nonfluency in aphasia. Role of the medial subcallosal fasciculus and other white matter pathways in recovery of spontaneous speech. Brain 112:1–38, 1989.

58. Benson DF and Geschwind N: Aphasia and related disorders: a clinical approach. In Mesulam MM

(ed). Principles of Behavioral Neurology. FA Davis, Philadelphia, 1985, pp 193–238.

59. Ross ED: Affective prosody and the aprosodias. In Mesulam MM (ed). Principles of Cognitive and Behavioral Neurology. Oxford University Press, New York, 2002, pp 316–331.

60. Weintraub S, Mesulam MM, and Kramer LL: Disturbances in prosody. Arch Neurol 38:742–744, 1981.

61. Buckingham HW: Mechanisms underlying aphasic transformations. In Ardila A and Ostrosky F (eds). Brain Organization of Language and Cognitive Processes. Plenum, New York, 1989, pp 123–145.

62. Albert ML, Yamadori A, Gardner H, and Howes D: Comprehension in alexia. Brain 96:317–328, 1973.

63. Stengel E: A clinical and psychological study of echo reactions. J Ment Sci 93:598–612, 1947.

64. Basso A, Taborelli A, and Vignolo LA: Dissociated disorders of speaking and writing in aphasics. J Neurol Neurosurg Psychiatry 41:556–563, 1978.

65. Goodglass H and Geschwind N: Language disturbance (aphasia). In Carterette EC and Friedman MP (eds). Handbook of Perception, Vol 7. Academic Press, New York, 1976, pp 389–428.

66. Price CJ, Moore CJ, Humphreys GW, et al.: The neural regions sustaining object recognition and naming. Proc R Soc Lond B Biol Sci 263:1501–1507, 1996.

67. Humphreys GW and Forde EM: Hierarchies, similarity, and interactivity in object recognition: "category-specific" neuropsychological deficits. Behav Brain Sci 24:453–476, 2001.

68. Geschwind N: The anatomy of acquired disorders of reading. In Money J (ed). Reading Disability: Progress and Research Needs in Dyslexia. Johns Hopkins University Press, Baltimore, 1962, pp 115–129.

69. Jackson JH: On affections of speech from diseases of the brain. Brain 1:304–330, 1878.

70. Bak TH, O'Donovan DG, Xuereb JH, Boniface S, and Hodges JR: Selective impairment of verb processing associated with pathological changes in Brodmann areas 44 and 45 in the motor neurone disease–dementia–aphasia syndrome. Brain 124:103–120, 2001.

71. Swinney D and Zurif E: Syntactic processing in aphasia. Brain Lang 50:225–239, 1995.

72. Sirigu A, Cohen L, Zalla T, et al.: Distinct frontal regions for processing sentence syntax and story grammar. Cortex 34:771–778, 1998.

73. Mohr JP, Pessin MS, Finkelstein S, et al.: Broca's aphasia: pathologic and clinical features. Neurology 28:311–324, 1978.

74. Schiff HB, Alexander MP, Naeser MA, and Galaburda AM: Aphemia: clinical-anatomical correlations. Arch Neurol 40:720–727, 1983.

75. Damasio AR: Aphasia. N Engl J Med 326:531–539, 1992.

76. Embick D, Marantz A, Miyashita Y, O'Neil W, and Sakai KL: A syntactic specialization for Broca's area. Proc Natl Acad Sci USA 97:6150–6154, 2000.

77. Kertesz A and Munoz DG: Frontotemporal dementia. Med Clin North Am 86:501–518, 2002.

78. Morris PL, Robinson RG, de Carvalho ML, et al.: Lesion characteristics and depressed mood in the stroke data bank study. J Neuropsychiatry Clin Neurosci 8:153–159, 1996.

79. Goldstein, K: Language and Language Disturbances. Grune and Stratton, New York, 1948.

80. Starkstein SE, Bryer JB, Berthier ML, et al.: Depression after stroke: the importance of cerebral hemisphere asymmetries. Clin Neurosci 3:276–285, 1991

81. MacHale SM, O'Rourke SJ, Wardlaw JM, and Dennis MS. Depression and its relation to lesion location after stroke. J Neurol Neurosurg Psychiatry 64: 371–374, 1998.

82. Lazar RM, Marshall RS, Prell GD, and Pile-Spellman J: The experience of Wernicke's aphasia. Neurology 55:1222–1224, 2000.

83. Godefroy O, Dubois C, Debachy B, Leclerc M, and Kreisler A: Vascular aphasias: main characteristics of patients hospitalized in acute stroke units. Stroke 33:702–705, 2002.

84. Martins IP: Childhood aphasias. Clin Neurosci 4: 73–77, 1997.

85. Van Hout A: Acquired aphasia in children. Semin Pediatr Neurol 4:102–108, 1997.

86. Mihailescu L: Communicative disorders in Wernicke's aphasics. Rom J Neurol Psychiatry 31:85–96, 1993.

87. Sevush S, Roeltgen DP, Campanella DJ, and Heilman KM: Preserved oral reading in Wernicke's aphasia. Neurology 33:916–920, 1983.

88. Semenza C, Cipolotti L, and Denes G: Reading aloud in jargon aphasia: an unusual dissociation in speech output. J Neurol Neurosurg Psychiatry 55:205–208, 1992.

89. Kirshner HS and Webb WG: Alexia and agraphia in Wernicke's aphasia. J Neurol Neurosurg Psychiatry 45:719–724, 1982.

90. Benson DF: Psychiatric aspects of aphasia. Br J Psychiatry 123:555–566, 1973.

91. Selnes OA, Knopman DS, Niccum N, and Rubens AB: The critical role of Wernicke's area in sentence repetition. Ann Neurol 17:549–557, 1985.

92. Alexander MP, Naeser MA, and Palumbo CL: Correlations of subcortical CT lesion sites and aphasia profiles. Brain 110:961–991, 1987.

93. Hillis AE, Wityk RJ, Tuffiash E, et al.: Hypoperfusion of Wernicke's area predicts severity of semantic deficit in acute stroke. Ann Neurol 50:561–566, 2001.

94. Kertesz A, Lau WK, and Polk M: The structural determinants of recovery in Wernicke's aphasia. Brain Lang 44:153–164, 1993.

95. D'Esposito M and Alexander MP: Subcortical aphasia: distinct profiles following left putaminal hemorrhage. Neurology 45:38–41, 1995.

96. Knight RT and Cooper J: Status epilepticus manifesting as reversible Wernicke's aphasia. Epilepsia 27:301–304, 1986.

97. Naeser MA and Palumbo CL: Neuroimaging and language recovery in stroke. J Clin Neurophysiol 11:150–174, 1994.

98. Albert ML and Bear D: Time to understand. A case study of word deafness with reference to the role of time in auditory comprehension. Brain 97:383–394, 1974.

99. Buchman AS, Garron DC, Trust-Cardamone JE, Wichter MD, and Schwartz M: Word deafness: one hundred years later. J Neurol Neurosurg Psychiatry 49:489–499, 1986.

100. Coslett HB, Brashear HR, and Heilman KM: Pure word deafness after bilateral primary auditory cortex infarcts. Neurology 34:347–352, 1984.
101. Pinard M, Chertkow H, Black S, and Peretz I: A case study of pure word deafness. Modularity in auditory processing? Neurocase 8:40–55, 2002.
102. Ardila A and Roselli M: Conduction aphasia and verbal apraxia. J Neurolinguistics 5:1–14, 1990.
103. Geschwind N. Carl Wernicke: The Breslau school and the history of aphasia. In Carterette EC (ed). Brain Function. Speech, Language, and Communication, Vol III. University of California Press, Berkeley, 1966, pp 1–16.
104. Mazzocchi F and Vignolo LA: Localization of lesions in aphasia: clinical CT-scan correlates in stroke patients. Cortex 15:627–653, 1979.
105. Damasio H and Damasio AR: The anatomical basis of conduction aphasia. Brain 103:337–350, 1980.
106. Anderson JM, Gilmore R, Roper S, Crosson B, Bauer RM, Nadeau S, et al.: Conduction aphasia and the arcuate fasciculus: a reexamination of the Wernicke-Geschwind model. Brain Lang 70:1–12, 1999.
107. Shuren JE, Schefft BK, Yeh HS, et al.: Repetition and the arcuate fasciculus. J Neurol 24:596–598, 1995.
108. Damasio A and Damasio H: The anatomical basis of pure alexia. Neurology 33:1573–1583, 1983.
109. Axer H, von Keyserlingk AG, Berks G, and von Keyserlingk DG: Supra- and infrasylvian conduction aphasia. Brain Lang 76:317–331, 2001.
110. Marshall RS, Lazar RM, Mohr JP, Van Heertum RL, and Mast H: "Semantic" conduction aphasia from a posterior insular cortex infarction. J Neuroimag 6:189–191, 1996.
111. Shuren J: Insula and aphasia. J Neurol 240:216–218, 1993.
112. Arnett PA, Rao SM, Hussain M, et al.: Conduction aphasia in multiple sclerosis: a case report with MRI findings. Neurology 47:576–578, 1996.
113. Metter EJ, Kempler D, Jackson C, Hanson WR, Mazziotta JC, and Phelps ME: Cerebral glucose metabolism in Wernicke's, Broca's, and conduction aphasia. Arch Neurol 46:27–34, 1989.
114. Mendez MF and Benson DF: Atypical conduction aphasia: a disconnection syndrome. Arch Neurol 42:886–891, 1985.
115. Quigg M and Fountain NB: Conduction aphasia elicited by stimulation of the left posterior superior temporal gyrus. J Neurol Neurosurg Psychiatry 66:393–396, 1999.
116. Kertesz A, Harlock W, and Coates R: Computed tomographic localization, lesion size, and prognosis in aphasia and nonverbal impairment. Brain Lang 8:34–50, 1979.
117. Saffran EM: Aphasia and the relationship of language and brain. Semin Neurol 20:409–418, 2000.
118. Pizzamiglio L, Galati G, and Committeri G: The contribution of functional neuroimaging to recovery after brain damage: a review. Cortex 37:11–31,2001.
119. Van Horn G and Hawes A: Global aphasia without hemiparesis: a sign of encephalopathy. Neurology 32:403–406, 1982.
120. Legatt AD, Rubin MJ, Kaplan LR, Healton EB, and Brust JCM: Global aphasia without hemipare-sis: multiple etiologies. Neurology 37:201–205, 1987.
121. Kumar R, Masih AK, and Pardo J: Global aphasia due to thalamic hemorrhage: a case report and a review of the literature. Arch Phys Med Rehabil 77:1312–1315, 1996.
122. Okuda B, Tanaka H, Tachibana H, Kawabata K, and Sugita M: Cerebral blood flow in subcortical global aphasia. Perisylvian cortical hypoperfusion as a crucial role. Stroke 25:1495–1499, 1994.
123. Hanlon RE, Lux WE, and Dromerick AW: Global aphasia without hemiparesis: language profiles and lesion distribution. J Neurol Neurosurg Psychiatry 66:365–369, 1999.
124. Hadano K, Nakamura H, and Hamanaka T: Effortful echolalia. Cortex 34:67–82, 1998.
125. Otsuki M, Soma Y, Koyama A, Yoshimura N, Furukawa H, and Tsuji S: Transcortical sensory aphasia following left frontal infarction. J Neurol 245:69–76, 1998.
126. Damasio AR and Van Hoesen GW: Emotional disturbances associated with focal lesions of the limbic frontal lobe. In Heilman KM and Satz P (eds). Neuropsychology of Human Emotion. Guilford Press, New York, 1983, pp 85–110.
127. Damasio AR and Damasio H: Aphasia and the neural basis of language. In Mesulam MM (ed). Principles of Cognitive and Behavioral Neurology. Oxford University Press, New York, 2002, pp 294–331.
128. Peraud A, Meschede M, Eisner W, Ilmberger J, and Reulen HJ: Surgical resection of grade II astrocytomas in the superior frontal gyrus. Neurosurgery 50:966–975, 2002.
129. Freedman M, Alexander MP, and Naeser MA: Anatomic basis of transcortical motor aphasia. Neurology 34:409–417, 1984.
130. Rubens AB: Transcortical motor aphasia. In Whitaker H and Whitaker HA (eds). Studies in Neurolinguistics, Vol 1. Academic Press, New York, 1976, pp 293–304.
131. Alexander MP, Benson DF, and Stuss DT: Frontal lobes and language. Brain 37:656–691, 1989.
132. McFarling D, Rothi LJ, and Heilman KM: Transcortical aphasia from ischaemic infarcts of the thalamus: a report of two cases. J Neurol Neurosurg Psychiatry 45:107–112, 1982.
133. Devinsky O. Behavioral Neurology: 100 Maxims. Edward Arnold, London, 1992, pp 114–118.
134. Kertesz A and McCabe P: Recovery patterns and prognosis in aphasia. Brain 100:1–18, 1977.
135. Kertesz A, Sheppard A, and MacKenzie R: Localization in transcortical sensory aphasia. Arch Neurol 39:475–478, 1982.
136. Godefroy O, Dubois C, Debachy B, Leclerc M, and Kreisler A: Lille Stroke Program. Vascular aphasias: main characteristics of patients hospitalized in acute stroke units. Stroke 33:702–705, 2002.
137. Boatman D, Gordon B, Hart J, Selnes O, Miglioretti D, and Lenz F: Transcortical sensory aphasia: revisited and revised. Brain 123:1634–1642, 2000.
138. Otsuki M, Soma Y, Koyama A, Yoshimura N, Furukawa H, and Tsuji S: Transcortical sensory aphasia following left frontal infarction. J Neurol 245:69–76, 1998.
139. Roebroek RM, Promes MM, Korten JJ, Lormans AC, and van der Laan RT: Transcortical sensory

aphasia in a right-handed patient following watershed infarcts in the right cerebral hemisphere: a 15–month evaluation of another case of crossed aphasia. Brain Lang 70:262–272, 1999.

140. Silveri MC and Colosimo C: Hypothesis on the nature of comprehension deficit in a patient with transcortical mixed aphasia with preserved naming. Brain Lang 49:1–26, 1995.

141. Alexander MP: Specific semantic memory loss after hypoxic–ischemic injury. Neurology 48:165–173, 1997.

142. Goodglass H and Wingfield A: Word-finding deficits in aphasia: brain–behavior relations and clinical symptomatology. In Goodglass H and Wingfield A (eds). Anomia: Neuroanatomical and Cognitive Correlates. Academic Press, San Diego, 1997, pp 3–27.

143. Yamadori A and Albert ML: Word category aphasia. Cortex 9:112–125, 1973.

144. Ferreira CT, Giusiano B, and Poncet M: Catagory specific anomia: implications of different neural networks in naming. Neuroreport 8:1595–1602, 1997.

145. Santori G and Job R: The oyster with four legs: a neuropsychological study of the interaction of visual and semantic information. Cogn Neuropsychol 5: 105–132, 1988.

146. Rapscak SZ, Comer JF, and Rubens AB: Anomia for facial expressions: neuropsychological mechanisms and anatomical correlates. Brain Lang 45:233–252, 1993.

147. Coslett HB, Saffran EM, and Schwoebel J: Knowledge of the human body: a distinct semantic domain. Neurology 59:357–363, 2002.

148. Hart J and Gordon B: Neural subsystems for object knowledge. Nature 359:60–64, 1992.

149. Silveri MC, Gainotti G, Perani D, Cappelletti JY, Carbone G, and Fazio F: Naming deficit for non-living items: neuropsychological and PET study. Neuropsychologia 35:359–367, 1997.

150. Tranel D, Damasio H, and Damasio AR: On the neurology of naming. In Goodglass H and Wingfield A (eds). Anomia: Neuroanatomical and Cognitive Correlates. Academic Press, San Diego, 1997, pp 65–90.

151. Damasio H, Grabowski TJ, Tranel D, Hichwa RD, and Damasio AR: A neural basis for lexical retrieval. Nature 380:499–505, 1996.

152. Semenza C and Zettin M: Evidence from aphasia for the role of proper names as pure referring expressions. Nature 342:678–679, 1989.

153. Damasio H, Grabowski TJ, Tranel D, Ponto LL, Hichwa RD, and Damasio AR: Neural correlates of naming actions and of naming spatial relations. Neuroimage 13:1053–1064, 2001.

154. Schwartz TH, Devinsky O, Doyle W, and Perrine K: Preoperative predictors of anterior temporal language areas. J Neurosurg 89:962–970, 1998.

155. Fukatsu R, Fujii T, Tsukiura T, Yamadori A, and Otsuki T: Proper name anomia after left temporal lobectomy: a patient study. Neurology 52:1096–1099, 1999.

156. Berndt RS, Haendiges AN, and Wozniak MA: Verb retrieval and sentence processing: dissociation of an established symptom association. Cortex 33:99–114, 1997.

157. Raymer AM, Foundas AL, Maher LM, et al.: Cognitive neuropsychological analysis and neu-

roanatomic correlates in a case of acute anomia. Brain Lang 58:137–156, 1997.

158. Ojemann JG, Ojemann GA, and Lettich E: Neuronal activity related to faces and matching in human right nondominant temporal cortex. Brain 115:1–13, 1992.

159. Karussis D, Leker RR, and Abramsky O: Cognitive dysfunction following thalamic stroke: a study of 16 cases and review of the literature. J Neurol Sci 172:25–29, 2000.

160. Mohr JP, Watters WC, and Duncan GW: Thalamic hemorrhage and aphasia. Brain Lang 2:3–17, 1975.

161. Damasio A, Damasio H, Rizzo M, et al.: Aphasia with nonhemorrhagic lesions in the basal ganglia and internal capsule. Arch Neurol 39:2–14, 1982.

162. Naeser MA, Alexander MP, Helm-Estabrooks N, Levine HL, Laughlin SA, and Geschwind N: Aphasia with predominantly subcortical lesion sites. Arch Neurol 39:2–14, 1982.

163. Graff-Radford N, Damasio H, Yamada T, et al.: Non-hemorrhagic thalamic infarctions: clinical, neurophysiological and electrophysiological findings in four anatomic groups defined by computerized tomography. Brain 108:485–516, 1985.

164. Watson RT and Heilman KM: Affect in subcortical aphasia. Neurology 32:102–103, 1982.

165. Bogousslavsky J, Regli F, and Uske A: Thalamic infarcts: clinical syndromes, etiology, and prognosis. Neurology 38:837–848, 1988.

166. Brunner RJ, Kornhuber HH, Seemuller E, et al.: Basal ganglia participation in language pathology. Brain Lang 16:281–299, 1982.

167. Fromm D, Holland AL, Swindell CS, and Reinmuth OM: Various consequences of subcortical stroke. Arch Neurol 42:943–950, 1985.

168. Mega MS and Alexander MP: Subcortical aphasia: the core profile of capsulostriatal infarction. Neurology 44:1824–1829, 1994.

169. Alexander GE, DeLong MR, and Strick PL: Parallel organization of functionally segregated circuits linking basal ganglia and cortex. Annu Rev Neurosci 9:357–381, 1986.

170. Caplan LR, Schmahmann JD, Kase CS, et al.: Caudate infarcts. Arch Neurol 47:133–143, 1990.

171. Nadeau SE and Crosson B: Subcortical aphasia. Brain Lang 58:355–402, 1997.

172. Ozaki I, Baba M, Narita S, Matsunaga M, and Takebe K: Pure dysarthria due to anterior internal capsule and/or corona radiata infarction: a report of five cases. J Neurol Neurosurg Psychiatry 49:1435–1437, 1986.

173. Lee MS, Lee SB, and Kim WC: Spasmodic dysphonia associated with a left ventrolateral putaminal lesion. Neurology 47:827–828, 1996.

174. Wolfe GI and Ross ED: Sensory aprosodia with left hemiparesis from subcortical infarction: right hemisphere analogue of sensory-type aphasia with right hemiparesis? Arch Neurol 44:668–671, 1987.

175. Starkstein SE, Federoff JP, Price TR, Leiguarda RC, and Robinson RG: Neuropsychological and neuroradiologic correlates of emotional prosody comprehension. Neurology 44:515–522, 1994.

176. Tuszynski MH and Petito CK: Ischemic thalamic aphasia with pathologic confirmation. Neurology 38: 800–802, 1988.

177. Nass R, Boyce L, Leventhal F, et al.: Acquired apha-

sia in children after surgical resection of left-thalamic tumors. Dev Med Child Neurol 42:580–590, 2000.

178. Maeshima S, Ozaki F, Okita R, et al.: Transient crossed aphasia and persistent amnesia after right thalamic haemorrhage. Brain Inj 15:927–933, 2001.

179. Karussis D, Leker RR, and Abramsky O: Cognitive dysfunction following thalamic stroke: a study of 16 cases and review of the literature. J Neurol Sci 172:25–29, 2000.

180. Murdoch BE: Subcortical brain mechanisms in speech and language. Folia Phoniatr Logop 53:233–251, 2001.

181. Hillis AE, Wityk RJ, Barker PB, et al.: Subcortical aphasia and neglect in acute stroke: the role of cortical hypoperfusion. Brain 125:1094–104, 2002.

182. Sodeyama N, Tamaki M, and Sugushita M: Persistant pure verbal amnesia and transient aphasia after left thalamic infarction. J Neurol 242: 289–294, 1995.

183. Boatman D, Freeman J, Vining E, et al.: Language recovery after left hemispherectomy in children with late-onset seizures. Ann Neurol 46:579–586, 1999

184. Satz P and Bullard-Bates C: Acquired aphasia in children. In Sarno MT (ed). Acquired Aphasia. Academic Press, New York, 1981, pp 299–426.

185. Connor LT, Albert ML, Tocco M, Fitzpatrick PM, and Albert ML: Effect of socioeconomic status on aphasia severity and recovery. Brain Lang 78:254–257, 2001.

186. Cameron RF, Currier RD, and Haerer AF: Aphasia and literacy. Br J Disord Commun 6:161–163, 1971.

187. Tzavaras A, Phocas C, Kaprinis G, and Karavatos A: Literacy and hemispheric specialization for language: dichotic listening in young functionally illiterate men. Percept Mot Skills 77:195–199, 1993.

188. Illes J, Francis WS, Desmond JE, et al.: Convergent cortical representation of semantic processing in bilinguals. Brain Lang 70:347–363, 1999.

189. Wuillemin D, Richardson B, and Lynch J: Right hemisphere involvement in processing later-learned languages in multilinguals. Brain Lang 46:620–636, 1994.

190. Kim KH, Relkin NR, Lee KM, and Hirsch J: Distinct cortical areas associated with native and second languages. Nature 388:171–174, 1997.

191. Ramamurthi B and Chari P: Aphasia in bilinguals. Acta Neurochir Suppl (Wien) 56:59–66, 1993.

192. Lambert W and Fillenbaum S: A pilot study of aphasia among bilinguals. Can J Psychol 13:28–34, 1959.

193. Martinell-Gispert-Sauch M, Gil Saladie D, and Delgado-Gonzalez M: Aphasia in a polyglot: description and neuropsychological course. Rev Neurol 25:562–565, 1997.

194. Yamadori A: Ideogram reading in alexia. Brain 98:231–238, 1975.

195. Obler LK and Albert ML: Influence of aging on recovery from aphasia in polyglots. Brain Lang 4:460–463, 1977.

196. Schwartz TH, Devinsky O, Doyle W, and Perrine K: Function-specific high-probability "nodes" identified in posterior language cortex. Epilepsia 40:575–583, 1999.

197. Devinsky O, Perrine K, Llinas R, Luciano DJ, and Dogali M: Anterior temporal language areas in patients with early onset of temporal lobe epilepsy. Ann Neurol 34:727–732, 1993.

198. Devinsky O, Perrine K, Hirsch J, McMullen W, Pacia S, and Doyle W: Relation of cortical language distribution and cognitive function in surgical epilepsy patients. Epilepsia 41:400–404, 2000.

199. Devinsky O, Kelly K, Yacubian EMT, et al.: Postictal behavior: a clinical and subdural electroencephalographic study. Arch Neurol 51:254–259, 1994.

200. Ficker DM, Shukla R, and Privitera MD: Postictal language dysfunction in complex partial seizures: effect of contralateral ictal spread. Neurology 56: 1590–1592, 2001.

201. Williamson PD, Thadani VM, French JA, et al.: Medial temporal lobe epilepsy: videotape analysis of objective clinical seizure characteristics. Epilepsia 39: 1182–1188, 1998.

202. Inoue Y, Mihara T, Fukao K, Kudo T, Watanabe Y, and Yagi K: Ictal paraphasia induced by language activity. Epilepsy Res 35:69–79, 1999.

203. Devinsky O, Vazquez B, Perrine K, and Luciano D: Ictal and postictal apraxia. Neuropsychiatry Neuropsychol Behav Neurol 6:256–259, 1993.

204. Aldenkamp AP, Overweg J, Gutter T, et al.: Effect of epilepsy, seizures and epileptiform discharges on cognitive functions. Acta Neurol Scand 93:253–259, 1996.

205. Aldenkamp AP: Effect of seizures and epileptiform discharges on cognitive function. Epilepsia 38(Suppl 1): S52–S55, 1997.

206. Croona C, Kihlgren M, Lundberg S, Eeg-Olofsson O, and Eeg-Olofsson KE: Neuropsychological findings in children with benign childhood epilepsy with centrotemporal spikes. Dev Med Child Neurol 41: 813–818, 1999.

206a. Deonna T, Zesiger P, Davidoff V, Maeder M, Mayor C, and Roulet E: Benign partial epilepsy: a longitudinal neuropsychological EEG study of cognitive function. Dev Med Child Neurol 42:595–603, 2000.

207. Nass R, Gross A, Wisoff J, and Devinsky O: Outcome of multiple subpial transections for autistic epileptiform regression. Pediatr Neurol 21:464–470, 1999.

208. Morrell F, Whisler WW, Smith MC, et al.: Landau-Kleffner syndrome. Treatment with subpial intracortical transection. Brain 118:1529–1546, 1995.

209. Lewine JD, Andrews R, Chez M, et al.: Magnetoencephalographic patterns of epileptiform activity in children with regressive autism spectrum disorders. Pediatrics 104:405–418, 1999.

210. Kaga M: Language disorders in Landau-Kleffner syndrome. J Child Neurol 14:118–122, 1999.

211. Tuchman RF: Acquired epileptiform aphasia. Semin Pediatr Neurol 4:93–101, 1997.

212. Jayakar PB and Seshia SS: Electrical status epilepticus during slow-wave sleep: a review. J Clin Neurophysiol 8:299–311, 1991.

213. De Negri M: Electrical status epilepticus during sleep (ESES). Different clinical syndromes: towards a unifying view? Brain Dev 19:447–451, 1997.

214. Radhakrishnan K, Silbert PL, and Klass DW: Reading epilepsy. An appraisal of 20 patients diagnosed at the Mayo Clinic, Rochester, Minnesota, between 1949 and 1989, and delineation of the epilepsy syndrome. Brain 118:75–89, 1995.

215. Singh B, Anderson L, al Gashlan M, al-Shahwan SA, and Riela AR: Reading-induced absence seizures. Neurology 45:1623–1624, 1995.

216. Ritaccio AL: Reflex seizures. In Devinsky O (ed). Epilepsy. II. Special issues. Neurol Clin 12:57–83, 1994.

217. Koutroumanidis M, Koepp MJ, Richardson MP, et al.: The variants of reading epilepsy. Brain 121:1409–1427, 1998.

218. Greener J, Enderby P, Whurr R, and Grant A: Treatment for aphasia following stroke: evidence for effectiveness. Int J Lang Commun Disord 33:158–161, 1998.

219. Albert ML, Sparks RW, and Helm NA: Melodic intonation therapy for aphasia. Arch Neurol 29:130–131, 1973.

220. Pollack MR and Disler PB: Rehabilitation of patients after stroke. Med J Aust 177:452–456, 2002.

221. Darley FL: Treatment of acquired aphasia. Adv Neurol 7:111–145, 1975.

222. Wertz RT, Weiss DG, Aten JL, et al.: Comparison of clinic, home, and deferred language treatment for aphasia. A Veterans Administration Cooperative Study. Arch Neurol 43:653–658, 1986.

223. David R, Enderby P, and Bainton D: Treatment of acquired aphasia: speech therapists and volunteers compared. J Neurol Neurosurg Psychiatry 45:957–961, 1982.

224. Lincoln NB, McGuirk E, Mulley GP, Lendrem W, Jones AC, and Mitchell JR: Effectiveness of speech therapy for aphasic stroke patients. A randomised controlled trial. Lancet 1:1197–2000, 1984.

225. Howard D, Patterson K, Franklin S, et al.: Treatment of word retrieval deficits in aphasia: a comparison of two therapy methods. Brain 108:817–829, 1985.

226. Robson J, Marshall J, Pring T, and Chiat S: Phonological naming therapy in jargon aphasia: positive but paradoxical effects. J Int Neuropsychol Soc 4:675–686, 1998.

227. Heiss WD, Kessler J, Thiel A, Ghaemi M, and Karbe H: Differential capacity of left and right hemispheric areas for compensation of poststroke aphasia. Ann Neurol 45:430–438, 1999.

228. Goodglass H and Kaplan E: The Assessment of Aphasia and Related Disorders, 2nd ed. Lea & Febiger, Philadelphia, 1983.

229. Kertesz A: Aphasia and associated disorders: taxonomy, localization, and recovery. Grune and Stratton, New York, 1979.

230. Spreen O and Benton AL: Neurosensory Center Comprehensive Examination for Aphasia, 2nd ed. University of Victoria, Victoria, 1977.

231. Porch BE: Multidimensional scoring in aphasia testing. J Speech Hear Res 14:776–792, 1971.

232. Holland AL: Communication Abilities in Daily Living. University Park Press, Baltimore, 1980.

233. Sarno MT: The Functional Communication Profile. New York University Press, New York, 1969.

234. Skelly R, Schinsky L, Smith R, Donaldson R, and Griffin J: American Indian sign, a gestural communication system for the speechless. Arch Phys Med Rehab 56:156–160, 1975.

235. Pring T, Whilet-Thomson M, Pound C, et al.: Picture/word matching tasks and word retrieval: some follow-up data and second thoughts. Aphasiology 4:479–483, 1990.

236. Holland AL: Treatment of aphasia after stroke. Stroke 10:475–477, 1979.

237. Sparks R, Helm N, and Albert M: Aphasia rehabilitation resulting from melodic intonation therapy. Cortex 10:303–316, 1974.

238. Basso A, Capitani E, and Vignolo L: Influence of rehabilitation on language skills in aphasic patients: a controlled study. Arch Neurol 36:190–196, 1979.

239. Helm-Estabrooks NA: Helm Elicited Language Program for Syntax Stimulation (HELPSS). Exceptional Resources, Austin, TX, 1981.

240. Helm-Estabrooks N, Fitzpatrick PM, and Baressi B: Visual action therapy for global aphasia. J Speech Hear Disord 47:385–389, 1982.

241. Benson DF, Brayton-Gerratt S, Dobkin BH, et al.: Melodic intonation therapy: report of the therapeutics and technology subcommittee. American Academy of Neurology, Minneapolis, 1994, pp 1–4.

242. Naeser MA, Baker EH, Palumbo CL, et al.: Lesion site patterns in severe, nonverbal aphasia to predict outcome with a computer-assisted treatment program. Arch Neurol 55:1438–1448, 1998.

243. Walker-Batson D, Curtis S, Natarajan R, et al.: A double-blind, placebo-controlled study of the use of amphetamine in the treatment of aphasia. Stroke 32:2093–2098, 2001.

244. Albert ML, Bachman DL, Morgan A, and Helm-Estabrooks N: Pharmacotherapy for aphasia. Neurology 38:877–879, 1988.

245. Bachman DL and Morgan A: The role of pharmacotherapy in the treatment of aphasia: preliminary results. Aphasiology 2:225–228, 1988.

246. Greener J, Enderby P, Whurr R, Grant A: Treatment for aphasia following stroke: evidence for effectiveness. Int J Commun Disord 33(Suppl.):158–161.

247. Wing AM: Motor control: mechanisms of motor equivalence in handwriting. Curr Biol 10:R245–R248, 2000.

248. Chedru F and Geschwind N: Writing disturbances in acute confusional states. Neuropsychologia 10:343–353, 1972.

249. Silveri MC, Misciagna S, Leggio MG, and Molinari M: Cerebellar spatial dysgraphia: further evidence. J Neurol 246:312–313, 1999.

250. Brust JC: Music and language: musical alexia and agraphia. Brain 103:367–392, 1980.

251. Tohgi H, Saitoh K, Takahashi S, et al.: Agraphia and acalculia after a left prefrontal (F1, F2) infarction. J Neurol Neurosurg Psychiatry 58:629–632, 1995.

252. Roeltgen DP and Heilman KM: Lexical agraphia: further support for the two-system hypothesis of linguistic agraphia. Brain 107:811–827, 1984.

253. Geschwind N and Kaplan EF: A human cerebral deconnection syndrome. Neurology 12:675–685, 1962.

254. Otsuki M, Soma Y, Arai T, Otsuka A, and Tsuji S: Pure apraxic agraphia with abnormal writing stroke sequences: report of a Japanese patient with a left superior parietal haemorrhage. J Neurol Neurosurg Psychiatry 66:233–237, 1999.

255. Alexander MP, Fischer RS, and Friedman R: Lesion localization in apractic agraphia. Arch Neurol 49:246–251, 1992.

256. Dubois J, Hecaen H, and Marcie P: L'agraphie pure. Neuropsychologia 7:271–286, 1969.

257. Rapcsak SZ, Arthur SA, and Rubens AB: Lexical

agraphia from focal lesions of the left precentral gyrus. Neurology 38:1119–1123, 1988.

258. Rosati G and De Bastiani P: Pure agraphia: a discrete form of aphasia. J Neurol Neurosurg Psychiatry 42:266–269, 1979.

259. Laine TN and Marttila RJ: Pure agraphia: a case study. Neuropsychologia 19:311–316, 1981.

260. Aiba E, Soma Y, Aiba T, et al.: Two cases of pure agraphia developed after thalamic hemorrhage. [in Japanese] Brain Nerve (Tokyo) 43:275–281, 1991.

261. Schomer DL, Pegna A, Matton B, et al.: Ictal agraphia: a patient study. Neurology 50:542–545, 1998.

262. Wilson SAK: Disorders of motility and muscle tone with special reference to the corpus striatum. Lancet 2:1–10, 1925.

263. Kim JS, Im JH, Kwon SU, Kang JH, and Lee MC: Micrographia after thalamo-mesencephalic infarction: evidence of striatal dopaminergic hypofunction. Neurology 51:625–627, 1998

264. Ibañez V, Sadato N, Karp B, Deiber MP, and Hallett M: Deficient activation of the motor cortical network in patients with writer's cramp. Neurology 53:96–105, 1999.

265. Silveri MC, Misciagna S, Leggio MG, and Molinari M: Spatial dysgraphia and cerebellar lesion: a case report. Neurology 48:1529–1532, 1997.

266. Van Vugt P, Paquier P, Kees L, and Cras P: Increased writing activity in neurological conditions: a review and clinical study. J Neurol Neurosurg Psychiatry 61:510–529, 1996.

267. Okamura T, Fukai M, Yamadori A, Hidari M, Asaba H, and Sakai T: A clinical study of hypergraphia in epilepsy. J Neurol Neurosurg Psychiatry 56:556–559, 1993.

268. Van Vugt P, Paquier P, Kees L, and Cras P: Increased writing activity in neurological conditions: a review and clinical study. J Neurol Neurosurg Psychiatry 61:510–514, 1996.

269. Gerstmann J: Zur symptomatologie der herderkrankungen in der ubergangsregion der unteren parietal-und mittleren okzipitalhirnwindung. Dtsch Z Nervenheilk 116:46–49, 1930.

270. Gerstmann J: Syndrome of finger agnosia, disorientation for right and left, agraphia and acalculia. Arch Neurol Psychiatry 44:398–408, 1940.

271. Mayer E, Martory MD, Pegna AJ, Landis T, Delavelle J, and Annoni JM: A pure case of Gerstmann syndrome with a subangular lesion. Brain 122:1107–1120, 1999.

272. Gold M, Adair JC, Jacobs DH, and Heilman KM: Right–left confusion in Gerstmann's syndrome: a model of body centered spatial orientation. Cortex 31:267–283, 1995.

273. Suresh PA and Sebastian S: Developmental Gerstmann's syndrome: a distinct clinical entity of learning disabilities. Pediatr Neurol 22:267–278, 2000.

274. Hodgson TL and Kennard C: Disorders of higher visual function and hemi-spatial neglect. Curr Opin Neurol 13:7–12, 2000.

275. Dehaene S, Tzourio N, Frak V, et al.: Cerebral activations during number multiplication and comparison: a PET study. Neuropsychologia 34:1097–1106, 1996.

276. Chochon F, Cohen L, van de Moortele PF, and Dehaene S: Differential contributions of the left and right inferior parietal lobules to number processing. J Cogn Neurosci 11:617–630, 1999.

277. Dehaene S, Spelke E, Pinel P, Stanescu R, and Tsivkin S: Sources of mathematical thinking: behavioral and brain-imaging evidence. Science 284:970–974, 1999

278. Boller F and Grafman J: Acalculia: historical development and current significance. Brain Cogn 2:205–223, 1983.

279. Delazer M and Benke T: Arithmetic facts without meaning. Cortex 33:697–710, 1997.

280. Smith A: The serial sevens subtraction test. Arch Neurol 17:77–80, 1967.

281. Dehaene S, Dehaene-Lambertz G, and Cohen L: Abstract representations of numbers in the animal and human brain. Trends Neurosci 21:355–361, 1998.

282. Caporali A, Burgio F, and Basso A: The natural course of acalculia in left-brain-damaged patients. Neurol Sci 21:143–149, 2000.

283. Basso A, Burgio F, and Caporali A: Acalculia, aphasia and spatial disorders in left and right brain-damaged patients. Cortex 36:265–280, 2000.

284. Grafman J, Passafiume D, Faglioni P, and Boller F: Calculation disturbances in adults with focal hemispheric damage. Cortex 18:37–49, 1982.

285. Levin HS, Scheller J, Rickard T, et al.: Dyscalculia and dyslexia after right hemisphere injury in infancy. Arch Neurol 53:88–96, 1996.

286. Dehaene S and Cohen L: Cerebral pathways for calculation: double dissociation between rote verbal and quantitative knowledge of arithmetic. Cortex 33:219–250, 1997.

287. Levy LM, Reis IL, and Grafman J: Metabolic abnormalities detected by ^{1}H-MRS in dyscalculia and dysgraphia. Neurology 53:639–641, 1999.

288. Gerstmann J: Some notes on the Gertsmann syndrome. Neurology 7:866–869, 1957.

289. Tucha O, Steup A, Smely C, and Lange KW: Toe agnosia in Gerstmann syndrome. J Neurol Neurosurg Psychiatry 63:399–403, 1997.

290. Ramachandran VS, Altschuler EL, and Hillyer S: Mirror agnosia. Proc R Soc Lond B Biol Sci 264:645–647, 1997.

291. Binkofski F, Buccino G, Dohle C, Seitz RJ, and Freund HJ: Mirror agnosia and mirror ataxia constitute different parietal lobe disorders. Ann Neurol 46:51–61, 1999.

292. McFie J and Zangwill O: Visual-constructive disabilities associated with lesions of the left cerebral hemisphere. Brain 83:243–260, 1960.

293. Benton AL: The fiction of the "Gertsmann syndrome." J Neurol Neurosurg Psychiatry 24:176–181, 1961.

294. Heimberger RF, DeMyer W, and Reitan RM: Implications of Gerstmann's syndrome. J Neurol Neurosurg Psychiatry 27:52–57, 1964.

295. Geschwind N and Strub RL: Gerstmann syndrome without aphasia: a reply to Poeck and Orgass. Cortex 11:296–298, 1975.

296. Wingard EM, Barrett AM, Crucian GP, Doty L, and Heilman KM: The Gerstmann syndrome in Alzheimer's disease. J Neurol Neurosurg Psychiatry 72:403–405, 2002.

297. Roeltgen DP, Sevush S, and Heilmann KM: Pure Gerstmann's syndrome from a focal lesion. Arch Neurol 40:46–47, 1983.

298. Morris HH, Luders H, Lesser RP, Dinner DS, and Hahn J: Transient neuropsychological abnormalities

(including Gerstmann's syndrome) during cortical stimulation. Neurology 34:877–883, 1984.

299. Riva D and Giorgi C: The cerebellum contributes to higher functions during development: evidence from a series of children surgically treated for posterior fossa tumours. Brain 123:1051–1061, 2000.

300. Van Dongen HR, Catsman-Berrevoets CE, and van Mourik M: The syndrome of "cerebellar" mutism and subsequent dysarthria. Neurology 44:2040–2046, 1994.

301. Bielamowicz S and Ludlow CL: Effects of botulinum toxin on pathophysiology in spasmodic dysphonia. Ann Otol Rhinol Laryngol 109:194–203, 2000.

302. Kent RD: Research on speech motor control and its disorders: a review and prospective. J Commun Disord 33:391–427, 2000.

303. Cohen L, Benoit N, Van Eeckhout P, Ducarne B, and Brunet P: Pure progressive aphemia. J Neurol Neurosurg Psychiatry 56:923–924, 1993.

304. Kremer M, Russell WR, and Smyth GE: A midbrain syndrome following head injury. J Neurol Neurosurg Psychiatry 10:49–60, 1947.

305. Schmahmann JD and Sherman JC: The cerebellar cognitive affective syndrome. Brain 121:561–579, 1998.

306. Wilson SAK: Neurology. Williams and Wilkins, Baltimore, 1940.

307. Weinstein EA and Keller NJS: Linguistic patterns of misnaming in brain injury. Neuropsychologia 1: 79–90, 1964.

308. Geschwind N: The varieties of naming errors. Cortex 3:97–112, 1967.

309. Blumenstein SE, Alexander MP, Ryalls JH, and Katz W: On the nature of the foreign accent syndrome: a case study. Brain Lang 31:215–244, 1987.

310. Gurd JM, Bessel NJ, Bladon AW, and Blamford JM: A case of foreign accent syndrome, with follow-up clinical, neuropsychological and phonetic descriptions. Neuropsychologia 26:237–251, 1988.

311. Takayama Y, Sugishita M, Kido T, et al.: A case of foreign accent syndrome without aphasia caused by a lesion of the precentral gyrus. Neurology 43:1361–1363, 1993.

312. Kurowski KM, Blumstein SE, and Alexander M: The foreign accent syndrome: a reconsideration. Brain Lang 54:1–25, 1996.

313. Reeves RR and Norton JW: Foreign accent-like syndrome during psychotic exacerbations. Neuropsychiatry Neuropsychol Behav Neurol 14:135–138, 2001.

314. Roy N and Bless DM: Personality traits and psychological factors in voice pathology: a foundation for future research. J Speech Lang Hear Res 43: 737–748, 2000.

315. Helm NA, Butler RB, and Benson DF: Acquired stuttering. Neurology 28:1159–1165, 1978.

316. Grant AC, Biousse V, Cook AA, and Newman NJ: Stroke-associated stuttering. Arch Neurol 56:624–627, 1999.

317. Carluer L, Marie RM, Lambert J, Defer GL, Coskun O, and Rossa Y: Acquired and persistent stuttering as the main symptom of striatal infarction. Mov Disord 15:343–346, 2000.

318. Yasuda Y, Akiguchi I, Ino M, Nabatabe H, and Kameyama M: Paramedian thalamic and midbrain infarcts associated with palilalia. J Neurol Neurosurg Psychiatry 53:797–799, 1990.

319. Serra-Mestres J, Shapleske J, and Tym E: Treatment of palilalia with trazodone. Am J Psychiatry 153:580–581, 1996.

320. Linetsky E, Planer D, and Ben-Hur T: Echolalia–palilalia as the sole manifestation of nonconvulsive status epilepticus. Neurology 55:733–734, 2000.

321. Cummings JL, Benson DF, Houlihan JP, and Gosenfeld LF: Mutism: loss of neocortical and limbic vocalization. J Nerv Ment Dis 171:255–259, 1983.

322. Alexander MP: Akinetic mutism after mesencephalic–diencephalic infarction: remediated with dopaminergic medications. Neurorehabil Neural Repair 15:151–156, 2001.

323. Devinsky O, Leeman W, Evans C, and Rottenberg DA: Akinetic mutism in a bone-marrow transplant recipient following whole-brain irradiation and amphotericin B: a PET and neuropathological study. Arch Neurol 44:414–417, 1987.

324. Laplane D, Talairach D, Meininger V, Bancaud J, and Bouchareine A: Motor consequences of motor area ablations in man. J Neurol Sci 31:29–49, 1977.

325. Fried I, Katz A, McCarthy G, et al.: Functional organization of human supplementary motor cortex studied by electrical stimulation. J Neurosci 11: 3656–3666, 1991.

326. Gerloff C, Corwell B, Chen R, Hallett M, and Cohen LG: Stimulation over the human supplementary motor area interferes with the organization of future elements in complex motor sequences. Brain 120:1587–1602, 1997.

327. Gelabert-Gonzalez M and Fernandez-Villa J: Mutism after posterior fossa surgery. Clin Neurol Neurosurg 103:111–114, 2001.

328. Leon-Carrion J, van Eeckhout P, and Dominguez-Morales MR: The locked-in syndrome: a syndrome looking for a therapy. Brain Inj 16:555–569, 2002.

329. Patterson JR and Grabois M: Locked-in syndrome: a review of 139 cases. Stroke 17:758–764, 1986.

330. Furst AL: Elective mutism: report of a case successfully treated by a family doctor. Isr J Psychiatry Relat Sci 26:96–102, 1989.

331. Kumpulainen K: Phenomenology and treatment of selective mutism. CNS Drugs 16:175–180, 2002.

332. Gordon N: Mutism: elective or selective, and acquired. Brain Dev 23:83–87, 2001.

Chapter 7

Motor System and Behavior

Behavioral output is expressed through movement and autonomic activity. Motor behavior varies from the hard-wired reflexes and species-specific responses to environmental stimuli to the creative genius of athletes and musicians. Many preprogrammed motor acts involve coordinated skeletomotor and autonomic responses. For example, the emotional expression of fear evokes a characteristic facial expression, as well as tachycardia and diaphoresis. Complex movements involve sequential planned actions that require widespread cortical and subcortical network interactions. Motor behavior is impaired by dysfunction at disparate sites ranging from cortical areas, such as the primary sensorimotor and sensorimotor association cortices, to subcortical areas, such as the basal ganglia and cerebellum.

Learning a motor task is effortful and can take months or years. This procedural knowledge (memory for skills) is not accessible to consciousness and utilizes neural systems dif-

ferent from declarative knowledge (memory for episodes and facts), which can be accessed by consciousness. Once acquired, a motor task can be skillfully performed with minimal effort, and attentional processes can simultaneously engage another task.

CORTICAL ANATOMY OF THE MOTOR SYSTEM

The cortex includes multiple motor areas. Like the sensory cortex, the primary motor cortex has the most direct connections to the periphery via corticospinal fibers. Unlike the sensory cortex, however, the primary motor cortex has its major efferents directed to the subcortical and spinal, not motor association, areas. Rather, information flows primarily from the prefrontal to motor association cortex to the primary motor cortex. The motor association cortex helps to prepare and initiate

226

movement, provide the motivational context for self-initiated and externally cued movements, and connect limbic and heteromodal association areas to modulate behavioral expression. Specialized motor areas mediate volitional eye movements and speech. The mosaic of frontal motor areas is anatomically and functionally interwoven with other cortical and subcortical areas. Frontal motor and parietal sensory areas are connected in a series of cir-

cuits that transform sensory data to action[1] and feedback action plans to sensory areas. Thalamic synchronization of activity in multiple motor areas, as well as related sensory, association, and subcortical areas, creates the unity and fluidity of movement (Figs. 7–1, 7–2). These sensory and motor hierarchies link the nervous system to the external environment, and the limbic hierarchy links the nervous system to the internal environment.

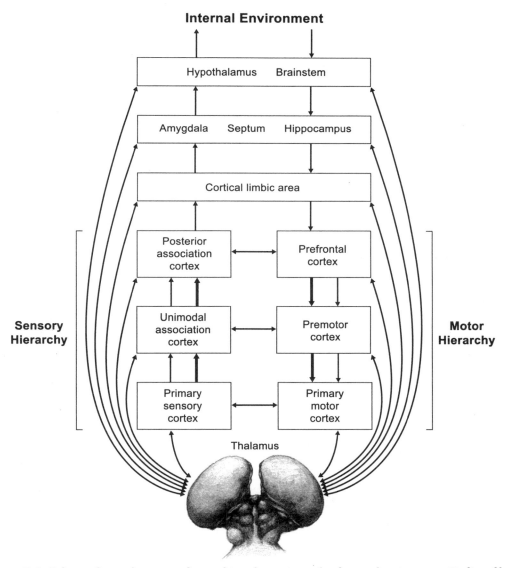

Figure 7–1. Relation of cortical sensory and motor hierarchies to external and internal environments. Binding of brain regions and integration of behavior occur through interconnections within hierarchies and thalamic synchronization (see Chapter 3).

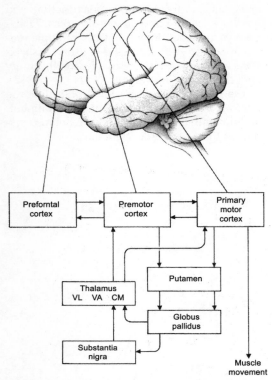

Figure 7–2. Overview of motor hierarchies; the relation of prefrontal, premotor, and primary motor cortex areas to each other and to subcortical motor areas. VL, ventral lateral; VA, ventral anterior; CM, centromedian nucleus.

Primary Motor Cortex

The primary motor cortex (M1, Brodmann's area [BA] 4), often simply called the motor cortex, executes skilled, voluntary, manipulative movements.[2] It is also activated during observation of actions made by others, as well as during action execution.[3] The cytoarchitecture of the primary motor cortex is unique: there are no granular cells in layer IV, and there is a dense giant pyramidal (Betz) cell population in layer V. An increased number of Betz cells in primate phylogeny correlates with a greater density of pyramidal tract terminations in the spinal cord ventral horn, greater dexterity, and a more persistent and severe motor deficit after M1 lesions.[4] Motor cortex input comes from the premotor cortex (PMC; M2, BA 6, posterior BA 8), cingulate motor area (CMA; M3, BA 23c, BA 24c), primary somatosensory and somatosensory association cortices (mainly proprioception), and thalamic nuclei (ventral

anterior, which connects to the basal ganglia; ventral lateral, which connects to the cerebellum).

The cortical motor map (homunculus) (Fig. 7–3) is a species-specific set of prewired neuronal connections. However, plasticity and learning occur throughout the life span, possibly mediated by horizontal neuronal connections.[5] The homunculus is an approximation as muscles within a limb are arranged in different sequences in different individuals.[6] The motor cortex has a large representation for laryngeal and tongue (speech) and finger (dexterity) muscles. Like their counterparts in primary somatosensory cortex (S1), the primate M1 hand and foot areas have no callosal connections.[7] The absence of callosal connections between the left and right hemisphere M1 and S1 hand and foot areas may be the anatomical foundation for hand and foot dominance.[8] In right-handed, and many left-handed, persons, the left hemisphere primary motor and motor association areas are dominant for skilled movements, including speech and fine single-finger movements. The motor-dominant hemisphere is the main repository of motor engrams for complex learned movements, such as writing.

After lesions of M1, which destroy motor neurons and their axons, humans can still per-

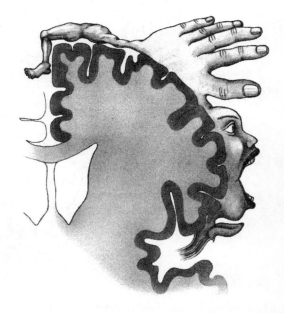

Figure 7–3. Cortical control of movement: the homunculus on the primary motor cortex.

form proximal movements, such as walking and extending an arm to break a fall; but fine finger and toe movements and some coarser movements of the wrist and ankle are lost. In humans, M1 lesions initially cause decreased tone, but this is followed by persistent increased tone and deep tendon reflexes and the Babinski sign.[9,10] Combined M1 and M2 medial lesions produce the grasp reflex, which is characterized by finger flexion after tactile contact of the palm.[9,11] After lesions of M1 (and motor association cortex), the impairment in strength, dexterity, initiation, and motivation-dependent utilization may partly result from hyperactivity of cortical inhibitory interneurons. This cortical hyperinhibition may result from damage to cortical afferents.[12] When M1 is isolated from bilateral motor association cortices, movement can be triggered by magnetic stimulation. In such cases, the patient's paralysis may result from failure to initiate movement.[13]

Motor Association Cortex

Motor association cortex consists of the lateral PMC (LPMC; M2, anterior BA 6, posterior BA 8), medial PMC (supplementary motor area, SMA; M2, BA6, posterior BA 8), and part of Broca's area (BA 44). The CMA (M3, BA 23c, BA 24c) shares cytoarchitectural and functional similarities with the motor association cortex. The architecture of the motor association cortex is transitional between the macropyramidal agranular (idiotypic) M1 and the granular (isocortical) prefrontal cortex. The cytoarchitectural transition from M1 to motor association areas is gradual. The functional border between M1 and motor association cortex is imprecise, varying between apes of the same species and within a given ape on different examinations. For example, in stimulation studies of apes, the border of M1 extended more anteriorly with mapping in a posterior-to-anterior direction than with mapping in an anterior-to-posterior direction.[14] Areas M1 and M2 form an integrated map representing different types of action made in different spatial regions.[15]

The motor and sensory association unimodal cortices have similar features. They connect M1 and S1 to other cortical areas and integrate sensorimotor functions, including fine and complex movements.[15] Motor association cortex receives input from parietal somatosensory association cortex (mainly proprioception) and the thalamus and reciprocally connects with M1 (Fig. 7–4). Motor association cortex projects to M1 and directly to subcortical and spinal areas in the corticospinal tract. The relative size of premotor compared to motor cortex increased during primate evolution.[16]

LATERAL PREMOTOR CORTEX

Motor association cortex provides instructions to M1, which executes movements. Fibers from other cortical association areas must synapse in motor association cortex to influence M1. Robust parietal–premotor connections are important for all phases of motor action. These topographically specific connections relate to different aspects of motor control, such as sensory guidance. Premotor cortex (LPMC and SMA) stores motor schemata (elementary motor acts) and retrieves them for externally cued movements. Together with prefrontal cortex, PMC prepares, initiates, selects, and learns movement patterns.[15,17–19] Motor association cortex is involved in the initial stage of working memory, in which information is temporarily stored for only seconds. In the left hemisphere, Broca's area, LPMC, and SMA are activated for the initial storage of verbal information in working memory; storage of spatial information activates the right LPMC.[20]

The LPMC and SMA are organized bilaterally with strong relations to axial musculature, as well as proximal and distal muscles. The SMA is concerned mainly with control of the proximal upper limb musculature, and the LPMC has greater distal limb representation; both areas have output influencing the entire limb.[21] The LPMC is critical for initiating movements to external cues, and the SMA plays a greater role in initiating movement based on internal cues.[4]

In monkeys, LPMC has dorsal and ventral components with distinct anatomy, connectivity, and function. Dorsal LPMC is involved in planning and controlling eye movements (supplementary eye field) and limb movements. The results of somatosensory and visual studies suggest that a critical function of dorsal LPMC is to monitor and control the arm while it moves toward a target, which is consistent with the in-

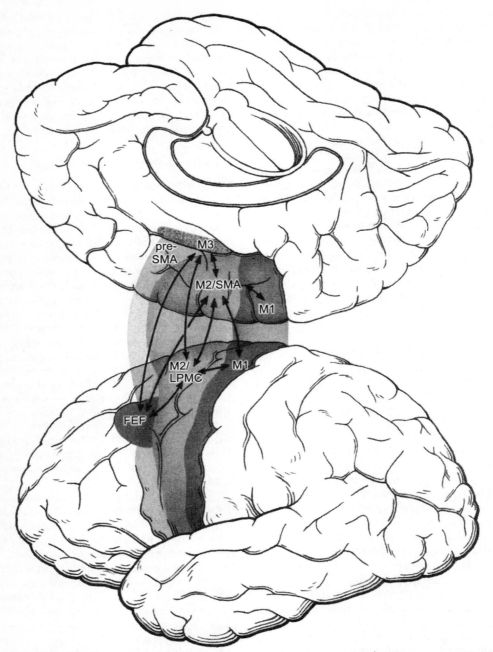

Figure 7–4. Cortical motor areas and their intraconnections. M1, primary motor cortex; M2, supplementary motor area (SMA); pre-SMA, presupplementary motor area; M3, cingulate motor area; LPMC, lateral premotor cortex; FEF, frontal eye field.

tense input from the superior parietal lobule to dorsal LPMC. Damage to this parietal area causes optic ataxia (see Chapter 5).

The function of neuronal groups in ventral LPMC of monkeys is threefold. First, they transform object locations into movements relative to *peripersonal space* (space as encoded into body part–centered coordinates whose center varies according to the type of movement).[22,23] Second, they transform the shape and representational memory of three-dimensional objects into appropriate hand movements,[24] provided that object size and shape are congruent with the prehension type coded by the neuron ("canonical" neurons).[1] Third, they discharge when the monkey observes hand actions performed by another animal, provided that the actions are similar to the motor action coded by the neurons ("mirror" neurons). In humans, similar neurons in Broca's area may be critical for learning mouth and tongue movements associated with speech. The juxtaposition of motor areas involved in planning hand movements that manipulate objects and movements that mirror another animal's actions may have linked praxis and motor dominance in monkeys. Mirroring of mouth and tongue movements may have linked language and motor dominance in humans.

In humans, LPMC lesions in either hemisphere impair motor tasks in conditioning paradigms,[15] bimanual and bibrachial interactions,[25,26] and sequential motor behaviors.[27] Lesions the LPMC spare strength but impair the speed, smoothness, and automaticity of movements.[28] Bilateral LPMC lesions cause postural and gait disorders, and unilateral lesions cause mild and usually transient proximal weakness, affecting shoulder and hip muscles.[27] Lesions of LPMC in the dominant hemisphere cause ideomotor apraxia in humans, and analogous defects of executing learned movements are observed in monkeys with unilateral LPMC lesions.[1,29–31] In monkeys, an area of ventral LPMC has neurons with oculomotor representation. In contrast to the fixed vector nature of saccades evoked by frontal eye field stimulation, the saccades evoked by stimulation of these neurons are goal-directed.[32,33] Together with the surrounding limb motor areas of the LPMC, this area may coordinate oculomotor and skeletomotor responses in goal-directed motor tasks.

Sequential movement tasks assess premotor and prefrontal function.[28] In the reciprocal coordination test, the patient holds one hand open with the palm down and the other hand in a fist. He or she must then simultaneously switch the hand positions. Marked impairment in this test with preserved strength suggests a lesion predominantly affecting the LPMC. A more challenging task, which may also be affected by prefrontal lesions, requires the patient to repeat a sequence of three hand movements (Fig. 9–10). Premotor lesions impair quick or smooth performance of these tasks, and prefrontal lesions cause out-of-sequence movements; lesions of either area can cause perseveration. Right-sided premotor and prefrontal lesions also cause *motor impersistence,* the inability to maintain an initiated voluntary movement, such as tongue protrusion, which normally can be performed briefly.[34]

SUPPLEMENTARY MOTOR AREA

The SMA helps to mediate spontaneous or self-initiated movements (based on internal cues), anticipatory postural adjustments, motor repetitions and sequences, motor reversals, and movements requiring motor cues.[35–38] The SMA consists of the SMA proper, lying immediately anterior to the medial M1, and the pre-SMA, lying anterior to the SMA (Fig. 7–4).[39,40] The SMA has a complete somatotopic body representation and a lower threshold for stimulation-evoked movement, and the pre-SMA has a motor representation for the arms, neck, and face at higher thresholds.[41] The SMA plays a major role in simple and practiced movements, and the pre-SMA helps mediate complex and novel movements.[42]

Representations for proximal and distal movements are not as well segregated in the SMA as in M1.[43] Electrical stimulation and spontaneous seizures involving the SMA evoke speech arrest and vocalizations, such as cries, grunts, and repeated syllables or words.[44,45] Stimulation of the SMA produces an urge to perform a movement or a feeling of anticipation that a movement is about to occur.[46,47] Because sensory symptoms are evoked by stimulating the SMA and motor responses by stimulating the postcentral mesial parietal cortex, the SMA may be a supplementary sensorimotor cortex extending across the medial precentral sulcus.[47] Alternatively, as with primary sensorimotor areas, robust interconnections cause motor responses with stimulation of S1 and sensory phenomena with stimulation of M1.

Bilateral SMA lesions cause akinetic mutism followed by persistent deficits in motor initiation. Unilateral SMA lesions initially cause global akinesia or bradykinesia, which is more prominent contralaterally. Muteness may follow SMA lesions of either hemisphere, but when the dominant hemisphere is involved, it can last weeks. Subacutely, spontaneous motor activity and facial emotional expression are impaired contralaterally. In the long term, patients have no residual effects or have mildly impaired motor spontaneity, rapid alternating hand movements and complex motor performance.[10,48–50] Lesions involving the SMA and anterior cingulate and prefrontal cortices cause a medial frontal form of the alien hand syndrome, which is characterized by reflex grasping, groping, and compulsive manipulation of tools by the dominant or, rarely, nondominant, hand (see Chapter 3).[51,52]

The pre-SMA forms a morphological and functional transition from the agranular, pyramidal cell-rich SMA to the granular, pyramidal cell-poor prefrontal areas. The pre-SMA is the only motor area in monkeys with very modest parietal inputs; it receives major inputs from prefrontal and anterior cingulate cortices. The pre-SMA helps to initiate movement. It is involved in more complex motor acts than the SMA.[42] The SMA, pre-SMA, and CMA provide motivational context for both self-initiated and externally cued movements.[31] The CMA may provide an emotional and drive-related context, and the pre-SMA may provide a greater cognitive context. Pre-SMA stimulation inhibits voluntary motor activity, most often causing speech arrest without associated language impairment.[53] The pre-SMA may be particularly related to the acquisition, rather than the storage or execution, of sequential motor tasks.[54] Blood flow in the pre-SMA and anterior globus pallidus, but not the SMA, correlates with the complexity of a learned finger movement sequence.[55]

FRONTAL EYE FIELD

The frontal eye field (BA 8) lies in the caudal middle frontal gyrus (Fig. 7–4), sending descending fibers to brain stem areas involved with eye movements, that is, the superior colliculi, interstitial nuclei of Cajal, medial longitudinal fasciculus, and pontine paramedian reticular formation. Although fibers do not directly stimulate brain stem motor nuclei controlling extraocular muscles, the frontal eye field is analogous to the primary motor cortex for eye movements. The supplementary eye field is formed by other portions of BA 8, which receive input from parietal and temporal sensory association cortices mainly concerned with

tactile (not proprioceptive), visual, and auditory inputs.[38] The frontal eye field is a center of voluntary eye movement, initiating purposeful saccades to behaviorally relevant targets. Frontal eye field stimulation causes contralateral conjugate eye deviation and fragments of attentive reactions such as pupillary dilatation and head rotation.[56,57]

The frontal eye field orients oculomotor behavior (looking), and the premotor and supplementary motor areas activate manipulative and vocal motor behavior.[38] The frontal eye field is the motor component of the visual attention system. Lesions of the frontal eye field (and usually other adjacent frontal areas) cause transient tonic deviation of the eyes to the side of the lesion and permanent impairments when looking to the contralateral side. These impairments include prolonged latency of saccades, impaired initiation of saccades to imagined targets, and impaired inhibition of inappropriate saccades to peripheral, visually attractive stimuli.[58]

BROCA'S AREA

Broca's area (the posterior portion of the inferior frontal gyrus, BA 44 and posterior BA 45 in the dominant hemisphere) is motor association cortex specialized for motor programming of laryngeal, tongue, and mouth movements during speech (see Chapter 6). Broca's area also contains neural codes for the sequential relationships underlying grammar. The rostroventral LPMC of monkeys is a possible early evolutionary form of Broca's area located in a similar region. Stimulation of Broca's area and its right hemisphere homologue evokes negative motor responses showing a somatotopic distribution.[53] Further, stimulation of Broca's area causes speech arrest and impaired fluency, as well as more subtle receptive language deficits.[53] BA 44 and BA 45 in the nondominant hemisphere may be important for the production of emotional intonation (a component of prosody) and singing.

Limbic Motor Areas

The limbic system influences motor activity through the anterior cingulate cortex (ACC), amygdala, and nucleus accumbens (see Chapter 10). Limbic motor activity is expressed through volitional and nonvolitional skeleto-motor and autonomic functions. The CMA and cingulate autonomic area provide higher levels of cortical processing for behavioral displays of such acts as laughter and blushing. These areas also provide emotional context and motivation for motor behavior. The amygdala–hypothalamic axis coordinates limbic output for such preprogrammed emotional displays as fear and rage. The ACC and amygdala also connect with cortical areas to provide emotional coloring of perception and cognition; that is, they infuse affect into sensory stimuli and thought. The ACC is active in early premotor functions that incorporate affective input and cognitive processing. The ACC helps to determine whether or not a movement is needed and the motivational relevance for the correct response pattern.

The contrast between limbic and cortical motor output is evident in the act of smiling. Spontaneous smiling triggered by emotional stimuli (limbic motor system) differs from volitional smiling to a command (pyramidal motor system). When asked by a photographer to smile, few persons—except politicians and actors—can imitate a natural smile. The limbic motor pathways for spontaneous smiling and other emotional expressions differ from those for volitional movements. Lesions of M1 and PMC impair volitional attempts to smile, and lesions of the limbic pathways for motor expression impair spontaneous smiling (Fig. 7–5). Clinical dissociations between these pathways are common, causing selective facial asymmetries for emotional or volitional displays.

The CMA (M3; BA 23c, 24c), located deep in the cingulate sulcus (Figs. 7–2, 7–4), contains corticospinal projection neurons.[59] In contrast to M1 and PMC, only CMA receives extensive inputs from prefrontal and limbic cortices. In monkeys, there are three CMAs: CMA-rostral (CMAr), CMA-dorsal (CMAd), and CMA-ventral (CMAv).[21] Electrical stimulation studies show that CMAd and CMAv contain more precise somatotopic maps than CMAr[21,42] consistent with the lower density of corticospinal fibers in the more rostral CMA. The CMAr is likely involved in more complex movements that reflect greater planning compared with CMAd and CMAv, which appear to play a greater role in simple, practiced movements.

Functional imaging studies suggest that humans have three CMAs,[42] with the same caudal–rostral division found in nonhuman primates but with one caudal zone and two rostral zones. The caudal zone shows greater activation during simple and nonfacial movements and relatively selective activation during somatosensory and painful stimuli.[42] The caudal CMA (CMAc) is strongly and selectively activated during the performance of simple and highly practiced, remembered sequences of movement.[21] The CMAc receives input for pain sensation, possibly mediating some higher level but simple motor responses to painful stimuli. The caudal–rostral (simple–complex movement) relative dichotomy of functions in nonhuman primates and humans parallels the pre-SMA (rostral) and SMA (caudal) functions. The rostral CMA (CMAr) appears to have both anterior (CMAra) and posterior (CMArp) divisions. Each of these divisions contains a focus related to oculomotor and speech tasks (face area) and a focus related to arm movements (see Chapter 10, Fig. 10–6).[42] The CMAra is activated by tasks that require an internally generated movement[60] or learning a new motor sequence.[42] The CMAra and CMArp are connected with the prefrontal cortex.

The SMA reciprocally connects with the CMA. These areas may act cooperatively to prepare and initiate movement.[36,61–63] The SMA and ACC are activated during sequential thumb–finger apposition movements.[64] Lesions involving both SMA and ACC severely impair early motor processing and may cause motor neglect or contribute to akinetic mutism.

In monkeys, the CMA is involved in vocalizations expressing internal states and in response to external stimuli. In humans, large lesions of the ACC and adjacent areas may cause mutism. Vocalization is rarely altered by ACC stimulation in humans,[65] but involuntary vocalization or speech arrest may occur with seizures arising from the ACC.[66] Studies in patients with epilepsy implicate the ACC in ictal laughter.[67,68]

The role of the ACC in motivation for movement is supported by studies that associate ACC abnormalities with obsessive–compulsive disorder at one end of the behavioral spectrum and abulia at the other end.[69,70] Increased metabolic activity in the ACC and orbitofrontal, caudate, and thalamic areas is found in idiopathic obsessive–compulsive disorder;[71] and ir-

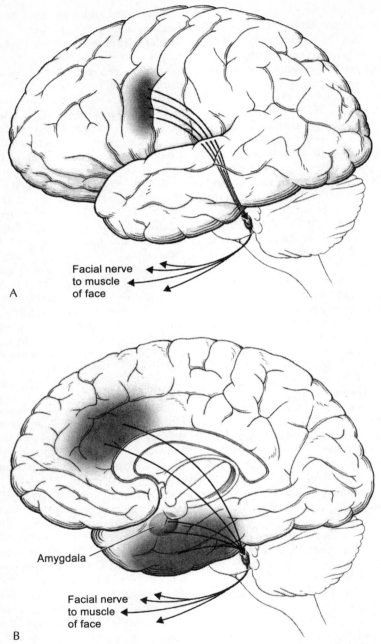

Figure 7–5. Areas and pathways involved in volitional (social) and spontaneous (emotional) smiling. Discrete lesions of the (A) primary motor area for the face or (B) the limbic area may selectively impair volitional (A) or emotional (B) smiling on the contralateral face.

ritative lesions of ACC may cause the disorder.[69] Abulia is most often caused by lesions of the dorsolateral frontal convexity. Akinetic mutism may be considered the most intense form of abulia.[72]

It occurs with bilateral frontal lesions (the cingulate and orbital gyri and the septal area)[73,74] and lesions of the paramedian reticular formation (diencephalon and midbrain).[75,76]

CORTICAL MOTOR CONTROL DISORDERS

Abulia

Abulia, a generalized slowing and decrease in behavioral activity, is produced from a variety of lesion sites and pathological processes (Table 7–1). The drive for behavioral output is reduced in abulia, and many patients appear depressed (pseudodepression) and unconcerned. Abulic patients show little spontaneous speech or motor activity; they may intermittently fail to respond to questions or commands for minutes at a time.[77] Responses are slow and apathetic. *Akinetic mutism* (see above), first reported in 1941 by Cairns et al.,[78] is a condition in which the patient appears to be awake and may fol-low the examiner with his or her eyes but spontaneous motor and verbal responses are absent, is incontinent of bowel and bladder, and responds incompletely to noxious stimuli.

Table 7–1. **Lesion Sites and Pathological Processes Associated with Abulia and Akinetic Mutism**

Focal Lesions

Unilateral (abulia, transient akinetic mutism)
  Medial prefrontal (cingulate gyrus, supplementary motor area)
  Lateral prefrontal (acute, large dorsolateral convexity)
Bilateral and central
  Thalamus
  Midbrain
  Medial forebrain bundle (ascending noradrenergic and dopaminergic fibers)
  Prefrontal
  Cerebellar hemisphere and dentate nuclei (rare, mutism only)
  Globus pallidus (rare)

Diffuse or Nonfocal Processes

Metabolic disorders (hypoxia, hypoglycemia, hepatic encephalopathy)

Traumatic brain injury

Hydrocephalus

Subarachnoid hemorrhage

Gliomatosis cerebri

Postictal state

Fat embolism

Creutzfeldt-Jakob disease

Leukoencephalopathy (e.g., 5-fluorouracil-induced)

Catatonic depression or schizophrenia

Apraxia

Apraxia, the inability to perform complex movements, results from the disconnection or destruction of motor association areas in the left hemisphere of right-handed persons. Language and praxis can be dissociated, especially in left-handed persons, in whom apraxia usually results from lesions of the right hemisphere.[79,80] Apraxia, by definition, cannot be explained by weakness, sensory loss, incoordination, poor comprehension, amnesia, or inattention. A mild deficit in neuromuscular, somatosensory, memory, attention, or other neurological function does not exclude apraxia; but for a definite diagnosis of apraxia, the impairment in motor performance must clearly exceed the deficit. Physicians may make a diagnosis of apraxia when the patient fails to produce a gesture to command, although the primary defect may be in transcoding language into motor action, not a motor deficit in ordinary life. However, damage to premotor regions and superior parietal lobules causes severe spontaneous higher-order motor deficits.[81] In right-handed patients, right-sided cerebral injuries have little or no effect on kinematics or praxis of right-handed movements, but left-sided cerebral injuries may severely impair kinematics and praxis of right- and left-handed movements.

Apraxia is common, often coexisting with Broca's and conduction aphasias, but may be overlooked unless specifically sought. Apraxia is usually considered only when the deficit involves learned or skilled movements. However, it includes such deficits as an inability to protrude the tongue on command, even though the ability to perform this motor act by imitation or spontaneous action (e.g., licking an ice cream cone) is preserved. *Parapraxia,* the cardinal feature of apraxia, is a motor defect affecting either the spatial course and final position or the temporal sequencing of a series of movements into a coherent motor act.[82–84] Spatial defects predominate over temporal defects, with impaired relations between the neural representations for the extrapersonal (spatial location) and intrapersonal (hand position) features of movement.[85] Patients with apraxia have deficits in the spatial plans for movement and in translating those plans into details of angular joint motions, even when actually manipulating a tool or object.[86] Parapraxias overlap with kinematic abnormalities, which are characterized by impaired trajectory and velocity of movement. However, there is no correlation between kinematic abnormalities and praxis errors.[84] This may partly reflect the functional and anatomical independence of kinematics and praxis, as well as the role of visual feedback in normalizing simple aiming movements in apraxic patients.[85] One primary defect in apraxic patients may be in the mental representation of a target position.[84]

Liepmann,[87] who introduced the term *apraxia,* correctly posited that the left hemisphere in right-handed persons contains a special repository for movement patterns or engrams. Support for Liepmann's hypothesis comes from functional neuroimaging and transcranial magnetic stimulation studies and observations of motor impairment in various disorders. Complex, but not simple, finger movements performed by the right hand activate only the left motor areas, but similar movements of the left hand activate bilateral motor areas.[88] Transcranial magnetic stimulation of the nondominant PMC impairs response selection only in the contralateral hand, but stimulation of the dominant side impairs motor activity in both hands.[89] In addition, some patients with Broca's aphasia or callosal lesions fail to imitate movements with their left arm or leg. Since such mimetic movements do not rely on transmission of verbal input from the left hemisphere to motor areas in the right hemisphere, this phenomenon demonstrates that disconnection of language and motor areas cannot account for all apraxic deficits.[90] Further, these patients probably would not display mimetic deficits if motor engram storage took place in the right hemisphere. A left hemisphere storehouse of acquired movements explains their deficits. Further support for this notion is found among patients with right-sided hemiplegia due to cortical lesions. When using left-sided limbs, these patients are often clumsy and very poor at acquiring new motor skills. In contrast, neurologically intact patients who have their right arm immobilized in a cast after injury may become dexterous with their

left arm. In this setting, the repository of motor skills in the left hemisphere assists right hemisphere motor control. Liepmann[91] theorized that the normal left hand might be even less dexterous than we think "because much of its skill may be borrowed from the left hemisphere across the corpus callosum." The extent of left hemisphere dominance for motor tasks is variable in individuals but more prominent for verbal than visuomotor tests of praxis.[92]

The left hemisphere may contain two repositories of motor engrams (Fig. 7–6), one in the parietal lobe supramarginal and angular gyri storing visuokinesthetic movement representations (formulas or "software programs" that integrate visual, tactile, and motor data needed to perform a complex sequence of movements) and possibly one in the SMA containing movement execution programs.[91,93] The SMA has a more vital role in motor execution than engram storage. In addition, right hemisphere frontoparietal areas are dominant for certain complex sequential movements.[94,95] The left angular gyrus is activated with transposition of a motor plan to the representation of the body schema.[96] Patients with SMA lesions in the left, or dominant, hemisphere have ideomotor apraxia of both arms (no buccofacial apraxia) but can comprehend and discriminate pantomimes.[97] Imitation and use of the actual object usually improve the movement. In contrast, patients with lesions in the supramarginal and angular gyri fail to pantomime to command, to discriminate between correct and incorrect movements by the examiner, and to understand the nature of the movement.[93,98] Patients with lesions in the deep parietal white matter can make the correct discrimination.[92,93] A possible third repository for motor engrams, especially for writing skills (Chapter 6), may be localized in the dominant superior parietal lobule.

Apraxia is commonly caused by subcortical lesions of the basal ganglia, extending to the peristriatal or periventricular white matter (e.g., superior longitudinal fasciculus) (Fig. 7–6); such lesions can also cause conduction aphasia.[99,100] Apraxia is a feature of pathological processes (e.g., stroke, tumor, inflammatory processes, cortical–basal ganglionic degeneration) associated with lesions of these areas. Lesions restricted to the putamen or thalamus (pulvinar and other lateral nuclei) rarely cause apraxia.[99,101–103]

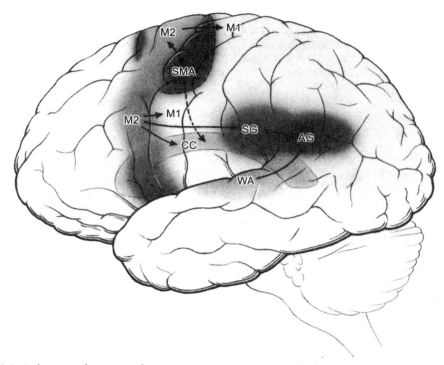

Figure 7–6. Pathways used in praxis. The premotor area communicates with the primary motor area, the corpus callosum (CC), and the supramarginal gyrus (SG) to initiate voluntary movement. Wernicke's area (WA) is necessary for comprehension of verbal praxis commands, and both the angular gyrus (AG) and the motor association cortex [supplementary motor area (SMA), M2] contribute when more complex motor sequences are attempted. Lesions of any of the shaded areas may cause some form of apraxia. M1, primary motor cortex.

Apraxia takes many forms. Ideomotor (motor) apraxia is the principal form and often is simply referred to as apraxia. Other forms are visuomotor apraxia, callosal ideomotor apraxia, disassociation apraxia, ideational apraxia, conduction apraxia, conceptual apraxia, constructional apraxia, limb-kinetic apraxia, gait apraxia, and dressing apraxia (see Chapter 3). Some "apraxias" are not true apraxias but apraxia-like neurological disorders, which are imprecisely characterized by the misnomer. For example, the so-called apraxia of eyelid opening is an extrapyramidal motor disorder with involuntary inhibition of the levator palpebrae, which may respond to botulinum toxin injection.[104,105] In addition, impaired dressing skills may be incorrectly identified as dressing apraxia (see Chapter 3).

LIMB APRAXIA

Assessment of limb apraxia is hierarchical. First, test the ability to pantomime by asking the patient to make a movement in response to a verbal command. Next, assess imitation ability by having the patient copy the examiner's movements. Finally, test the patient's ability to perform the movement with a physical object or tool (e.g., blow out a lit match). Test both transitive movements, involving an object or tool, and intransitive movements, not involving an object or tool (e.g., "Blow a kiss"). Instruct the patient not to use a body part as a tool but, rather, to hold the tool in the hand. The severity of ideomotor apraxia is graded mild (pantomime deficit to verbal command), moderate (failure to imitate the movement), or severe (failure to perform transitive or intransitive movement with the actual object).

Limb apraxia involves the upper or lower limbs and may be unilateral. Therefore, test all four extremities. Assess pantomime ability by having the patient "Salute with your left hand," "Put out a cigarette with your left foot," "Kick a ball with your right foot," and "Brush your teeth holding an imaginary toothbrush with your right hand." Praxis errors include the use of a finger for the toothbrush or failure to open the mouth. In subsequent tasks, vary the commands for each side as visual cues can artificially enhance performance. However, if the patient fails to perform a task, repeat the task with the contralateral extremity after an interval of at least several minutes.

Limb apraxia is typically manifested by errors of production, not content.[106] Thus, when patients are asked to pantomime (e.g., hammer a nail), their failed attempts usually reveal the correct goal and core movement, not a well-executed alternative movement (e.g., use of a screwdriver). Production errors in limb apraxia result from using the body part as a tool,[107] spatial errors, and timing errors.[106,108] Spatial errors include failure to position the limb correctly, orient body parts, and move the limb through space in the correct trajectory and sequence of actions. Patients with limb apraxia may show a prolonged delay before initiating a movement and fail to make a smooth, continuous movement. Instead, their actions are a series of "stuttering," often clumsy, movements. This disruption in the temporal organization of movement is the hallmark of ideational apraxia but may also occur in limb apraxia.

BUCCOFACIAL AND TRUNCAL APRAXIA

Test apraxia of the buccal and facial muscles by having the patient imitate various motor acts, such as "Blow out a match," "Drink with a straw," or "Stick out your tongue." The patient may pretend to hold the match or straw, but discourage this behavior as it makes the task easier. Observe the patient for incomplete, unrelated, or opposite motor acts, such as inhaling while blowing out the imaginary match. Test truncal apraxia with commands such as "Bow" or "Stand like a boxer." Axial movements are typically preserved in apraxic patients, probably because these movements may be mediated through nonpyramidal pathways.[90]

VISUOMOTOR APRAXIA

Visuomotor apraxia, characterized by the failure to use visual information when performing a target-directed movement, is typically associated with occipitoparietal lesions that disconnect cortical visual and motor areas. How-

ever, a right-sided thalamic lesion can also cause visuomotor apraxia.[109]

CALLOSAL IDEOMOTOR APRAXIA

Callosal ideomotor apraxia results from lesions of the anterior corpus callosum that disconnect the dominant, left hemisphere motor area from the right hemisphere.[110,111] Since the motor engrams are almost exclusively in the left hemisphere, patients with callosal ideomotor apraxia cannot pantomime and, in many cases, imitate or use tools correctly with their left hand.[92] In these cases, visual cueing may occur if the patient first performs the task with the right limb and is subsequently asked to perform the same task with the left limb. Patients with callosal dissociation apraxia may have impaired constructional skills of the right hand as left hemisphere motor areas are disconnected from right hemisphere visuospatial–motor centers.[112]

DISASSOCIATION APRAXIA

Disassociation (disconnection) apraxia results from other white matter lesions that disconnect pathways between Wernicke's area, motor engram storage areas in the left parietal and frontal lobes, and motor areas of the left hemisphere.[111,113–115] Patients with disassociation apraxia are unable to make meaningful movements to verbal command but, unlike those with ideomotor apraxia, are able to imitate perfectly the examiner's movements or use an object. Other patients can pantomime to verbal command but not in response to visual or tactile stimuli.[111]

IDEATIONAL APRAXIA

Ideational apraxia refers to "a disruption in the logical and harmonious succession of separate elements,"[116] which impairs the ability to perform nonverbal motor sequences that are not initiated after the verbal command,[117,118] such as spontaneously lighting a cigarette. Patients with ideational apraxia may successfully perform individual components of a complex motor sequence but fail to execute the correct series of actions. Ideational apraxia usually results from parietal lesions in the left, or dominant, hemisphere and is often associated with fluent aphasia and components of Gerstmann's syndrome.[115,119] Prominent comprehension deficits confound the diagnosis. Ideational apraxia is difficult to distinguish from the impaired planning and sequencing behaviors observed after prefrontal lesions. In general, patients with prefrontal lesions have greater difficulty with complex, multistep tasks, such as making dinner or planning a vacation, and those with ideational apraxia fail at simple sequential behaviors, such as boiling water. The following experience of a patient with an oligodendroglioma of the left parietal lobe (Fig. 7–7) is a vivid illustration of ideational apraxia:

The patient, a 40–year-old right-handed man, had seizures in which he was unable to manipulate tools. During the seizures, his strength and sensation were normal or near normal. During one seizure, he was carving a roast and suddenly looked down at the meat, holding the knife in his right hand, and had "no idea what to do with the knife. My inner voice said 'Cut the damn meat,' but my hand was clueless. It held the knife but was unable to cut the meat."

CONDUCTION APRAXIA

Conduction apraxia is characterized by greater impairment of movement with imitation than to command.[120] This contrasts with the usual pattern in ideomotor apraxia. Patients with conduction apraxia comprehend the examiner's pantomime and gesture (*intact input praxicon*) and produce the correct movement to verbal command (*intact output praxicon*).[121] Their deficit results from impaired communication between the input and the output praxicons,[122] which is analogous to the defect in conduction aphasia. The location of the lesion remains uncertain.

CONCEPTUAL APRAXIA

Conceptual apraxia results from impaired knowledge of what tools and objects are needed to perform a skilled movement. In contrast to the production errors of ideomotor apraxia, patients with conceptual apraxia make content errors, being unable to recall the relationship between objects and specific actions.[123,124] This form of apraxia is common in Alzheimer's disease.[125]

CONSTRUCTIONAL APRAXIA

Constructional apraxia refers to impaired spatial manipulation of objects and may represent visuospatial agnosia,[126–128] especially for those deficits caused by injury of the right hemisphere.[129,130] The lesions that cause constructional apraxia are usually parietal and are right-sided in two-thirds of patients.[131,132]

Test for constructional apraxia by having the patient copy or spontaneously draw figures, arrange blocks in patterns, and construct or mentally manipulate three-dimensional structures. Patients with right-sided lesions often demonstrate left-sided neglect and, when copying and constructing, produce replicas that lack the original's general outline, or gestalt. In contrast, patients with left-sided lesions often make impoverished copies that lack detail but preserve the outline and general structure. In addition, visual cues are of greater benefit to patients with left-sided lesions. Indeed, the constructional deficits in patients with left-sided lesions may be more aptly described as an executive motor disorder than as constructional apraxia.

LIMB-KINETIC APRAXIA

Limb–kinetic apraxia refers to the loss of fine, skilled movements following premotor or corticospinal lesions. Patients are clumsy, slow, and awkward in executing motor tasks that were performed rapidly and precisely prior to the cerebral insult. Since corticospinal tract lesions cause identical deficits in monkeys,[133] this disorder is not true apraxia.

SUBCORTICAL ANATOMY OF THE MOTOR SYSTEM

Basal Ganglia

The basal ganglia are intimately related to movement and robustly connected to cortical and subcortical motor areas. In turn, cortical motor areas project to motor-related neurons throughout the neuraxis. The basal ganglia do not directly project to the spinal cord but influence motor activity and behavior through a series of parallel loop circuits linking the basal ganglia with the frontal lobes and thalamus.

Basal ganglia and cortical motor association areas are involved in the learning and automatic execution of motor programs.[38,134] The basal

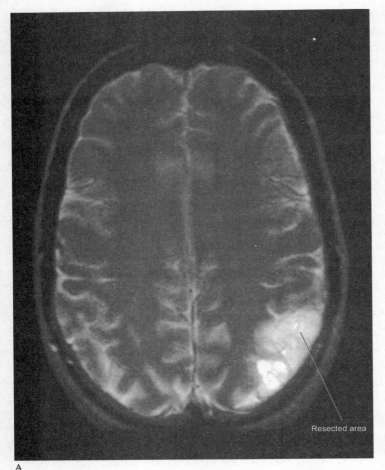

Resected area

A

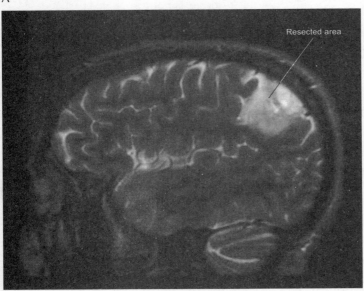

Resected area

B

Figure 7–7. Magnetic resonance image of a patient with a left superior parietal tumor and ictal apraxia. *A:* Axial view. *B:* Sagittal view.

ganglia are vital for acquiring and automatizing new procedures (procedural learning) and activating motor skills and overlearned behaviors.[135] This procedural knowledge includes complex response habits strategically adapted to environmental needs. The basal ganglia influence cognitive, affective, and motivational behavior. Working with cortical–subcortical networks, basal ganglia help to generate, maintain, alternate, and mix behavioral repertoires involving cognition, emotion, and movement. In part, the basal ganglia may have evolved as a central switching mechanism to control access to limited motor and cognitive resources.[136] The connections of these nuclei underlie their role in motor and nonmotor behavior.

The basal ganglia comprise five principal nuclei and two closely related brain stem nuclei. The basal ganglia nuclei consist of the caudate nucleus (associative or "cognitive" striatum), putamen (sensorimotor striatum), nucleus accumbens (limbic striatum), globus pallidus (GP), and subthalamic nucleus. The brain stem nuclei consist of the substantia nigra and the pedunculopontine nucleus.

STRIATUM

The striatum is the main receptive component of the basal ganglia (Fig. 7–8) (see Chapter 8, Fig. 8–5a). The dorsal striatum, formed by the caudate and putamen, receives massive excitatory (glutaminergic) input from the cerebral cortex, mainly from multimodal association cortex (caudate), primary somatosensory and motor cortices, and motor association cortex (putamen). Cortical input is somatotopically organized to striatal cell clusters (*martisomes*). The striatum receives a rich supply of dopaminergic fibers from the substantia nigra pars compacta (SNpc, excitatory on D_1 receptors and inhibitory on D_2 dopamine receptors) and glutaminergic fibers from the thalamic intralaminar nucleus (excitatory). The striatum sends inhibitory γ-aminobutyric acid-ergic (GABAergic) fibers to the GP and substantia nigra pars reticularis (SNpr). The ventral, or limbic, striatum,[137,138] formed by the nucleus accumbens and olfactory tubercle, receives input from cortical and limbic areas. The ventral striatum receives a large dopaminergic supply

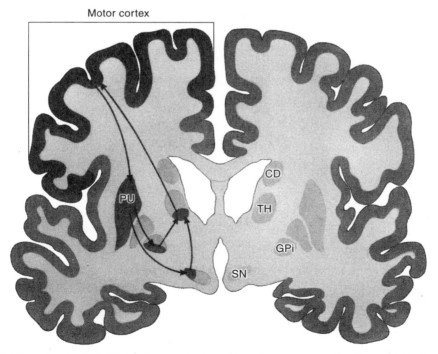

Figure 7–8. The motor circuit that links primary motor (as well as primary sensory and motor association) cortex to corresponding subcortical components. Information passes from the cortex to the putamen (PU) to the ventral globus pallidus interna (GP$_i$) and substantia nigra (SN, pars reticularis) to the ventrolateral nucleus of the thalamus (TH) to the primary motor cortex. CD, caudate nucleus.

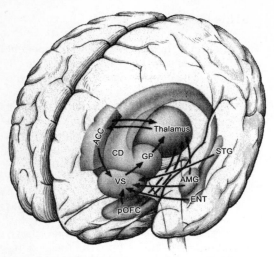

Figure 7–9. The limbic circuit links cortical limbic areas to the ventral striatum (nucleus accumbens and olfactory tubercle), ventral pallidum, and medial dorsal nucleus of the thalamus. This circuit helps to initiate movement based on emotion or motivation. Anterior cingulate cortex (ACC), caudate nucleus (CD), globus pallidus (GP), ventral striatum (VS), posterior orbitofrontal cortex (pOFC), entorhinal cortex (ENT), and amygdala (AMG), superior temporal gyrus (STG).

from the ventral tegmental area and projects inhibitory GABAergic fibers to the ventral GP (paralleling dorsal striatal fibers to dorsal pallidal fibers) (Figs. 7–8, 7–9) and the ventral tegmental area. Striatal martisomes that receive afferents from one cortical area project to the same regions in the GP and SNpr. Cortical data diverge in the striatum but reconverge in the pallidum.[139]

The predominant neuronal type in the striatum (nearly 90%) is the medium spiny GABAergic neuron that projects to basal ganglia output regions. A small population of large cholinergic (aspiny) interneurons that have dense D_2 receptors are tonically active and involved in learning.[140]

GLOBUS PALLIDUS

The GP consists of two major regions: a dorsal region, which is divided into interna (GPi, medial) and externa (GPe, lateral) segments, and a ventral (subcommissural) region. Input to the pallidum comes mainly from the striatum (inhibitory, GABAergic) and subthalamic nucleus (excitatory, glutaminergic). Dorsal striatal efferents project to the dorsal GP, and ventral

striatal efferents project to the ventral GP. The GPe sends a large excitatory (glutaminergic) projection to the subthalamic nuclei, with other efferents supplying the GPi, SNpr, SNpc, and striatum (inhibitory). The GPi and SNpr are the major output nuclei of the basal ganglia, sending a prominent inhibitory GABAergic projection to the ventral thalamus (ventral anterior [VA], ventral lateral [VL]), with smaller projections to the thalamus (medial dorsal [MD], reticular nuclei) and brain stem nuclei. The excitatory (glutaminergic) ventral thalamocortical pathways maintain topographic relationships. Thus, cortical areas projecting to the striatum eventually receive fibers back from these same striatal regions (maristomes) via the loop that connects these regions with the GP and ventral thalamus (Figs. 7–8, 7–9).

SUBTHALAMIC NUCLEI

The subthalamic nuclei connect reciprocally with GPe and receive afferents from cortical motor areas and the pedunculopontine nucleus (cholinergic). The subthalamic nucleus modifies basal ganglia outflow, its efferent fibers passing to the two major output centers: GP and SNpr. Subthalamic nuclei may alter the membrane potential or modulate synaptic transmission in these outflow centers prior to striatal inputs.[141]

SUBSTANTIA NIGRA PARS RETICULARIS AND PEDUNCULOPONTINE NUCLEI

The SNpr receives input from GPe and sends inhibitory GABAergic fibers to thalamic nuclei (VA, VL, MD) and pedunculopontine nuclei. The pedunculopontine nuclei receive input from the cerebellum and SNpr and send efferents to the SNpc, VL thalamus (cholinergic fibers), and striatum. Pedunculopontine nuclei, like VL thalamus, interface between cerebellar and basal ganglia and cortical motor systems.

Parallel Cortical–Subcortical Circuits

Five parallel circuits connect the frontal lobes, basal ganglia, and thalamus (Figs. 7–8, 7–9).[142–144] These independent loops, distinguished by their connectivity, modulate different aspects of motor, cognitive, and affective behavior. The neuronal nodes within these circuits have independent afferent and efferent connections, additionally influencing the loop functions. For example, in motor tasks requiring fine tuning based on sensory data, there is a significant correlation of output from the cerebellum with the SMA and output from the basal ganglia with M1 activity.[145]

Each of the five major frontal–subcortical loops can be further divided according to discrete anatomical and functional modules. For example, the "motor circuit" arising from the GPi projects to the primary motor (movement parameters), premotor (externally guided movements), and supplementary motor (internally guided movements) regions.[146] The motor circuit links sensorimotor and motor association cortices (S1, M1, and M2) to the putamen to the dorsal GP to the thalamus (VA, VL) to the M1–M2–S1. This circuit coordinates movement and contributes to motor planning and learning. The oculomotor circuit links the frontal eye fields (BA 8) and dorsal parietal visuomotor cortex (BA 7) to the caudate to the dorsal GP to the thalamus (MD, VA) to BA 8. Three circuits link prefrontal cortical areas with subcortical areas: dorsolateral, orbital, and medial (see Chapter 9, Figs. 9–7, and 9–8). The limbic circuit mediates working memory, planning, and temporal sequencing of behavior. It links limbic areas of the prefrontal, temporal, and insular regions to the ventral striatum (nucleus accumbens and olfactory tubercle) to the ventral pallidum to the MD nucleus of the thalamus (Fig. 7–9). It helps to initiate movement in response to motivationally or emotionally significant stimuli, as well as other diverse limbic functions.[142,147]

The notion of parallel loops extends beyond the basal ganglia to include discrete areas of the substantia nigra and cerebellum. These nigral and cerebellar output channels, like pallidal output channels, form loops with the thalamic and cortical areas involved with similar sensory, motor, oculomotor, cognitive, and behavioral tasks.[146] The properties and functional responsiveness of neurons within these subcortical circuits are similar to those cortical neurons in the same loop. Thus, distinct behavioral functions are served by parallel circuits connecting the cortex not only with the basal ganglia and thalamus but also with the substantia nigra and thalamus as well as the cerebellum and thalamus.[146]

Direct and Indirect Motor Circuits

The basal ganglia facilitate motor programs. Simplistically, this function is accomplished by two circuits acting simultaneously. The direct motor circuit disinhibits a small thalamic area that facilitates a desired action. The indirect motor circuit inhibits a wide region surrounding the thalamus that suppresses undesired actions. Although the anatomy and pathology of these pathways are best defined for the motor system, similar parallel pathways facilitate cognition and emotion.

In the direct motor circuit (Fig. 7–10A), cortical efferents excite striatal GABAergic neurons, which then inhibit the GPi and SNpr. These latter structures send inhibitory fibers to the thalamus, disinhibiting cell groups and thereby facilitating a motor program.[148,149] Striatal neurons in this pathway use D_1 receptors, which stimulate striatal neurons. The direct circuit provides positive feedback between the basal ganglia and the thalamus. Bradykinesia in Parkinson's disease and Huntington's disease results from the loss of dopaminergic input to the striatum or the loss of striatal cells, which affects the direct motor circuit, impairing the initiation and maintenance of motor programs.[149]

In the indirect motor circuit (Fig. 7–10B), excitatory cortical output stimulates striatal GABAergic and enkephalinergic neurons that inhibit the GPe. Since the GPe inhibits the subthalamic nucleus, GPi, and SNpr, striatal inhibition of the GPe disinhibits these three subcortical nuclei. In addition, the subthalamic nucleus projects excitatory fibers to the GPi and SNpr, further enhancing activity in certain GPi and SNpr neurons. These neurons inhibit ventral thalamic motor nuclei. Activating the indirect motor circuit thereby suppresses unwanted motor programs and actions.[148,149] Striatal neurons in the indirect motor circuit use D_2 receptors, which inhibit striatal neurons. The indirect circuit provides negative feedback between the basal ganglia and the thalamus. In Parkinson's disease, decreased inhibition of the indirect circuit excessively suppresses unwanted movements. In Huntington's disease, the effects are more complex, with progressive loss of different striatal neuronal populations (e.g., GABA and enkephalin before GABA and substance P).

Direct Motor Circuit   **Indirect Motor Circuit**

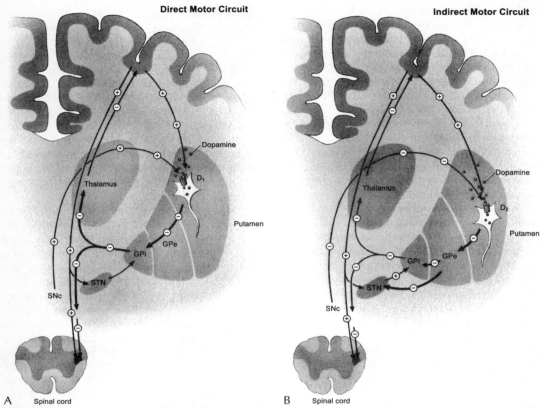

Figure 7–10. Direct *A* and indirect *B* motor pathways. GPi/GPe, globus pallidus interna and externa, respectively; D$_1$/D$_2$, dopamine receptors; SNc, substantia nigra pars compacta; STN, subthalamic nucleus.

SUBCORTICAL MOTOR CONTROL DISORDERS

Lesions of the basal ganglia cause "negative" and "positive" motor symptoms. Functional deficits include loss of motor spontaneity and initiative *(akinesia),* impaired postural reflexes, lack of motor planning, and hypokinesia or bradykinesia. *Procedural learning,* the acquisition of a motor or perceptual skill through repeated exposure, is impaired by lesions of the caudate (mirror reading, serial reaction time task) or putamen (pursuit rotor task).[136] Positive symptoms, resulting mainly from disinhibition of cortical or subcortical motor areas, include rigidity, tremor, dystonia, dyskinesia, chorea, athetosis, and ballismus.

Basal ganglia lesions also cause negative and positive cognitive and behavioral symptoms. In monkeys, striatal lesions impair selective attention, behavioral control, rule acquisition,

and working memory.[136] In humans, negative symptoms include mental inertia and lack of spontaneity, psychomotor slowing, attentional and memory retrieval deficits, impaired development and maintenance of behavioral sets, reduced affective range, and inability to formulate plans and strategies.[135,136,150] Following bilateral GP or caudate infarcts, profound behavioral inertia, or "idling" (psychic akinesia, loss of psychic self-activation), may develop. Patients will spend large blocks of time doing and thinking about nothing. When incited to action by others, they can actively participate in sports or challenging puzzles. One patient lay in bed for 30 minutes with an unlit cigarette in his mouth, waiting for a light.[151] A patient with postencephalitic parkinsonism was found "frozen," lying next to a bathtub overflowing with water. When touched, she snapped from her lapse and asked the doctor what had happened. When asked "What do you think happened?" she replied "I turned the water on for a bath, and a moment later you just touched me" (Oliver Sacks, personal communication). Depression often follows basal ganglia lesions (Parkinson's disease, Huntington's disease), with symptoms such as behavioral withdrawal, apathy, emotional disinterest, anhedonia, hopelessness, and sadness.

Positive behavioral symptoms include obsessive–compulsive phenomena, irritability, aggressiveness, sexual promiscuity, delusions, and hallucinations in somatosensory, auditory, and visual modalities.[135,152,153] The basal ganglia help to initiate and activate behavior but also suppress automatic stereotypical behaviors. Bilateral caudate or GP lesions are often associated with repetitive and compulsive behaviors.[136,151,152,154] Stereotypical and obsessive–compulsive behaviors associated with basal ganglia lesions include ritual checking, counting, repeating sentences, shouting, coprolalia, finger movements, and repetition of an active motor program.[136,152] The "sign of applause" is tested by asking patients to clap their hands three times quickly. The sign is positive when they cannot stop clapping. They begin applauding in a prolonged and rapid series of claps, a marker of basal ganglia lesions.[136] Patients with obsessive–compulsive symptoms produced by basal ganglia lesions often do not exhibit features of the idiopathic disorder (i.e., ritualistic behavior, incorporation of preventive maneuvers into obsessive thoughts or compulsive actions to form more complex phenomena, and anxiety when suppressing their behavior).

Basal Ganglia Vascular Lesions

Discrete basal ganglia lesions produce deficits similar to those caused by lesions in cortical areas projecting to the basal ganglia area.[152,155–157] The behavioral effects of caudate and prefrontal lesions are similar,[152] with particular difficulty initiating and maintaining a behavioral set. Bilateral caudate or pallidal lesions causing prominent behavioral changes but minimal motor symptoms are associated with prefrontal hypometabolism and hypoperfusion.[152,158] Lesions of the dorsal caudate, which receives input from the dorsolateral prefrontal cortex, cause confusion and impair interest.[153] Lesions of the ventral caudate, which receives input from orbitofrontal and limbic areas,

cause socially inappropriate and disinhibited behavior, often with euphoria. Both dorsal and ventral caudate lesions impair attention, memory, set shifting (as in the Wisconsin Card Sorting Test), and complex problem solving.[153] Bilateral ventral–rostral GP lesions associated with carbon monoxide intoxication cause apathy, indifference, and placidity, with loss of internal drive and motivation but without motor or cognitive deficits.[158] Blood flow may be reduced in the frontal lobes, with maximal involvement in the medial (ACC, SMA) region.

The most severe and enduring behavioral manifestations follow bilateral striatal lesions.[159] Bilateral caudate lesions profoundly change personality, motivation, affect, and cognition. Patients may exhibit verbal and physical aggression, easy frustration, impulsivity, emotional flattening or lability, hypersexuality, vulgarity and socially inappropriate behavior (e.g., shoplifting, exposing oneself), poor hygiene, and impairment of memory, attention, and executive functions.[160] Unilateral caudate lesions may cause abulia, agitation, and hyperactivity. Right-sided caudate lesions may cause left-sided sensory or motor neglect, and left-sided caudate lesions may produce language disorders.[161–164] Hypokinesia of the left limb after right-sided caudate lesions is increased with bilateral simultaneous movements, resulting in motor extinction.[161] Aphasia after left-sided caudate lesions, with the typical hypophonia and festinating features of subcortical aphasias, may result from adjacent white matter lesions.[143]

Emotional Incontinence and Pseudobulbar Palsy

Emotional incontinence is characterized by inappropriate or excessive (pathological) crying or laughing. In many cases, the two expressions paradoxically appear simultaneously or follow one another. These emotional expressions are rarely accompanied by the experience of a congruent emotion and are often triggered by a trivial stimulus, such as the doctor entering the room. These emotional paroxysms appear to result from disinhibition of brain stem reflexes.

Emotional incontinence is an element of pseudobulbar palsy, together with other features such as dysarthria and dysphasia. Pseudobulbar palsy results from bilateral upper motor neuron lesions, usually in subcortical white matter pathways supplying the cranial nerve nuclei.[165] Pseudobulbar palsy involves a dramatic dissociation between impaired voluntary movement of muscles innervated by motor cranial nerves of the lower pons and medulla (e.g., swallowing, moving the tongue or smiling, opening the mouth to command) and preserved or accentuated movement of the same muscles in spontaneous (e.g., yawning or coughing) or evoked (e.g., gag and jaw jerk) reflexes. Some patients with emotional incontinence have a misdiagnosis of depression because of excessive crying or of frontal disinhibition because of inappropriate laughter.

Pseudobulbar palsy most often occurs with bilateral lacunar strokes, amyotrophic lateral sclerosis, progressive supranuclear palsy, multiple sclerosis, cerebral palsy, and traumatic brain injury.[166] In a developmental syndrome with bilateral perisylvian cortical malformations, the pseudobulbar state is often accompanied by seizures, developmental delay, and weakness.[167] Paroxysmal crying and laughing, unrelated to pseudobulbar palsy, may occur in partial epilepsy of temporal, frontal, or hypothalamic origin. Many patients with emotional incontinence respond well to selective serotonin reuptake inhibitors (SSRIs) or tricyclic antidepressants (e.g., fluoxetine, sertraline, paroxetine, imipramine, or nortriptyline),[168,169] and others improve with levodopa, methylphenidate, and amantadine.[170,171]

Degenerative and Other Basal Ganglia Disorders

Degenerative, metabolic, genetic, and toxic basal ganglia disorders cause motor, behavioral, and cognitive problems (Table 7–2).[172] Defining the contribution of specific anatomical structures within and outside the basal ganglia to neurobehavioral symptoms is often difficult as these disorders can involve brain stem nuclei with widespread cortical and subcortical projections, as well as the hypothalamus, thalamus, and cortex. Neuroimaging helps to define the structural and functional anatomy of neurodegenerative disorders (Table 7–3). In treating movement disorders, the selection of target symptoms is key. Cognitive, emotional, and behavioral symptoms, rather than motor disorders, are frequently the focus of treatment. Neuropsychiatric symptoms are important determinants of mortality and disease progression, as well as quality of life and disease course, caregiver distress, and nursing home admission. For example, SSRIs improve the mood, obsessive–compulsive symptoms, and anxiety associated with several different movement disorders. The atypical antipsychotic agents often effectively treat hallucinations and psychotic symptoms without worsening the movement disorders.[173,174]

PARKINSON'S DISEASE

Parkinson's disease is often accompanied by depression and cognitive impairment. In his 1817 essay on "the shaking palsy," James Parkinson[175] incorrectly stated that intellectual functions are unaltered until delirium intervenes shortly before death. Parkinson's disease is an idiopathic disorder characterized by parkinsonism, a common neurological syndrome of progressive slowness of movement, rigidity, prominent tremor at rest, and abnormal posture and gait. Several other disorders cause symptoms that overlap with those of Parkinson's disease (Table 7–4). Pathologically, Parkinson's disease is characterized by degeneration of the dopaminergic substantia nigra and ventral tegmental region and other pigmented brain stem nuclei (noradrenergic locus ceruleus, serotonergic dorsal raphe). Other causes of parkinsonism, such as antipsychotic drugs, encephalitis, and carbon monoxide poisoning, either destroy the dopaminergic nigral cells or basal ganglia nuclei upon which they terminate or block the postsynaptic dopamine receptors. Dopaminergic drugs, such as levodopa and bromocriptine, improve the bradykinesia, rigidity, and gait but are less effective for tremor. Indeed, responsiveness to levodopa is required for the diagnosis of Parkinson's disease. The movement disorder largely results from decreased dopaminergic activity.

Bradykinesia is often the most troubling symptom of Parkinson's disease. Patients lack spontaneity and have difficulty initiating and executing movements. Rigidity predominates in flexor muscles of the limbs and trunk. As in other extrapyramidal disorders, increased tone is equal throughout passive limb excursion, a condition called *lead-pipe rigidity,* and is not accompanied by increased tendon reflexes.

Cogwheel rigidity is the ratchet-like interruptions in passive movements from tremor superimposed on rigidity. The coarse parkinsonian tremor is most prominent during rest and diminishes with voluntary movements. The trunk flexes over the waist, and walking is difficult to initiate, with small steps and decreased arm swing. Postural instability causes some patients to accelerate their shuffling gait, called *festination,* with difficulty stopping. Expressionless facial features, diminished voice volume, dysarthria, small handwriting *(micrographia),* sleep disorder, oily seborrheic skin, excessive salivation, and constipation are other features.

The most common neuropsychiatric symptoms in Parkinson's disease are depression, cognitive impairment, apathy, anxiety, and psychosis. The affective and cognitive disorders of Parkinson's disease must be distinguished from psychological adjustment, impaired motor performance, somatic complaints, and medication effects.[176] Antiparkinsonian therapy either alleviates or exacerbates these symptoms, and psychotropic medications may affect movement. Reactive components of neuropsychiatric symptoms may improve with maximization of antiparkinsonian therapy. Further, fluctuations in dopamine may be directly tied to the neuropsychiatric symptoms of Parkinson's disease. Mood and motoric fluctuations may occur together with the "on–off" phenomenon, but motor disability is usually more severe than the behavioral changes.[177,178] Occasionally, dysphoria, anxiety, and panic attacks are the most prominent features of the "off" state.[179–183]

A common treatment dilemma is balancing the negative and positive effects of dopaminergic therapy. The medical history and selection of target symptoms help to identify a patient's most disabling symptoms. Hallucinations with retained insight are rarely an indication for treatment.

Psychosis is common in advanced Parkinson's disease and most often associated with dopaminergic therapy. Because dopamine agonists are more likely to induce psychosis than levodopa,[184] consider withdrawing or reducing the dose of these agents in the psychotic patient. Sleep disturbance is linked to psychosis; improving sleep hygiene and low doses of a sedative, such as a tricyclic antidepressant or a benzodiazepine, at bedtime is helpful.[185] Antipsychotic agents, often in low doses, are effective for treating psychosis in Parkinson's disease. The antipsychotics quetiapine and clozapine (see Chapter 11) are least likely to worsen parkinsonian symptoms; quetiapine is usually the first-line choice as clozapine can cause agranulocytosis and requires frequent blood tests.[186,187] Low-dose clozapine therapy effectively treats psychosis and prevents recurrent psychotic episodes;[188] it also improves depression, anxiety, hypersexuality, sleep disturbance, and akathisia.[189] Olanzapine, risperidone, and quetiapine also help to treat psychosis without the risk of agranulocytosis associated with clozapine,[173] although, as mentioned later, olanzapine and risperidone may worsen motor disability.

Depression affects approximately 40% (range 12%–90%) of patients with Parkinson's disease.[176,190–192] Prominent anxiety may accompany the depression or occur independently.[193,194] Bradykinesia and *bradyphrenia* (mental slowing) simulate depression by slowed thought and action and facial expression betraying little emotion. It is important to search specifically for the cognitive and vegetative features of depression. In Parkinson's disease, depression is accompanied by decreased drive and motivation, excessive health concerns and somatic complaints, pessimism, and hopelessness. Suicidal thoughts are common, but suicide is rare.

In patients with Parkinson's disease, depression results from psychosocial adjustment and neurological changes.[195] Patients may have depression scores that are similar to or higher than those of patients with a chronic disabling physical illness.[196,197] The relation between the severity of the depression and the severity of the motor disorder varies.[159,195] Further, unlike the locomotor disability, the mood state and cognitive abilities of patients without dementia are largely unrelated to striatal dopaminergic depletion and may result from dysfunction of extrastriatal dopaminergic systems or other mechanisms.[198] A contribution of serotonergic deficiency to affective changes in Parkinson's disease is supported by decreased levels of the serotonin metabolite 5-hydroxytryptamine in the cerebrospinal fluid of depressed Parkinson's disease patients.[199,200] Depression is treated with tricyclic antidepressants or SSRIs, but controlled studies of their efficacy in Parkinson's disease are lacking.[201]

Table 7–2. **Basal Ganglia Disorders**

Disorder	Etiology	Age at Onset	Cognitive Dysfunction	Behavioral Dysfunction	Motor Dysfunction
Vascular					
Unilateral caudate	Ischemic infarction, hemorrhage	>40 yr	Attention, memory, set shifting, complex problem solving, language abnormalities (dominant), neglect (nondominant)	Abulia, hyperactivity, agitation, psychosis, depression, anxiety	Contralateral hypokinesia; speech initiation, hypophonia, nasality (dominant side); dysarthria
Dorsal	As above	>40 yr	Attention, memory, set shifting, complex problem solving apathy, disinterest, confusion	Abulia, apathy	As above
Ventral	As above	>40 yr	Attention, memory, set shifting, complex problem solving	Disinhibition, euphoria, inappropriateness, impulsivity	Mild akinesia
Bilateral caudate	As above	>40 yr	Psychic akinesia (marked abulia)	Impulsivity, lability, hypersexuality, flat affect, vulgarity, aggression, frustration	Akinesia
Globus pallidus	Ischemic infarction, hemorrhage, carbon monoxide intoxication	>40 yr	Thought content and initiative, memory, set shifting, organization	Behavioral inertia and withdrawal, apathy, depression, anhedonia, indifference, placidity, obsessions and compulsions	Akinesia
Putamen	Hemorrhage, ischemic infarction	>40 yr	Executive function (minor), verbal paraphasia (dominant), neglect (nondominant), short-term memory	None, minor	Hypophonia, hemidystonia, hemichorea
Basal Ganglia Calcification					
Fahr's syndrome, high serum calcium, lead poisoning, AIDS, radiation, idiopathic		Third to seventh decade	Executive function, fluency, learning, visuospatial, subcortical dementia	Psychosis, euphoria, depression, obsessions, compulsions	Parkinsonism, chorea, athetosis

Disorder	Etiology	Age of onset	Cognitive features	Psychiatric features	Motor/neurological features
Huntington's Disease	Autosomal dominant with trinucleotide CAG repeat on chromosome 4p16.3	First to eighth decade	Executive function, memory, dementia, motor sequencing, visuospatial, fluency	Depression, apathy, euphoria, psychosis, irritability, impulsivity, aggression, lability	Chorea, athetosis, dysarthria, dyskinesia, abnormal saccades, ataxia
Parkinson's Disease	Idiopathic, dopaminergic, substantia nigra degeneration	Fifth to seventh decade	Executive function, visuospatial, fluency, construction, memory, bradyphrenia, subcortical dementia	Depression, anxiety, suicidal ideation, euphoria, psychosis (usually side effect of therapy)	Rigidity, shuffling gait, resting tremor, postural instability, bradykinesia, masked face, micrographia
Sydenham's Chorea	Probable autoimmune reaction following group A streptococcal pharyngitis	Any, usually childhood	Attention deficit	Psychosis, depression, euphoria, compulsions, irritability, delirium, aggression	Chorea of face, tongue, and extremities; "milk-maid's" sign, ataxia, tics, seizures
Wilson's Disease	Autosomal recessive defect in hepatic copper excretion; chromosome 13	Second to third decade	Thought content and initiative, subcortical dementia	Anxiety, personality change, irritability, incongruity, depression, psychosis	Resting tremor, dystonia, bradykinesia, chorea, dysarthria, rigidity, catatonia, dysphagia
Progressive Supranuclear Palsy	Idiopathic degenerative disorder	Fifth to eighth decade	Subcortical dementia, prefrontal-like syndrome, dyslexia, dysgraphia	Emotional lability, apathy, personality change, confusion, depression, psychosis	Vertical gaze palsy, axial dystonia, dysarthria, parkinsonism
Tourette's Syndrome	Idiopathic and genetic, possible autoimmune reaction to group A streptococcal infection	<20 yr	Executive function, attention, planning, conceptualization, learning	Depression, attention deficit, hyperactivity, obsessions, compulsions	Motor and vocal tics, simple or complex
Diffuse Lewy Body Disease	Idiopathic degenerative disorder	Sixth to eighth decade	Rapid dementia, visuospatial, memory, confusion	Psychosis, depression, agitation, visual hallucinations	Extrapyramidal signs, rigidity, ataxia, postural instability, tremor (infrequently)

In nonprogressive basal ganglia disorders, deficits are often transient or improve markedly. AIDS, acquired immunodeficiency syndrome.

Table 7–3. Results of Structural and Functional Imaging in Neurodegenerative Disorders

Disorder	Structural Imaging	Functional Imaging*
Parkinson's disease	Nonspecific cerebral atrophy, narrowing between red nucleus and substantia nigra pars reticularis on T_2 images, shrunken substantia nigra pars compacta	Basal ganglia, reduced blood flow/metabolism in posterior putamen and caudate, usually asymmetrical; normal number of D_2 receptors in caudate on raclopride PET
Multiple system atrophy[†]	Hypointensity in striatum (more in putamen than caudate), focal atrophy of cerebellum and brachium pontis in OPCA	Reduced blood flow/metabolism in striatum, more symmetrical, less putamen-to-caudate gradient than in Parkinson's; decrease (equal) in fluorodopa uptake in anterior and posterior putamen
Progressive supranuclear palsy	Decreased T_2 signal in putamen, midbrain atrophy	Reduced blood flow/metabolism in medial frontal cortex, thalamus, and midbrain
Cortical–basal ganglionic degeneration	Posterior frontal and parietal atrophy, usually asymmetrical	Reduced blood flow/metabolism in striatum, thalamus, posterior frontal, inferior parietal, and lateral temporal cortex, usually asymmetrical
Huntington's disease	Atrophy of caudate and putamen more than pallidum, diffuse cerebral and cerebellar atrophy, lateral ventriculomegaly ("boxcar ventricle"), increased T_2 signal in caudate	Blood flow/metabolism markedly decreased in caudate nuclei, possibly asymmetrical
Alzheimer's disease	Progressive cerebral atrophy on serial scans, greatest in medial temporal region; selective hippocampal atrophy on MRI morphometry; basal ganglia preserved	Reduced blood flow/metabolism in bilateral posterior temporoparietal regions with relative sparing of basal ganglia, somatosensory cortex, and cerebellum
Pick's disease	Frontal and/or temporal atrophy, sparing posterior two-thirds of superior temporal gyrus; "knife edge" cortical gyri	Reduced blood flow/metabolism in frontal and temporal areas
Binswanger's disease[‡]	Cortical and subcortical infarcts of various ages, white matter disease, nonspecific cerebral atrophy	Reduced blood flow/metabolism corresponding with areas of multiple infarcts
Normal-pressure hydrocephalus	Ventricular enlargement disproportionate to sulcal prominence	Nonspecific, diffuse reduction in blood flow/metabolism

*Hypoperfusion on single photon emission tomography or hypometabolism on positron emission tomography (PET).
[†]Comprises parkinsonism, striatonigral degeneration, sporadic olivopontocerebellar atrophy (OPCA), and Shy-Drager syndrome.
[‡]Multi-infarct dementia.
D_2, dopamine receptor; MRI, magnetic resonance imaging.

Table 7–4. Clinical Features of Syndromes with Parkinsonian Symptoms

Syndrome	Age at Onset (yr)	Disease Duration (yr)	Levodopa Response	Rigidity	Tremor	Bradykinesia	Dystonia	Autonomic Symptoms	Cerebellar Symptoms	Supranuclear Palsy and Gaze Disorders	Vocal Cord Paralysis	Dementia	Cortical Signs	Postural Instability	Gait
Parkinson's disease	60–70	10–20	Very good	++, appendicular	++	+	Late°	Late, mild	Uncommon	None	Late	Late, mild subcortical	Rare	Late	Festinating
Striatonigral degeneration	45–55	7–10	Poor	+	+	++	Early, neck	Mild	Absent	None	Present, with stridor	Mild, subcortical	Rare	Late	Festinating
Shy-Drager syndrome	45–55	5–10	Poor	++	+	−	Uncommon	Early, severe	Absent	None	Present, with stridor	Mild	Rare	Early	Festinating
Sporadic olivoponto-cerebellar atrophy	50–55	5–15	Poor severe	±	+	±	Facial	Mild	Severe	Oculomotor disturbances	Uncommon	Severe in familial type	Rare	Early, severe	Wide-based
Progressive supranuclear palsy	65–70	5–10	Poor	+, axial	−	+	Facial	Moderate	Mild	Early downgaze palsy, eyelid apraxia, square-wave jerks	Uncommon	Severe	Rare	Early falls	Broad-based
Cortical-basal ganglionic degeneration	50–60	4–7	Poor	+	−	+	Limb, often painful	Mild	Mild	Supranuclear palsy, late; eyelid apraxia, occasionally	Uncommon	Late	Alien limb, neglect, apraxia, aphasia, cortical focal myoclonus, corticospinal involvement	Early loss of postural reflexes	Spastic

+, present; ++, strongly present; ±, occasionally present; −, absent.
°Dystonia develops in response to levodopa therapy.

The serotonin syndrome resulting from a combination of selegiline, a selective monoamine oxidase-B inhibitor, and an SSRI or tricyclic antidepressant makes their coadministration potentially dangerous.[202] The serotonin syndrome is characterized by the triad of altered mental status (e.g., delirium), autonomic dysfunction (e.g., tachycardia), and neuromuscular abnormalities (e.g., bizarre movements or myoclonus). Levodopa may improve the depression and anxiety of some Parkinson's disease patients but not those with multiple system atrophy.[183,203] Electroconvulsive therapy (ECT) may be used in depressed patients who are refractory to medication, but post-therapy confusion or delusions and delayed cognitive impairment are potential side effects.[204]

Psychiatric complications from medications used to treat Parkinson's disease are common, especially among the elderly. Levodopa and dopaminergic receptor agonists such as bromocriptine may cause hallucinations, paranoia, mania, insomnia, anxiety, nightmares, hypersexuality, and depression.[205,206] Obsessive behaviors involving the collection, categorization, and handling of objects may occur with levodopa therapy.[207] Mania rarely complicates Parkinson's disease, except as an adverse reaction to dopaminergic drugs. Traditional and some atypical antipsychotic drugs (e.g., risperidone, with high D_2 receptor binding, and olanzapine)[208] may exacerbate the motor symptoms of Parkinson's disease. Anticholinergic drugs, including transdermal preparations, cause delirium, confusion, lethargy, hallucinations, and other behavioral reactions. Simplify treatment regimens to avoid toxic confusional states that exacerbate cognitive impairment.

Cognitive impairments are common in Parkinson's disease, ranging from mild problems with executive function (e.g., planning, organization), visuospatial skills, or memory skills to dementia in approximately 25% of patients.[209] No therapy effectively prevents the cognitive deficits in Parkinson's disease. However, acetylcholinesterase inhibitors may improve the cognitive and psychiatric symptoms. For instance, in a small open-label study, rivastigmine had beneficial effects.[210] Motor deficits correlate poorly with cognitive deficits,[211,212] and time-limited or motor-dependent tests of cognition are biased against patients with movement disorders. Although neuropsychological tests show cognitive and emotional processing deficits in most Parkinson's disease patients, the deficits are often mild and do not interfere with daily living.[213]

Visuospatial functions, facial recognition, and incidental learning of verbal material are impaired early in Parkinson's disease.[214–216] Cognitive problems mimic those associated with prefrontal lesions, including perseverative errors, impaired set shifting and verbal fluency, bradyphrenia, and impaired planning and execution of constructional tasks.[214,217–219] Language functions are relatively preserved in patients with Parkinson's disease and dementia. Emotional processing deficits in patients with Parkinson's disease include impaired ability to produce emotional prosody, to discriminate affectively colored speech, and to detect humor in sketches.[220]

Dementia with memory impairment is more common in older Parkinson's disease patients and those with depression or other neurological problems.[209] Cognitive problems and dementia are delayed, and progress more slowly, in younger patients.[221] The origin of dementia in Parkinson's disease is primarily subcortical, but cortical impairment also contributes. Cognitive impairment is correlated with the density of Lewy neurites in the hippocampus.[222] Parkinson's disease with dementia is now considered part of the spectrum of Lewy body syndromes.[223] Anticholinergic drugs, such as scopolamine, may cause impaired memory storage or exacerbate memory impairment in patients with Parkinson's disease. Although cognitive symptoms, especially bradyphrenia, may improve with dopaminergic therapy, the benefits are usually mild and transient.

PROGRESSIVE SUPRANUCLEAR PALSY

Progressive supranuclear palsy (PSP) is a degenerative disorder causing supranuclear ophthalmoplegia affecting mainly vertical gaze, dystonic rigidity of the neck and upper trunk, and pseudobulbar palsy with prominent dysarthria. It usually begins at age 45–75 (mean 63) years, presenting as a gait change or falls (60%) or a behavioral change (20%).[224] It affects approximately 5% of patients with parkinsonism at tertiary care centers; there is a 2:1 male predominance. Death ensues 5–10 years after the initial symptoms.

Early diagnosis of PSP eludes most clinicians

since the initial complaints, including fatigue, headaches, pains, depression, memory loss, unsteadiness, slowed movement, or visual changes, are nonspecific. Parkinson's disease is often misdiagnosed until the poor response to dopaminergic agonists, lack of resting tremor, and presence of vertical gaze palsy and neck dystonia are recognized. The diagnosis is often quite delayed when gaze palsy develops late or dementia dominates the early course. Early oculomotor findings include slow, hypometric, and defective vertical saccades; gaze impersistence; and hesitancy initiating eye movements to command. Other features that help to distinguish PSP from other parkinsonian syndromes are normal autonomic function, symmetrical motor symptoms, prominent gait impairment with tendency to fall, and the "astonished" facial expression.[225] Magnetic resonance imaging (MRI) reveals selective midbrain atrophy.[226]

Vertical gaze impairment is the cardinal feature of PSP, usually affecting downgaze more than upgaze, making it difficult for patients to navigate stairs. The spared vestibulo-ocular and caloric reflexes led to the supranuclear designation. Other oculomotor disorders include diplopia, impaired pursuit and willed eye movements, impaired convergence, unilateral or bilateral internuclear ophthalmoplegia, and blepharospasm.[227] Other motor features of PSP mimic parkinsonism, with bradykinesia, masked facies, postural instability and falls, mild resting tremor, and mental slowing. In addition to the gaze palsy, cerebellar and pyramidal signs distinguish PSP from Parkinson's disease.

Behavioral changes in PSP include personality changes, emotional incontinence from pseudobulbar palsy, confusional episodes, apathy, depression, and disinhibition.[228] Personality changes include introversion, withdrawal from social activities, and diminished motivation. Patients with Parkinson's disease are more likely to develop hallucinations, delusions, and major depression than PSP patients.[228]

The cognitive changes in PSP led to the concept of "subcortical dementia."[229] The cognitive changes include slowing of mental processes, impairment of sustained and divided attention, forgetfulness and impaired working memory, increased sensitivity to interference, poor manipulation of acquired knowledge, limited access to long-term memory for strategic planning, and decline in premorbid intelli-

gence quotients, both verbal and performance.[230–232] Many of these deficits mimic the executive impairments associated with prefrontal lesions. Evidence from studies of prefrontal hypometabolism in PSP supports the tenet that loss of subcortical inputs to prefrontal cortex contributes to prefrontal dysfunction. Memory deficits are mild. Patients with PSP and other subcortical dementias "forget to remember;" although they cannot retrieve on free recall, they can recognize learned materials.[229,233] Language is largely preserved in PSP patients, although speech is slow and dysarthric and handwriting is labored and clumsy. Some patients experience visual dyslexia, constructional dysgraphia, and naming errors, possibly resulting from visual misperception.[234] Ideomotor apraxia occurs but is milder than in cortical–basal ganglionic degeneration.[235]

Dementia develops in 30%–60% of PSP patients. Relative preservation of speech, memory, and praxis helps to distinguish subcortical from cortical dementia syndromes. Except for severely impaired verbal fluency, linguistic aspects of speech, comprehension, repetition, confrontation naming, reading, and writing are partly or completely spared.

The lesions are localized to the upper brain stem, thalamus, GP, and cerebellar dentate gyrus; the cerebral cortex is relatively spared. Maximal cell loss occurs in the midbrain reticular formation, where neurofibrillary tangles also predominate.[236] Prominent filamentous τ inclusions and brain degeneration without β-amyloid deposits are found in PSP, as well as cortical–basal ganglionic degeneration, Pick's disease, and hereditary frontotemporal dementia and parkinsonism linked to chromosome 17.[237]

Treatment of PSP is disappointing, with only mild and transient responses to dopaminergic agents. Measures to minimize aspiration and falling are often very helpful. Treatment of depression or anxiety with SSRIs or buspirone may be helpful. Agitation and confusion is managed with the short-term use of a short-acting benzodiazepine (e.g., lorazepam) or an antipsychotic medication (e.g., olanzapine, quetiapine). Motor symptoms and depression may respond to ECT, but post-treatment confusion limits its value.[238] Donepezil provides minimal, but clinically insignificant, cognitive benefits but impairs daily activities and mobility.[239,240]

MULTIPLE SYSTEM ATROPHY

Multiple system atrophy is a degenerative disorder with combinations of extrapyramidal, cerebellar, autonomic, and pyramidal dysfunction. Falling under the umbrella of this disorder are striatonigral degeneration, sporadic olivopontocerebllar atrophy (OPCA), and Shy-Drager syndrome (Table 7–5).[241,242] All of these disorders share the feature of intracytoplasmic glial inclusion bodies. Extrapyramidal symptoms include bradykinesia, rigidity, postural instability, and hypokinetic speech. Prominent tremor is infrequent. Levodopa responsiveness is absent or mild and unsustained. Cerebellar dysfunction causes ataxia of gait, limb movements, speech, and eye movements. Autonomic disorders include orthostatic hypotension, urinary incontinence or retention, constipation, and impaired sweating.

In most patients with this disorder, overall scores on intelligence tests are in the average or mildly impaired range,[243–245] although dementia may complicate the late course (especially in familial OPCA, which is not considered part of the disorder's spectrum). During the initial stages of multiple system atrophy, deficits in executive functions are common and include impaired set shifting, sequencing, sustained attention, and motor organization and planning.[243,246] Verbal fluency and praxis may also be affected. Depression and emotional lability frequently occur. A rapid eye movement sleep disorder may complicate multiple system atrophy and Parkinson's disease.[247] Apneas and hypopneas are common in the sleep of patients with multiple system atrophy.[248]

Pathological changes involve neuronal loss and gliosis in the substantia nigra, locus ceruleus, pons, inferior olivary nucleus, cerebellar cortex, lateral GP, and autonomic brain stem nuclei. Dementia may be associated with degeneration in the cholinergic basal nucleus in some patients with OPCA.[249] Many cognitive and behavioral changes result from damage to the cerebellum and its connections, as well as cells that provide ascending catecholaminergic input to the basal ganglia and cortex. In addition, progressive cerebral atrophy likely contributes to the behavioral changes in multiple system atrophy.[250]

CORTICAL–BASAL GANGLIONIC DEGENERATION

First described by Rebei and colleagues in 1968,[251] cortical–basal ganglionic degeneration begins at age 55–75 years, and death occurs within a decade. Initial symptoms include a combination of rigidity, clumsiness, akinesia, and ideomotor apraxia. The symptoms and signs are often strikingly asymmetrical.[252] Symptoms often developing after 1–2 years but also possibly occurring initially include dystonia, myoclonus, cortical sensory impairment, corticospinal tract dysfunction, dysarthria, depression, alien hand phenomenon, and impaired sustained attention and verbal fluency. Executive dysfunction, aphasia, memory impairment, and dementia may complicate later stages but rarely dominate the presentation.[233,253,254]

The diagnosis of cortical–basal ganglionic degeneration may be difficult. Rigidity and akinesia suggest Parkinson's disease. Rigidity, akinesia, and impaired initiation of voluntary saccades suggest PSP. Early predominance of cognitive and behavioral symptoms suggests Alzheimer's disease or frontotemporal dementia. In contrast with all these disorders, cortical–basal ganglionic degeneration is often accompanied, early on, by the alien hand phenomenon and prominent ideomotor apraxia. Unlike patients with mild Alzheimer's disease, patients with this disorder have better memory

Table 7–5. Syndromes of Multiple System Atrophy

Syndrome	Parkinsonian Symptoms	Cerebellar Symptoms	Autonomic Insufficiency	Corticospinal Symptoms
Striatonigral degeneration	+°	−	−	−
Olivopontocerebellar atrophy	+	+	−	±
Shy-Drager syndrome	+	−°°	+	−

+, usually present; ±, occasionally present; −, absent; °without tremor; °°ataxia may occur.

but more prominent deficits in praxis, finger tapping, motor programming, and mood.[255] The absence of characteristic tremor and true supranuclear palsy helps to distinguish cortical–basal ganglionic degeneration from Parkinson's disease and PSP. Action-induced and stimulus-sensitive focal reflex myoclonus may be confused with tremor.[256] Functional neuroimaging helps to distinguish cortical–basal ganglionic degeneration from PSP, Parkinson's disease, and Alzheimer's disease (Table 7–3).

The praxis deficit in cortical–basal ganglionic degeneration involves executing learned skilled movements with relatively preserved comprehension and identification of pantomimed actions.[257] This pattern suggests predominant dysfunction in the SMA rather than parietal lobe praxis areas. However, impaired ability to correct praxis errors is associated with hypometabolism in superior parietal and frontal areas.[258] Apraxia is misdiagnosed when clumsiness from rigidity, bradykinesia, and dystonia impair performance of skilled movements.[259] Apraxia in cortical–basal ganglionic degeneration is often asymmetrical.

The alien limb phenomenon (see Chapter 3) develops in half of cortical–basal ganglionic degeneration patients.[260] The alien limb phenomenon often manifests as compulsive, nonvolitional approach behavior with manipulation or groping. These symptoms are most often seen with prefrontal strokes (affecting the orbitofrontal area, anterior cingulate, SMA, or corpus callosum) but may occur with Alzheimer's disease and Creutzfeldt-Jakob disease. In contrast with the alien limb phenomenon, levitation and related limb movements are simpler and nonpurposeful (e.g., elevation of an arm from a resting position) with contralateral parietal lesions and PSP.[260–262]

Cognitive impairments affect executive function, sustained attention, psychomotor speed, planning, integration (e.g., initiation, bimanual coordination, temporal organization), memory (free recall with relatively preserved cued recall and recognition memory), and language (anomia, paraphasia, verbal fluency).[233,253–255] Perseveration is common. As the disorder progresses, a more global dementia, depression, and personality changes (e.g., decreased motivation, irritability, aggressiveness) may develop.

Treatment of cortical–basal ganglionic degeneration is palliative and symptom-based, with progressive degeneration being the rule. Dopaminergic agents offer limited improvement of rigidity and bradykinesia in a third of patients[263] but may evoke motor and behavioral symptoms, necessitating assessment of benefit. Myoclonus may respond to clonazepam, levetiracetam and zonisamide, but not valproate.[260] Botulinum toxin injection inconsistently improves dystonia.

Pathological changes are maximal in superficial layers of frontoparietal cortex, substantia nigra, locus ceruleus, lentiform nucleus, thalamus, and other subcortical areas. Cell loss, gliosis, and swollen and poorly staining neurons (i.e., "ballooned neurons" or Pick cells) are found in the cortex and substantia nigra. Initially considered pathognomic of Pick's disease, ballooned neurons are found in cortical–basal ganglionic degeneration and, occasionally, PSP, Alzheimer's disease, and Creutzfeldt-Jakob disease. Biochemical analysis shows severe, diffuse striatal dopamine deficiency.[252]

HUNTINGTON'S DISEASE

Changes in personality and affect are often the first signs of Huntington's disease. The principal feature of the disease was described by Huntington[264] in 1872 as "insanity with a tendency to suicide." The emotional and intellectual deterioration in Huntington's disease, an autosomal dominant disorder, is often more disabling and feared than the motor symptoms, which are commonly choreiform movements, dyskinesia, dysarthria, and ataxia. Early in the course of Huntington's disease, chorea appears as "piano-playing" finger movements, usually while walking, or as slight facial grimaces or twitches. These movements grow more severe but plateau after a decade. In the Westphal variant, which usually begins in childhood, rigidity predominates.[265] Voluntary movement is impaired, affecting gait, speech, rapid alternating movements, and saccadic pursuits and tracking, and progressively worsens during the course of the illness.

Like other disorders affecting the caudate, Huntington's disease commonly causes personality changes, psychosis, impulsivity, and sexual disorders.[266] Patients are "hard to get along with," impulsive, erratic, and prone to rage or despondency. The premorbid personality may be exaggerated or reversed.[265] For instance, quiet individuals may become introverted and apathetic, and extroverts may become boisterous, irritable, and aggressive, or vice versa. Sleep and appetite changes often develop early. Impaired functioning at home and work is common, with diminished spontaneity, lack of insight and initiative, emotional lability, impulsiveness, irritability, and impaired judgment.[267] Sexual promiscuity, verbal and physical aggression, and antisocial behavior, including criminal acts, may be early features of Huntington's disease.[268,269] Behavioral disorders become more severe as the disease progresses. Situational apathy, marked by inactivity and impaired spontaneous emotional and motor expression, modifiable by environmental stimulation, often develops early and progressively worsens.[270] Irritability may respond to SSRIs.

Depression occurs in 40% of Huntington's disease patients and precedes the onset of chorea or dementia by an average of 5 years.[270,271] Apathy is a prominent feature of depression in Huntington's disease. Chorea often decreases with depression and increases with mania.[272,273] Nearly 10% of patients experience manic episodes.[271] Although psychological and social factors may contribute to the depression in Huntington's disease, affective disorders are primarily organic in origin as many patients who experience these symptoms are unaware of their genetic risk for the disease. The neurobiological origin of the symptoms is further evidenced by the manic episodes, which are rare in reactive depressions, and the vegetative symptoms, such as anorexia and sleep disorders.[273] Suicide is common. The confirmed or suspected diagnosis of Huntington's disease can devastate patients and their relatives, and genetic counseling is mandatory.

Depression in Huntington's disease responds to SSRIs and tricyclic antidepressants; the latter should be started at low doses in elderly or demented patients.[274] Antidepressants often improve the somatic signs of depression without affecting the patient's dysphoric outlook.[270,272,273] Mania responds to neuroleptics, lithium carbonate, and carbamazepine and other antiepileptic drugs; the latter are preferred because Huntington's disease patients are at increased risk of lithium toxicity.[270] Aggressiveness may respond to β-blockers, neuroleptics, or SSRIs.[275]

Psychosis occurs in nearly 10% of Hunting-

ton's disease patients and more frequently in younger ones; it can develop at any stage of the illness.[276] Paranoid delusions are a prominent feature, and auditory and visual hallucinations also occur. Neuroleptics, including the newer atypical antipsychotics, are used to treat the psychosis, aggression, and involuntary movements but may worsen apathy and executive disorders. Neuroleptics may also exacerbate rigidity in patients with the Westphal variant.

Neuropsychological deficits for attentional set shifting and semantic verbal fluency are present in preclinical Huntington's disease.[277] Cognitive deficits are usually mild in the early stages, although dementia complicates many moderate and advanced cases. The most frequent impairments are on measures of memory acquisition, cognitive flexibility and abstraction, planning and sequence generation, manual dexterity, attention and concentration, performance skill, and verbal fluency.[278,279] Memory disturbance is often the first cognitive deficit observed by family members. Cognitive function is correlated with reduced striatal D_1 and D_2 receptor binding, especially D_2 binding.[278]

SYDENHAM'S CHOREA

Sydenham's (rheumatic) chorea, a complication of rheumatic fever, is now uncommon. Chorea occurs with or without joint, skin, and cardiac symptoms. Although chorea is the most common and prominent symptom of central nervous system involvement, the initial stage of the disease may be complicated by delirium, irritability, hallucinations, seizures, depression, mania, paranoia, psychosis, catatonia, compulsive behavior, tics, or aggressiveness.[280] The antiepileptic valproate or antipsychotic drugs are used to treat acute symptoms. Long-term sequelae, affecting personality and emotion, are common and may result in obsessive-compulsive disorder (OCD), chorea gravidarum, and possibly of Tourette's syndrome.[280,281] Sydenham's chorea is probably the result of striatal and other extrapyramidal inflammatory changes and neuronal loss, possibly mediated by antineuronal antibodies.[282] Pediatric autoimmune neuropsychiatric disorders may, in certain children with streptococcal autoimmunity, cause OCD and Tourette's syndrome instead of Sydenham's chorea[283] (see Tourette's Syndrome, below).

WILSON'S DISEASE

Wilson's disease, hepatolenticular degeneration, is an autosomal recessive disorder of copper metabolism. The defective gene is located on chromosome 13.[284] Defective hepatic copper excretion leads to the pathogenic accumulation of copper in the liver, brain, and other organs.[285] The onset of neuropsychiatric, hepatic, ocular, renal, or joint disorders usually occurs between 10 and 30 years of age. The pathognomonic Kayser-Fleischer (gold-brown corneal) rings are present on slit-lamp examination when neuropsychiatric features are present. Asymptomatic elevation of liver enzymes, jaundice, hepatitis, or cirrhosis may be present.

Neurological disturbances may be the initial symptoms and include tremor (wing-beating tremor develops later), catatonia, chorea, dystonia, bradykinesia, dysarthria, and dysphagia.[286] Rigidity, expressionless face, and cognitive decline leading to dementia occur as the disease advances. Cognitive impairment is maximal for tasks requiring perceptual and mental speed, reasoning and manipulation of acquired knowledge, memory, and performance with interfering stimuli.[287-289] As with other subcortical disorders, aphasia, apraxia, and agnosia are typically absent in Wilson's disease. Generalized atrophy, putaminal lesions with bilateral symmetrical concentric laminar hyperintensity, and involvement of the SNpc, periaqueductal gray matter, pontine tegmentum, and thalamus are shown on MRI.[290]

Psychiatric features, common at presentation, include personality and mood changes, irritability, anxiety, social and behavioral problems at school or work, antisocial behavior (such as criminality and alcohol or drug abuse), and incongruous behavior (that is, dissociation between environmental cues and behavior).[291,292] Depression and psychosis are common, and suicide may occur. Chelation therapy may improve cognition and incongruous behavior.[292]

DIFFUSE LEWY BODY DISEASE

Lewy bodies are spherical inclusions found in the cytoplasm near the nucleus of neurons. They were first identified in the pigmented brain stem nuclei of patients with Parkinson's disease. Diffuse Lewy body disease is a syndrome of severe, rapidly evolving dementia associated with cortical Lewy bodies and senile plaques.[293] In addition to the cognitive problems, relatively specific clinical features of diffuse Lewy body disease include marked variability in symptom intensity (e.g., fluctuating attention), extrapyramidal signs and symptoms, and psychiatric symptoms, such as visual hallucinations.[294] The cholinergic deficit is profound, and anticholinesterase therapy (e.g., rivastigmine) improves the neuropsychiatric symptoms.[295] Distinguishing diffuse Lewy body disease from Alzheimer's disease is often difficult on clinical grounds alone, although the relatively early onset of hallucinations and rapidly progressive extrapyramidal symptoms and signs suggest diffuse Lewy body disease.[293]

TOURETTE'S SYNDROME

Tourette's syndrome of chronic motor and vocal tics is associated with neuropsychiatric features that include attention-deficit hyperactivity disorder (ADHD) and OCD. Tourette's syndrome often has a genetic basis, but the inheritance pattern is uncertain. Multiple tics usually begin before the age of 21 years. There is a 3:1 male predominance. Tourette's syndrome is usually a lifelong disorder, but the intensity of symptoms varies. The social stigma may be severe; vocal tics may limit social and employment opportunities. Reactive depression is often overlooked. Social and professional adaptation is better in adults than children, who often have disabling behavioral and educational problems.

Tics are classified as simple or complex. Simple motor tics include eye blinks, grimaces, and head or arm jerks. Complex motor tics merge imperceptibly with compulsions, ranging from grooming behaviors and sequential reaching or touching of objects and body parts to aggressive acts. Tics may fuse with functional acts to produce bizarre concatenations of voluntary and involuntary movements, such as lunging one's open hand forward to greet someone. Simple vocal tics include grunts, throat clearing, clicking, snorting, and animal sounds such as barking or quacking. Complex vocal tics consist of words and phrases that may be repeated; these include obscenities (*coprolalia*), which occur in a third of patients and often describe sexual or excretory functions. The repertoire of tics forms a fragmented and bizarre archive of life experiences, analogous to dreams, which may combine meaningless bits of a conversation from years before with a recent image to evoke a complex motor–vocal tic that becomes a stable tic pattern for months.[296]

Tic disorders form a continuous spectrum from isolated tics in neurologically intact persons under stress (mannerisms or habits) to Tourette's syndrome. Transient tic disorder, found in up to 15% of children and adolescents, is characterized by simple motor or vocal tics lasting less than a year. Eye blinks and sudden head movements are most common. The tics may briefly recur during adulthood, especially during periods of stress. In chronic motor tic disorder, tics last longer than a year and occur almost every day but do not include vocal tics.

Tics occur in other disorders, including Huntington's chorea, dystonia musculorum deformans, neuroacanthocytosis, and brain infections or postinfectious states, such as encephalitis or Sydenham's chorea. Tics can be caused by medications, including central nervous system stimulants, cocaine, levodopa, carbamazepine, and phenytoin. Tardive tics, developing after medication is discontinued, can complicate the use of dopamine-blocking agents. Tics may follow traumatic brain injury, stroke, carbon monoxide poisoning, static perinatal encephalopathy, and degenerative disorders.

Tourette's syndrome provides a rare, albeit distorted, view of relations between emotion, drive, motivation, unconscious thought, inhibition, and motor behavior. Many patients report that thinking of the tic evokes the tic, which is perhaps a model of neural mechanisms by which some thoughts are translated into actions. Patients often describe an irresistible "itch to tic."[297] Like an itch, tics can be suppressed at the cost of increased mental tension; when a flurry of tics are later unleashed, the tension resolves. Coprolalia and other "forbidden" words may occur at uniquely inappropriate times. For example, a patient with Tourette's syndrome may shout "F——ing oink-oink" when passing a policeman or "Holy big tits, holy big tits" upon seeing a woman with large breasts. Such thoughts may pass through the mind of other persons, but for a person with Tourette's syndrome, the inhibition that marks social intercourse evaporates, exposing the "dirty" world where our minds may flow, hidden from those around us. Coprolalia is often the most socially disabling symptom.

Patients with Tourette's syndrome usually have normal intelligence[298] but an increased incidence of ADHD and learning disorders affecting reading, writing, or arithmetic.[299] Adults with Tourette's syndrome may show impaired shifting of the attentional focus and inhibition of environmental stimuli.[300] Obsessions and compulsions occur in roughly half of patients with Tourette's syndrome and may worsen during adolescence. Patients often exhibit emotional incontinence and are unable to inhibit sexual and aggressive impulses.

Other disorders associated with Tourette's syndrome include sleep disorder, *palilalia* (repeating of one's own sounds or words, most often the last or first syllable, with increasing speed), *echolalia* (repeating of sounds or words from an external source), *echopraxia* (repeating movements made by another person), and *copropraxia* (obscene gestures such as simulating masturbation or gesturing with the middle finger extended). Many patients have an altered sense of personal space, often failing to respect the traditional boundaries for entering another's space. This is expressed as lunges of an extremity or the head, nearly touching another person's face, or movement of the car toward or away from another car on the highway.

Persons with persistent neurological disorders often experience a doubleness of life in which the "it" of the disorder coexists with the prior self. In Tourette's syndrome, the "it" assumes unusual vitality, bringing its own set of demands and expressions.[296] Most importantly, the it has its own will, an independent consciousness that can lie at rest, dominate over mental and motor behavior, or comingle with the native self. The person created by the union of the native and alien will is often unwilling to relinquish the "symptomatic" side, for it becomes a part of the person, especially when present since early childhood. Patients with Tourette's syndrome may decline neuroleptic therapy because it removes a part of themselves that they enjoy and loathe at the same time.

Tics are often exacerbated by stress, anxiety, or fatigue and diminished during mental concentration and sleep. Patients are often tic-free during periods of attentive interest. Then, as a lull occurs in the stream of thought, the mind and body shift from the "normal" to the "Tourette:" the smooth flow of speech, thought, and movement becomes accelerated, staccato, impulsive, and compulsive.

Tics in Tourette's syndrome may result from excessive dopaminergic stimulation of the dorsal striatum. The mechanisms of obsessions and compulsions are even less certain, but excessive dopaminergic stimulation of the ventral striatum and limbic prefrontal cortex may contribute. Involvement of the ACC may accelerate response selection and more closely link thought and affect without the usual inhibitions. Relative orbitofrontal hypoactivity during tics may impair the inhibition of socially taboo visceral functions, such as sex or bowel and bladder function, and controversial topics, such as racial differences.[301] Imaging studies reveal striatal hypermetabolism[302] and reduced basal ganglia volumes.[303] Anatomical attention focuses on the striatum, although the midbrain as well as the ACC and orbitofrontal cortex, which receive dopaminergic innervation, may also be involved.[304]

Some cases of Tourette's syndrome, ADHD, and OCD may result from an autoimmune reaction against streptococcal antigens in susceptible children.[283,305] Children with specific human leukocyte antigen types (D8/17) are more likely than other children to acquire tic disorders, OCD, or Sydenham's chorea after exposure to streptococcal infections. It remains uncertain what these findings mean for the treatment of Tourette's syndrome patients in general and for the use of antibiotics or other therapy in children with neuropsychiatric symptoms first developing or worsening after streptococcal infections.[305] However, plasmapharesis or γ-globulin may be beneficial in selected pediatric patients.[306]

Antidopaminergic agents, such as haloperidol, olanzepine, risperidone, quetiapine, and pimozide, effectively treat tics but are of little benefit for obsessive–compulsive phenomena.[307] The adverse effects of these medications, including sedation, weight gain, dysphoria, acute dystonia, akathisia, and impaired school or work performance, must be weighed against their therapeutic benefits. Tardive movement disorders are uncommon among Tourette's syndrome patients. Clonidine helps to treat vocal tics, and clonazepam may lessen motor tics. Dopamine-depleting agents, such as reserpine and tetrabenazine, may control the tics; and SSRIs reduce obsessions and compulsions.[307,308] Unfortunately, the treatment of ADHD with central nervous system stimulants often exacerbates the tics but may be used judiciously. Selegiline, a selective monoamine oxidase-B inhibitor, improves ADHD symptoms, with fewer than 10% of patients experiencing increased tics.[309] Behavioral therapies may be mildly beneficial.[310]

BASAL GANGLIA CALCIFICATION

Calcification of the basal ganglia, an extrapyramidal disorder, causes motor and behavioral symptoms. Dense calcifications develop in the basal ganglia, mainly the putamen and caudate, pulvinar nucleus of the thalamus, and cerebellar dentate gyrus.[311,312] Perivascular ferrocalcific deposits are found in affected gray matter structures.[311] Basal ganglia calcifications may develop as a familial disorder (Fahr's syndrome) or other phosphocalcific metabolic disorders and may be caused by carbon monoxide and lead intoxication, birth anoxia, radiation exposure, methotrexate therapy, chronic antiepileptic drug toxicity, inflammatory disorders, and acquired immune deficiency syndrome.[313,314]

Calcification of the basal ganglia usually begins between 20 and 60 years of age with affective disorder, obsessive–compulsive symptoms, psychosis, or motor symptoms (e.g., rigidity, bradykinesia, choreoathetosis, impaired dexterity).[314–316] Neuropsychological assessment reveals impaired motor programming and executive functions, verbal and figural fluency, auditory learning, and visuospatial skills.[314] Subcortical dementia may develop later in life.

Treatment of basal ganglia calcification symptoms is problematic. Parkinsonism is treated with dopaminergic agents, which often provoke or exacerbate psychosis and other behavioral symptoms. Affective and obsessive–compulsive symptoms may respond to SSRIs. Lithium carbonate, antiepileptic drugs and SSRIs help to treat thought and affective disorders.[317] Psychosis may respond partially to neuroleptics or ECT, but symptoms often recur and prove difficult to control. Neuroleptics often cause disabling extrapyramidal effects.

THE CEREBELLUM

Functional Anatomy

Cerebellar function is topographically organized (Fig. 7–11). The archicerebellum (flocculonodular lobe), vermis, and fastigial nucleus

Cerebellum

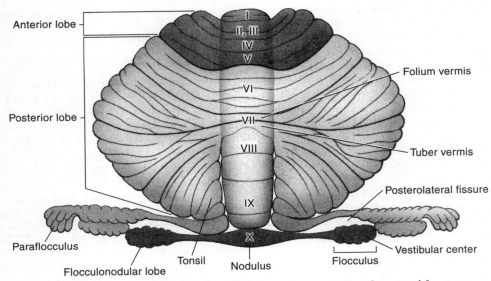

Figure 7–11. Anatomy of the cerebellum. Shaded areas have cognitive and emotional functions.

are involved in gait and balance (anterior vermis), saccadic eye movements (dorsal vermis), autonomic functions (vermis, fastigial nucleus), and affect and emotional memories (posterior vermis) (Table 7–6). Sensorimotor functions are predominantly located in the paleocerebellum (anterior lobe, lobules I–V), with additional representation in the posterior lobe (lobules VIII and IX). Cognitive functions are located mainly in the neocerebellum (posterior lobe, lobules VI and VII). The cerebellar hemisphere and dentate nucleus have a role in executive, visuospatial, linguistic, learning, and memory functions.

The cerebellum was traditionally viewed as a motor center for maintaining posture, coordinating movements of speech, as well as axial (e.g., walking) and appendicular (e.g., writing) musculature, executing sequential movements, and executing complex smooth pursuit movements when tracking a moving target. These functions and the cerebellar connections that support them (e.g., with spinal cord, brain stem, thalamus, and cortical areas related to vestibular, proprioceptive, and motor systems) are well documented. The inferior cerebellar peduncle carries input from the ipsilateral spinal cord, inferior olive, and vestibular nuclei. The corticopontine fibers synapse on the

pontine nuclei, which in turn send fibers to the contralateral cerebellum in the middle cerebellar peduncle. Cerebellar output flows through the superior cerebellar peduncle to the contralateral red nucleus and VL and ventral posterolateral (VPL) thalamic nuclei. The VL and VPL nuclei project to primary sensorimotor and sensorimotor association areas. The vast majority of cerebellar outflow passes to VL nuclei, which in turn project to motor areas. Corticopontine fibers arising from motor areas complete the cortical–pontine–cerebellar–thalamic loop. Cerebellar injuries cause ipsilateral motor symptoms, reflecting the cerebellum's connections with ipsilateral areas of the spinal cord and body and contralateral motor areas of the cerebrum.

The role of the massive corticopontine fibers was relatively neglected in the classic literature on the cerebellum. Most of these fibers (and cerebellar inputs via pontine nuclei) arise from association cortices in all four lobes and serve cognitive functions, and others arise in limbic areas and serve affective functions.[318] The cerebral cortex is said to "beat down" upon the cerebellum, instilling the message that the cerebellum has a subtle but complex and broad role in cognitive and affective behavior.

The strength of cerebellar–cortical relations

Table 7–6. **Localization of Cerebellar Signs and Symptoms**

Signs and Symptoms	Lesion Site	Mechanism
Motor and Coordination		
Truncal ataxia	Anterior vermis, lateral hemisphere	Impaired postural reflexes
Limb and hand ataxia	Lateral hemisphere and dentate nucleus	Muscle asynergy and impaired context-dependent movement
Ocular dysmetria	Dorsal vermis	Impaired scaling of saccadic amplitude
Dysarthria	Posterior left hemisphere and vermis	Muscle asynergy and impaired context-dependent movement
Limb action tremor	Deep nuclei or cerebellar outflow to ventral thalamus	Impaired damping of oscillations in posture and movement
Titubation (body or head tremor)	Anterior vermis and deep nuclei	Impaired damping of oscillations in posture and movement
Palatal and rest tremor	Dentate nucleus	Hyperactivity of inferior olive
Myoclonus	Dentate nucleus	Brain stem or cortical hyperexcitability
Autonomic dysfunction	Vermis or fastigial nucleus	Impaired tuning of autonomic reflexes
Affect and Behavior		
Flattened or(?) inappropriate affect and mood	Posterior vermis	Scaling of emotional responses
Impaired cognition°	Neocerebellum (posterior lobe, lobules VI and VII, dentate nucleus)	Impaired context-dependent modulation of thought and action (dysmetria of thought)

°Impaired planning, reasoning, attention, response time, set shifting, working memory, time estimation, verbal fluency, spatial functions.

is reflected in *diaschisis*, dysfunction in brain areas remote from a destructive lesion, originally described in 1914 by von Monakow.[319] Cerebellar lesions produce diffuse contralateral cerebral hypometabolism. Similarly, frontal lesions cause contralateral cerebellar hypometabolism and, later, cerebellar atrophy through the loss of transsynaptic trophic effects.[320] The cerebellum may globally modulate central nervous system activity, in a fashion analogous to brain stem–cortical modulation, and subserve specific functions mediated by discrete connections between cerebellum, thalamus, and cortex.

The comparative evolution of the cerebellum sheds insight into its role in humans. Initially, in early vertebrates, the protocerebellum primarily facilitated motor coordination by temporally sequencing the activation–inactivation cycle of agonist–antagonist muscle groups by means of sensory feedback, providing a rhythm and fluidity to directed motion. In lower vertebrates, the red nucleus correlated cerebellar and striatal activity, a function that was supplanted by VL nuclei in higher vertebrates. The robust anatomical connections between the cerebellum and the basal ganglia are paralleled by functional similarities. Like the basal ganglia, the cerebellum is activated more by movements related to problem solving than by similar movements divorced from mental challenge.[321] Like the basal ganglia, the cerebellum funnels a wide flow of input from all cortical regions and outputs via the thalamus in a focused stream influencing frontal areas.[322] Patients with cerebellar and basal ganglia lesions often display motor, cognitive, and behavioral changes similar to those seen after premotor and prefrontal lesions. In higher mammals, the cerebellum modulates and coordinates action plans based on diverse inputs and provides outputs that influence movement as well as cognitive and affective behaviors related to those action plans. The relatively large cerebellar hemispheres in the whale, which has atrophic extremities and limited fine motor skills, support the nonmotor role of the cerebellum in behavior.[323]

Functional neuroimaging studies of healthy subjects indicate a role of the cerebellum in diverse behaviors. For example, the cerebellum is active during tasks that tap executive functions, such as cognitive planning, abstract reasoning, searching for responses, set shifting, working memory, time estimation,[324–328] and mental processing speed.[329] In addition, the cerebellum is involved in learning and recognition memory,[330,331] as well as spatial orientation and spatial cognition. The cerebellum responds to visual motion in the environment, influencing stability and equilibrium. It blends sensory and motor information with cutaneous and kinesthetic feedback to facilitate learning of visuomotor skills and smooth execution of movements.[332] The cerebellum participates in perceiving and expressing symbolic visuomotor actions, including gestures. Finally, the cerebellum supports cognitive functions such as spatial reasoning and recall, visual imagery, attention, and abstract visual thought.[333–335] Conclusions regarding the visuospatial role of the cerebellum must be tempered because many findings are confounded by the motor component of constructional tasks used to assess these functions.

Cerebellar Diseases

Stroke, tumor, degenerative disorders, and many other neurological disorders associated with cognitive and affective changes involve the cerebellum (e.g., OPCA, cerebellar agenesis) (Table 7–7). Studies of patients with autism show abnormalities in the cerebellar circuits and limbic system.[336,337] However, cerebellar disease is not a consistent feature of autism. A morphometric MRI study of 46 boys with ADHD revealed significant loss of cerebellar volume, mainly involving the posterior inferior lobe.[338] Dysfunction in a cerebello-thalamo-prefrontal circuit impairs motor control, inhibitory functions, and executive functions in ADHD.

The role of the cerebellum in cognitive and affective behavior was explored by anatomical, neuroimaging, bedside mental status, neurological, and neuropsychological examinations

in 20 patients with various cerebellar disorders.[339] These patients had variable impairments of executive functions, visuospatial cognition involving visuospatial organization and memory, and language function with dysprosodia, agrammatism, and mild anomia, as well as "frontal" personality changes characterized by blunting of affect or disinhibited and inappropriate behavior. Arousal and alertness were normal, and remote episodic and semantic memory were preserved. Learning was only mildly impaired. Isolated cerebellar lesions usually cause mild to moderate cognitive and affective changes, and may interfere with rehabilitation for motor cerebellar functions.[340]

The contribution of the cerebellum to cognition and affect appears primarily one of modulation rather than generation. The cerebellum likely prevents and detects errors and corrects cognitive and behavioral actions. Cerebellar lesions impair context-dependent modulation of thought and action, *dysmetria of thought*. Therefore, lesions in the posterior lobe and vermis appear critical, but the relation between the site of cerebellar involvement and behavior must be precisely defined for a fuller understanding of the cerebellum's role in motor functions.

SUMMARY

The human motor system is the principal route for behavioral expression. The primary motor cortex executes motor commands. The premotor area (LPMC, SMA, pre-SMA) links cognition and movement, playing a critical role in preparing, initiating, selecting, and learning movement patterns. Motor association areas also store motor schemata (elementary motor patterns) for limb and trunk, speech (Broca's area), and volitional eye movements (frontal eye fields). The dominant hemisphere stores motor engrams (learned patterns for motor sequences and spatial patterns) for speech, fine motor skills (praxis), and writing. CMAs help to link affect and movement, providing motivational context for self-initiated movements. Subcortical areas, including the basal ganglia, specific thalamic and brain stem nuclei, and cerebellum, are critical components of the motor system. Four parallel circuits connect the basal ganglia, thalamus, and frontal lobes. These circuits modulate different aspects of

Table 7-7. **Pathological Features of Cerebellar Disorders**

Disorder	Principal Site	Comment
Hemorrhage	Dentate	Hypertension a major risk factor
Infarction	Hemisphere	Anterior inferior cerebellar artery, basilar artery
Tumor		
Medulloblastoma	Midline, 4th ventricle	Children
Ependymoma	Midline, 4th ventricle	Children
Astrocytoma (cystic)	Hemisphere	Children
Metastatic	All regions	Adults
Hemangioblastoma	Paramedian hemisphere	Adults, 25% with von Hippel-Lindau disease
Abscess	Hemisphere	Bacterial, tuberculosis, toxoplasmosis
Viral encephalitis and postinfectious cerebellitis	Midline and hemisphere	Mumps, Epstein-Barr virus, varicella infection, vaccination
Drug toxicity	Midline and hemisphere	Ethanol, antiepileptics, cardiac medications, lithium, chemotherapeutics
Toxins	Midline and hemisphere	Thallium, methylmercury, methylbromide, bismuth, toluene
Vitamin or mineral deficiency	—	Vitamins B_{12}, B_1, E; zinc
Multiple sclerosis	White matter, inflow/outflow tracts	—
Paraneoplastic disorders		
Anti-Purkinje cell antibody	Anti-Yo antibody: breast, ovarian, and adnexal carcinoma; anticytoplasmic antibody: Hodgkin's lymphoma	Anti-Yo autoantibody assay
Antineuronal cell antibody (anti-Hu)	Small cell lung, breast, and prostate carcinoma; neuroblastoma (with opsoclonus)	Anti-Hu antibody assay
Familial periodic ataxia	Calcium channel defect	Acetazolamide-responsive

Continued on the following page

Table 7-7—continued

Disorder	Principal Site	Comment
Autosomal dominant cerebellar ataxia		
Types I–IV	Gene defect: various chromosomal locations	Spinocerebellar ataxia with other features
Cerebral cortical atrophy	Gene defect: unknown gene(s)	—
Dentato-rubro-pallidoluysian atrophy	Chromosome 12p	Most often found in Japan, resembles Huntington's disease
Gerstmann-Straussler-Scheinker disease	Chromosome 20p	Prion
Creutzfeldt-Jakob disease	Chromosome 20p	Prion
Recessive or maternally inherited degenerative disorders		
Olivopontocerebellar atrophy	Gene defect: unknown gene(s)	—
Adrenoleukodystrophy (X-linked)	Gene defect: unknown gene(s)	Very-long-chain fatty acids increased
Friedreich's ataxia	Chromosome 9q	DNA analysis for diagnosis
α-Tocopherol (vitamin E) transfer protein deficiency	Chromosome 8, missense mutation	Resembles Friedreich's ataxia, serum vitamin E level for diagnosis
Sporadic degenerative disorders		
Multiple system atrophy (sporadic OPCA)	Unknown	Extrapyramidal, pyramidal, autonomic features
Mitochondrial encephalomyopathy	Nuclear or mitochondrial DNA	Resembles OPCA with peripheral neuropathy, atrophy, hearing loss

OPCA, olivopontocerebellar atrophy.

motor, cognitive, and affective behavior. Synchronization of activity in cortical and subcortical motor areas provides for the unity and fluidity of movement.

Cortical and subcortical lesions can impair the learning, planning, initiation, organization, and execution of movement. Apraxia may include deficits in performing a complex movement to verbal command, imitation, or use of a supplied tool or instrument. Apraxia usually results from cortical lesions in the dominant hemisphere inferior parietal lobe (supramarginal and angular gyri). Subcortical lesions in motor areas can cause positive symptoms (e.g., rigidity, tremor, dystonia, dyskinesia) or negative symptoms (e.g., loss of motor spontaneity and initiative, hypokinesia, bradykinesia).

Lesions of subcortical motor areas, including the basal ganglia and related brain stem nuclei, give rise to several degenerative disorders. These disorders are often associated with cognitive changes characterized by prominent mental slowing with relative preservation of language, memory, and praxis. Depression often complicates these disorders. Subcortical motor abnormalities can also cause nonprogressive disorders, such as stroke or Tourette's syndrome.

The cerebellum modulates cognition and affect based on the internal and environmental context. Massive corticopontine fibers robustly link cortical and limbic areas with the cerebellum. Cognitive functions are located mainly in the neocerebellum. Affect and emotional functions are located mainly in the posterior vermis. Many genetic and acquired cerebellar disorders impair cognition and behavior.

REFERENCES

1. Rizzolatti G and Fadiga L: Grasping objects and grasping action meanings: the dual role of the monkey rostroventral premotor cortex (area F5). Novartis Found Symp 218:81–95, 1998.
2. Gerloff C, Corwell B, Chen R, et al.: The role of the human motor cortex in the control of complex and simple finger movement sequences. Brain 121:1695–1709, 1998.
3. Hari R, Forss N, Avikainen S, et al.: Activation of human primary motor cortex during action observation: a neuromagnetic study. Proc Natl Acad Sci USA 95: 15061–15065, 1998.
4. Passingham RE: Functional specialization of the supplementary motor area in monkeys and humans. Adv Neurol 70:105–116, 1996.
5. Sanes JN and Donoghue JP: Plasticity and primary motor cortex. Annu Rev Neurosci 23:393–415, 2000.
6. Penfield W and Boldrey E: Somatic motor and sensory representation in the cerebral cortex of man as studied by electrical stimulation. Brain 60:389–443, 1937.
7. Karol EA and Pandya DN: The distribution of the corpus callosum in the rhesus monkey. Brain 94:471–486, 1971.
8. Mesulam MM: Principles of Behavioral Neurology. FA Davis, Philadelphia, 1985, p 14.
9. Denny-Brown D: The Cerebral Control of Movement. Liverpool University Press, Liverpool, 1966.
10. Laplane D, Talairach D, Meninger V, Bancard J, and Bouchareine A: Motor consequences of motor area ablations in men. J Neurol Sci 31:29–49, 1977.
11. Shahani B, Burrows PT, and Whitty CW: The grasp reflex and perseveration. Brain 93:181–192, 1970.
12. Classen J, Schnitzler A, Binkofski F, et al.: The motor syndrome associated with exaggerated inhibition within the primary motor cortex of patients with hemiparetic stroke. Brain 120:605–619, 1997.
13. Sakai K, Kojima E, Suzuki M, et al.: Primary motor cortex isolation: complete paralysis with preserved primary motor cortex. J Neurol Sci 155:115–119, 1998.
14. Sherrington C: On the motor area of the cerebral cortex. In Denny-Brown D (ed).: Selected Writings of Sir Charles Sherrington. Hamilton, London, 1939, pp 397–439.
15. Graziano MS, Taylor CS, Moore T, and Cooke DF: The cortical control of movement revisited. Neuron 36:349–362, 2002.
16. Blinkov SM and Gleser II: The Human Brain in Figures and Tables: A Quantitative Handbook. Plenum, New York, 1968.
17. Halsband U and Passingham RE: Premotor cortex and the conditions for movement in the monkey. Exp Brain Res 18:269–276, 1985.
18. Petrides M: The effect of periarcuate lesions in the monkey on the performance of symmetrically and asymmetrically reinforced visual and auditory go, no-go tasks. J Neurosci 6:2054–2063, 1986.
19. Deiber MP, Passingham RE, Colebatch JG, Friston KJ, Nixon PD, and Frackowiak RSJ: Cortical areas and the selection of movement: a study with positron emission tomography. Exp Brain Res 84:393–402, 1991.
20. Smith EE and Jonides J: Storage and executive processes in the frontal lobes. Science 283:1657–1661, 1999.
21. Strick PL, Dum RP, and Picard N: Motor areas on the medial wall of the hemisphere. Novartis Found Symp 218:64–80, 104–108, 1998.
22. Rizzolatti G, Fadiga L, Fogassi L, and Gallese V: The space around us. Science 277:190–191, 1997.
23. Rizzolatti G, Luppino G, and Matelli M: The organization of the cortical motor system: new concepts. Electroencephalogr Clin Neurophysiol 106:283–296, 1998.
24. Jeannerod M, Arbib MA, Rizzolatti G, and Sakata H: Grasping objects: the cortical mechanisms of visuomotor transformation. Trends Neurosci 18:314–320, 1995.
25. Halsband U, Ito N, Tanji J, and Freund H-J: The role of premotor cortex and the supplementary motor area in the temporal control of movement in man. Brain 116:243–266, 1993.
26. Gerloff C and Andres FG. Bimanual coordination

and interhemispheric interaction. Acta Psychol 110: 161–186, 2002.

27. Freund HJ and Hummelsheim H: Lesions of premotor cortex in man. Brain 108:697–733, 1985.

28. Luria AR: The functional organization of the brain. Sci Am 222:66–72, 1970.

29. Picard N and Strick PL. Imaging the premotor areas. Curr Opin Neurobiol 11:663–672, 2001.

30. Hlustik P, Solodkin A, Gullapalli RP, Noll DC, and Small SL: Functional lateralization of the human premotor cortex during sequential movements. Brain Cogn 49:54–62, 2002.

31. Hoshi E and Tanji J. Integration of target and body-part information in the premotor cortex when planning action. Nature 408:466–470, 2000.

32. Fujii N, Mushiake H, and Tanji J: Intracortical microstimulation of bilateral frontal eye field. J Neurophysiol 79:2240–2244, 1998.

33. Fujii N, Mushiake H, and Tanji J: An oculomotor representation area within the ventral premotor cortex. Proc Natl Acad Sci USA 95:12034–12037, 1998.

34. Maeshima S, Nakai K, Itakura T, et al.: Exploratory-motor task to evaluate right frontal lobe damage. Brain Inj 11:211–217, 1997.

35. Jankelowitz SK and Colebatch JG: Movement-related potentials associated with self-paced, cued and imagined arm movements. Exp Brain Res 147: 98–107, 2002.

36. Jurgens U: Neural pathways underlying vocal control. Neurosci Biobehav Rev 26:235–258, 2002.

37. Massion J: Movement, posture and equilibrium: interaction and coordination. Prog Neurobiol 38:35–56, 1992.

38. Passingham R: The Frontal Lobes and Voluntary Action. Oxford University Press, Oxford, 1993, pp 93–95.

39. Zilles K, Schlaug G, Geyer S, Luppino G, Matelli M, Qu M, et al.: Anatomy and transmitter receptors of the supplementary motor areas in the human and nonhuman primate brain. Adv Neurol 70:29–43, 1996.

40. Rizzolatti G, Luppino G, and Matelli M: The classic supplementary motor area is formed by two independent areas. Adv Neurol 70:45–56, 1996.

41. Matsuzaka Y, Aizawa H, and Tanji J: A motor area rostral to the supplementary motor area (presupplementary motor area) in the monkey: neuronal activity during a learned motor task. J Neurophysiol 68:653–662, 1992.

42. Picard N and Strick PL: Motor areas of the medial wall: a review of their location and functional activation. Cereb Cortex 6:342–353, 1996.

43. Russo GS, Backus DA, Ye S, and Crutcher MD: Neural activity in monkey dorsal and ventral cingulate motor areas: comparison with the supplementary motor area. J Neurophysiol 88:2612–2629, 2002.

44. Penfield W and Roberts L: Speech and Brain Mechanisms. Princeton University Press, Princeton, 1959.

45. Morris HH 3rd, Dinner DS, Luders H, Wyllie E, and Kramer R: Supplementary motor seizures: clinical and electroencephalographic findings. Neurology 38: 1075–1082, 1988.

46. Fried I, Katz A, McCarthy G, Sass KJ, Williamson P, Spencer SS, et al.: Functional organization of human supplementary motor cortex studied by electrical stimulation. J Neurosci 11:3656–3666, 1991.

47. Lim SH, Dinner DS, and Luders HO: Cortical stimulation of the supplementary sensorimotor area. Adv Neurol 70:187–197, 1996.

48. Pai MC: Supplementary motor area aphasia: a case report. Clin Neurol Neurosurg 101:29–32, 1999.

49. Bleasel A, Comair Y, and Luders HO: Surgical ablations of the mesial frontal lobe in humans. Adv Neurol 70:217–235, 1996.

50. Burton DB, Chelune GJ, Naugle RI, and Bleasel A: Neurocognitive studies in patients with supplementary sensorimotor area lesions. Adv Neurol 70:249–261, 1996.

51. Feinberg TE, Schindler RJ, Flanagan NG, and Haber LD: Two alien hand syndromes. Neurology 42:19–24, 1992.

52. Trojano L, Crisci C, Lanzillo B, Elefante R, and Caruso G: How many alien hand syndromes? Follow-up of a case. Neurology 43:2710–2712, 1993.

53. Lim SH, Dinner DS, Pillay PK, Luders H, Morris HH, Klem G, et al.: Functional anatomy of the human supplementary sensorimotor area: results of extraoperative electrical stimulation. Electroencephalogr Clin Neurophysiol 91:179–193, 1994.

54. Nakamura K, Sakai K, and Hikosaka O: Effects of local inactivation of monkey medial frontal cortex in learning of sequential procedures. J Neurophysiol 82: 1063–1068, 1999.

55. Boecker H, Dagher A, Ceballos-Baumann AO, et al.: Role of the human rostral supplementary motor area and the basal ganglia in motor sequence control: investigations with H_2 ^{15}O PET. J Neurophysiol 79: 1070–1080, 1998.

56. Wagman IH and Mehler WR: Physiology and anatomy of the cortico-oculomotor mechanism. Prog Brain Res 37:619–635, 1972.

57. Blanke O, Morand S, Thut G, et al.: Visual acuity in the human frontal eye field. Neuroreport 10:925–930, 1999.

58. Schall JD: The neural selection and control of saccades by the frontal eye field. Philos Trans R Soc Lond B Biol Sci 357:1073–1082, 2002.

59. Dum RP and Strick PL: Medial wall motor areas and skeletomotor control. Curr Opin Neurobiol 2:836–839, 1992.

60. Petrides M, Alivisatos B, Meyer E, and Evans AC: Functional activation of the human frontal cortex during performance of verbal working memory tasks. Proc Natl Acad Sci USA 90:873–877, 1993.

61. Verfaellie M and Heilman KM: Response preparation and response inhibition after lesions of the medial frontal lobe. Arch Neurol 44:1265–1271, 1987.

62. Morecraft RJ and Van Hoesen GW: Cingulate input to the primary and supplementary motor cortices in the rhesus monkey: evidence for somatotopy in areas 24c and 23c. J Comp Neurol 322:471–489, 1992.

63. Bates JF and Goldman-Rakic PS: Prefrontal connections of medial motor areas in the rhesus monkey. J Comp Neurol 336:211–228, 1993.

64. Schlaug G, Knorr U, and Seitz R: Inter-subject variability of cerebral activations in acquiring a motor skill: a study with positron emission tomography. Exp Brain Res 98:523–534, 1994.

65. Meyer G, McElhaney M, Martin W, and McGraw CP: Stereotactic cingulotomy with results of acute stimulation and serial psychological testing. In Laitinen LV and Livingston KE (eds). Surgical Approaches in Psychiatry. University Park Press, Baltimore, 1973, pp 39–58.

66. Devinsky O, Morrell MJ, and Vogt BA: Contributions of anterior cingulate cortex to behaviour. Brain 118:279–306, 1995.

67. Arroyo S, Lesser RP, Gordon B, Uematsu S, Hart J, Schwerdt P, Andreasson K, and Fisher RS: Mirth, laughter and gelastic seizures. Brain 116:757–780, 1993.

68. Sammaritano MR, Adam C, Giard N, and Saint-Hillaire JM: Frontal lobe origin of gelastic seizures [Abstract]. Epilepsia 34(Suppl 6):132, 1993.

69. Levin B and Duchowny M: Childhood obsessive–compulsive disorder and cingulate epilepsy. Biol Psychiatry 30:1049–1055, 1991.

70. Stein DJ, Shoulberg N, Helton K, and Hollander E: The neuroethological approach to obsessive–compulsive disorder. Compr Psychiatry 33:274–281, 1992.

71. Saxena S, Brody AL, Schwartz JM, and Baxter LR: Neuroimaging and frontal-subcortical circuitry in obsessive–compulsive disorder. Br J Psychiatry Suppl 35:26–37, 1998.

72. Fisher CM: Abulia minor vs agitated behavior. Clin Neurosurg 31:9–31, 1983.

73. Nielsen JM and Jacobs LL: Bilateral lesions of the anterior cingulate gyri: report of a case. Bull Los Angeles Neurol Soc 16:231–234, 1951.

74. Freemon FR: Akinetic mutism and bilateral anterior cerebral artery occlusion. J Neurol Neurosurg Psychiatry 34:693–698, 1971.

75. Cravioto H, Silberman J, and Feigin I: A clinical and pathologic study of akinetic mutism. Neurology 10:10–21, 1960.

76. Kemper TL and Romanul FC: State resembling akinetic mutism in basilar artery occlusion. Neurology 17:74–80, 1967.

77. Fisher CM: Intermittent interruption of behavior. Trans Am Neurol Assoc 93:209–210, 1968.

78. Cairns H, Oldfield RC, Pennybacker JB, et al.: Akinetic mutism with an epidermoid cyst of the third ventricle. Brain 64:273–290, 1941.

79. Heilman K, Coyle JM, Gonyea EF, and Feschwind N: Apraxia and agraphia in a left-hander. Brain 96:21–28, 1973.

80. Valenstein E and Heilman KM: Apraxic agraphia with neglect induced paragraphia. Arch Neurol 36:506–508, 1979.

81. Marsden CD: The apraxias are higher-order defects of sensorimotor integration. Novartis Found Symp 218:308–331, 1998.

82. Liepmann H: Drei Aufsatze aus dem Apraxiegebiet. Karger, Berlin, 1908.

83. Poeck K: The two types of motor apraxia. Arch Ital Biol 120:361–369, 1982.

84. Hermsdorfer J, Mai N, Spatt J, Marquardt C, Veltkamp R, and Goldenberg G: Kinematic analysis of movement imitation in apraxia. Brain 119:1575–1586, 1996.

85. Haaland KY, Harrington DL, and Knight RT: Spatial deficits in ideomotor limb apraxia. A kinematic analysis of aiming movements. Brain 122:1169–1182, 1999.

86. Poizner H, Clark MA, Merians AS, Macauley B, Rothi LJG, and Heilman KM: Joint coordination deficits in limb apraxia. Brain 118:227–242, 1995.

87. Liepmann H: Das Krankheitsbild der Apraxie ("motorischen Asymbolie"). Karger, Berlin, 1900.

88. Rao SM, Binder JR, Bandettini PA, et al.: Functional magnetic resonance imaging of complex human movements. Neurology 43:2311–2318, 1993.

89. Schluter ND, Rushworth MF, Passingham RE, and Mills KR: Temporary interference in human lateral premotor cortex suggests dominance for the selection of movements. A study using transcranial magnetic stimulation. Brain 121:785–799, 1998.

90. Geschwind N: The apraxias: neural mechanisms of disorders of learned movements. Am Sci 63:188–195, 1975.

91. Liepmann H: The syndrome of apraxia (motor asymboly) based on a case of unilateral apraxia. Bohne WHO (translator). Monatschr Psychiatrie Neurol 8:15–44, 1900.

92. Graff-Radford NR, Welsh K, and Godersky J: Callosal apraxia. Neurology 37:100–105, 1987.

93. Heilman KM, Rothi LJ, and Valenstein E: Two forms of ideomotor apraxia. Neurology 32:342–346, 1982.

94. Sadato N, Campbell G, Ibanez V, Deiber M, and Hallett M: Complexity affects regional cerebral blood flow change during sequential finger movements. J Neurosci 16:2691–2700, 1996.

95. Catalan MJ, Honda M, Weeks RA, Cohen LG, and Hallett M: The functional neuroanatomy of simple and complex sequential finger movements: a PET study. Brain 121:253–264, 1998.

96. de Jong BM, Willemsen AT, and Paans AM: Brain activation related to the change between bimanual motor programs. Neuroimage 9:290–297, 1999.

97. Watson RT, Fleet WS, Rothi LG, and Heilman KM: Apraxia and the supplementary motor area. Arch Neurol 43:787–792, 1986.

98. Rothi LJG, Heilman KM, and Watson RT: Pantomime comprehension and ideomotor apraxia. J Neurol Neurosurg Psychiatry 48:207–210, 1985.

99. Pramstaller PP and Marsden CD: The basal ganglia and apraxia. Brain 119:319–340, 1996.

100. Benson DF, Sheremata WA, Bouchard R, Segarra JM, Price D, and Geschwind N: Conduction aphasia. A clinicopathological study. Arch Neurol 28:339–346, 1973.

101. Della Sala S, Basso A, Laiacona M, and Papagno C: Subcortical localization of ideomotor apraxia: a review and experimental study. In Vallar G, Cappa SF, and Wallesch CW (eds): Neuropsychological Disorders Associated with Subcortical Lesions. Oxford University Press, Oxford, 1992, pp 357–380.

102. Nadeau SE, Roeltgen DP, Sevush S, Ballinger WE, and Watson RT: Apraxia due to a pathologically documented thalamic infarction. Neurology 44:2133–2137, 1994.

103. Shuren JE, Maher LM, and Heilman KM: Role of the pulvinar in ideomotor praxis. J Neurol Neurosurg Psychiatry 57:1282–1283, 1994.

104. Piccione F, Mancini E, Tonin P, and Bizzarini M: Botulinum toxin treatment of apraxia of eyelid opening in progressive supranuclear palsy: report of two cases. Arch Phys Med Rehabil 78:525–529, 1997.

105. Defazio G, Livrea P, Lamberti P, et al.: Isolated so-called apraxia of eyelid opening: report of 10 cases and a review of the literature. Eur Neurol 39:204–210, 1998.

106. Rothi LJG, Mack L, Verfaellie M, et al.: Ideomotor apraxia: error pattern analysis. Aphasiology 2:381–387, 1988.

107. Goodgalss H and Kaplan E: Disturbance of gesture and pantomime in aphasia. Brain 86:703–720, 1963.

108. Poizner H, Mack L, Verfaellie M, et al.: Three dimensional computer graphic analysis of apraxia. Brain 113:85–101, 1990.

109. Classen J, Kunesch E, Binkofski F, et al.: Subcortical origin of visuomotor apraxia. Brain 118:1365–1374, 1995.

110. Liepmann H and Mass O: Fall von linksseitiger agraphie und apraxiebei rechsseitiger lahmung. Z Psychol Neurol 10:214–227, 1907.

111. Heilman KM, Watson RT, and Rothi LG: Disorders of skilled movements: limb apraxia. In Feinberg TE and Farah MJ (eds). Behavioral Neurology and Neuropsychology. McGraw-Hill, New York, 1996, pp 227–235.

112. Marangolo P, De Renzi E, Di Pace E, et al.: Let not thy left hand know thy right hand knoweth. The case of a patient with an infarct involving the callosal pathways. Brain 121:1459–1467, 1998.

113. Geschwind N: Disconnection syndromes in animals and man. Brain 88:237–294, 1965.

114. Heilman KM: Ideational apraxia—a re-definition. Brain 96:861–864, 1973.

115. DeRenzi E, Faglioni F, and Sargata P: Modality specific and supramodal mechanisms of apraxia. Brain 105: 301–312, 1982.

116. Hecaen H and Albert M: Human Neuropsychology. John Wiley & Sons, New York, 1978.

117. Marcuse H: Apraktiscke Symotome bein linem Fall von seniler Demenz. Zentralbl Mervheik Psychiatr 27:737–751, 1904.

118. Pick A: Studien uber Motorische Apraxia und ihre Mahestenhende Erscheinungen. Deuticke, Leipzig, 1905.

119. Lehmkuhl G and Poeck K: A disturbance in the conceptual organization of actions in patients with ideational apraxia. Cortex 17:153–158, 1981.

120. Ochipa C, Rothi LJG, and Heilman KM: Conduction apraxia. J Clin Exp Neuropsychol 12:89, 1990.

121. Heilman KM and Rothi LJG: Apraxia. In Heilman KM and Valenstein E (eds). Clinical Neuropsychology, 3rd ed. Oxford University Press, New York, 1993, pp 141–163.

122. Rothi LJG, Ochipa C, and Heilman KM: A cognitive neuropsychological model of limb praxis. Cogn Neuropsychol 8:443–458, 1991.

123. DeRenzi E and Lucchelli F: Ideational apraxia. Brain 113:1173–1188, 1988.

124. Ochipa C, Rothi LJG, and Heilman KM: Ideational apraxia: a deficit in tool selection and use. Ann Neurol 25:190–193, 1989.

125. Ochipa C, Rothi LJG, and Heilman KM: Conceptual apraxia in Alzheimer's disease. Brain 115:1061–1071, 1992.

126. McFie J, Piercy MF, and Zangwill OL: Visual spatial agnosia associated with lesions of the right hemisphere. Brain 73:167–190, 1950.

127. Oxbury JM, Campbell DC, and Oxbury SM: Unilateral spatial neglect and impairments of spatial analysis and visual perception. Brain 97:551–565, 1974.

128. Yim Y, Morrow L, Passafiume D, and Boller F: Visuoperceptual and visuomotor abilities and locus of lesion. Neuropsychologia 22:177–185, 1984.

129. Ratcliff G: Spatial thought, mental rotation and the right cerebral hemisphere. Neuropsychologia 17:49–54, 1979.

130. Warrington EK, James M, and Kinsbourne M: Drawing disability in relation to laterality of cerebral lesion. Brain 89:53–82, 1966.

131. Arrigoni G and DeRenzi E: Constructional apraxia and hemispheric locus of lesion. Cortex 1:170–194, 1964.

132. Black FW and Strub RL: Constructional apraxia in patients with discrete missile wounds of the brain. Cortex 2:212–220, 1976.

133. Lawrence DG and Kuypers HGJM: The functional organization of the motor system in the monkey. Brain 91:1–36, 1968.

134. Marsden CD: Functions of the basal ganglia. Rinsho Shinkeigaku 22:1093–1094, 1982.

135. Dubois B, Defontaines B, Deweer B, Malapani C, and Pillon B: Cognitive and behavioral changes in patients with focal lesions of the basal ganglia. Adv Neurol 65:29–41, 1995.

136. Redgrave P, Prescott TJ, and Gurney K: The basal ganglia: a vertebrate solution to the selection problem? Neuroscience 89:1009–1023, 1999.

137. Heimer L, Zaborszky L, Zahm DS, and Alheid GF: The ventral striatopallidothalamic projection: I. The striatopallidal link originating in the striatal parts of the olfactory tubercle. J Comp Neurol 255:571–591, 1987.

138. Haber SN and Fudge JL: The primate substantia nigra and VTA: integrative circuitry and function. Crit Rev Neurobiol 11:323–342, 1997.

139. Flaherty AW and Graybiel AM: Output architecture of the primate putamen. J Neurosci 13:3222–3237, 1993.

140. Graybiel AM, Aosaki T, Flaherty AW, and Kimura M: The basal ganglia and adaptive motor control. Science 265:1826–1831, 1994.

141. Parent A and Hazrati LN: Functional anatomy of the basal ganglia. II. The place of subthalamic nucleus and external pallidum in basal ganglia circuitry. Brain Res Brain Res Rev 20:128–154, 1995.

142. Heimer L, Switzer RD, and Van Hoesen GW: Ventral striatum and ventral pallidum: components of the motor system? Trends Neurosci 5:83–87, 1982.

143. Alexander GE, Crutcher MD, and DeLong MR: Basal ganglia-thalamocortical circuits: parallel substrates for motor, oculomotor, "prefrontal" and "limbic" functions. Prog Brain Res 85:119–146, 1990.

144. Tekin S and Cummings JL. Frontal-subcortical neuronal circuits and clinical neuropsychiatry: an update. J Psychosom Res 53:647–654, 2002.

145. Liu Y, Gao JH, Liotti M, et al.: Temporal dissociation of parallel processing in the human subcortical outputs. Nature 400:364–367, 1999.

146. Middleton FA and Strick PL: Basal ganglia and cerebellar loops: motor and cognitive circuits. Brain Res Brain Res Rev 31:236–250, 2000.

147. Kretschmer BD and Koch M: The ventral pallidum mediates disruption of prepulse inhibition of the acoustic startle response induced by dopamine agonists, but not by NMDA antagonists. Brain Res 798:204–210, 1998.

148. Rouse ST, Marino MJ, Bradley SR, Awad H, Wittmann M, and Conn PJ: Distribution and roles of metabotropic glutamate receptors in the basal ganglia motor circuit: implications for treatment of Parkinson's disease and related disorders. Pharmacol Ther 88:427–435, 2000.

149. Young AB and Penney JB: Biochemical and functional organization of the basal ganglia. In Jankovic J and Tolosa E (eds). Parkinson's Disease and Movement Disorders. Lippincott Williams & Wilkins, Philadelphia, 1998, pp 1–13.
150. Saint-Cyr JA, Taylor AE, and Nicholson K: Behavior and the basal ganglia. Adv Neurol 65:1–28, 1995.
151. Ali-Cherif A, Royere ML, Gosset A, Poncet M, Salamon G, and Khalil R: Behavior and mental activity disorders after carbon monoxide poisoning. Bilateral pallidal lesions [in French]. Rev Neurol (Paris) 140:401–405, 1984.
152. Laplane D, Levasseur M, Pillon B, Dubois B, Baulac M, Mazoyer B, et al.: Obsessive–compulsive and other behavioural changes with bilateral basal ganglia lesions. A neuropsychological, magnetic resonance imaging and positron tomography study. Brain 112:699–725, 1989.
153. Mendez MF, Adams NL, and Lewandowski KS: Neurobehavioral changes associated with caudate lesions. Neurology 39:349–354, 1989.
154. Laplane D, Baulac M, Widlocher D, and Dubois B: Pure psychic akinesia with bilateral lesions of basal ganglia. J Neurol Neurosurg Psychiatry 47:377–385, 1984.
155. Exner C, Koschack J, and Irle E: The differential role of premotor frontal cortex and basal ganglia in motor sequence learning: evidence from focal basal ganglia lesions. Learn Mem 9:376–386, 2002.
156. Saint-Cyr JA, Taylor AE, and Nicholson K: Behavior and the basal ganglia. Adv Neurol 65:1–28, 1995.
157. Chikama M, McFarland NR, Amaral DG, and Haber SN: Insular cortical projections to functional regions of the striatum correlate with cortical cytoarchitectonic organization in the primate. J Neurosci 17:9686–9705, 1997.
158. Mori E, Yamashita H, Takauchi S, and Kondo K: Isolated athymhormia following hypoxic bilateral pallidal lesions. Behav Neurol 9:17–23, 1996.
159. Devinsky O, Sato S, Conwit RA, and Schapiro MB: Relation of EEG alpha background to cognitive function, brain atrophy, and cerebral metabolism in Down's syndrome. Age-specific changes. Arch Neurol 47:58–62, 1990.
160. Richfield EK, Twyman R, and Berent S: Neurological syndrome following bilateral damage to the head of the caudate nuclei. Ann Neurol 22:768–771, 1987.
161. Valenstein E and Heilman KM: Unilateral hypokinesia and motor extinction. Neurology 31:445–448, 1981.
162. Weiller C, Willmes K, Reiche W, Thron A, Isensee C, Buell U, et al.: The case of aphasia or neglect after striatocapsular infarction. Brain 116:1509–1525, 1993.
163. Caplan LR, Schmahmann JD, Kase CS, Feldmann E, Baquis G, Greenberg JP, Gorelick PB, Helgason C, and Hier DB: Caudate infarcts. Arch Neurol 47:133–143, 1990.
164. Kumral E, Evyapan D, and Balkir K: Acute caudate vascular lesions. Stroke 30:100–108, 1999.
165. Tilney F and Morrison JF: Pseudobulbar palsy, clinically and pathologically considered, with the clinical report of five cases. J Nerv Ment Dis 39:505, 1912.
166. Kim JS and Choi-Kwon S: Poststroke depression and emotional incontinence: correlation with lesion location. Neurology 54:1805–1810, 2000.
167. Gropman AL, Barkovich AJ, Vezina LG, Conry JA, Dubovsky EC, and Packer RJ: Pediatric congenital bilateral perisylvian syndrome: clinical and MRI features in 12 patients. Neuropediatrics 28:198–203, 1997.
168. Nahas Z, Arlinghaus KA, Kotrla KJ, Clearman RR, and George MS: Rapid response of emotional incontinence to selective serotonin reuptake inhibitors. J Neuropsychiatry Clin Neurosci 10:453–455, 1998.
169. Muller U, Murai T, Bauer-Wittmund T, and von Cramon DY: Paroxetine versus citalopram treatment of pathological crying after brain injury. Brain Inj 13:805–811, 1999.
170. Udaka T, Yamao ZS, Nagata H, Nakamura S, and Kameyama M: Pathological laughing and crying treated with levodopa. Arch Neurol 41:1095–1096, 1984.
171. Arciniegas DB and Topkoff J: The neuropsychiatry of pathologic affect: an approach to evaluation and treatment. Semin Clin Neuropsychiatry 5:290–306, 2000.
172. Lauterbach EC: External globus pallidus in depression. J Neuropsychiatry Clin Neurosci 11:515–516, 1999.
173. Aarsland D, Larsen JP, Lim NG, and Tandberg E: Olanzapine for psychosis in patients with Parkinson's disease with and without dementia. J Neuropsychiatry Clin Neurosci 11:392–394, 1999.
174. Tesei S, Antonini A, Canesi M, Zecchinelli A, Mariani CB, and Pezzoli G: Tolerability of paroxetine in Parkinson's disease: a prospective study. Mov Disord 15:986–989, 2000.
175. Parkinson J: An Essay on the Shaking Palsy. Sherwood, Neely, and Jones, London, 1817.
176. Levin BE, Llabre MM, and Weiner WJ: Parkinson's disease and depression: psychometric properties of the Beck Depression Inventory. J Neurol Neurosurg Psychiatry 51:1401–1404, 1988.
177. Girotti F, Carella F, Grassi MP, Soliveri P, Marano R, and Caraceni T: Motor and cognitive performances of parkinsonian patients in the on and off phases of the disease. J Neurol Neurosurg Psychiatry 49:657–660, 1986.
178. Quinn NP: Classification of fluctuations in patients with Parkinson's disease. Neurology 51(Suppl 2):S25–S29, 1998.
179. Cantello R, Gilli M, Riccio A, and Bergamasco B: Mood changes associated with "end-of-dose deterioration" in Parkinson's disease: a controlled study. J Neurol Neurosurg Psychiatry 49:1182–1190, 1986.
180. Nissenbaum H, Quinn NP, Brown RG, Toone B, Gotham AM, and Marsden CD: Mood swings associated with the "on–off" phenomenon in Parkinson's disease. Psychol Med 17:899–904, 1987.
181. Menza MA, Sage J, Marshall E, Cody R, and Duvoisin R: Mood changes and "on-off" phenomena in Parkinson's disease. Mov Disord 5:148–151, 1990.
182. Vazquez A, Jimenez-Jimenez FJ, Garcia-Ruiz P, and Garcia-Urra D: "Panic attacks" in Parkinson's disease. A long-term complication of levodopa therapy. Acta Neurol Scand 87:14–18, 1993.
183. Fentoni V, Loliveri P, Monza D, et al.: Affective symptoms in multiple system atrophy and Parkinson's disease: response to levodopa therapy. J Neurol Neurosurg Psychiatry 66:541–544, 1999.
184. Rascol O: The pharmacological therapeutic manage-

ment of levodopa-induced dyskinesias in patients with Parkinson's disease. J Neurol 247:1151–1157, 2000.

185. Juncos JL: Management of psychotic aspects of Parkinson's disease. J Clin Psychiatry 60:42–53, 1999.

186. Menza MM, Palermo B, and Mark M: Quetiapine as an alternative to clozapine in the treatment of dopamimetic psychosis in patients with Parkinson's disease. Ann Clin Psychiatry 11:141–144, 1999.

187. Dewey RB Jr and O'Suilleabhain PE: Treatment of drug-induced psychosis with quetiapine and clozapine in Parkinson's disease. Neurology 55:1753–754, 2000.

188. Factor SA and Brown D: Clozapine prevents recurrence of psychosis in Parkinson's disease. Mov Disord 7:125–131, 1992.

189. Trosch RM, Friedman JH, Lannon MC, Pahwa R, Smith D, Seeberger LC, et al.: Clozapine use in Parkinson's disease: a retrospective analysis of a large multicentered clinical experience. Mov Disord 13:377–382, 1998.

190. Mayeux R: Depression in the patient with Parkinson's disease. J Clin Psychiatry 51:24–25, 1990.

191. Sano M, Stern Y, Williams J, Cote L, Rosenstein R, and Mayeux R: Coexisting dementia and depression in Parkinson's disease. Arch Neurol 46:1284–1286, 1989.

192. Cummings JL: Depression and Parkinson's disease: a review. Am J Psychiatry 149:443–454, 1992.

193. Schiffer RB, Kurlan R, Rubin A, and Boer S: Evidence for atypical depression in Parkinson's disease. Am J Psychiatry 145:1020–1022, 1988.

194. Stein MB, Heuser IJ, Juncos JL, and Uhde TW: Anxiety disorders in patients with Parkinson's disease. Am J Psychiatry 147:217–220, 1990.

195. Poewe W and Luginger E: Depression in Parkinson's disease: impediments to recognition and treatment options. Neurology 52(Suppl 3):S2–S6, 1999.

196. Gotham AM, Brown RG, and Marsden CD: Depression in Parkinson's disease: a quantitative and qualitative analysis. J Neurol Neurosurg Psychiatry 49:381–389, 1986.

197. Horn S: Some psychological factors in parkinsonism. J Neurol Neurosurg Psychiatry 37:27–31, 1974.

198. Broussolle E, Dentresangle C, Landais P, et al.: The relation of putamen and caudate nucleus ^{18}F-Dopa uptake to motor and cognitive performances in Parkinson's disease. Neurol Sci 166:141–151, 1999.

199. Kostic VS, Djuricic BM, Covickovic-Sternic N, Bumbasirevic L, Nikolic M, and Mrsulja BB: Depression and Parkinson's disease: possible role of serotonergic mechanisms. J Neurol 234:94–96, 1987.

200. Mayeux R, Stern Y, Sano M, Williams JB, and Cote LJ: The relationship of serotonin to depression in Parkinson's disease. Mov Disord 3:237–244, 1988.

201. Zesiewicz TA, Gold M, Chari G, and Hauser RA: Current issues in depression in Parkinson's disease. Am J Geriatr Psychiatry 7:110–118, 1999.

202. Tom T and Cummings JL: Depression in Parkinson's disease. Pharmacological characteristics and treatment. Drugs Aging 12:55–74, 1998.

203. Evans DL, Staab JP, Petitto JM, Morrison MF, Szuba MP, Ward HE, et al.: Depression in the medical setting: biopsychological interactions and treatment considerations. J Clin Psychiatry 60:40–56, 1999.

204. Wengel SP, Burke WJ, Pfeiffer RF, et al.: Mainte-

nance electroconvulsive therapy for intractable Parkinson's disease. Am J Geriatr Psychiatry 6:263–269, 1998.

205. Yahr MD: Overview of present day treatment of Parkinson's disease. J Neural Transm 43:227–238, 1978.

206. Lang AE, Quinn N, Brincat S, Marsden CD, and Parkes JD: Pergolide in late-stage Parkinson disease. Ann Neurol 12:243–247, 1982.

207. Fernandez HH and Friedman JH: Punding on L-dopa. Mov Disord 14:836–838, 1999.

208. Fahn S: The spectrum of levodopa-induced dyskinesias. Ann Neurol 47:S2–S11, 2000.

209. Aarsland D, Tandberg E, Larsen JP, and Cummings JL: Frequency of dementia in Parkinson disease. Arch Neurol 53:538–542, 1996.

210. Reading PJ, Luce AK, and McKeith IG: Rivastigmine in the treatment of parkinsonian psychosis and cognitive impairment: preliminary findings from an open trial. Mov Disord 16:1171–1174, 2001.

211. Mortimer JA, Piroolo FJ, Hansch EC, and Webster DD: Relationship of motor symptoms to intellectual deficits in Parkinson disease. Neurology 32:133–137, 1982.

212. Taylor AE, Saint-Cyr JA, and Lang AE: Idiopathic Parkinson's disease: revised concepts of cognitive and affective status. Can J Neurol Sci 15:106–113, 1988.

213. Stocchi F and Brusa L: Cognition and emotion in different stages and subtypes of Parkinson's disease. J Neurol 247(Suppl 2):II114–II121, 2000.

214. Lees AJ and Smith E: Cognitive deficits in the early stages of Parkinson's disease. Brain 106:257–270, 1983.

215. Montse A, Pere V, Carme J, Francesc V, and Eduardo T: Visuospatial deficits in Parkinson's disease assessed by judgment of line orientation test: error analyses and practice effects. J Clin Exp Neuropsychol 23:592–598, 2001.

216. Ivory SJ, Knight RG, Longmore BE, and Caradoc-Davies T: Verbal memory in non-demented patients with idiopathic Parkinson's disease. Neuropsychologia 37:817–828, 1999.

217. Mentis MJ, McIntosh AR, Perrine K, Dhawan V, Berlin B, Feigin A, et al.: Relationships among the metabolic patterns that correlate with mnemonic, visuospatial, and mood symptoms in Parkinson's disease. Am J Psychiatry 159:746–754, 2002.

218. Pillon B, Dubois B, Cusimano G, Bonnet AM, Lhermitte F, and Agid Y: Does cognitive impairment in Parkinson's disease result from non-dopaminergic lesions? J Neurol Neurosurg Psychiatry 52:201–206, 1989.

219. Savage CR: Neuropsychology of subcortical dementias. Psychiatr Clin North Am 20:911–931, 1997.

220. Benke T, Bosch S, and Andree B: A study of emotional processing in Parkinson's disease. Brain Cogn 38:36–52, 1998.

221. Levy G, Schupf N, Tang MX, Cote LJ, Louis ED, Mejia H, et al.: Combined effect of age and severity on the risk of dementia in Parkinson's disease. Ann Neurol 51:722–729, 2002.

222. Churchyard A and Lees AJ: The relationship between dementia and direct involvement of the hippocampus and amygdala in Parkinson's disease. Neurology 49:1570–1576, 1997.

223. McKeith IG: Spectrum of Parkinson's disease,

Parkinson's dementia, and Lewy body dementia. Neurol Clin 18:865–902, 2000.

224. Golbe LI, Davis PH, Schoenberg BS, and Duvoisin RC: Prevalence and natural history of progressive supranuclear palsy. Neurology 38:1031–1034, 1988.

225. Kimber J, Mathias CJ, Lees AJ, Bleasdale-Barr K, Chang HS, Churchyard A, and Watson L: Physiological, pharmacological and neurohormonal assessment of autonomic function in progressive supranuclear palsy. Brain 123:1422–1430, 2000.

226. Soliveri P, Monza D, Paridi D, Radice D, Grisoli M, Testa D, et al.: Cognitive and magnetic resonance imaging aspects of corticobasal degeneration and progressive supranuclear palsy. Neurology 53:502–507, 1999.

227. Maher ER and Lees AJ: The clinical features and natural history of the Steele-Richardson-Olszewski syndrome (progressive supranuclear palsy). Neurology 36:1005–1008, 1986.

228. Aarsland D, Litvan I, and Larsen JP: Neuropsychiatric symptoms of patients with progressive supranuclear palsy and Parkinson's disease. J Neuropsychiatry Clin Neurosci 13:42–49, 2001.

229. Albert ML, Feldman RG, and Willis AL: The "subcortical dementia" of progressive supranuclear palsy. J Neurol Neurosurg Psychiatry 37:121–130, 1974.

230. Pillon B, Dubois B, Ploska A, and Agid Y: Severity and specificity of cognitive impairment in Alzheimer's, Huntington's, and Parkinson's diseases and progressive supranuclear palsy. Neurology 41:634–643, 1991.

231. Litvan I, Grafman J, Gomez C, and Chase TN: Memory impairment in patients with progressive supranuclear palsy. Arch Neurol 46:765–767, 1989.

232. Esmonde T, Giles E, Gibson M, and Hodges JR: Neuropsychological performance, disease severity, and depression in progressive supranuclear palsy. J Neurol 243:638–643, 1996.

233. Pillon B, Gouider-Khouja N, Deweer B, Vidailhet M, Malapani C, Dubois B, et al.: Neuropsychological pattern of striatonigral degeneration: comparison with Parkinson's disease and progressive supranuclear palsy. J Neurol Neurosurg Psychiatry 58:174–179, 1995.

234. Podoll K, Schwarz M, and Noth J: Language functions in progressive supranuclear palsy. Brain 114:1457–1472, 1991.

235. Pharr V, Uttl B, Stark M, Litvan I, Fantie B, and Grafman J: Comparison of apraxia in corticobasal degeneration and progressive supranuclear palsy. Neurology 56:957–963, 2001.

236. Morris HR, Wood NW, and Lees AJ: Progressive supranuclear palsy (Steele-Richardson-Olszewski disease). Postgrad Med J 75:579–584, 1999.

237. Lee VM, Goedert M, and Trojanowski JQ: Neurodegenerative tauopathies. Annu Rev Neurosci 24:1121–1159, 2001.

238. Barclay CL, Duff J, Sandor P, and Lang AE: Limited usefulness of electroconvulsive therapy in progressive supranuclear palsy. Neurology 46:1284–1286, 1996.

239. Fabbrini G, Barbanti P, Bonifati V, Colosimo C, Gasparini M, Vanacore N, et al.: Donepezil in the treatment of progressive supranuclear palsy. Acta Neurol Scand 103:123–125, 2001.

240. Litvan I, Phipps M, Pharr VL, Hallett M, Grafman J, and Salazar A: Randomized placebo-controlled trial of donepezil in patients with progressive supranuclear palsy. Neurology 57:467–473, 2001.

241. Fahn S: The freezing phenomenon in parkinsonism. Adv Neurol 67:53–63, 1995.

242. Gilman S, Low P, Quinn N, Albanese A, Ben-Shlomo Y, Fowler C, et al.: Consensus statement on the diagnosis of multiple system atrophy. American Autonomic Society and American Academy of Neurology. Clin Auton Res 8:359–362, 1998.

243. Robbins TW, James M, Lange KW, Owen AM, Quinn NP, and Marsden CD: Cognitive performance in multiple system atrophy. Brain 115:271–291, 1992.

244. Testa D, Fetoni V, Soliveri P, Musicco M, Palazzini E, and Girotti F: Cognitive and motor performance in multiple system atrophy and Parkinson's disease compared. Neuropsychologia 31:207–210, 1993.

245. Monza D, Soliveri P, Radice D, Fetoni V, Testa D, Caffarra P, et al.: Cognitive dysfunction and impaired organization of complex motility in degenerative parkinsonian syndromes. Arch Neurol 55:372–378, 1998.

246. Meco G, Gasparini M, and Doricchi F: Attentional functions in multiple system atrophy and Parkinson's disease. J Neurol Neurosurg Psychiatry 60:393–398, 1996.

247. Olson EJ, Boeve BF, and Silber MH: Rapid eye movement sleep behaviour disorder: demographic, clinical and laboratory findings in 93 cases. Brain 123:331–339, 2000.

248. Manni R, Morini R, Martignoni E, Pacchetti C, Micieli G, and Tartara A: Nocturnal sleep in multisystem atrophy with autonomic failure: polygraphic findings in ten patients. J Neurol 240:249–250, 1993.

249. Kish SJ, Schut L, Simmons J, Gilbert J, Chang LJ, and Rebbetoy M: Brain acetylcholinesterase activity is markedly reduced in dominantly-inherited olivopontocerebellar atrophy. J Neurol Neurosurg Psychiatry 51:544–548, 1988.

250. Horimoto Y, Aiba I, Yasuda T, Ohkawa Y, Katayama T, Yokokawa Y, et al.: Cerebral atrophy in multiple system atrophy by MRI. J Neurol Sci 173:109–112, 2000.

251. Rebeiz JJ, Kolodny EH, and Richardson EP: Corticodentatonigral degeneration with neuronal achromasia. Arch Neurol 18:20–33, 1968.

252. Riley DE, Lang AE, Lewis A, Resch L, Ashby P, Hornykiewicz O, and Black S: Cortical-basal ganglionic degeneration. Neurology 40:1203–1212, 1990.

253. Bergeron C, Pollanen MS, Weyer L, Black SE, and Lang AE: Unusual clinical presentations of corticalbasal ganglionic degeneration. Ann Neurol 40:893–900, 1996.

254. Grimes DA, Lang AE, and Bergeron CB: Dementia as the most common presentation of cortical-basal ganglionic degeneration. Neurology 53:1969–1974, 1999.

255. Massman PJ, Kreiter KT, Jankovic J, and Doody RS: Neuropsychological functioning in cortical-basal ganglionic degeneration: differentiation from Alzheimer's disease. Neurology 46:720–726, 1996.

256. Thompson PD, Day BL, Rothwell JC, Brown P, Britton TC, and Marsden CD: The myoclonus in corticobasal degeneration. Evidence for two forms of cortical reflex myoclonus. Brain 117:1197–1207, 1994.

257. Leiguarda R, Lees AJ, Merello M, Starkstein S, and Marsden CD: The nature of apraxia in corticobasal

degeneration. J Neurol Neurosurg Psychiatry 57: 455–459, 1994.

258. Peigneux P, Salmon E, Garraux G, Laureys S, Willems S, Dujardin K, et al.: Neural and cognitive bases of upper limb apraxia in corticobasal degeneration. Neurology 57:1259–1268, 2001.

259. Okuda B and Tachibana H: The nature of apraxia in corticobasal degeneration. J Neurol Neurosurg Psychiatry 57:1548–1549, 1994.

260. Kumar R, Bergeron C, Pollanen MS, and Lang AE: Cortical basal ganglionic degeneration. In Jankovic J and Tolosa E (eds). Parkinson's Disease and Movement Disorders. Williams & Wilkins, Baltimore, 1998, pp 297–316.

261. Denny-Brown D, Meyer JS, and Horenstein S: The significance of perceptual rivalry from parietal lobe lesions. Brain 75:433–471, 1952.

262. Gunal DI, Agan K, and Aktan S: A case of spontaneous arm levitation in progressive supranuclear palsy. Neurol Sci 21:405–406, 2000.

263. Goetz CG and Diederich NJ: There is a renaissance of interest in pallidotomy for Parkinson's disease. Nat Med 2:510–514, 1996.

264. Huntington G: On chorea. Med Surg Rep 26:320–321, 1872.

265. Hayden MR: Huntington's Chorea. Springer-Verlag, New York, 1981, pp 72–74.

266. Lauterbach EC, Cummings JL, Duffy J, et al.: Neuropsychiatric correlates and treatment of lenticulostriatal diseases: a review of the literature and overview of research opportunities in Huntington's, Wilson's, and Fahr's diseases. J Neuropsychiatry Clin Neurosci 10:249–266, 1998.

267. Paulsen JS, Ready RE, Hamilton JM, Mega MS, and Cummings JL: Neuropsychiatric aspects of Huntington's disease. J Neurol Neurosurg Psychiatry 71:310–314, 2001.

268. Naarding P, Kremer HP, and Zitman FG: Huntington's disease: a review of the literature on prevalence and treatment of neuropsychiatric phenomena. Eur Psychiatry 16:439–445, 2001.

269. Rosenblatt A and Leroi I: Neuropsychiatry of Huntington's disease and other basal ganglia disorders. Psychosomatics 41:24–30, 2000.

270. Leroi I and Michalon M: Treatment of the psychiatric manifestations of Huntington's disease: a review of the literature. Can J Psychiatry 43:933–940, 1998.

271. Folstein S, Abbott MH, Chase GA, Jensen BA, and Folstein MF: The association of affective disorder with Huntington's disease in a case series and in families. Psychol Med 13:537–542, 1983.

272. Whittier J, Haydu G, and Crawford J: Effect of imipramine on depression and hyperkinesia in Huntington's disease. Am J Psychiatry 146:246–249, 1961.

273. McHugh PR and Folstein MF: Psychiatric syndromes of Huntington's chorea. In Benson DF and Blumer D (eds). Psychiatric Aspects of Neurologic Disease. Grune and Stratton, New York, 1975, pp 275–285.

274. Como PG, Rubin AJ, O'Brien CF, et al.: A controlled trial of fluoxetine in nondepressed patients with Huntington's disease. Mov Disord 12:397–401, 1997.

275. Ranen NG, Lipsey JR, Treisman G, and Ross CA: Sertraline in the treatment of severe aggressiveness in Huntington's disease. J Neuropsychiatry Clin Neurosci 8:338–340, 1996.

276. Cummings JL: Behavioral and psychiatric symptoms associated with Huntington's disease. Adv Neurol 65:179–186, 1995.

277. Lawrence AD, Hodges JR, Rosser AE, et al.: Evidence for specific cognitive deficits in preclinical Huntington's disease. Brain 121:1329–1341, 1998.

278. Lawrence AD, Weeks RA, Brooks DJ, et al.: The relationship between striatal dopamine receptor binding and cognitive performance in Huntington's disease. Brain 121:1343–1355, 1998.

279. Zakzanis KK: The subcortical dementia of Huntington's disease. J Clin Exp Neuropsychol 20:565–578, 1998.

280. Moore DP: Neuropsychiatric aspects of Sydenham's chorea: a comprehensive review. J Clin Psychiatry 57:407–414, 1996.

281. Swedo SE, Rapoport JL, Cheslow DL, Leonard HL, Ayoub EM, Hosier DM, et al.: High prevalence of obsessive–compulsive symptoms in patients with Sydenham's chorea. Am J Psychiatry 146:246–249, 1989.

282. Kotby AA, El Badawy N, El Sokkary S, Moawad H, and El Shawarby M: Antineuronal antibodies in rheumatic chorea. Clin Diagn Lab Immunol 5:836–839, 1998.

283. Swedo SE, Leonard HL, Mittleman BB, et al.: Identification of children with pediatric autoimmune neuropsychiatric disorders associated with streptococcal infections by a marker associated with rheumatic fever. Am J Psychiatry 154:110–112, 1997.

284. Frydman M: Genetic aspects of Wilson's disease. J Gastroenterol Hepatol 5:483–490, 1990.

285. Wilson SA: Progressive lenticular degeneration: a familial nervous disease with cirrhosis of the liver. Brain 34:295–509, 1912.

286. Davis EJ and Borde M: Wilson's disease and catatonia. Br J Psychiatry 162:256–259, 1993.

287. Medalia A, Isaacs-Glaberman K, and Scheinberg IH: Neuropsychological impairment in Wilson's disease. Arch Neurol 45:502–504, 1988.

288. Lang C: Is Wilson's disease a dementing condition? J Clin Exp Neuropsychol 11:569–570, 1989.

289. Lang C, Muller D, Claus D, and Druschky KF: Neuropsychological findings in treated Wilson's disease. Acta Neurol Scand 81:75–81, 1990.

290. Saatci I, Topcu M, Baltaoglu FF, et al.: Cranial MR findings in Wilson's disease. Acta Radiol 38:250–258, 1997.

291. Dening TR and Berrios GE: Wilson's disease: clinical groups in 400 cases. Acta Neurol Scand 80:527–534, 1989.

292. Dening TR and Berrios GE: Wilson's disease: a longitudinal study of psychiatric symptoms. Biol Psychiatry 28:255–265, 1990.

293. Luis CA, Barker WW, Gajaraj K, et al.: Sensitivity and specificity of three clinical criteria for dementia with Lewy bodies in an autopsy-verified sample. Int J Geriatr Psychiatry 14:526–533, 1999.

294. McKeith IG, Perry RH, Fairbairn AF, Jabeen S, and Perry EK: Operational criteria for senile dementia of Lewy body type (SDLT). Psychol Med 22:911–922, 1992.

295. McKeith IG, Grace JB, Walker Z, Byrne EJ, Wilkinson D, Stevens T, et al.: Rivastigmine in the treatment of dementia with Lewy bodies: preliminary findings from an open trial. Int J Geriatr Psychiatry 15:387–392, 2000.

296. Sacks O: An Anthropologist on Mars. Alfred A. Knopf, New York, 1995.
297. Bliss J: Sensory experiences of Gilles de la Tourette syndrome. Arch Gen Psychiatry 37:1343–1347, 1980.
298. Shapiro AK, Shapiro ED, Brunn RD, et al.: Gilles de la Tourette Syndrome. Raven Press, New York, 1978, pp 115–145.
299. Jankovic J and Rohaidy H: Motor, behavioral and pharmacologic findings in Tourette's syndrome. Can J Neurol Sci 14:541–546, 1987.
300. Georgiou N, Bradshaw JL, Phillips JG, et al.: The Simon effect and attention deficits in Gilles de la Tourette's syndrome and Huntington's disease. Brain 118:1305–1318, 1995.
301. Devinsky O: A mind that tics. Arch Gen Psychiatry 57:753, 2000.
302. Robertson MM and Stern JS: The Gilles de la Tourette syndrome. Crit Rev Neurobiol 11:1–19, 1997.
303. Castellanos FX, Giedd JN, Hamburger SD, et al.: Brain morphometry in Tourette's syndrome: the influence of comorbid attention-deficit/hyperactivity disorder. Neurology 47:1581–1583, 1996.
304. Devinsky O: Neuroanatomy of Gilles de la Tourette's syndrome. Possible midbrain involvement. Arch Neurol 40:508–514, 1983.
305. Kurlan R: Tourette's syndrome and "PANDAS:" will the relation bear out? Neurology 50:1530–1534, 1998.
306. Perlmutter SJ, Leitman SF, Garvey MA, et al.: Therapeutic plasma exchange and intravenous immunoglobulin for obsessive–compulsive disorder and tic disorders in childhood. Lancet 354:1153–1158, 1999.
307. Peterson BS: Considerations of natural history and pathophysiology in the psychopharmacology of Tourette's syndrome. J Clin Psychiatry 57(Suppl 9): 24–34, 1996.
308. Kurlan R, Como PG, Deeley C, McDermott M, and McDermott MP: A pilot controlled study of fluoxetine for obsessive–compulsive symptoms in children with Tourette's syndrome. Clin Neuropharmacol 16:167–172, 1993.
309. Jankovic J: Deprenyl in attention deficit associated with Tourette's syndrome. Arch Neurol 50:286–288, 1993.
310. Peterson AL, Campise RL, and Azrin NH: Behavioral and pharmacological treatments for tic and habit disorders: a review. J Dev Behav Pediatr 15:430–441, 1994.
311. Moskowitz MA, Winickoff RN, and Heinz ER: Familial calcification of the basal ganglions: a metabolic and genetic study. N Engl J Med 285:72–77, 1971.
312. Trautner RJ, Cummings JL, Read SL, and Benson DF: Idiopathic basal ganglia calcification and organic mood disorder. Am J Psychiatry 145:350–353, 1988.
313. Fenelon G, Gray F, Paillard F, et al.: A prospective study of patients with CT detected pallidal calcifications. J Neurol Neurosurg Psychiatry 56:622–625, 1993.
314. Lopez-Villegas D, Kulisevsky J, Deus J, Junque C, Pujol J, Guardia E, and Grau JM: Neuropsychological alterations in patients with computed tomography–detected basal ganglia calcification. Arch Neurol 53:251–256, 1996.
315. Francis AF: Familial basal ganglia calcification and schizophreniform psychosis. Br J Psychiatry 135: 360–362, 1979.
316. Cummings JL, Gosenfeld LF, Houlihan JP, and McCaffrey T: Neuropsychiatric disturbances associated with idiopathic calcification of the basal ganglia. Biol Psychiatry 18:591–601, 1983.
317. Munir KM: The treatment of psychotic symptoms in Fahr's disease with lithium carbonate. J Clin Psychopharmacol 6:36–38, 1986.
318. Schmahmann JD and Sherman JC: The cerebellar cognitive affective syndrome. Brain 121:561–579, 1998.
319. von Monakow C: Die lokalisation im grosshirn. The mechanism of vision. XVIII. Effects of destroying the visual "associative areas" of the monkey. Genet Psychol Monogr 37:107–166, 1914.
320. Chung HD: Retrograde crossed cerebellar atrophy. Brain 108:881–895, 1985.
321. Kim JS, Lee JH, and Lee MC: Small primary intracerebral hemorrhage. Clinical presentation of 28 cases. Stroke 25:1500–1506, 1994.
322. Mesulam M: Brain, mind, and the evolution of connectivity. Brain Cogn 42:4–6, 2000.
323. Jansen JK, Nicolaysen K, and Walloe L: The firing pattern of dorsal spinocerebellar tract neurones during inhibition. Acta Physiol Scand 77:68–84, 1969.
324. Grafman J, Litvan I, Massaquoi S, Stewart M, Sirigu A, and Hallett M: Cognitive planning deficit in patients with cerebellar atrophy. Neurology 42:1493–1496, 1992.
325. Klein D, Milner B, Zatorre RJ, Meyer E, and Evans AC: The neural substrates underlying word generation: a bilingual functional-imaging study. Proc Natl Acad Sci USA 92:2899–2903, 1995.
326. Nichelli P, Alway D, and Grafman J: Perceptual timing in cerebellar degeneration. Neuropsychologia 34: 863–871, 1996.
327. Hallett M and Grafman J: Executive function and motor skill learning. In Schmahmann JD (ed). The Cerebrum and Cognition. Academic Press, New York, 1997, pp 297–323.
328. Desmond JE, Gabrieli JD, and Glover GH: Dissociation of frontal and cerebellar activity in a cognitive task: evidence for a distinction between selection and search. Neuroimage 7:368–376, 1998.
329. Tachibana H, Kawabata K, Tomino Y, and Sugita M: Prolonged P3 latency and decreased brain perfusion in cerebellar degeneration. Acta Neurol Scand 100: 310–316, 1999.
330. Drepper J, Timmann D, Kolb FP, and Diener HC: Non-motor associative learning in patients with isolated degenerative cerebellar disease. Brain 122:87–97, 1999.
331. Kim JJ, Andreasen NC, O'Leary DS, et al.: Direct comparison of the neural substrates of recognition memory for words and faces. Brain 122:1069–1083, 1999.
332. Lalonde R: Visuospatial abilities. In Schmahmann JD (ed). The Cerebrum and Cognition. Academic Press, New York, 1997, pp 191–230.
333. Doyon J, Gaudreau D, Laforce R Jr, et al.: Role of the striatum, cerebellum, and frontal lobes in the learning of a visuomotor sequence. Brain Cogn 34: 218–245, 1997.
334. Schmahmann JD: Rediscovery of an early concept. In Schmahmann JD (ed). The Cerebrum and Cognition. Academic Press, New York, 1997, pp 3–27.

335. Thomas KM, King SW, Franzen PL, et al.: A developmental functional MRI study of spatial working memory. Neuroimage 10:327–338, 1999.

336. Bauman M and Kemper TL: Histoanatomic observations of the brain in early infantile autism. Neurology 35:866–874, 1985.

337. Courchesne E, Yeung-Courchesne R, Press GA, Hesselink JR, and Jernigan TL: Hypoplasia of cerebellar lobules VI and VII in autism. N Engl J Med 318:1349–1354, 1988.

338. Berquin PC, Giedd JN, Jacobsen LK, et al.: Cerebellum in attention-deficit hyperactivity disorder: a morphometric MRI study. Neurology 50:1087–1093, 1998.

339. Schmahmann JD and Sherman JC: Cerebellar cognitive affective syndrome. Int Rev Neurobiol 41:433–440, 1997.

340. Chafetz MD, Friedman AL, Kevorkian CG, and Levy JK: The cerebellum and cognitive function: implications for rehabilitation. Arch Phys Med Rehabil 77:1303–1308, 1996.

Chapter 8

Memory and Memory Disorders

Memory is a gift of nature, the ability of living organisms to retain and to utilize acquired information or knowledge. . . . Owners of biological memory systems are capable of behaving more appropriately at a later time because of their experiences at an earlier time . . .

E. TULVING (1995)[1]

Understanding of the neural basis of memory function has advanced rapidly during the past few decades. Numerous neuropsychological and neurophysiological studies of memory function reveal a system of dissociable processes, not a unitary system. Anatomical studies in humans and other primates map these dissociable processes onto distributed neural networks. Neuropharmacological studies reveal that different neurotransmitter systems play distinct roles in the various memory processes. Memory is not localized to one brain region or restricted to one neurotransmitter system. The theoretical distinctions of memory functions developed by psychologists and neuroscientists provide a meaningful framework for understanding the symptoms of memory disorders. New therapies will likely arise from advances in understanding

the neuroanatomical and neurochemical underpinnings of memory function.

THEORETICAL MODELS OF MEMORY

The most common theoretical classification of memory distinguishes short-term and long-term memory. In clinical practice, *short-term* and *long-term* memory are used imprecisely to describe memory processes. Many clinicians describe recently acquired information (e.g., what you had for breakfast) as short-term memory and memories from the distant past (e.g., what you did during your last vacation) as long-term memory. However, this sensible distinction does not conform to experimentally derived models of memory function.[2]

Short-Term and Long-Term Memory

Short-term memory is properly defined as the ability to store information temporarily (for seconds) before it is consolidated into long-term memory. Short-term memory is examined with a test such as Digit Span (e.g., "Repeat these digits immediately back to me: 4, 3, 7, 1, 5, 0, 6"). The average span of neurologically healthy subjects is usually six to seven digits.[3] Chapter 9 contains a more extensive discussion of short-term memory and the modern notion of the function called *working memory*.

Long-term memory is properly defined as the ability to learn new information and recall this information after some time has passed. Long-term memory is tested by asking the patient to learn items that must be retrieved after an interval with distraction (e.g., recall of three items—cat, apple, table—after 1 minute of performing some other task). The term *amnesic syndrome* refers to the loss of long-term memory only. *Remote memory*, a form of long-term memory, is information that was consolidated in the past. It can be tested by asking the subject to remember past public events (e.g., "When did the first person land on the moon?") or personal events (e.g., "Where did you go on your last vacation?"). Neurologically healthy subjects should easily recall three items after a short distracted delay or accurately recall events from their recent or distant past.

Declarative and Procedural Memory

Several subdivisions of long-term memory have been proposed (Fig. 8–1). A widely accepted dichotomous classification is declarative and procedural memory.[2] *Declarative memory* represents memories of episodes and facts that can be consciously accessed, and *procedural memory* represents memory for skills. Unlike declarative memory, procedural memory is not available to consciousness. Procedural memories can be motor skills or mental procedures, such as performing complex arithmetic. Declarative memory may be further subdivided into episodic and semantic memory.[4] *Episodic memory* represents specific, personally experienced episodes. In contrast, *semantic memory* represents facts (e.g., information about objects, people, and events), principles, and rules that make up our general knowledge of the world. For example, London is a city in England, and dolphins are mammals. Semantic memories may evolve from specific episodes when such information is first encountered, but with the passage of time these episodes lose their temporal context.[5] These distinctions are illustrated by our experience with a bicycle:[6] we may recall when we last rode a bicycle (episodic memory), know what a bicycle is (semantic memory), or know how to ride a bicycle (procedural memory).

Explicit and Implicit Memory

Another proposed classification is explicit and implicit memory.[7] *Explicit memory* includes the conscious recollection of any memory encompassing both episodic and semantic memories. *Implicit memory* does not require conscious recollection and includes procedural memory as well as priming and classical conditioning. *Priming* is the phenomenon that previously encountered information has an increased probability of being recalled later, even if there is no explicit recall of the earlier ("priming") experience.[8] For example, in a prototypical priming experiment, the subject is first presented with a list of words to read (e.g., *motel, abstain, house*). Subsequently, the subject is given three-letter stems (e.g., *mot–*) and asked to produce the first word that comes to mind. The probability of generating a previously encountered word (e.g., *motel*) is greater than with words not on the original list (e.g., *mother*).

FUNCTIONAL NEUROANATOMY OF MEMORY PROCESSES

Episodic Memory

The report of patient H.M. in 1957 demonstrated conclusively that the medial temporal

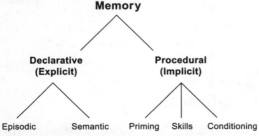

Figure 8–1. Proposed divisions of long-term memory.

lobe is critical for episodic long-term memory.[9] Patient H.M. had intractable epilepsy and underwent bilateral surgical excision of the hippocampus and amygdala. A magnetic resonance imaging (MRI) scan, performed many years after his operation, showed the extent of the lesion (Fig. 8–2). Following surgery, H.M. suffered a dense and isolated impairment in episodic memory, which persisted for decades.[10]

Experimental lesion studies in nonhuman primates support the importance of the medial temporal lobe in episodic memory.[11,12] These studies and correlative lesion studies in humans

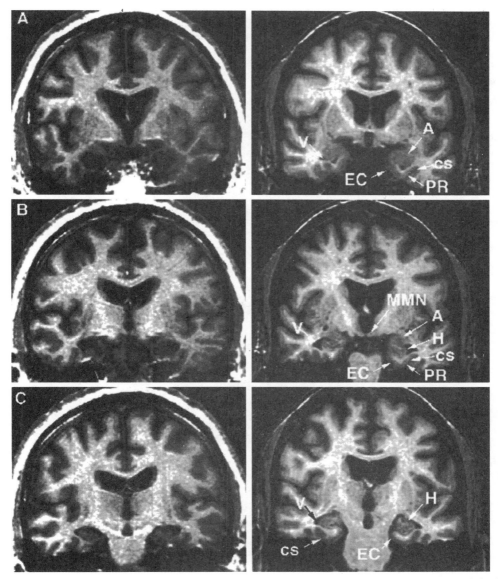

Figure 8–2. Coronal slices from a magnetic resonance imaging scan from rostral (A) to caudal (C) of H.M. (left) showing the extent of bilateral hippocampal ablation compared to an age-matched control (from Corkin et al.[10]). Note that the amygdala, hippocampus, and entorhinal cortex anterior to the level of the mamillary bodies are removed with relative sparing of the posterior perirhinal cortex in the banks of the collateral sulcus. H, hippocampus, A, amygdala, EC, entorhinal cortex, CS, collateral sulcus, PR, perirhinal cortex, V, temporal horn of lateral ventricle, MMN, medial mamillary nucleus.

show that the hippocampus and amygdala are part of a critical neural network for episodic memories (Fig. 8–3).[13] This memory network has two anatomical loops, or circuits.[14,15] The first circuit includes the hippocampus, which projects via the fornices to the mamillary bodies. Via the mamillothalamic tract, the mamillary bodies project to the anterior nuclei of the thalamus, which in turn send projections to the posterior cingulate cortex. The circuit is completed by projections from the cingulate to the hippocampal formation. Within this circuit are also important reciprocal connections between the hippocampus and the septal nuclei via the fornix. The second circuit includes the amygdala, thalamus, and frontal lobe. The amygdala projects to the dorsomedial nucleus of the thalamus via amygdalofugal pathways. The dorsomedial nucleus projects to the prefrontal cortex, which reciprocally connects with the amygdala, completing the loop. All critical structures and pathways comprising these parallel memory circuits can be grouped into three main brain areas: the medial temporal lobes, the thalamus, and the basal forebrain. A lesion anywhere within these brain areas or connecting pathways can impair episodic memory.

MEDIAL TEMPORAL LOBES

The hippocampal formation, parahippocampal gyrus, and amygdala form the medial temporal lobes. The hippocampal formation is a three-layered cortex containing the hippocampus with prominent pyramidal cells (cornu ammonis, CA1–4) and dentate gyrus with prominent granule cells, one of the few nonprimary sensory cortices with this feature (Fig. 8–4). At the hippocampal fissure, the subiculum and entorhinal cortex of the parahippocampal gyrus gradually transition from three- to six-layered cortex. The hippocampal formation and parahippocampal gyrus contain a closed-loop circuit.[16] The subiculum and entorhinal cortex are essential links between the hippocampal formation and both the subcortical and cortical areas. The major input into the hippocampus is excitatory, arising from entorhinal cortex and subiculum, which relay extensive midline thalamic, limbic, and neocortical inputs, and from cholinergic

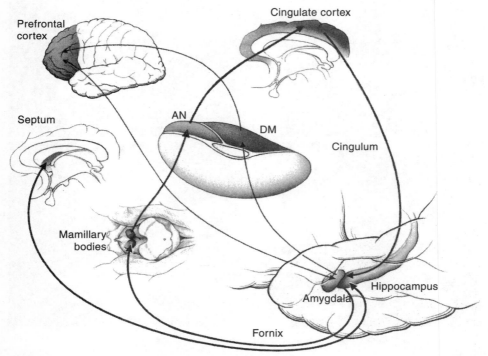

Figure 8–3. The neuroanatomical structures involved in episodic long-term memory function. Black arrows interconnect regions that are part of the *hippocampal* circuit and gray arrows interconnect regions that are part of the *amygdala* circuit. AN, anterior nucleus; DM, dorsomedial nucleus of the thalamus.

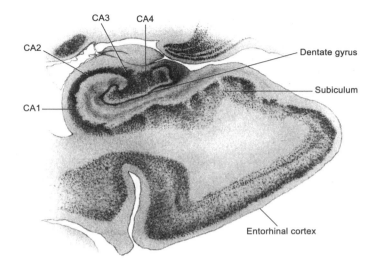

A

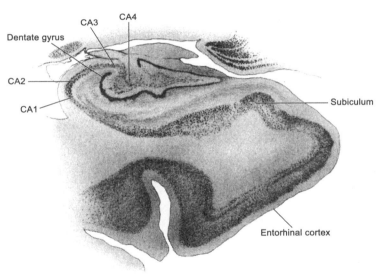

B

Figure 8–4. (A) Normal anatomy of the hippocampal formation and related structures within the medial temporal lobes. (B) Hippocampal formation after hypoxia, showing severe cell loss in CA1, CA3, and CA4.

septal fibers. Inhibitory input arises from the contralateral hippocampus. The hippocampus also receives strong dopaminergic, noradrenergic, and serotonergic inputs. The fornix is the major output from the hippocampus, carrying largely glutaminergic excitatory fibers from the hippocampus, subiculum, and entorhinal cortex to the septum, mamillary bodies, thalamic nuclei (anterior, dorsolateral, and intralaminar), amygdala, nucleus accumbens, posterior orbitofrontal cortex, and cingulate cortex.[17] Hippocampal efferents also reach widespread cortical areas via the entorhinal cortex.[18]

Several distinctive physiological attributes of the hippocampus may contribute to its unique role in memory, as well as its vulnerability to disease. For example, large pyramidal cells in the hippocampal CA1 sector (Sommer's sector) are metabolically very active and have a dense covering of N-methyl-D-aspartate receptors, but their exquisite sensitivity to hypoxia (Fig. 8–4B) accounts for the amnesic syndrome after cardiac arrest. A patient with severe anterograde amnesia (patient R.B.) had a lesion restricted to the CA1 region of the hippocampus on autopsy.[19] Brief, repetitive stimulation of dentate or hippocampal afferents led to a three-fold to fourfold potentiation of single stimuli along the same fibers for up to 2 hours.[20] Long-term potentiation of synaptic transmission exemplifies synaptic memory and plasticity and may partly underlie the hippocampal formation's role in memory[21] as well as its unusually low threshold for seizure activity.[22]

Behavioral studies of patients with bilateral hippocampal formation damage (i.e., the hippocampus and entorhinal cortex) advanced our notion of how these brain regions serve memory function. Since patients with extensive hippocampal lesions can recall information from before their injury (i.e., relatively preserved retrograde memory), it is unlikely that memories are stored in the hippocampus[23] Rather, the hippocampal formation likely builds "directories/address books" to bind and find fragments of experience.[24] Once learned, such memory representations are distributed throughout the neocortex.[23] These representations, both episodic (e.g., attending a recent musical concert) and semantic (e.g., the name of the last recording by your favorite musical artist), continue to consolidate over time. The hippocampal formation is critical not only for encoding new facts and experiences by establishing "initially sparse and fragile linkages, nurturing them, and inserting them into a matrix of existing knowledge" but also probably for accessing them.[25]

Although the hippocampus is now synonymous with memory, as more components of the medial temporal lobe system are damaged, the severity of episodic memory impairment increases. For example, damage restricted to the hippocampus proper, the dentate gyrus, and the subicular region causes less severe memory impairment than when damage extends to the entorhinal, perirhinal, and parahippocampal cortex.[26] Fornix lesions, interrupting projections from the hippocampus to medial mamillary nuclei, cause persistent episodic memory dysfunction in humans.[27–28]

Although the amygdala has extensive reciprocal projections with the hippocampus, its role in memory remains unclear since bilateral amygdalectomy in humans does not typically cause significant memory disturbance.[29] The amygdala appears critical in forming long-term emotional memories,[30] but it lacks a general role in memory (see Chapter 10). The amygdala bonds a stimulus with its emotional con-notation but cannot alter this association. It helps to mediate the influence of emotional valence on learning[31] and encode the emotional valence of an experience.[32]

FRONTAL LOBES

Episodic memory impairments in patients with prefrontal cortex damage clearly differ from those with medial temporal damage. Hecaen and Albert[33] summarized an enormous literature on frontal lobe memory deficits and concluded that impairments were due to inefficiencies caused by poor attention or poor executive function (see Chapter 9). Patients with prefrontal lesions show consistent impairment in multiple trial list learning tasks,[34] failing on recall measures but generally performing normally on recognition measures. This suggests defective retrieval, a function requiring strategy and effort, as opposed to normal storage, a more passive function.[35]

Patients with frontal lobe lesions also have defective recall of temporal order (i.e., recalling the context of learned items), even when they can remember these items.[36] Frontal lobe lesions impair *meta-memory*, one's knowledge and self-report of memory ability (i.e., they are very poor judges of "how well they know something").[37] In summary, patients with prefrontal cortex damage are impaired in "the process involved in planning, organization and other strategic aspects of learning and memory that may facilitate encoding and retrieval of information."[35]

Depending on the specific site of the frontal lobe lesion, the effects on episodic memory are substantially different.[38] Patients with left dorsolateral frontal lobe lesions are particularly impaired on list learning, which is highly correlated with deficits in lexicosemantic capacity measured by verbal fluency and naming tasks. Patients with right frontal lobe damage are particularly prone to perseverative errors in recall tasks. All of these patients are defective in applying strategies to improve learning.

Confabulation,[39] the production of fabricated verbal responses, usually occurs in patients with combined deficits in autobiographical (episodic) memory,[40] self-monitoring,[41] false recognition,[42] and temporal ordering.[43] The confabulatory responses produced by patients are described as "spontaneous" when they occur without any apparent motivation or "provoked" when they occur in response to questions from others. It is proposed that provoked confabulations depend on a patient's search in his or her deficient memory, whereas spontaneous confabulations are based on a failure to recognize the temporal order of stored information, resulting in erroneous recollection of elements of memory that do not belong together.[43]

Frontal lobe lesions, especially affecting posterior medial orbitofrontal cortex and its connections to the basal forebrain, lead to confabulation.[44–46] Such damage is typically seen after traumatic brain injury or rupture of an anterior communicating aneurysm.[45] In Korsakoff's amnesia, functional imaging studies reveal bilateral medial frontal and diencephalic hypometabolism. The amnesia persists, but the confabulation resolves as the frontal lobe abnormalities resolve,[41] providing additional evidence for a link between the frontal lobes and confabulation.

Confabulation, a verbal disorder, may also be considered the product of a left hemisphere "interpreter mechanism" that creates narrative explanations for actions of the disconnected right hemisphere.[47] Normal individuals typically recall many aspects of new experiences but, when questioned, often claim to remember details that were not part of the experience. When callosotomy patients are tested in the same paradigm, false recollections are generated by the left, but not the right, hemisphere; the right hemisphere provides a much more accurate account of the experience.[48]

THALAMUS

The critical structures within the thalamus for memory are the dorsomedial and anterior nuclei. The best-studied example of a memory disorder due to damage of these nuclei is Korsakoff's syndrome, which causes damage to both the mamillary bodies (which project to the anterior nucleus) and the dorsomedial nucleus of the thalamus.[49] Although these two structures are commonly implicated in causing episodic memory impairments, the specific thalamic lesion that is sufficient to cause memory dysfunction is still unclear. Two comprehensive clinicopathological studies of four cases of Korsakoff's syndrome showed that the site of damage was within the mamillary bodies and in an area of the medial thalamus

adjacent to the dorsomedial nucleus of the thalamus.[50,51]

Several factors limit brain–behavior correlations derived from Korsakoff's syndrome. First, because the cause is usually chronic alcoholism, many patients have diffuse cortical atrophy with prominent frontal lobe involvement, have had numerous mild traumatic brain injuries, and may have had recurrent seizures.[52,53] Second, damage to the dorsomedial thalamus (and its secondary effect on the prefrontal cortex, its projection site) can impair executive functions that modify the clinical appearance of memory impairments, as already mentioned.

The major differences between patients with Korsakoff's syndrome and patients with bilateral medial temporal lobe lesions concern retrograde amnesia and performance on several complex memory measures. Patients with Korsakoff's syndrome have a more severe retrograde amnesia, often showing a temporal gradient with better recall of more remote information.[54] Patients with Korsakoff's syndrome also perform poorly on the Brown-Peterson Task, a measure of long-term memory in the face of significant interference; exhibit increased sensitivity to proactive interference; and perform poorly on tasks that require memory for context. Performance on these memory measures is related to performance on "frontal" cognitive measures.[55,56] Patients with medial temporal lobe lesions perform much better on all of these memory tasks. Thus, in Korsakoff's syndrome, the pattern of memory impairment on these tasks is similar to that of patients with frontal lobe lesions. Patients with Korsakoff's syndrome often confabulate.

Other causes of damage to the thalamus provide a clearer understanding of this brain region's role in causing memory impairment. For example, careful study of amnesia following small thalamic infarcts defined the critical structures.[57,58] The mamillothalamic tract (originate in the mamillary bodies) and the ventral portion of the internal medullary lamina, which includes amygdala–thalamic connections (at the ventrolateral boundary of the dorsomedial nucleus of the thalamus), are the critical lesion sites for causing memory dysfunction. Thus, pathway lesions can be as important as nuclear lesions.[59]

Patients with bilateral thalamic infarcts initially have a depressed level of consciousness, ranging from a drowsy state to a deep coma.[60,61]

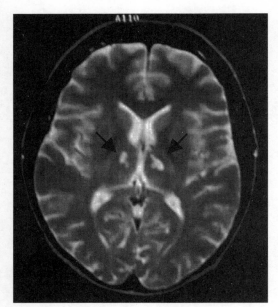

Figure 8–5. Magnetic resonance imaging scan of patient with bilateral medial thalamic infarcts.

These cells provide cholinergic input to the amygdala and to paralimbic and neocortical regions. Similar cells in the neighboring structures also provide cholinergic input: medial septal nucleus to the hippocampus and diagonal band nuclei to the olfactory cortex.[62] Together, these cells encompass a relatively broad area spanning from the septum anteriorly to the midbrain posteriorly, from which the entire cortex receives cholinergic innervation. These cells are similar to the substantia nigra–ventral tegmental area for dopaminergic innervation, the raphe nuclei for serotonergic innervation, and the locus ceruleus for noradrenergic innervation to the cortex. The substantia innominata also projects to the reticular nucleus of the thalamus[62] and may thereby indirectly influence the cortex since the reticular nucleus regulates thalamic transmission.[61] The substantia innominata also contains γ-aminobutyric acid-ergic (GABAergic) neurons and receives its input from the hypothalamus, amygdala, and limbic cortices.

Damage to the basal forebrain occurs most commonly after rupture of an anterior communicating artery aneurysm and may result in severe episodic memory dysfunction.[64] The minimal lesion in this region that produces memory dysfunction is unknown. It may be as small as damage to the septal nucleus (Fig. 8–7) or isolated damage to the diagonal band of Broca.[65,66] Irle and colleagues[67] studied memory function in a large group of patients with rupture of an anterior communicating artery aneurysm who were selected because of lesions in the ventromedial frontal lobe or striatum. The relation between lesion site and severity of memory dysfunction was clear: patients with combined lesions in the basal forebrain and striatum or the basal forebrain, striatum, and frontal lobes had a severe memory deficit, and patients with lesions in the basal forebrain or striatum alone had essentially no deficit. Patients with Alzheimer's disease also have early and profound episodic memory loss and a marked reduction of neurons in the nucleus basalis.[68,69]

Early neuroimaging may not reveal the infarctions (Fig. 8–5), which sometimes leads to a misdiagnosis. The period of hypoarousal may be brief, lasting a few days, or quite prolonged, lasting several weeks to months; but all patients eventually awaken. Following this hypersomnolent state, patients can have serious cognitive impairments. In particular, despite regaining alertness, they exhibit marked impairments in attention and mental control. Patients respond very slowly when attempting to perform tasks that test these cognitive functions and are easily distractable. Even after their attention improves, patients show deficits in executive function. They are initially disoriented, and memory testing reveals impairments in anterograde and retrograde memory. The pattern of memory deficits can be quite similar to the pattern found in Korsakoff's syndrome.

BASAL FOREBRAIN

The basal forebrain comprises the septal nuclei, diagonal band of Broca, and substantia innominata. Situated directly below the anterior commissure (Fig. 8–6), the substantia innominata is a group of loosely organized cells, including the clusters of large basophilic neurons comprising the basal nucleus of Meynert.

Semantic Memory

The limbic and cortical networks supporting semantic and episodic memory systems overlap but also contain separate circuits. Both

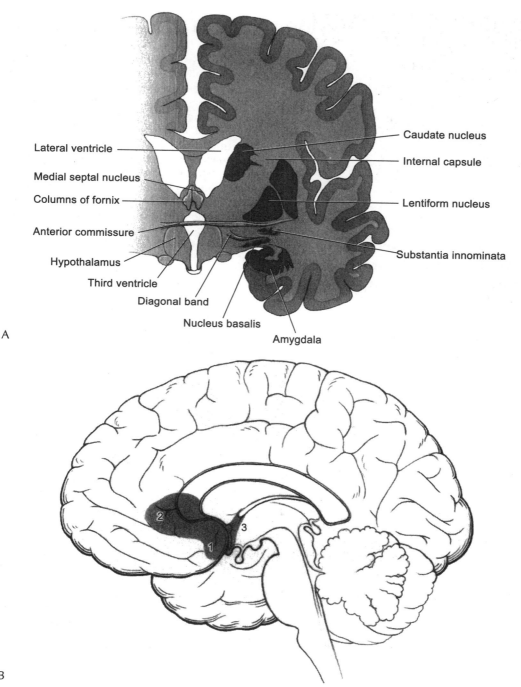

Figure 8–6. Anatomy of the basal forebrain. (A) Coronal view. (B) Sagittal view. Shaded area depicts the distribution of the circulation of the anterior communicating artery perforators. 1. basal forebrain. 2. anterior cingulate. 3, hypothalamus. Adapted from Alexander et al.[64]

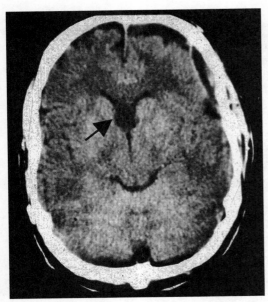

Figure 8–7. Computed tomographic scan of a patient with a septal infarction which resulted following rupture of an anterior communicating aneurysm. Arrow points to an area of infarction (hypodensity).

types of memory can become deeply embedded in the knowledge matrix through extensive links and repetitive exposure or a single, very strong emotional exposure. Once consolidated into the matrix of knowledge, semantic memories become independent of limbic connections, while episodic memories for personal experiences remain tethered to limbic areas. For semantic memories, the unimodal and heteromodal cortical areas are repositories for general knowledge regarding facts about our world.

Patients with degenerative disease, such as Pick's disease, can present with a selective impairment of semantic memory,[70–72] the syndrome of "semantic dementia." Despite being relatively good on most tasks of language and cognition, these patients do poorly on tasks that require intact semantic memory. Such tasks include confrontation naming, word–picture matching, and naming or answering questions about presented pictures (e.g., showing a picture of a bottle of wine and asking if it contains alcohol). When attempting to name a picture, patients with semantic dementia often make semantic paraphasic errors; that is, they will produce a related word, such as *fork* for *spoon*. In a naming task, patients will not typically benefit from being provided with a phonemic cue, such as *spo-* when shown a picture of a spoon.

Thus, on language testing, these patients can have normal phonology as well as syntax. The hallmark of this syndrome is that patients appear to have intact recall of past autobiographical information, and their day-to-day memory seems unaffected.

Neurodegenerative disorders and focal lesions causing semantic dementia typically affect the left temporal or frontal lobes.[73] This pattern of brain damage suggests that semantic knowledge, especially for nouns and semantic representations of living things, is distributed mainly in the lateral temporal lobe. In contrast, the medial temporal lobes are crucial for episodic memory. In addition to frontotemporal dementia, other neurological disorders that selectively affect the lateral temporal lobes and severely impair semantic memory include herpes encephalitis[74] and traumatic brain injury.[75] In patients with these disorders, where damage to the temporal lobes may be more restricted than in patients with degenerative disease, impairments may remarkably be limited to certain categories of semantic knowledge. For example, patients may show a disproportionate impairment in the knowledge of living things (e.g., animals) compared with nonliving things.[74] Other patients have a disproportionate deficit in knowledge of nonliving things.[76] These observations led to the notion that the semantic memory system is subdivided into different sensorimotor modalities.[74,77] For instance, living things, compared with nonliving things, are represented by their visual and other sensory attributes (e.g., a banana is yellow), while nonliving things are represented by their function (e.g., a hammer is a tool but comes in many different visual forms). In addition, distinct neural substrates may serve different categories of semantic knowledge. The small number of patients with these deficits, and often large lesions, limits precise anatomical–behavioral relationships. However, functional neuroimaging studies in normal subjects reveal that distinct regions within the neocortex are activated during retrieval of different categories of semantic knowledge[78] (see Chapter 6, Fig. 6–8).

Procedural Memory

Procedural memory is the acquisition of sensorimotor, perceptual, or cognitive skills. Skill learning is measured by improved accuracy or speed with practice. Once acquired, procedural memories are often difficult or impossible to access consciously (see Chapter 3). For example, riding a bicycle or typing is easier to do than describing the skills knowledge required to perform such a task. Although optimal performance of skills requires neocortical systems, skill learning relies heavily on basal ganglia and cerebellar functions.[79] The subcortical systems involved in procedural memory vary by task.[80,81]

Patients with dense amnesias often exhibit dramatic dissociation for episodic and semantic information and normal skill learning. Thus, patients with bilateral medial temporal lobe lesions in Alzheimer's disease or after encephalitis may be unable to learn a list or recall what they ate for breakfast that day but show intact learning of mirror tracing, rotary pursuit, or serial reaction time.[82] Similarly, amnestic patients can learn perceptual skills (e.g., read mirror-reversed text) or cognitive skills (e.g., Tower Tasks that require problem solving and planning, probabilistic classification problems). In contrast, patients with basal ganglia disorders, such as Huntington's disease and Parkinson's disease, perform at or near normal on declarative memory tasks but exhibit moderate to severe impairment on these sensorimotor, perceptual, and cognitive skill learning tasks.[83] Cerebellar lesions impair sensorimotor procedural memories,[84] with less well-studied effects on perceptual and cognitive procedural memories.

Working (Short-Term) Memory

Working memory refers to the short-term storage of information that is inaccessible in the environment and the processes that keep this information active for later use in behavior.[85,86] For example, holding in mind a telephone number given to you by the operator while you are searching for a pencil and paper requires working memory. Both animal and human studies show that the prefrontal cortex is critical for working memory. For example, prefrontal neurons exhibit persistent activity when a monkey temporarily maintains information in memory,[87,88] and prefrontal lesions impair working memory.[89,90] Working memory impairments occur in humans following restricted prefrontal cortex damage,[91–93] and prefrontal cortex is activated on functional neuroimaging

studies of normal subjects during working memory tasks (for a review, see D'Esposito).[94] Chapter 9 includes an in-depth discussion of working memory and the role of the frontal lobes in this cognitive ability.

MEMORY DYSFUNCTION PATTERNS IN NEUROLOGICAL DISORDERS

The nature of the memory deficit in various neurological disorders depends on the extent and location of the cortical and subcortical damage. As previously discussed, several different brain networks support memory function, and each memory process (e.g., episodic vs. semantic memory) is supported by distinct but overlapping networks. Thus, focal brain damage will cause a pattern of memory impairment that will affect some memory processes and leave others intact. For example, with bilateral medial temporal lesions, short-term memory is normal, as in patient H.M., who had a normal digit span,[10] but long-term episodic memory is severely impaired. Semantic memory is generally preserved, although acquisition of new semantic knowledge is deficient,[95] and retrieval of general semantic knowledge may be subtly defective after medial temporal lobe damage.[96] Remote memory of personal events (retrograde amnesia) is variably affected, but in cases with damage limited to the hippocampus, the retrograde deficit is usually restricted to a brief period (weeks to a few years) before the injury.[10,97] All implicit memory tasks are performed normally.[98,99] Notably, patients with restricted medial temporal lobe damage, such as H.M., do not suffer a decline in intellect, as measured by the intelligence quotient (IQ). Other cognitive skills, such as reading, writing, and visuoperception, mediated by other areas of the cerebral cortex, are not affected.

Although memory is supported by distinct neural networks, lesions in brain regions critical for any aspect of information processing produce learning deficits that depend on that process. For example, aphasic patients will have learning and memory deficits for material that requires encoding of specific language processes. These learning and memory impairments are specific to disturbed language processes.[100,101] Patients with phonological deficits are impaired in verbal short-term memory (i.e., they have a reduced digit span), and patients with lexical–semantic deficits are impaired in verbal long-term memory (i.e., they are impaired at learning new verbal information). The same phenomenon occurs in patients with perceptual deficits for visual memory. Many patients complain of memory problems that are due to processing deficits and not impaired memory per se. Thus, neuropsychological tests showing a "verbal memory problem" in mildly aphasic patients may shed little light on a patient's real experiential memory capacity.

MEMORY DISORDERS

Acute Memory Disorders

TRANSIENT GLOBAL AMNESIA

Originally reported by Bender,[102] the clinical features of transient global amnesia were expanded and the name coined by Fisher and Adams[103] in 1958. Since then, comprehensive reviews of transient global amnesia have been published.[104] Transient global amnesia occurs in middle-aged and elderly adults (usually around age 60) who present with confusion, anxiety, mild or moderate agitation, and amnesia. The patient typically repeats questions concerning location ("Where am I?" "How did I get here?"), objects in the environment ("Whose car is that?"), and time. Episodes begin abruptly and last from 30 minutes to 24 hours but usually 2–4 hours. During the attack, patients retain personal identity and can recall remote memories but cannot store or retrieve newly acquired information (i.e., episodic memories). Thus, when patients are told the location and date, they will often repeat the question a minute later, having remembered neither the previous question nor the answer. During the attack, performance of complex motor tasks is preserved, and the patient may skillfully drive a car or throw a ball (i.e., procedural memories).

After the attack of transient global amnesia has resolved, there may be retrograde amnesia spanning minutes to hours (patients cannot recall events before the onset of the episode), as well as anterograde amnesia lasting hours.[105] In many cases, attacks follow specific precipitating factors. Physical exertion, sexual intercourse, emotional stress, physical symptoms (e.g., pain, nausea, vomiting), and exposure to

cold temperatures are the most frequent precipitants, in order of decreasing frequency.[106] Although the episodes are usually single, recurrences affect about 15% of patients.[104]

Caplan[107] proposed four criteria for transient global amnesia: (1) onset of the attack is witnessed, (2) dysfunction during the attack is limited to repetitive queries and amnesia, (3) no other major neurological signs and symptoms, and (4) transient memory loss, usually lasting hours or up to a day. When these criteria are met, the diagnosis of transient global amnesia is certain, and a good prognosis can almost always be assured. The incidence of subsequent transient ischemic attacks and strokes is not significantly different from that in the general population of the same sex and similar age.[104] Hodges and Warlow[108] added a fifth criterion for a benign outcome: duration of attack longer than 1 hour. In their study of 153 cases of transient global amnesia, when attacks lasted less than 1 hour and were rapidly recurrent, the disorder was often epilepsy. When historical information is fragmentary or if the medical history or neurological examination reveals other signs or symptoms, the disorder is often not classic transient global amnesia but another disorder associated with amnesia.

The pathophysiology of transient global amnesia is uncertain, and in 60%–70% of 114 cases studied by Hodges and Warlow,[108] the underlying etiology was not clear after a complete work-up. Multiple mechanisms have been implicated, including migraine,[109], Leão's spreading depression,[110] cerebral ischemia in the posterior cerebral artery distribution,[111] and partial epilepsy.[112]

Patients with transient global amnesia have a dysfunction of the medial temporal lobes or diencephalon or both, which disappears after recovery.[113,114] Transient global amnesia likely results from mainly limbic–hippocampal dysfunction, but evidence for this specific mechanism is lacking.[115] Although most attacks are not migraines, transient global amnesia may represent another brain state to which migraine patients are susceptible. An epileptic cause seems unlikely since the electroencephalogram (EEG) is almost always normal, both during and between attacks.[116,117] Further, transient global amnesia is not common in young patients with migraine or epilepsy. Diffusion-weighted MRIs in patients with transient global amnesia[118,119] have supported a spreading depression[110] rather than an ischemic origin. Also, an MRI spectroscopy study of a patient during and 2 weeks after a transient global amnesia episode showed no evidence of ischemia, indirectly supporting a spreading depression mechanism.[120]

OTHER ACUTE MEMORY IMPAIRMENTS

Memory can be acutely impaired by a variety of conditions (Table 8–1). Traumatic brain injury is a very common cause; in some cases, relatively minor injuries trigger prominent memory impairment. However, when traumatic brain injury causes memory impairment, the injury is often significant, with loss of consciousness, and associated with other neurological signs and symptoms (see Chapter 9). Migraine may cause memory impairment with or without other neurological abnormalities.[121,122] Multiple attacks in a patient suggest an epileptic basis for transient memory impairment.[112] Complex partial seizures always impair memory during the episode, and patients may repetitively utter the same phrase or question or speak in full sentences (usually with right temporal lobe foci.[123] However, the unresponsiveness (i.e., the inability to answer such questions as "What is your name?") and automatisms clearly distinguish most complex partial seizures from transient global amnesia.[124] Pure amnestic seizures are characterized by impaired memory retention for what occurs during the seizure despite preservation of other cognitive skills and normal interactions with the physical and social environments.[125–127] Pure amnestic seizures never represent the only type of seizures. Such seizures are hypothesized to result from bilateral mesial temporal lobe involvement with sparing of the neocortex in the temporal and other lobes.[128]

Focal cortical damage from stroke can acutely impair memory. Cerebral ischemia in the posterior cerebral artery (PCA) territory, involving the thalamus or hippocampus or both, transiently or permanently impairs memory.[129,130] Damage to either the right or the left PCA territory can cause memory impairment restricted to a single material (e.g., verbal deficit after left PCA infarct or spatial deficit after right PCA infarct)[131] or a single modality (e.g., visual or tactile).[132,133] Transient ischemic attacks can also cause transient memory impairment. Other neurological disorders that can cause focal damage to the medial temporal lobes, resulting in severe memory impairments, include herpes encephalitis[134] (Fig. 8–8) and cerebral anoxia (Fig. 8–4B).[135,136]

Hypoglycemia often causes episodic confusion and memory impairment.[137] Intoxication with alcohol ("blackouts"), benzodiazepines, or anticholinergics produces transient amnesia. (Anticholinergics are sometimes given in a "pharmacological mugging" attack: the mugger puts some scopolamine in a drink and the victim never remembers the drink or the hours before the drink.) Dissociative disorders, including multiple personality disorder, psychogenic fugue, and psychogenic amnesia, are characterized by disturbances of self and memory.[131] Loss of personal identity in these patients distinguishes these disorders from transient global amnesia. Another clue may be the disproportionate deficit in retrograde memory function and the ability to use information that is not recalled.[138]

Table 8–1. **Disorders Associated with Acute Onset of Amnesia**

Cerebral ischemia

Drug intoxication (benzodiazepines, scopolamine, alcohol)

Epilepsy

Herpes encephalitis

Hypoglycemia

Migraine

Psychiatric disorders

Transient global amnesia

Traumatic brain injury

Chronic Memory Disorders

Dementia, the global deterioration of cognitive and intellectual functions, is usually associated with personality changes severe enough to impair personal or occupational performance. The cardinal and often presenting feature of dementia is impaired memory, accompanied by impairments in at least two other cognitive abilities, such as language, visuoperception, or executive function. In most dementias, the loss

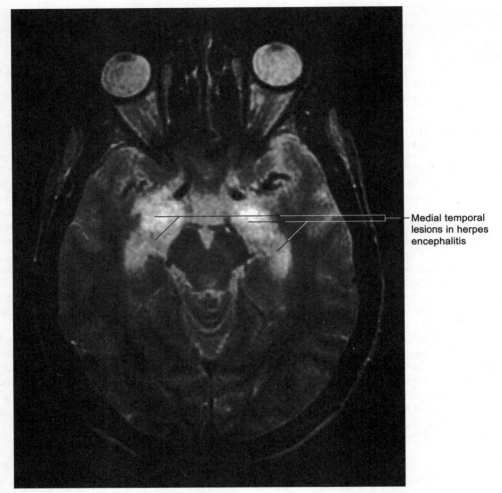

Medial temporal lesions in herpes encephalitis

Figure 8–8. Magnetic resonance imaging scan of a patient with bilateral medial temporal lesions caused by acute herpes encephalitis.

of mental functions is progressive, occurring steadily or gradually, as in Alzheimer's disease, or in discrete steps, as in multi-infarct or vascular dementia.

ALZHEIMER'S DISEASE

Alzheimer's disease (AD) probably accounts for more than half of all cases of dementia.[139] The landmark case report by Alois Alzheimer described the silver-staining neuropathological neurofibrillary tangles and neuritic plaques in a 55-year-old woman with progressive dementia.[140] The diagnosis of AD was initially restricted to cases of "presenile dementia" in patients younger than 65 years. However, the clinical and pathological features of degenerative dementia starting before or after age 65 years are indistinguishable,[141] and AD is now diagnosed without an age limit. The incidence and prevalence of AD increases with age, with rare cases in the fourth decade. One representative epidemiological study found that incidence rates rise from 2.8 per 1000 person-years in the age group 65–69 years to 56.1 per 1000 person-years in the older than 90-year age group.[142]

Although AD usually occurs sporadically, familial AD is linked to mutations in the amyloid precursor protein *(APP)* gene on chromosome 21,[143,144] the presenilin 1 gene on chromosome 14,[145] and the presenilin 2 gene on chromosome 1.[146] A common polymorphism in the apolipoprotein E (*APOE*) gene is linked to the more common late-onset form of the disease, greatly increasing the risk of developing AD.[147,148] Further, studies implicate at least four additional genes other than *APOE* in late-onset AD. One of these may make a greater contribution to variation in age at onset than the *APOE* ϵ4 allele.[149] Most cases of AD may be hereditary, but delayed disease expression until age 80 years or later prevents recognition of familial patterns.[150]

Pathologically, AD is characterized by neuronal loss, large extracellular β-amyloid plaques, neuritic plaques, and τ-containing intraneuronal neurofibrillary tangles scattered in the brain's frontal, parietal, and temporal association cortices, limbic areas, and subcortical regions, including the basal nucleus of Meynert, locus ceruleus, raphe nucleus, and hypothalamus. There is relative sparing of primary motor, somatosensory, and visual cortices, as well as the basal ganglia.[151]

The β-amyloid in plaques is a metabolite of the APP that forms from alternative (β-secretase and then γ-secretase) enzymatic pathways.[152] Mutations in the *APP* gene may contribute to AD by modulating APP metabolism. Theories of neuronal death in AD include direct toxicity of Aβ in plaques, intracellular events during APP processing, or extraneuronal preplaque Aβ oligomers. The severity of dementia in AD is more closely related to the degree of the associated neuronal and synaptic loss.[152]

The slow, progressive course of intellectual and behavioral deterioration is the most characteristic clinical feature of AD. The first stage (years 1–4) is marked by an insidious loss of episodic long-term memory. Patients forget information, misplace objects, annoyingly repeat questions or stories, and commonly get lost in new places. Patients are often brought to medical attention when relatives become concerned over their failing memory. At first, patients are unable to learn new information. Even in mild cases, recent memory is impaired for bits of information that exceed digit span. Initially, there is a prominent dissociation between preserved recall of autobiographical information and remote memories and impaired recall of recently acquired information. However, as the disease advances, remote memory progressively worsens. Early cognitive problems include word-finding difficulty during spontaneous speech and diminished abstract thought and planning. In most cases, the patient is unaware of or vigorously denies any problem. However, the patient may realize his or her brain is failing and respond with irritability, withdrawal, and sadness. Occasionally, AD presents as delirium in a patient with a medical illness such as pneumonia. When the pneumonia and delirium resolve, the patient is no longer the same: dementia is finally recognized. Mildly demented patients can live independently with reasonable hygiene, nutrition, and judgment despite significant impairment in cognitive, social, or work activities.

As the disease progresses to the second stage (years 4–10), the cognitive and behavioral symptoms worsen and the spectrum of impaired functions widens. Memory for both recent and remote events is severely impaired. Patients cannot recall their addresses or phone numbers. They may misplace the list that allayed amnesia in the first stage or, worse still, forget to make it. However, even in moderately advanced stages of the disease, inappropriate insertions of fragments from a conversation 10–30 minutes before can occur, demonstrating that some information does "get in."[153] Spatial disorientation causes the patient to get lost in the neighborhood. A dangerous combination of cognitive deficits, slowed reaction time, and impaired vision and hearing makes motor vehicle accidents more likely.[154] Fluent aphasia with circumlocution and empty speech, diminished auditory and written comprehension, and difficulty with even simple calculations develop.[155]

During the second stage of AD, personality changes that were annoying during the initial stage move to the forefront, causing great difficulty for family, friends, and support persons. Apathy, indifference, and rigidity intensify. Premorbid personality traits may be grossly exaggerated or reversed. Patients become fearful, paranoid, and delusional. They accuse their spouses of infidelity, blame nursing aides for losing their misplaced items, or want police called to remove imaginary burglars and enemies from the house. Stubborn insistence on their wants and opinions often provokes disagreements and, in some cases, agitated and aggressive behaviors.[153,156] Patients refuse to participate in or allow others to provide basic care. They become restless, impatient, and argumentative. Rudeness extends from embarrassing comments to undressing, passing flatus, and urinating in public. Patients in this stage are not safe in a completely unsupervised setting. They are likely to ignore important aspects of hygiene, eat a very limited diet, drive unsafely, and have difficulty with finances, which makes them vulnerable to aggressive salespeople. Severely demented patients function at an extremely low level, making activities of daily living (e.g., shopping, eating, or bathing) difficult or impossible. They require continuous supervision.

The third and terminal stage of AD (years 7–14) is a near-vegetative existence as the patient becomes more akinetic and mute. After 6–12 years of illness, intellect and memory deteriorate to the point that patients no longer recognize spouses or children. Personal hygiene and nutrition are ignored. Sphincter control is lost, and a progressive gait disorder with smaller and less certain steps, rigidity, and flexed extremities causes the patient to become bedridden. Seizures may occur. Death commonly comes from infection and trauma.[157]

PICK'S DISEASE

Pick's disease, or frontotemporal dementia, is a degenerative dementia affecting the frontal and temporal lobes.[158] Pick's disease occurs in adulthood, with a peak between 55 and 65 years, which is typically earlier than in AD. There is a slight female predominance. In most cases, the disease is inherited as an autosomal dominant trait, although the cause is unknown. There is approximately one case of Pick's disease for every 75–100 cases of AD.[159] Patients present with personality changes typical of the frontal lobe syndrome: disinhibition, loss of social graces, jocularity, and apathy punctuated by irritability. Difficulty with concentration and language dysfunction is common during the early stages, with reduced verbal output and word-finding difficulty (anomic aphasia). Temporal involvement may predominate early on, with transcortical or fluent aphasias and isolated semantic memory impairments, as discussed earlier. For an in-depth discussion of Pick's disease and other frontotemporal dementias, see Chapter 9.

During the initial stages of illness, prototypical cases of Pick's disease—with prominent personality changes but relatively preserved memory, visuospatial skills, and praxis—can be

recognized as distinct from AD, in which memory, language, and visuospatial impairments predominate. However, as Pick's disease progresses, it may become more difficult to distinguish from AD.

NONPROGRESSIVE AND PSEUDODEMENTIA

Acute or subacute nonprogressive dementia may occur after such insults as encephalitis, anoxia, traumatic brain injury, stroke, or massive demyelination. For example, patients with Wernicke's aphasia due to a left middle cerebral artery stroke superficially appear confused or demented. These patients make no sense when they speak and cannot comprehend spoken or written language. This is a common misinterpretation of the patient's clinical problem, especially among family members or friends who first encounter the patient after the stroke. The lack of motor or sensory signs may contribute to a misdiagnosis. Acute confusional states are due to a deficit in attention (see Chapter 4), rather than a deficit in language, the salient feature of Wernicke's aphasia (see Chapter 6). Delirium, the most common acute confusional state (see Chapter 4), must be considered before dementia is diagnosed. Dementia is usually not associated with a clouded sensorium and is not transient. In contrast, an attentional deficit is always present in delirium.

Psychiatric disorders may also be confused with dementia caused by neurological disease. Kiloh (1961)[160] introduced the term pseudodementia to describe patients in whom the diagnosis of dementia was considered but "abandoned because of the subsequent course of the illness." His patients were ultimately diagnosed with depression, conversion disorder, malingering, mania, paraphrenia (late-life psychosis), or Ganser syndrome (a dissociative disorder in which patients give "approximate answers" to questions and amnesia and disorientation are often present). Kiloh recognized that the term pseudodementia is "purely descriptive and carries no diagnostic weight." Depression is the most common psychiatric cause of pseudodementia.[161] In people of all ages, depression causes psychological symptoms (e.g., sadness, helplessness, hopelessness, and worthlessness) and vegetative symptoms (e.g., sleep disturbance, especially early morning awakening, diminished appetite, and impaired libido).

In the elderly, however, intellectual dysfunction is a prominent feature: 10%–20% of older depressed patients have serious cognitive deficits.[162] Thus, some patients initially diagnosed with dementia are later found to have primary depression.

The clinical features that distinguish primary degenerative dementia from depressive pseudodementia are shown in Table 8–2. Demented patients are often unaware of or offer only modest complaints of cognitive impairment, while depressive patients may exaggerate or focus on cognitive problems. Bedside mental status testing reveals stable or progressive deficits in dementia and variable performance in pseudodementia. The dissociation between mild cognitive deficits on mental status testing and presentation of severe functional disability suggests pseudodementia. Neuropsychological testing early in the course of dementia will show deficits in cognitive abilities that reflect the nature of the disease. For example, patients with early AD have language, memory, and visuospatial deficits but sparing of other abilities. In contrast, depressed patients often show some impairment across all cognitive domains. In some pseudodementia patients, the attentional deficit or poor cooperation on neuropsychological tests may falsely indicate profound cognitive losses. Retesting often shows dramatic fluctuations in certain cognitive functions, reflecting variability in effort. A meta-analysis of neuropsychological studies of depression found that, relative to healthy control subjects, depressed patients

were more impaired on speed-dependent tasks and vigilance tasks (i.e., effortful tasks).[163] Impairment on both effortful and noneffortful tasks suggests dementia, not pseudodementia. Depressive pseudodementia is best differentiated from dementia by observing improved affective and cognitive symptoms with antidepressant therapy and no progressive intellectual decline after at least 1 year of follow-up.

Other psychiatric disorders that may present as pseudodementia in the elderly include personality disorders, late-life psychosis, conversion disorder, somatization disorder, dissociative disorders, and paranoid disorder. Paranoia is common among the elderly and results from life stresses (e.g., social isolation, loss of loved ones, or loss of employment), physical deterioration, and sensory deprivation, as well as psychopathological processes. In many older persons, paranoia is combined with delusions and hallucinations.[164]

DIFFERENTIAL DIAGNOSIS OF DEMENTIA

In the work-up of patients with dementia, treatable causes must be excluded. Such causes include depression, hypothyroidism, normal pressure hydrocephalus, neurosyphilis, or other metabolic derangements such as hypercalcemia. Serological studies and neuroimaging can easily rule out these possibilities. Commonly, however, the results of the dementia work-up are equivocal, with for example, *(1)* hydrocephalus "in between" ex vacuo

Table 8–2. **Differential Diagnosis of Dementia versus Pseudodementia**

Feature	Dementia	Pseudodementia
Onset	Often insidious	Usually acute or subacute
Progression	Usually slow, early changes often missed	Usually rapid
Symptom duration at presentation	Long	Short
Psychiatric history or recent life crisis	Uncommon	Common
Extensive self-report of mental impairment	Uncommon	Common
Mental status or psychometric testing	Progressive decline	Variable, effort-related
Memory impairment	Common, most severe for recent events	Common, often selective amnesia, inconsistent deficits over time
Affective changes	Apathy, shallow emotions	Depression common
Nocturnal exacerbation of symptoms	Common	Uncommon

(atrophy) and occult (normal pressure); (2) a small area of encephalomalacia or multiple, small, unidentified bright objects on imaging studies; or (3) a moderately elevated serum calcium level. Under these circumstances, conservative therapeutic trials, such as a tap test for hydrocephalus or judicious hydration for hypercalcemia, may be helpful.

There are currently no biochemical tests or histological findings in readily accessible tissue that permit a definitive diagnosis of AD or other related neurodegenerative disorders causing dementia. For AD, the demonstration of plaques and tangles in the brain is the only absolute criterion for diagnosis. Brain biopsy is not indicated, however, because of its risks and the lack of curative treatment for AD. Furthermore, the chances of discovering a treatable disorder by brain biopsy are exceeding low when other diagnostic studies are negative. Cerebrospinal fluid (CSF) biomarkers are not currently used to diagnose AD as the improvement over clinical diagnostic tests may be only 10%.[165] However, recent advances in the specificity and sensitivity of diagnostic markers, such as CSF levels of paired-helical-filament τ protein and the ratio of amyloid β proteins 40 and 42 ($A\beta40/A\beta42$), suggest that the technique may soon be useful in some cases.[166–168] In a small study, the ratio of ventricular CSF 8-hydroxyguanine levels in intact DNA to free levels showed a marked difference between all AD patients and all control subjects.[169] If confirmed in lumbar CSF, this test could offer a very sensitive and specific diagnostic tool for AD.

After excluding treatable causes of dementia, a mental status examination remains the most useful tool for distinguishing the dementias. For example, AD typically presents with memory difficulties followed by difficulties in language and visuospatial abilities, reflecting the predominantly posterior (temporal and parietal) involvement of early disease. In contrast, Pick's disease (frontotemporal dementia) affects the frontal and anterior temporal lobes and initially presents with personality changes, impairments in executive abilities, and language disability. Functional neuroimaging studies, such as positron emission tomography (PET) or single-photon emission computed tomography (SPECT),[170] are useful adjunctive diagnostic tests, often revealing hypometabolism. In AD, hypometabolism is first detected

in the posterior cingulate and precuneus, followed by broader parietotemporal association cortex. In the frontal variant of frontotemporal dementia, hypometabolism first appears in the ventromedial frontal region, followed by prefrontal and anterior temporal regions. In semantic dementia (temporal variant of frontotemporal dementia), metabolic or blood flow changes are first detected in one or both temporal lobes.[171]

MEMORY REHABILITATION

There are two general approaches to improving memory after neurological injury: pharmacological therapy and cognitive remediation therapy. Neither approach has profoundly impacted the recovery and rehabilitation of memory disorders, perhaps because both therapies remain primitive. Pharmacological interventions aim at simple replacement or augmentation of a neurotransmitter that is considered critical in memory function. Cognitive remediation interventions attempt to "exercise" the weakened memory system. Critical appraisal of these approaches guides investigators to novel, innovative ways of treating memory disorders.

Pharmacological Therapy

EPISODIC MEMORY

The neurotransmitter most closely linked to long-term episodic memory function is acetylcholine. Early studies observed that healthy young subjects had reduced immediate and delayed free recall of word lists after administration of the anticholinergic scopolamine.[172,173] Further, anticholinergics impair episodic memory only, leaving semantic, procedural, and short-term memory intact.[174] This pattern of memory deficits in normal subjects mimics that observed in dementia and could be alleviated by physostigmine, a cholinesterase inhibitor, which prolongs acetylcholine action within the synapse.[174,175] This observation led to numerous investigations of acetylcholine replacement and augmentation therapy for memory enhancement in dementia patients, especially AD, where the dominant cognitive impairment is amnesia.[177] Several observations support cholinergic therapy for memory loss in AD: the synthetic enzyme choline acetyltransferase is markedly reduced in the amygdala, hippocampus, and neocortex;[178] also, enzyme reduction is correlated with senile plaque formation and mental status test scores, and there is severe neuronal loss in the nucleus basalis of Meynert, the major source of cholinergic input to the cortex.[68]

Overall, clinical trials with cholinergic medications in AD have been disappointing since improvement in memory function was neither dramatic nor sustained.[179,180] Three such medications have been approved by the Food and Drug Administration: tacrine, donepezil, and rivastigmine (see Chapter 11). These medications are anticholinesterase inhibitors, which increase the synaptic levels of acetylcholine in the brain. Clinical trials of these medications (e.g., donepezil) produced modest improvement in some patients, and more than 80% of patients showed no decline over 6 months of therapy.[181] A handful of single-case studies reported on cholinergic drugs administered to patients with memory impairments due to acute brain injury. Two patients with temporal lobe damage, one from herpes encephalitis and one from a penetrating injury, showed improvement on long-term memory tasks with cholinergic agonists.[182,183] In an open trial involving a patient with a lesion limited to the diagonal band of Broca in the basal forebrain after surgical resection of a low-grade glioma, physostigmine produced modest improvement in immediate recall of a word list. However, physostigmine was of no benefit during a 6-day double-blind, placebo-controlled trial[184] in which SPECT showed decreased blood flow in the medial temporal region ipsilateral to the lesion during the baseline study and increased blood flow in this region after a physostigmine dose.

WORKING MEMORY

Few studies have addressed pharmacological therapeutic intervention in working memory impairments. The frontal lobes, critical for working memory, contain the highest concentration of dopaminergic receptors in the cortex.[185] Further, in animal studies, depletion of dopamine in the frontal lobes or pharmacological blockade of dopamine impaired working memory function.[184,185] Dopaminergic drugs reversed the working memory impairments in these animals.[186,188]

Dopamine is also linked to working memory function in humans (see Chapter 9). Healthy young human subjects given dopaminergic agonists, such as bromocriptine[189] or pergolide,[190] performed better on working memory tasks than with placebo. In both of these studies, the dopaminergic medication specifically affected working memory since it had no effects on other cognitive measures such as attention or sensorimotor function.

Another study of bromocriptine and working memory in healthy young subjects found that the effect varied by subject, interacting with the individual's short-term memory capacity.[191] Subjects with lower baseline working memory abilities tended to show cognitive improvement while on the drug, and subjects with higher baseline working memory abilities worsened. Thus, there may be an optimal level of dopamine necessary for working memory abilities.

These investigations in humans and other primates faintly outline an initial pharmacological model of memory and possibly provide a foundation for developing pharmacological therapies to improve cognition. Acetylcholine may be critical for episodic long-term memory, and dopamine may modulate working memory. Extensive animal studies draw a much more complex picture. Many other neurotransmitters, such as GABA, serotonin, and norepinephrine, also play a role in memory function.[192] Neuromodulators, such as neuropeptides (e.g., opioids and vasopressin), also influence memory processes.[193] The operation of memory systems involves the interaction of multiple neurochemicals. Treatment directed at a single neurotransmitter is unlikely to affect memory significantly. Altering several neurotransmitter systems, especially systems that are less affected but involved in memory processes, offers an innovative approach for improving memory. For example, rats have a high concentration of GABA receptors in the basal forebrain, and GABA agonists (e.g., benzodiazepines) decrease acetylcholine release and impair memory. In contrast, GABA agonists reverse the amnesic effects of anticholinergics.[194] In another study, low-dose cholinergic and noradrenergic agonists improved memory performance in rats depleted of acetylcholine and norepinephrine.[195] Low doses of either agonist alone could not improve memory. This finding challenges the monotherapy approach commonly practiced in current clinical trials that attempt to improve cognition. Clinical trials using drug combinations that affect different neurotransmitter systems may be fruitful.

Questions about the influence of different lesion sites on treatment parallel the uncertainties about the critical mix of neurotransmitters involved in memory processing. Extensive bilateral damage to the hippocampus may leave little substrate for pharmacological therapy to influence. Lesions that damage pathways (e.g., fornix, cingulate bundle, collateral isthmus) might respond better to drug treatment because receptor neurons are intact. Future investigations must choose specific neurochemical agents, study specific cognitive processes, and control for extent and location of brain damage to discover and dissociate the different neurochemical substrates from the different components and mechanisms of memory.

Cognitive Remediation Therapy

Cognitive remediation for memory rehabilitation developed along three general lines: (1) retraining a damaged memory system through exercises and drills, (2) using compensatory strategies such as memory aids and mnemonics, and (3) tapping residual learning abilities.

MEMORY RETRAINING

The notion that practice improves memory led to the early domination of retraining techniques in memory rehabilitation programs. However, repetitive practice does not effectively apply to real-life situations despite numerous hours of intensive training.[196,197] A dramatic illustration is the case of a man who increased his digit span from 7 to 80 by repetitive practice, but when switched to a memory span task using letters, his performance dropped to 7 items, the average span performance.[198] Unlike a weakened muscle, damaged memory processes show little recovery through repetition training. The proliferation of inexpensive software for personal computers that allows endless memory drills increases the likelihood that patients will be exposed to memory rehabilitation paradigms without therapeutic value.[199,200]

COMPENSATORY STRATEGIES

The alternative to repetition retraining is to develop compensatory strategies for impaired memory abilities. Memory rehabilitation does not seek to restore the unrestorable but to produce improvements that allow patients to understand and cope with these difficulties, thereby facilitating a more normal life.[201] One popular compensatory strategy for memory impairment is to use visual imagery to organize information during learning to facilitate later recall; the assumption is that broader encoding enhances recall. Experimental evidence shows improvement in memory recall when learned items are linked with visual images. For example, patients with left hemisphere damage showed improved verbal memory after being trained to link each word on a list of 10 items with a ridiculous but vivid visual image. For example, *teacup* is linked with *radio* by imagining drinking tea from a radio instead of a cup.[202] Training to link a list of verbal paired associates with a visual image improved verbal recall in patients with left temporal lobectomy but was of no benefit in patients with right temporal lobectomy.[203] Thus, an intact right medial temporal lobe system may use image-mediated verbal learning to compensate for verbal learning deficits following left medial temporal lobe damage. Unfortunately, patients with more severe memory disturbances due to bilateral lesions, including patient H.M., do not benefit from visual imagery. These patients are unable even to remember the images taught during initial learning to enhance memory recall.

Optimism generated from these techniques must be tempered by their limitations when they are used outside of the laboratory. First, elaborative encoding by visual imagery or other mnemonics places excessive demands on brain-damaged patients with limited processing capacities.[204] Second, even if amnesic patients can use these strategies, many patients are unaware of their memory deficits and therefore unmotivated to use them spontaneously. Third, even subjects with normal memory may not use these mnemonic techniques when attempting to recall past learned information.[200] Finally, mental imagery may help amnesic patients to learn a short shopping list, but it would be just as useful to teach the patient to write the items down on a piece of paper, the ultimate compensatory strategy.[6]

A simple compensatory technique that can effectively help memory-impaired patients is the use of memory prostheses. External memory aids reduce reliance on defective memory. Notebooks, diaries, personal digital assistants, name tags, posted signs containing useful information in critical areas around a person's living environment, or simply relying on a spouse are all useful.[205] Patients and families are often given too little instruction in the use of these aids, causing patients to reject the memory books or not use them correctly. Memory rehabilitation programs must be designed to train patients with memory disorders to use these external aids. One well-designed program takes at least 2 months to train patients to use a memory book spontaneously.[206] Many patients with memory disorders have other cognitive problems, such as alexia (from PCA strokes) or poor motivation (from thalamic and frontal lesions), that make them poor candidates for external aids. We find that external aids are valuable only for "forgetful" patients (e.g., most traumatic brain injury patients and frontal lesion patients) but not for densely amnesic patients.

"Memory manuals" for patients with mild memory disturbances can complement memory aids. These manuals address typical day-to-day problems that patients will likely face and offer strategies for dealing with them.[207] Many centers that treat patients with memory disorders also provide memory support groups to emphasize and reinforce the strategies. Rather than actually improving memory performance, these groups reduce anxiety and depression and provide social contacts.[208]

TAPPING RESIDUAL MEMORY ABILITIES

Tapping residual memory capacities is another type of compensation for memory difficulties. For instance, the technique of "vanishing cues" takes advantage of preserved implicit memory in patients with a severe episodic memory disturbance after bilateral medial temporal lobe lesions.[209] The aim is to teach amnesic patients complex domain-specific knowledge that enhances their day-to-day functioning. Glisky and colleagues[209] taught dense amnesic patients

the vocabulary necessary to use a personal computer and carry out simple programs. In this procedure, a definition was presented and the patient was given as many letters as were needed to elicit the correct word. In subsequent learning trials, letters were gradually withdrawn from the cues until the patient produced the correct word without the letter cues. The amnesic patients could eventually generate the definitions of each word without letter cues, and this knowledge was retained across a 6–week interval. This technique produced faster learning and better retention than techniques without given cues.

In a follow-up study using the same technique, memory-impaired patients were taught to manipulate information on a computer screen and execute simple computer programs.[210] Further, this knowledge was retained for up to 9 months.[205] Finally, a patient with severely amnesic encephalitis was taught to enter data into a computer and demonstrate these skills in the workplace.[211] Unfortunately, this technique is profoundly limited since the knowledge learned is "hyperspecific" (i.e., only accessible when the original conditions are reintroduced). This suggests that neither the information nor the procedure of learning generalizes. When the patients who were successful in the workplace were presented with novel situations, learning slowed dramatically.[199] In addition, as a practical treatment matter, these methods take an inordinate amount of time and effort for a result with little generalization.

SUMMARY

Memory impairments are a common manifestation of many neurological disorders. Persistent memory difficulties greatly reduce functional independence and limit return to work, school, and leisure activities. Memory function comprises several processes, and different subcomponents of memory may become impaired following brain damage. For instance, despite the inability to learn new episodic information (i.e., dense anterograde amnesia), the ability to learn new motor skills (i.e., procedural memory) is preserved. The qualitatively different patterns of amnesia found in patients depend on the location of brain damage within the network of brain regions that support memory function.

Clinicians who care for patients with memory disorders will find that knowledge of the psychological functions and neuroanatomical, neurophysiological, and neurochemical bases for memory processes will facilitate appropriate assessment and classification of the disorder, enhance understanding of the underlying pathophysiology, and clarify the role of neuroimaging studies to inform the prognosis. Neuropsychological assessment that pinpoints cognitive strengths may provide a route for compensation with memory therapy. Cognitive theories of memory may lead to new therapeutic approaches. Pharmacological therapy targets specific components of memory and uses specific neurochemical mediators. Cognitive remediation therapy must abandon the idea that repeated practice and drills will strengthen the weakened "memory muscle" and must use compensatory strategies for overcoming memory impairments. As severe memory impairments are rarely reversible, our attempts to help patients must strive for long-term effects across their disabled life span.

REFERENCES

1. Tulving E: Memory: Introduction. In Gazzaniga M. (ed). The Cognitive Neurosciences. MIT Press, Cambridge, MA, 1995, p 751.
2. Squire LR: Memory and Brain. Oxford University Press, New York, 1987.
3. Lezak M: Neuropsychological Assessment, 3rd ed. Oxford University Press, New York, 1995.
4. Tulving E: How many memory systems are there? Am Psychol 40:385–398, 1985.
5. Cermak LS: The episodic–semantic distinction in amnesia. In Squire LS, Butters N (eds). Neuropsychology of Memory. Guilford Press, New York, 1984, pp 55–62.
6. Parkin A: Memory: Phenomenon, Experiment and Theory. Blackwell, Oxford, 1993.
7. Schacter D: Implicit memory: history and current status. J Exp Psychol Learn Mem Cogn 13:501–518, 1987.
8. Tulving E and Schacter DL: Priming and human memory systems. Science 247:301–306, 1990.
9. Scoville WB and Milner B: Loss of recent memory after bilateral hippocampal lesions. Neuropsychologia 20:11–21, 1957.
10. Corkin S: Lasting consequences of bilateral medial temporal lobectomy: clinical course and experimental findings in H.M. Semin Neurol 4:249–259, 1984.
11. Zola SM, Squire LR, Teng E, et al.: Impaired recognition memory in monkeys after damage limited to the hippocampal region. J Neurosci 20:451–463, 2000.
12. Zola SM and Squire LR: Relationship between magnitude of damage to the hippocampus and impaired recognition memory in monkeys. Hippocampus 11:92–98, 2001.
13. Zola-Morgan S and Squire LR: Neuroanatomy of memory. Ann Rev Neurosci 16:547–563, 1993.
14. Mishkin M: Memory in monkeys severely impaired by combined but not separate removal of the amygdala and hippocampus. Nature 273:297–298, 1978.
15. Mishkin M: A memory system in the monkey. Philos Trans R Soc Lond B Biol Sci 298:85–92, 1982.
16. Schwartzkroin PA, Scharfman HA, and Sloviter RS: Similarities in circuitry between Ammon's horn and dentate gyrus: local interactions and parallel processing. Prog Brain Res 83:269–286, 1990.
17. Creutzfeldt OD: Performance, Structural and Functional Organization of the Cortex. Oxford University Press, New York, 1995.
18. Rosene DL and Van Hoesen GW: Hippocampal efferents reach widespread areas of cerebral cortex and amygdala in the rhesus monkey. Science 198:315–317, 1977.
19. Zola-Morgan S, Squire LR, and Amaral DG: Human amnesia and the medial temporal region: enduring memory impairment following bilateral lesions limited to field CA1 of the hippocampus. J Neurosci 6:2950–2967, 1976.
20. Silva AJ. Molecular and cellular cognitive studies of the role of synaptic plasticity in memory. J Neurobiol 54:224–237, 2003.
21. Martin SJ, Grimwood PD, and Morris RG: Synaptic plasticity and memory: an evaluation of the hypothesis. Annu Rev Neurosci 23:649–711, 2000.
22. Engel J Jr: Mesial temporal lobe epilepsy: what have we learned? Neuroscientist 7:340–352, 2001.
23. Alvarez P and Squire LR: Memory consolidation and the medial temporal lobe: a simple network model. Proc Natl Acad Sci USA 91:7041–7045, 1994.
24. Mesulam M: Brain, mind, and the evolution of connectivity. Brain Cogn 42:4–6, 2000.
25. Mesulam M-M: From sensation to cognition. Brain 121:1013–1052, 1998.
26. Zola-Morgan S, Squire LR, and Ramus SJ: Severity of memory impairment in monkeys as a function of locus and extent of damage within the medial temporal lobe system. Hippocampus 4:483–494, 1994.
27. D'Esposito M, Verfaellie M, Alexander MP, et al.: Amnesia following traumatic bilateral fornix transection. Neurology 45:1546–1550, 1995.
28. Gaffan D and Gaffan EA: Amnesia in man following transection of the fornix: a review. Brain 114:2611–2618, 1991.
29. Small IF, Hemiburger RF, Small JG, et al.: Follow-up of stereotaxic amygdalotomy for seizure and behavior disorders. Biol Psychiatry 12:401–411, 1977.
30. Cahill L: Neurobiological mechanisms of emotionally influenced, long-term memory. Prog Brain Res 126:29–37, 2000.
31. McGaugh JL, Cahill L, and Roozendaal B: Involvement of the amygdala in memory storage: interaction with other brain systems. Proc Natl Acad Sci USA 93:13508–13514, 1996.
32. Bechara A, Tranel D, Damasio H, et al.: Double dissociation of conditioning and declarative knowledge relative to the amygdala and hippocampus in humans. Science 269:1115–1118, 1995.
33. Hecaen H and Albert ML: Human Neuropsychology. John Wiley & Sons, New York, 1978.

34. Janowsky JS, Shimamura AP, Kritchevsky M, et al.: Cognitive impairment following frontal lobe damage and its relevance to human amnesia. Behav Neurosci 103:548–560, 1989.

35. Shimamura AP, Janowsky JS, and Squire LS: What is the role of frontal lobe damage in memory disorders? In Levin H, Eisenberg H, and Benton A (eds). Frontal Lobe Function and Dysfunction. Oxford University Press, New York, 1991, pp 173–195.

36. Shimamura AP, Janowsky JS, and Squire LR: Memory for the temporal order of events in patients with frontal lobe lesions and amnesic patients. Neuropsychologia 28:803–813, 1990.

37. Jurado MA, Junque C, Vendrell P, et al.: Overestimation and unreliability in "feeling-of-doing" judgements about temporal ordering performance: impaired self-awareness following frontal lobe damage. J Clin Exp Neuropsychol 20:353–364, 1998.

38. Stuss DT, Alexander MP, Palumbo CL, et al.: Organizational strategies of patients with unilateral or bilateral frontal lobe injury in word list learning tasks. Neuropsychology 8:355–373, 1994.

39. Johnson MK, Hayes SM, D'Esposito M, et al.: Confabulation. In Cermak LS (ed). Handbook of Neuropsychology, 2nd ed, Vol 2. Elsevier, Amsterdam, 2001, pp 359–383.

40. Burgess PW and Shallice T: Confabulation and the control of recollection. Memory 4:359–411, 1996.

41. Benson DF, Djenderedjian A, Miller BL, et al.: Neural basis of confabulation. Neurology 46:1239–1243, 1996.

42. Schacter DL, Dodson CS: Misattribution, false recognition and the sins of memory. Philos Trans R Soc Lond B Biol Sci 356:1385–1393, 2001.

43. Schnider A, von Daniken C, and Gutbrod K: The mechanisms of spontaneous and provoked confabulations. Brain 119:1365–1375, 1996.

44. Stuss DT, Alexander MP, Lieberman A, et al.: An extraordinary form of confabulation. Neurology 28:1166–1172, 1978.

45. Fischer RS, Alexander MP, D'Esposito M, et al.: Neuropsychological and neuroanatomical correlates of confabulation. J Clin Exp Neuropsychol 17:20–28, 1995.

46. Schnider A: Spontaneous confabulation, reality monitoring, and the limbic system—a review. Brain Res Brain Res Rev 36:150–160, 2001.

47. Phelps EA and Gazzaniga MS: Hemispheric differences in mnemonic processing: the effects of left hemisphere interpretation. Neuropsychologia 30:293–297, 1992.

48. Gazzaniga MS: The split brain revisited. Sci Am 279:50–55, 1998.

49. Victor M, Adams RD, and Collins GH: The Wernicke-Korsakoff syndrome. FA Davis, Philadelphia, 1971.

50. Mayes AR, Meudell R, Mann D, et al.: Location of lesions in Korsakoff's syndrome: neuropsychological and neuropathological data on two patients. Cortex 24:367–388, 1987.

51. Mair WGP, Warrington EK, and Weiskrantz L: Memory disorder in Korsakoff's psychosis: a neuropathological and neuropsychological investigation of two cases. Brain 102:749–783, 1979.

52. Lishman W: Cerebral disorder in alcoholism: syndromes of impairment. Brain 104:1–20, 1981.

53. Butters N: Alcohol Korsakoff's syndrome: an update. Semin Neurol 4:226–244, 1984.

54. Albert MA, Butters N, and Levin JA: Temporal gradients in the retrograde amnesia of patients with alcoholic Korsakoff's disease. Arch Neurol 36:211–216, 1979.

55. Leng NR and Parkin AJ: Aetiological variation in the amnesic syndrome: comparisons using the Brown-Peterson task. Cortex 25:251–259, 1989.

56. Squire LR: Comparisons between forms of amnesia: some deficits are unique to Korsakoff's syndrome. J Exp Psychol Learn Mem Cogn 8:560–571, 1982.

57. von Cramon DY, Hebel N, and Schuri U: A contribution to the anatomical basis of thalamic amnesia. Brain 108:993–1008, 1985.

58. Graff-Radford NR, Tranel D, Van Hoesen GW, and Brandt JP: Diencephalic amnesia. Brain 113:1–25, 1990.

59. Delay J and Brion S: Le Syndrome de Korsakoff. Masson, Paris, 1969.

60. Katz D, Alexander M, and Mandell A: Dementia following strokes in the mesencephalon and diencephalon. Arch Neurol 44:1127–1133, 1987.

61. Szirmai I, Vastagh I, Szombathelyi E, et al.: Strategic infarcts of the thalamus in vascular dementia. J Neurol Sci 203–204:91–97, 2002.

62. Mesulam M-M, Mufson EJ, Levey AI, et al.: Cholinergic innervation of the cortex by the basal forebrain: cytochemistry and cortical connections of the septal area, diagonal band nuclei, nucleus basalis (substantia innominata) and hypothalamus in the rhesus monkey. J Comp Neurol 214:170–197, 1983.

63. Jones EG: Some aspects of the organization of the thalamic reticular complex. J Comp Neurol 162:285–308, 1975.

64. Alexander MP and Freedman M: Amnesia after anterior communicating artery aneurysm. Neurology 34:752–757, 1984.

65. Morris M, Bowers D, Chatterjee A, et al.: Amnesia following a discrete lesion of the basal forebrain. Brain 115:1827–1847, 1992.

66. Phillips S, Sangalang V, and Sterns G: Basal forebrain infarction. Arch Neurol 44:1184–1190, 1987.

67. Irle E, Wowra B, Kunert HJ, et al.: Memory disturbance following anterior communicating artery rupture. Ann Neurol 31:473–480, 1992.

68. Whitehouse PJ, Price DL, Clark AW, et al.: Alzheimer's disease: evidence for selective loss of cholinergic neurons in the nucleus basalis. Ann Neurol 10:122–126, 1981.

69. Coyle J, Price DL, and DeLong MR: Alzheimer's disease, a disorder of cortical cholinergic innervation. Science 219:1184–1190, 1983.

70. Hodges JR, Patterson K, Oxbury S, et al.: Semantic dementia. Brain 115:1783–1806, 1992.

71. Snowden JS, Goulding PJ, and Neary D: Semantic dementia: a form of circumscribed cerebral atrophy. Behav Neurol 2:167–182, 1992.

72. Warrington EK: The selective impairment of semantic memory. Q J Exp Psychol 27:635–657, 1975.

73. Martin A and Chao LL: Semantic memory and the brain: structure and processes. Curr Opin Neurobiol 11:194–201, 2001.

74. Warrington EK and Shallice T: Category specific semantic impairments. Brain 107:829–854, 1984.

75. Wilson BA: Semantic memory impairments following non-progressive brain injury: a study of four cases. Brain Inj 11:259–269, 1997.

76. Warrington EK and McCarthy R: Categories of knowledge: further fractionations and an attempted explanation. Brain 110:1273–1296, 1987.

77. Allport DA: Distributed memory, modular subsytems and dysphasia. In Newman S and Epstein R (eds). Current Perspectives in Dysphasia. Churchill Livingstone, Edinburgh, 1985, pp 32–60.

78. Thompson-Schill SL: Neuroimaging studies of semantic memory: inferring "how" from "where." Neuropsychologia 41:280–292, 2003.

79. Packard MG and Knowlton BJ: Learning and memory functions of the basal ganglia. Annu Rev Neurosci 25:563–593, 2002.

80. Poldrack RA, Prabhakaran V, Seger CA, et al.: Striatal activation during acquisition of a cognitive skill. Neuropsychology 13:564–574, 1999.

81. Poldrack RA and Gabrieli JD: Characterizing the neural mechanisms of skill learning and repetition priming: evidence from mirror reading. Brain 124:67–82, 2001.

82. Eldridge LL, Masterman D, and Knowlton BJ: Intact implicit habit learning in Alzheimer's disease. Behav Neurosci 116:722–726, 2002.

83. Knowlton BJ, Mangels JA, and Squire LR: A neostriatal habit learning system in humans. Science 273:1399–1402, 1996.

84. Sanes JN, Dimitrov B, and Hallett M: Motor learning in patients with cerebellar dysfunction. Brain 113:103–120, 1990.

85. Fuster J: The Prefrontal Cortex: Anatomy, Physiology, and Neuropsychology of the Frontal Lobes, 3rd ed. Raven Press, New York, 1997.

86. Goldman-Rakic PS: Circuitry of the prefrontal cortex and the regulation of behavior by representational memory. In Plum F and Mountcastle V (eds). Handbook of Physiology. The Nervous System, Sect 1, Vol 5. American Physiological Society, Bethesda, MD, 1987, pp 373–417.

87. Fuster JM and Alexander GE: Neuron activity related to short-term memory. Science 173:652–654, 1971.

88. Funahashi S, Bruce CJ, and Goldman-Rakic PS: Mnemonic coding of visual space in the monkey's dorsolateral prefrontal cortex. J Neurophysiol 61:331–349, 1989.

89. Funahashi S, Bruce CJ, and Goldman-Rakic PS: Dorsolateral prefrontal lesions and oculomotor delayed-response performance: evidence for mnemonic "scotomas." J Neurosci 13:1479–1497, 1993.

90. Bauer RH and Fuster JM: Delayed-matching and delayed-response deficit from cooling dorsolateral prefrontal cortex in monkeys. J Comp Physiol Psychol 90:293–302, 1976.

91. Verin M, Partiot A, Pillon B, et al.: Delayed response tasks and prefrontal lesions in man—evidence for self generated patterns of behavior with poor environmental modulation. Neuropsychologia 31:1379–1396, 1993.

92. Ptito A, Crane J, Leonard G, et al.: Visual–spatial localization by patients with frontal-lobe lesions invading or sparing area 46. Neuroreport 6:1781–1784, 1995.

93. Pierrot-Deseilligny C, Rivaud S, Gaymard B, et al.: Cortical control of memory-guided saccades in man. Exp Brain Res 83:607–617, 1991.

94. D'Esposito M: Working memory. In Cabezza R and Kingstone A (eds). Handbook of Functional Neuroimaging of Cognition. MIT Press, Cambridge, MA, 2001, pp 293–327.

95. Gabrieli JDE, Cohen NJ, and Corkin S: The impaired learning of semantic knowledge following bilateral medial temporal-lobe resection. Brain 7:157–177, 1988.

96. Barr WB, Goldberg E, Wasserstein J, et al.: Retrograde amnesia following unilateral temporal lobectomy. Neuropsychologia 28:243–255, 1990.

97. Marslen-Wilson WD and Teuber HL: Memory for remote events in anterograde amnesia: recognition of public figures from news photos. Neuropsychologia 13:353–364, 1975.

98. Corkin S: Acquisition of a motor skill after bilateral medial temporal lobe excision. Neuropsychologia 6:255–265, 1968.

99. Cohen N and Squire LR: Preserved learning and retention of pattern-analyzing skill in amnesia: dissociation of knowing how and knowing that. Science 210:207–210, 1980.

100. Ween JE, Verfaellie M, and Alexander MP: Verbal memory function in mild aphasia. Neurology 47:795–801, 1996.

101. Risse GL, Rubens AB, and Jordan LS: Disturbances in long-term memory in aphasic patients. Brain 107:605–617, 1984.

102. Bender MB: Syndrome of isolated episode of confusion with amnesia. J Hillside Hosp 5:212–215, 1956.

103. Fisher CM and Adams RD: Transient global amnesia. Trans Am Neurol Assoc 83:143–146, 1958.

104. Hodges JR and Warlow CP: The aetiology of transient global amnesia. A case-control study of 114 cases with prospective follow-up. Brain 113:639–657, 1990.

105. Kritchevsky M, Squire LR, and Zouzounis JA: Transient global amnesia: characterization of anterograde and retrograde amnesia. Neurology 38:213–219, 1988.

106. Fisher CM: Transient global amnesia. Precipitating activities and other observations. Arch Neurol 39:605–608, 1982.

107. Caplan LR: Transient global amnesia: criteria and classification. Neurology 36:441, 1986.

108. Hodges JR and Warlow CP: Syndromes of transient amnesia: towards a classification. A study of 153 cases. J Neurol Neurosurg Psychiatry 53:834–843, 1990.

109. Caplan L, Chedru F, Lhermitte F, et al.: Transient global amnesia and migraine. Neurology 31:1167–1170, 1981.

110. Olesen J and Jorgensen MB: Leao's spreading depression in the hippocampus explains transient global amnesia. A hypothesis. Acta Neurol Scand 73:219–220, 1986.

111. Jensen TS and De Fine Olivarius B: Transient global amnesia as a manifestation of transient cerebral ischemia. Acta Neurol Scand 61:115–124, 1980.

112. Kapur N: Transient epileptic amnesia—a clinical update and a reformulation. J Neurol Neurosurg Psychiatry 56:1184–1190, 1993.

113. Schmidtke K, Reinhardt M, and Krause T: Cerebral perfusion during transient global amnesia: findings with HMPAO SPECT. J Nucl Med 39:155–159, 1998.

114. Eustache F, Desgranges B, Petit-Taboue MC, et al.: Transient global amnesia: implicit/explicit memory dissociation and PET assessment of brain perfusion and oxygen metabolism in the acute stage. J Neurol Neurosurg Psychiatry 63:357–367, 1997.

115. Pantoni L, Lamassa M, and Inzitari D: Transient global amnesia: a review emphasizing pathogenic aspects. Acta Neurol Scand 102:275–283, 2000.

116. Rowan AJ and Protass LM: Transient global amnesia: clinical and electroencephalographic findings in 10 cases. Neurology 29:869–872., 1979.

117. Miller JW, Petersen RC, Metter EJ, et al.: Transient global amnesia: clinical characteristics and prognosis. Neurology 37:733–737, 1987.

118. Huber R, Aschoff AJ, Ludolph AC, et al.: Transient global amnesia: evidence against vascular ischemic etiology from diffusion weighted imaging. J Neurol 249:1520–1524, 2002.

119. Strupp M, Bruning R, Wu RH, et al.: Diffusion-weighted MRI in transient global amnesia: elevated signal intensity in the left mesial temporal lobe in 7 of 10 patients. Ann Neurol 43:164–170, 1998.

120. Zorzon M, Longo R, Mase G, et al.: Proton magnetic resonance spectroscopy during transient global amnesia. J Neurol Sci 156:78–82, 1998.

121. Calandre EP, Bembibre J, Arnedo ML, et al.: Cognitive disturbances and regional cerebral blood flow abnormalities in migraine patients: their relationship with the clinical manifestations of the illness. Cephalalgia 22:291–302, 2002.

122. Le Pira F, Zappala G, Giuffrida S, et al.: Memory disturbances in migraine with and without aura: a strategy problem? Cephalalgia 20:475–478, 2000.

123. Leung LS, Ma J, and McLachlan RS: Behaviors induced or disrupted by complex partial seizures. Neurosci Biobehav Rev 24:763–775, 2000.

124. Theodore WH, Porter RJ, and Penry JK: Complex partial seizures: clinical characteristics and differential diagnosis. Neurology 33:1115–1121, 1983.

125. Mendes MH: Transient epileptic amnesia: an underdiagnosed phenomenon? Three more cases. Seizure 11:238–242, 2002.

126. Kapur N: Transient epileptic amnesia—a clinical update and a reformulation. J Neurol Neurosurg Psychiatry 56:1184–1190, 1993.

127. Palmini AL, Gloor P, and Jones-Gotman M: Pure amnestic seizures in temporal lobe epilepsy. Definition, clinical symptomatology and functional anatomical considerations. Brain 115:749–769, 1992.

128. Palmini A, Andermann F, Tampieri D, et al.: Epilepsy and cortical cytoarchitectonic abnormalities: an attempt at correlating basic mechanisms with anatomoclinical syndromes. Epilepsy Res Suppl 9: 19–29, 1992.

129. Gorelick PB, Amico LL, Ganellen R, et al.: Transient global amnesia and thalamic infarction. Neurology 38:496–499, 1988.

130. Benson DF, Marsden CD, and Meadows JC: The amnesic syndrome of posterior cerebral artery occlusion. Acta Neurol Scand 50:133–145, 1974.

131. De Renzi E, Lucchelli F, Muggia S, et al.: Is memory loss without anatomical damage tantamount to a psychogenic deficit? The case of pure retrograde amnesia. Neuropsychologia 35:781–794, 1997.

132. Ross ED: Sensory-specific and fractional disorders of recent memory in man. I. Isolated loss of visual recent memory. Arch Neurol 37:193–200, 1980.

133. Ross ED: Sensory-specific and fractional disorders of recent memory in man. II. Unilateral loss of tactile recent memory. Arch Neurol 37:267–272, 1980.

134. Damasio AR, Eslinger PJ, Damasio H. et al.: Multi-modal amnesic syndrome following bilateral temporal and basal forebrain damage. Arch Neurol 42:252–259, 1985.

135. Zola-Morgan S, Squire LR, and Amaral DG: Human amnesia and the medial temporal region: enduring memory impairment following a bilateral lesion limited to field CA1 of the hippocampus. J Neurosci 6:2950–2967, 1986.

136. Caine D and Watson JD: Neuropsychological and neuropathological sequelae of cerebral anoxia: a critical review. J Int Neuropsychol Soc 6:86–99, 2000.

137. Chalmers J, Risk MT, Kean DM, et al.: Severe amnesia after hypoglycemia. Clinical, psychometric, and magnetic resonance imaging correlations. Diabetes Care 14:922–925, 1991.

138. Barbarotto R, Laiacona M, and Cocchini G: A case of simulated, psychogenic or focal pure retrograde amnesia: did an entire life become unconscious? Neuropsychologia 34:575–585, 1996.

139. Cummings JL and Cole G: Alzheimer disease. JAMA 287:2335–2338, 2002.

140. Alzheimer A: Uber eine eigenartige Erkangkung der Hirnrinde. All Z Psychiatr 64:146–148, 1907.

141. Blessed G, Tomlinson BE, and Roth M: The association between quantitative measures of dementia and of senile change in the cerebral grey matter of elderly subjects. Br J Psychiatry 114:797–811, 1968.

142. Kukull WA, Higdon R, Bowen JD, et al.: Dementia and Alzheimer disease incidence: a prospective cohort study. Arch Neurol 59:1737–1746, 2002.

143. St George-Hyslop PH, Haines JL, Farrer LA, et al.: Genetic linkage studies suggest that Alzheimer's disease is not a single homogeneous disorder. FAD Collaborative Study Group. Nature 347:194–197, 1990.

144. Goate A, Chartier-Harlin MC, Mullan M, et al.: Segregation of a missense mutation in the amyloid precursor protein gene with familial Alzheimer's disease. Nature 349:704–706, 1991.

145. Schellenberg GD: Genetic dissection of Alzheimer disease, a heterogeneous disorder. Proc Natl Acad Sci USA 92:8552–8559, 1995.

146. Rogaev EI, Sherrington R, Rogaeva EA, et al.: Familial Alzheimer's disease in kindreds with missense mutations in a gene on chromosome 1 related to the Alzheimer's disease type 3 gene. Nature 376:775–778, 1995.

147. Roses AD: Apolipoprotein E and Alzheimer's disease. A rapidly expanding field with medical and epidemiological consequences. Ann NY Acad Sci 802: 50–57, 1996.

148. Mayeux R, Saunders AM, Shea S, et al.: Utility of the apolipoprotein E genotype in the diagnosis of Alzheimer's disease. Alzheimer's Disease Centers Consortium on Apolipoprotein E and Alzheimer's Disease. N Engl J Med 338:506–511, 1998.

149. Bertram L and Tanzi RE: Of replications and refutations: the status of Alzheimer's disease genetic research. Curr Neurol Neurosci Rep 1:442–450, 2001.

150. Fitch N, Becker R, and Heller A: The inheritance of Alzheimer's disease: a new interpretation. Ann Neurol 23:14–19, 1988.

151. Terry RD and Katzman R: Senile dementia of the Alzheimer type. Ann Neurol 14:497–506, 1983.

152. Carter J and Lippa CF: Beta-amyloid, neuronal death and Alzheimer's disease. Curr Mol Med 1:733–737, 2001.

153. Fisher CM: Neurologic fragments. I. Clinical observations in demented patients. Neurology 38:1868–1873, 1988.
154. Friedland RP, Koss E, Kumar A, et al.: Motor vehicle crashes in dementia of the Alzheimer type. Ann Neurol 24:782–786, 1988.
155. Cummings JL, Benson F, Hill MA, et al.: Aphasia in dementia of the Alzheimer type. Neurology 35:394–397, 1985.
156. Petry S, Cummings JL, Hill MA, et al.: Personality alterations in dementia of the Alzheimer type. Arch Neurol 45:1187–1190, 1988.
157. Chandra V, Bharucha NE, and Schoenberg BS: Conditions associated with Alzheimer's disease at death: case-control study. Neurology 36:209–211, 1986.
158. Hodges JR: Frontotemporal dementia (Pick's disease): clinical features and assessment. Neurology 56:S6–S10, 2001.
159. Neary D, Snowden JS, Northen B, et al.: Dementia of frontal lobe type. J Neurol Neurosurg Psychiatry 51:353–361, 1988.
160. Kiloh LG: Pseudodementia. Acta Psychiatr Scand 37:336–351, 1961.
161. Dobie DJ: Depression, dementia, and pseudodementia. Semin Clin Neuropsychiatry 7:170–186, 2002.
162. Reynolds CF and Hoch CC: Differential diagnosis of depressive pseudodementia and primary degenerative dementia. Psychiatric Ann 17:743–749, 1988.
163. Christensen H, Griffiths K, and MacKinnon A: A quantitative review of cognitive deficits in depression and Alzheimer's-type dementia. J Int Neuropsychol Soc 3:631–651, 1997.
164. Miller BL, Read SL, Mahler ME, et al.: Altered mental status in the elderly. Prim Care 11:653–665, 1984.
165. Knopman D: Cerebrospinal fluid beta-amyloid and tau proteins for the diagnosis of Alzheimer disease. Arch Neurol 58:349–350, 2001.
166. Diaz-Arrastia R and Baskin F: New biochemical markers in Alzheimer disease. Arch Neurol 58:354–356, 2001.
167. Shoji M, Matsubara E, Murakami T, et al.: Cerebrospinal fluid tau in dementia disorders: a large scale multicenter study by a Japanese study group. Neurobiol Aging 23:363–370, 2002.
168. Shoji M: Cerebrospinal fluid Abeta40 and Abeta42: natural course and clinical usefulness. Front Biosci 7:997–1006, 2002.
169. Lovell MA and Markesbery WR: Ratio of 8–hydroxyguanine in intact DNA to free 8–hydroxyguanine is increased in Alzheimer disease ventricular cerebrospinal fluid. Arch Neurol 58:392–396, 2001.
170. Matsuda H: Cerebral blood flow and metabolic abnormalities in Alzheimer's disease. Ann Nucl Med 15:85–92, 2001.
171. Garrard P and Hodges JR: Semantic dementia: clinical, radiological and pathological perspectives. J Neurol 247:409–422, 2000.
172. Crow TJ and Grove-White IG: An analysis of the learning deficit following hyoscine administration to man. Br J Pharmacol 49:322–327, 1973.
173. Crow TJ, Grove-White I, and Ross DG: The specificity of the action of hyoscine on human learning. Br J Clin Pharmacol 2:367P–368P, 1975.
174. Koppleman MD: The cholinergic neurotransmitter system in human memory and dementia: a review. Q J Exp Psychol 38A:535–573, 1986.
175. Drachman DA and Leavitt JL: Human memory and the cholinergic system: a relationship to aging? Arch Neurol 30:113–121, 1974.
176. Drachman DA: Memory and cognitive function in man: does the cholinergic system have a specific role. Neurology 27:783–790, 1977.
177. Thal L: Pharmacological treatment of memory disorders. In Boller F and Grafman J (eds). Handbook of Neuropsychology. Elsevier, New York, 1991, pp 247–267.
178. Davies P and Mahoney AJ: Selective loss of central cholinergic neurons in Alzheimer's disease. Lancet 2:1403, 1976.
179. Knopman D: Pharmacotheraphy for Alzheimer's disease. Curr Neurol Neurosci Rep 1:428–434, 2001.
180. Bullock R: New drugs for Alzheimer's disease and other dementias. Br J Psychiatry 180:135–139, 2002.
181. Shigeta M and Homma A: Donepezil for Alzheimer's disease: pharmacodynamic, pharmacokinetic, and clinical profiles. CNS Drug Rev 7:353–368, 2001.
182. Peters B and Levin H: Memory enhancement after physostigmine treatment in the amnesic syndrome. Arch Neurol 34:215–219, 1977.
183. Goldberg E, Gerstman L, Mattis S, et al.: Effects of cholinergic treatment on posttraumatic anterograde amnesia. Arch Neurol 34:581, 1982.
184. Chatterjee A, Morris M, Bowers D, et al.: Cholinergic treatment of an amnestic man with a basal forebrain lesion: theoretical implications. J Neurol Neurosurg Psychiatry 56:1282–1289, 1993.
185. Brown RM, Crane AM, and Goldman PS: Regional distribution of monoamines in the cerebral cortex and subcortical structures of the rhesus monkey: concentrations and in vitro synthesis rates. Brain Res 168:133–150, 1979.
186. Brozoski TJ, Brown RM, Rosvold HE, et al.: Cognitive deficit caused by regional depletion of dopamine in prefrontal cortex of rhesus monkey. Science 205:929–932, 1979.
187. Sawaguchi T and Goldman-Rakic PS: D_1 dopamine receptors in prefrontal cortex: involvement in working memory. Science 251:947–950, 1991.
188. Arnsten KT, Cai JX, Murphy BL, et al.: Dopamine D_1 receptor mechanisms in the cognitive performance of young adult and aged monkeys. Psychopharmacology 116:143–151, 1994.
189. Luciana M, Depue RA, Arbisi P, et al.: Facilitation of working memory in humans by a D_2 dopamine receptor agonist. J Cogn Neurosci 4:58–68, 1992.
190. Müller U, Pollmann S, and von Cramon DY: D_1 versus D_2-receptor stimulation of visuo-spatial short-term memory. J Neurosci 18:2720–2728, 1998.
191. Kimberg DY, D'Esposito M, Farah MJ: Effects of bromocriptine on human subjects depend on working memory capacity. NeuroReport 8:3581–3585, 1997.
192. Altman HJ and Normile HJ: What is the nature of the role of the serotonergic nervous system in learning and memory: prospects for development of an effective treatment strategy for senile dementia. Neurobiol Aging 9:627–638, 1988.
193. Zager EL and Black PM: Neuropeptides in human memory and learning processes. Neurosurgery 17:355–369, 1985.
194. Sarter M and Schneider HH: High density of benzodiazepine binding sites in the substantia innominata of the rat. Pharmacol Biochem Behav 30:679–682, 1988.

195. Haroutunian V, Santucci AC, and Davis KL: Implications of multiple transmitter system lesions for cholinomimetic therapy in Alzheimer's disease. Prog Brain Res 84:333–346, 1990.
196. Prigatano G, Fordyce D, Zeiner H, et al.: Neuropsychological rehabilitation after closed head injury in young adults. J Neurol Neurosurg Psychiatry 47:505–513, 1984.
197. Godfrey H and Knight R: Cognitive rehabilitation of memory functioning in amnesic alcoholics. J Clin Exp Neuropsychol 8:292–312, 1985.
198. Erickson R and Chase W: Acquisition of a memory skill. Science 208:1181–1182, 1980.
199. Glisky E and Schacter D: Models and methods of memory rehabilitation. In Boller F and Grafman J (eds). Handbook of Neuropsychology. Elsevier, New York, 1991, pp 233–246.
200. O'Connor M and Cermak LS: Rehabilitation for Organic Memory Disorders. Guilford Press, New York, 1987.
201. Wilson B: Rehabilitation of memory disorders. In Squire L and Butters N (eds). Neuropsychology of Memory, 2nd ed. Guilford Press, New York, 1993, pp 315–321.
202. Patten BM: The ancient art of memory. Usefulness in treatment. Arch Neurol 26:25–31, 1972.
203. Jones MK: Imagery as a mnemonic aid after left temporal lobectomy: contrast between material-specific and generalized memory disorders. Neuropsychologia 12:21–30, 1974.
204. Baddeley A: Amnesia: a minimal model and interpretation. In Cermak L (eds). Human Amnesia. Lawrence Erlbaum, Hillsdale, NJ, 1982, pp 305–336.
205. Harris J: External memory aids. In Gruneberg M, Morris P, and Sykes R (eds). Practical Aspects of Memory. Academic Press, London, 1978, pp 172–179.
206. Sohlberg MM and Mateer CA: Training use of compensatory memory books: a three stage behavioural approach. J Clin Exp Neuropsychol 11:871–891, 1989.
207. Kapur N: The Wessex Memory Manual. 1989.
208. Evans J and Wilson B: A memory group for individuals with brain injury. Clin Rehabil 6:75–81, 1992.
209. Glisky E, Schacter D, and Tulving E: Learning and retention of computer-related vocabulary in memory-impaired patients: method of vanishing cues. J Clin Exp Neuropsychol 3:292–312, 1986.
210. Glisky EL and Schacter DL: Long-term memory retention of computer learning by patients with memory disorders. Neuropsychologia 26:173–178, 1988.
211. Glisky EL and Schacter DL: Extending the limits of complex learning in organic amnesia: computer training in a vocational domain. Neuropsychologia 27:107–120, 1989.

Chapter 9

Executive Function and the Frontal Lobes

At one time, the most anterior portion of the frontal lobes, the prefrontal cortex, was considered "silent" because moderate-sized lesions of this region produced few or no abnormalities on the neurological examination and electrical stimulation rarely altered behavior.[1] Moreover, following prefrontal resections of the dominant hemisphere, patients had normal memory and an intelligence quotient (IQ) of 150 or more.[2] Although behavioral and cognitive changes challenge clinical measurement at the bedside, most families of patients with bilateral frontal lobe damage recognize them as "very different." For example, these patients may drive past stop signs, fail to show concern when a kettle is boiling over, become slovenly and unkempt, joke about someone's physical deformity in front of him or her, become violent after a minor provocation and quickly return to their previous calm state, urinate on the street, or leave a baby unattended to watch tel-

evision. Such observations led prominent psychologists and neuroscientists to characterize function of the frontal lobes as a "riddle"[3] and "mystifying."[4] Subsequently, elegant investigations in humans and other species began to solve the enigma of frontal lobe function.

ANATOMY OF THE FRONTAL LOBES

The frontal lobes are enormous and comprise more than one-third of the human cerebral cortex. This region is anatomically complex, with diverse connections to most other cortical and subcortical regions. Most knowledge of connections derives from nonhuman primate studies; data on humans are limited. However, understanding frontal lobe function depends on knowledge of frontal lobe anatomy.

Anatomically, the frontal lobes are bounded

by the central sulcus (separating them from the parietal lobes), the sylvian fissure (separating them from the temporal lobes), and the corpus callosum (separating them from subcortical structures). The frontal lobes are divided into two major functional subdivisions: the motor and premotor cortex and the prefrontal cortex (Fig. 9–1). The two major subdivisions are further subdivided.

Motor and Premotor Cortex

The anatomy of the primary motor cortex (Brodmann's area [BA] 4), lateral premotor

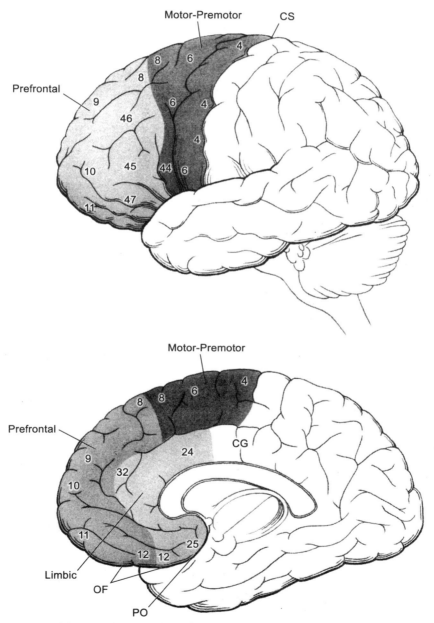

Figure 9–1. Functional divisions of the frontal lobes. Lateral (*A*) and medial (*B*) views shown. CS, central sulcus; CG, cingulate gyrus; OF, orbitofrontal area; PO, posterior orbitofrontal area.

cortex (BA 6), supplementary motor area (medial BA 6), and the frontal eye fields (BA 8) is reviewed in Chapter 7. Broca's area (BAs 44, 45), lying within the inferior frontal gyrus (and sometimes called the frontal operculum because it is the cortex covering the insula), is described in Chapter 6. Broca's area can also be considered a motor association area, supporting language production.

Prefrontal Cortex

The prefrontal cortex lies anterior to the motor and premotor areas and consists of heteromodal (or multimodal) association cortex (dorsolateral convexity and anteromedial surface) as well as limbic cortex (anterior cingulate and posterior orbitofrontal area). The prefrontal cortex is divided into three regions: (1) lateral prefrontal cortex (dorsal, or superior [BAs 9, 46, 10], and ventral, or inferior [BAs 44, 45, 47]), (2) orbitofrontal cortex [BAs 11, 12], and (3) basomedial cortex, which includes the anterior cingulate cortex (BAs 24, 25, 32). The cytoarchitecturally less differentiated agranular–dysgranular cortex of the basomedial areas connects mainly with limbic and lateral prefrontal areas. The more differentiated granular areas of the lateral prefrontal cortex connect extensively with parietal and temporal heteromodal association areas, thus receiving information that originated in primary somatic, auditory, visual, olfactory, and gustatory areas. All prefrontal areas connect reciprocally with the dorsomedial thalamic nucleus.

LATERAL PREFRONTAL CORTEX

The lateral prefrontal cortex, at a minimum, is organized along a dorsal–ventral axis. The dorsolateral and medial prefrontal cortices receive somatosensory and visual inputs from parietal heteromodal association cortex, concerning peripheral vision, motion, spatial orientation, and tactile sensations from the trunk and extremities. This input contributes to the identification of an object's spatial location as part of the "where" system.[5] Foveal input from temporal visual association cortices, facial tactile input, and auditory inputs project to the ventrolateral prefrontal convexity. This input helps to identify an object's form as part of the "what" sys-

tem. Receiving segregated projections about spatial and object features from posterior association cortex, the frontal lobes integrate this information.[6,7]

Prefrontal cortex is relatively unique, projecting to the subcortical monoaminergic and cholinergic sources (ventral tegmental area, dorsal raphe, locus ceruleus, basal nucleus of Meynert).[8] These projections permit prefrontal cortex to influence more global behavioral patterns such as attention and arousal. Thus, impaired motivation, initiation of actions, and affect after prefrontal lesions may partly result from this area's failure to activate the diffusely projecting subcortical modulatory systems. Like the anterior cingulate, lateral prefrontal cortex has extensive, but mainly indirect, limbic connections via the anterior cingulate and posterior orbital cortex; receives highly transformed and integrated sensory data from other heteromodal association cortices; and is involved in premotor planning and response selection with robust motor connections to M1, M2, M3, the striatum (mainly the caudate), the superior colliculus (eye movements), and the pons (corticopontocerebellar system).

ORBITOFRONTAL CORTEX

The orbitofrontal cortex is divided into an anterior granular region, a posterior agranular region that forms part of the limbic system (see Chapter 10), and a transitional dysgranular segment in between.[9–12] The posterior agranular and dysgranular cortices strongly connect to the brain stem reticular formation, limbic cortices (entorhinal and anterior cingulate cortices), amygdala, and midline thalamic nuclei. The anterior granular cortex strongly connects to association cortex and thalamic association nuclei.[13] The lateral regions of orbitofrontal cortex receive input from taste areas, and the medial portions receive olfactory inputs. Thus, the orbitofrontal cortex is a convergence zone for afferents from limbic and heteromodal association areas.[14]

ANTERIOR CINGULATE CORTEX

The anterior cingulate cortex (ACC) is the largest component of the limbic system (see Chapter 10), extending above the corpus callosum on the medial hemisphere. The ACC encircles the callosal rostrum, continuing inferiorly as the subcallosal area (BA 25). The ACC is part of a large structural–functional matrix within the limbic system, including the amygdala, periaqueductal gray, ventral striatum, and orbitofrontal and anterior insular cortices. It also connects extensively with the posterior cingulate cortex, which lies above the callosal splenium and continues inferiorly and caudally as the retrosplenial area and retrocalcarine area (BAs 29 and 30). Both anterior and posterior cingulate cortices connect with heteromodal association and limbic cortices. The ACC lacks a layer IV, has stronger connections with the amygdala and temporal pole, and receives more diverse thalamic inputs than the posterior cingulate, which receives greater input from sensory association cortices.

In summary, the prefrontal cortex has afferent and efferent connections to most areas of association cortex in the parietal, temporal, and occipital lobes. In addition, it connects to the premotor cortex (and therefore has indirect connections to primary motor cortex); the limbic cortex (including the cingulate gyrus, amygdala, and hippocampus); the basal ganglia (the caudate and putamen); the thalamus (predominantly the dorsomedial nucleus); the hypothalamus; and the midbrain. Many intrafrontal connections exist, but these pathways are still poorly understood. Thus, the human prefrontal cortex is privileged to communicate with almost every brain area (sensory, motor, and limbic systems) and plays a vital role in diverse cognitive and behavioral function.

CLINICAL CHARACTERISTICS OF THE PREFRONTAL SYNDROME

The function of the human prefrontal cortex and the identity of the specific subdivisions within this region have been determined from studying patients with focal lesions of the frontal lobes.[15,16] Valuable information is imparted by functional neuroimaging studies, including positron emission tomography (PET) and functional magnetic resonance imaging (fMRI) (see Chapter 2), and by electrophysiological studies, namely, event-related potentials (ERPs), of healthy, young individuals performing cognitive tasks. These studies reveal

that the signs of prefrontal damage do not lend themselves easily to quantitative analysis in the laboratory. Nevertheless, significant progress has been made in understanding the behavioral, cognitive, and neurological deficits after prefrontal damage (Table 9–1).

Behavior and the Prefrontal Cortex

Damage to the prefrontal cortex can produce many behavioral alterations. Such damage usually results in socially inappropriate behavior and difficulty in taking actions that require decisions and planning. When making any determination of impairment, consider the normal variation and range of human behavior as well as the patient's age, educational level, social and cultural group, and previous achievements. Many behavioral alterations overlap with the range of normal behavior, and large frontal lobe lesions may go undetected unless the patient's present state is compared with the premorbid state. The diverse and idiosyncratically expressed behavioral changes associated with

Table 9–1. **Behavioral, Cognitive, and Motor Changes after Prefrontal Lesions**

Behavioral
  Lack of appreciation of social roles and
    restrictions
  Flat affect, blunted emotional response, and
    decreased drive
  Lack of self-awareness
  Imitation and utilization behavior
  Separation of action from knowledge
Cognitive
  Impaired "in real-life" intelligence
  Impaired executive function
    Inability to alter behavior in response to
      changing rules
    Inability to plan and handle multistep,
      sequential behaviors
    Inability to inhibit responses
    Perseveration
  Impaired working memory
  Impaired language
Motor
  Primitive reflexes (e.g., grasp, groping, snout,
    palmomental)

frontal lobe damage can occur in any combination in any single patient.

SOCIAL RULES AND RESTRICTIONS

A lack of appreciation and disregard of social rules and restrictions may result in impulsivity, disinhibition, and sometimes episodic dyscontrol (short periods of anger or rage). The paradigmatic case of the frontal lobe syndrome, Phineas Gage, reported in 1868 by Dr. Harlow,[17] exemplifies these behavioral changes. The energetic, reliable, and effective foreman accidentally blasted a pointed, 3-foot-long and 1-inch-wide tamping iron through his frontal lobes (Fig. 9–2). Phineas survived but was changed after his accident.

Prior to his accident he was a religious, family-loving, honest and hard working man who was described after his frontal injury as "fitful, irreverent, indulging at times in the grossest profanity . . . impatient of restraint or advice when it conflicts with his desires . . . obstinate, devising many plans of operation, which are no sooner arranged than they are abandoned in turn for others appearing more feasible.

Benson (1994)[18]

EMOTIONAL RESPONSE AND DRIVE

Frontal lobe damage can cause a flat affect, blunted emotional response, and a decrease in drive. The loss of spontaneity and willpower is called *abulia*.[19] Since the clinical characteristics of abulia are difficult to measure and vary considerably among normal individuals throughout the life span, it is easy to miss. For example, many children are hyperactive and overly spontaneous, while many elderly are slow, make few extraneous movements, and are generally aspontaneous. When you walk into the room, the abulic patient lies there, silent and motionless. He sees you enter, understands who you are, comprehends your questions, hesitates, seems to ignore you, or gives yes-or-no answers to your questions. In some cases, abulia is extreme: patients do not speak unless spoken to and do not move unless very hungry or ready to void. They are often incontinent because they cannot energize themselves to go to the bathroom or do not care about the consequences of voiding in the bed or chair. An example of this behavior is evident in a patient with a frontal lobe lesion.

He was quiet, did not initiate conversation, and appeared remote and withdrawn. Although frequently incontinent, he was unconcerned and almost never initiated an attempt to remedy the status.

Benson (1994)[18]

SELF-AWARENESS

Patients with frontal lobe lesions may be unaware that their cognitive abilities, behavior, or expression or appreciation of emotion has changed from their preinjury state. Moreover, they seem unable to "evaluate the conse-

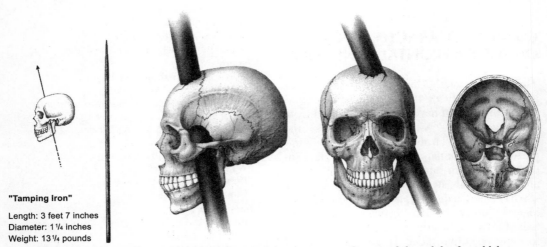

"Tamping Iron"

Length: 3 feet 7 inches
Diameter: 1 ¼ inches
Weight: 13 ¼ pounds

Figure 9–2. The skull wound of Phineas Gage and the tamping iron that passed through his frontal lobes.

quences and implications of their own behavior."[20] An example of this inability to monitor one's own behavior is evident in the description of a patient with frontal lobe damage.

If asked directly, he denied any disability and insisted that he could return to work at any time, although he never requested discharge or even a weekend pass and was totally unconcerned about his wife and children or the fact that they no longer visited him.

Benson (1994)[18]

If a hierarchy exists among the functions linked to the frontal lobes, self-awareness may be one of the frontal lobe's highest functions.[21,22] A related phenomenon is *anosognosia,* the denial of one's illness (see Chapter 3). Patients with anosognosia typically have right hemisphere lesions. These patients' behavior may range from being unconcerned about their deficit to frank delusions and paranoia.

IMITATION AND UTILIZATION BEHAVIOR

Patients with frontal lobe lesions may display a remarkable tendency to imitate the examiner's gestures and behaviors, even without instruction to do so and even when this imitation entails considerable personal embarrassment.[23–25] The mere sight of an object may elicit the compulsion to use it, although there was no request to use it and the context is inappropriate, as in a patient who sees a tongue depressor and proceeds to give the physician a checkup or who puts on a pair of glasses despite having a pair on already (Fig. 9–3). According to one theory,[23,24] these symptoms comprise the "environmental dependency syndrome," and the frontal lobes may promote distance from the environment and the parietal lobes foster approach toward one's environment. Therefore, a lesion that impairs frontal inhibition may result in overactivity of the parietal lobes. Without frontal inhibition, autonomy from the environment and abstract thinking are impaired or impossible. A given stimulus automatically calls up a predetermined response regardless of the context.

SEPARATION OF ACTION FROM KNOWLEDGE

Although cognitive functions such as language and visuoperception are relatively preserved in patients with prefrontal lesions, effective employment of these skills may be limited. This problem is illustrated in a case history.

While being evaluated for the presence of diabetes insipidus, the patient was instructed, "Don't drink any water; don't go near the water fountain." Within a few minutes he was observed having a drink at the water fountain. When asked by the examiner what he had just been told, he immediately replied: "Don't drink any water; don't go near the water fountain."

Benson (1994)[18]

The patient understood and remembered the instructions, but this knowledge could not modulate his actions.

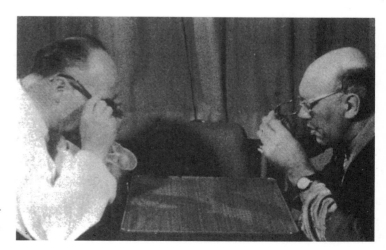

Figure 9–3. Photograph of a patient with imitation behavior. The patient on the right puts on a pair of glasses despite already wearing a pair.[24]

Cognition and the Prefrontal Cortex

INTELLIGENCE

Intelligence can be considered "a global capacity to engage in adaptive, goal directed behavior," which is not necessarily what is measured by IQ tests performed during routine neuropsychological testing.[20] Thus, although the frontal lobes are likely critical for human intelligence, damage to them may not be captured by the performance of these patients on tests of the abilities measured by intelligence. Thus, patients with frontal damage can score normally on the Wechsler Adult Intelligence Scale–Revised (WAIS-R), which is the most common intelligence test used by neuropsychologists (see Chapter 1). For example, a group of 44 Vietnam veterans who suffered penetrating unilateral frontal injuries scored within the average range on the WAIS-R.[26] In the well-studied patient E.V.R.,[27] who had resection of a large orbitofrontal meningioma, the WAIS revealed a verbal IQ of 125 (95th percentile) and a performance IQ of 124 (94th percentile) despite a significant change in his behavior after surgery leading to his inability to hold a job or maintain his marriage. Patient E.V.R. is a paradigmatic example of the dissociation between intelligence measured in the laboratory and the lack of intelligent behavior in real life by patients with frontal lobe injury.[27]

Patients with frontal lobe lesions may fail in real life because they are unable to succeed in open-ended, multiple subgoal situations that require them to maintain goals and intentions and plan ahead.[28] For instance, patients with frontal lobe damage were assessed on their ability to carry out multiple errands during which minor unforeseen events might occur. Most of the errands were simple (e.g., buy a loaf of bread), but one of them required the subject to be at a certain place 15 minutes after he started, which was not enough time to complete all of the errands. Despite fully understanding the instructions, the patients made numerous errors, such as not using the most effective strategy (e.g., entering a shop more than once); broke rules (e.g., left a shop with a newspaper without paying); misinterpreted instructions; did not carry out the task; or did not complete it satisfactorily.[28]

Intelligence as measured by standard psychometric tests clearly does not fully predict life success. A complex and changing world demands other, less easily measured faculties such as mental flexibility, adaptability, quickness, the ability to creatively solve novel problems, the ability to obey social rules, and judgment of the behavioral relevance of environmental events. The prefrontal cortex is critical for many of the faculties that are necessary for success in life.

EXECUTIVE FUNCTION

Under the rubric of "executive function," the clinical neuropsychological literature includes a wide range of cognitive processes, such as focused and sustained attention, fluency and flexibility of thought in the generation of solutions to novel problems, and planning and regulating adaptive and goal-directed behavior.[29] Executive function captures a wide spectrum of high-level cognitive abilities.[21] Such abilities are difficult to define and difficult to measure, especially at the bedside, prompting the development of many clinical and experimental neuropsychological tests to tap this function.[29,30] Despite its elusive testability, executive function is vital for daily function. Many impairments characterize executive dysfunction.

ALTERATION OF BEHAVIOR IN RESPONSE TO CHANGING RULES

The inability of patients with frontal lobe damage to alter their behavior in response to changing rules is reflected by poor performance on a commonly administered neuropsychological measure called the Wisconsin Card Sorting Test.[31] During this test, four stimulus cards (one with a red triangle, one with two green stars, one with three yellow crosses, and one with four blue circles) are placed in front of the patient. The patient is then given a deck of response cards, each containing from one to four identical figures (stars, triangles, crosses, or circles) in one of four colors. The patient is instructed to place each response card next to one of the four stimulus cards according to *one* of the stimulus dimensions (i.e., color, form, or number). However, the patient is not told the correct sorting principle but, rather, must infer this from the examiner's feedback after each response. For example, if the patient sorts by color and the examiner says "incorrect," the patient is prompted to sort by form or number with the next card. After 10 correct sorts by the patient, the examiner changes the sorting principle without warning by saying "incorrect" to previously correct trials. This procedure continues until five shifts of the sorting category are completed or 128 cards are sorted. Almost invariably, patients with frontal lobe lesions understand what they are supposed to do and can repeat the rules of the test ("I am supposed to arrange these by color, shape, or number"). Moreover, since four stimulus cards are always visible, patients do not have to remember the sorting principles. However, frontal lobe patients are unable to follow them or use knowledge of incorrect performance based on feedback to alter their behavior.[27,32] Patients with frontal lobe lesions make both random errors and perseverative errors on the Wisconsin Card Sorting Test.[33] Perseverative errors are traditionally viewed as failure to inhibit a previous response pattern, as discussed later, and on this test in particular as failure to shift set using a new sorting criterion. A random error occurs when a patient is sorting correctly and switches to a new, incorrect sorting category without any prompt from the examiner; this is viewed as a transient failure in maintaining the goal at hand.

MULTISTEP SEQUENTIAL BEHAVIOR

Simple daily tasks require many steps. To make spaghetti and sauce, one must find the spaghetti and pot, fill the pot with water, turn the stove on, put the pot on the stove, allow the water to boil, put the spaghetti in the pot, note the time, get out the sauce and another small pot, and so on. Superimposed upon that sequence may be the phone ringing, a television show in the background, and a child running through the house. We need to plan behavior in relation to the environment, start it, switch actions within a task, stop and attend to another distracting stimulus, and return to the plan until the goal is complete. A simple but interrupted behavioral sequence can be an insurmountable task for patients with frontal lobe lesions. As the behavioral sequence requires greater creativity and complexity and the interruptions increase (integration over discontinuous time periods), the performance of patients with frontal lobe lesions becomes worse.

Notably, patients with frontal lobe lesions often do not have difficulty with the individual steps that are necessary to complete a sequential task. For example, these patients can easily perform the basic operations (e.g., adding and subtracting) required to complete complex arithmetical tasks. However, when given more complex problems requiring multiple steps, the patient responds impulsively to an early stimulus and fails to analyze or execute the component steps required for problem solution. The following task is almost impossible for patients with frontal lobe lesions, even though they can perform the direct arithmetical task of multiplying 6 by 31 with ease: "The price of canned peas is two cans for 31 cents. What is the price of one dozen cans?" Similar errors occur in routine, everyday tasks that require a series of simple steps, such as wrapping a present or making a sandwich.[34]

Grafman[35] argued that managerial knowledge units are the predominant type of information unit represented in the human frontal lobe. These units are overlearned sequences of events or "scripts" that are retrieved automatically and have a chronological sequence with a beginning and an end. Managerial knowledge units are analogous to software programs that are written and modified by the brain through experience. These programs allow us to put certain functions on "autopilot" so that, for example, we can make spaghetti while talking on the telephone and focus on the conversation. It is proposed that patients with frontal lobe lesions have lost their scripts and therefore pause to recall the next line; during this pause, they may completely lose their train of thought if another stimulus comes into consciousness and causes the original script to be abandoned. Thus, patients with frontal lobe lesions are impaired at formulating and executing plans of action.[36] Moreover, fMRI studies of healthy subjects have shown activation of prefrontal cortex during tasks that require the processing of sequences of a script.[37,38]

PERSEVERATION

Perseveration is abnormal repetition of a specific behavior.[39] It can occur after frontal lobe damage in a wide range of tasks, including motor acts, verbalizations, sorting tests, drawing, or writing. Perseverative responses may be mistaken for impaired comprehension, praxis, and

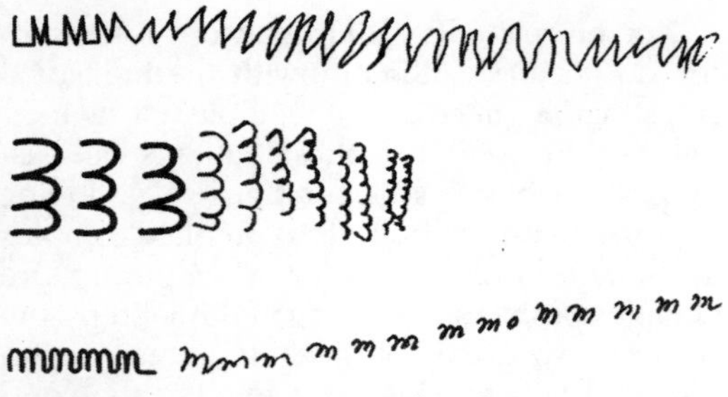

Figure 9–4. Patient examples of perseveration.

visuospatial and other cognitive functions. Perseveration takes three different forms: *(1) recurrent perseveration* is a repetition of a previous response to a subsequent stimulus, *(2) stuck-in-set perseveration* is an inability to shift a cognitive set, and *(3) continuous* or *compulsive perseveration* is a prolongation of ongoing activity.[40,41] Perseverative behavior is illustrated in Figure 9–4.

REGULATION OF SENSORY INFORMATION

The inability to inhibit prepotent responses and filter out distracting information can be revealed with a neuropsychological measure called the Stroop paradigm.[42] This test is based on the observation that it takes less time to read color names (e.g., blue, green, red, yellow) printed in black type than to read color names printed in ink of a different color (e.g., the word *green* printed in red). This effect is exaggerated in patients with frontal lobe lesions, especially with damage to superior medial regions,[43,44] presumably owing to an impaired ability to inhibit the interference created by reading color names printed in an incongruent ink color.

Animal research first provided evidence for a prefrontal–thalamic inhibitory system that regulates the flow of sensory information from the external world to the cerebral cortex. For example, cooling the prefrontal cortex in the cat increased the amplitudes of evoked electrophysiological responses recorded from primary cortex in all sensory modalities.[45] Conversely, stimulation of specific thalamic regions (i.e., nucleus reticularis thalami) that surround the sensory relay thalamic nuclei suppresses activity in primary sensory cortex.[46] Thus, these findings support an inhibitory pathway from prefrontal cortex that regulates the flow of sensory information through thalamic relay nuclei. This prefrontal–thalamic inhibitory system provides a mechanism for modality-specific suppression of irrelevant inputs in early sensory processing.

Human data support prefrontal inhibitory control on other cortical and subcortical regions. For example, in patients with focal prefrontal damage, primary auditory and somatosensory ERPs are enhanced, suggesting disinhibition of sensory flow to these regions. In a series of ERP experiments, task-irrelevant auditory and somatosensory stimuli (monaural clicks or brief electric shocks to the median nerve) were presented to patients with comparably sized lesions in lateral prefrontal cortex, the temporal–parietal junction, or lateral parietal cortex. Unlike damage in temporal and parietal regions, lateral prefrontal cortical damage resulted in enhanced ERP amplitudes in both primary auditory and somatosensory components.[47–49] Spinal cord and brain stem potentials were not affected by lateral prefrontal cortex damage, suggesting that the amplitude enhancements result from abnormalities in either a prefrontal–thalamic or a prefrontal–sensory cortex mechanism.

Several functional neuroimaging studies in healthy young subjects also link lateral prefrontal cortical function and inhibitory control.[50–54] For example, inhibitory control was investigated with the go–no go task. In this task, during go trials, a green square is presented and subjects must respond by promptly pushing a button. In no go trials, a red square is presented and subjects are instructed not to respond. During this type of task, patients with frontal lesions typically respond to no go trials despite being told repeatedly not to do so. During fMRI scanning, normal healthy subjects exhibit greater activity within prefrontal cortex during no go trials than go trials, suggesting that prefrontal cortex inhibits inherent response tendencies. Thus, functional neuroimaging in normals and electrophysiological studies in patients with prefrontal lesions provide powerful evidence that the human prefrontal cortex provides net inhibitory regulation of early sensory transmission.[55]

MEMORY

Working memory is the short-term storage of information that is not accessible in the environment and the set of processes that keep this information active for later use in behavior.[56] This system is important in cognition, providing a critical physiological infrastructure for such functions as reasoning, language comprehension, planning, and spatial processing. Evidence for the neural basis of working memory was initially provided from animal studies (for a review, see Fuster[57]). Electrophysiological studies of awake, behaving monkeys often use delayed-response tasks to study working memory. In these tasks, the monkey must keep in mind, or actively maintain, a stimulus over a short delay. During such tasks, neurons within the lateral prefrontal cortex are persistently activated during the delay period of a delayed-response task when the monkey is maintaining information in memory prior to making a motor response.[58,59] The necessity of this region actively to maintain information over short delays was demonstrated in monkeys with lateral prefrontal lesions who were severely impaired on these tasks.[60,61] Thus, the prefrontal cortex may integrate events separated in time and utilize stored representational knowledge to guide an appropriate motor response.[57,62]

Human studies provide converging evidence that working memory is subserved in part by the prefrontal cortex. Working memory impairments occur in humans following restricted prefrontal damage[63–66] or in normal subjects when virtual frontal lesions are produced by transcranial magnetic stimulation.[67–69] In addition, functional neuroimaging studies of working memory in healthy young adults empirically link working memory and prefrontal cortex (for a review, see D'Esposito et al.[70,71]).

In contrast with this severe impairment in working memory, patients with frontal lobe lesions have little impairment on tasks of information storage over longer periods of time. (This process, long-term memory, is discussed extensively in Chapter 8.) However, despite preserved memory capacity on neuropsychological testing, these patients may show severe impairments when using these abilities in real-life situations. Thus, patients appear "forgetful" to family members. This impairment may result from inefficiencies caused by poor attention or poor executive function. This type of memory deficit is due to defective retrieval, a function that requires strategy and effort, as opposed to normal storage, a more passive function. There are several other interesting features of these real-life memory difficulties. They are defective in recall of temporal order, that is, recalling the context of learned items, even when they can remember these items. For example, a patient instructed to remember words spoken by either a male or a female speaker may later recall or recognize most of the words but cannot correctly identify the speaker. In addition, patients with frontal lobe lesions do poorly at tasks requiring them to judge the probability that they would recognize the correct answer to a multiple-choice question (e.g., a feeling of knowing), reflecting deficient self-monitoring abilities.[72] In summary, patients with prefrontal lesions are impaired in the processes involved in planning, organizing, and other strategic aspects of learning and memory that facilitate the encoding and retrieval of information.

LANGUAGE

Damage to the posterior frontal Broca's area causes nonfluent aphasia with impaired naming and repetition and preserved comprehension (see Chapter 6). However, many language difficulties are observed in patients with frontal lobe lesions, sparing Broca's area (for review, see Alexander[73,74]). Although these patients are not aphasic, their use of language is abnormal. Those with left frontal lesions exhibit reduced formulation of responses and impoverished discourse. For example, these patients are impaired at speech initiation, making little effort to speak and often showing a delay before a verbal response is uttered. These patients are poor at producing well-formulated and structured language output despite normal articulation. They produce unelaborated, sparse utterances and are impaired in abstract language ability and verbal reasoning.[74] For example, in verbal fluency tasks that require patients to produce a list of words belonging to a given category (e.g., animals, words beginning with the letter S), patients with left frontal lobe lesions show a marked reduction of responses. These patients also have difficulty comprehending complex syntax of spoken and written language. Right prefrontal lesions alter narrative discourse, understanding of sarcasm and humor, prosody, and other paralinguistic functions (see Chapter 3). Thus, even when patients with frontal lobe damage appear to have normal language abilities in conversational speech, further testing may reveal significant abnormalities.

Neurological Deficits and the Prefrontal Cortex

Several findings on the neurological examination are consistent with prefrontal damage. These findings together with the typical behavioral and cognitive changes described above aid in making the bedside diagnosis of prefrontal damage. Many of these signs may be subtle, and identifying them is not as easy as detecting loss of strength or a visual field cut. However, all clinicians in a position to diagnose frontal lobe injury must be skilled in these aspects of the neurological examination.

Prefrontal damage can lead to the emergence, or "release," of several reflexes that are typically present in infancy but later disappear with normal development. Inhibition by the frontal lobes results in the normal loss of these reflexes, and their reappearance after frontal lobe injury likely reflects loss of this inhibitory control. The presence of these reflexes after 1–2 years of age is abnormal. These include the grasp, groping, snout, sucking, rooting, and palmomental reflexes (Fig. 9–5). The grasp reflex, found in the hand or foot, may be unilateral or bilateral. It appears as a forced grasp when the patient's palm or sole of the foot comes in contact with an object such as the examiner's hand. Even if instructed to release the grasp, the patient may be unable to do so. The groping reflex is elicited when the patient's hands or eyes involuntarily follow objects that are moved in front of the face. The sucking reflex is easily elicited by gently tapping the patient's lips with a reflex hammer. The palmomental reflex is contraction of the lip when the patient's palm is scratched. Any one or all of these reflexes may be present in a patient with a frontal lobe lesion.

Frontal lobe lesions can also cause abnormalities in appendicular movements, muscle tone, and gait. In the most extreme case, patients may be akinetic (typically accompanied by mutism), but they more commonly appear to move normally until careful observation reveals a paucity of spontaneous motor behavior. The movement abnormality may be limited to one side and is not due to diminished strength or power but to decreased initiation of movements.

Patients with right frontal lobe lesions may exhibit *motor impersistence*, the inability to sustain a motor act.[75] These patients can perform a requested motor act for brief periods but then spontaneously cease. Despite repeated requests by the examiner, the patient cannot persist in keeping the eyes closed, tongue protruded, or arms up. This deficit may be related to the impairments in sustained attention commonly exhibited by patients with right frontal lobe lesions.[76–79] Another deficit encountered after right frontal lobe lesions is motor, or intentional, neglect.[80,81] Unlike attentional neglect occurring after right parietal lobe lesions (see Chapter 4), motor neglect is characterized by impaired initiation and execution of extremity or ocular movements into the left side of space. These patients exhibit left-sided hypokinesia, bradykinesia, and *hypometria* (reduced motor amplitude).

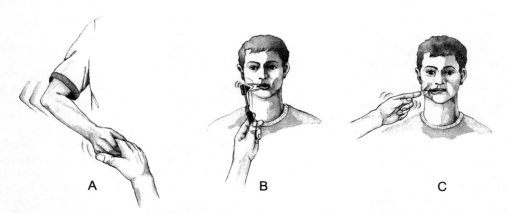

Figure 9–5. Frontal release signs. *A:* The grasp reflex. *B:* The snout reflex. *C:* The rooting reflex.

Examination of muscle tone reveals gegen-halten rigidity or paratonia. This is elicited when the examiner passively moves the patient's arm or leg and the patient resists with a movement in the opposite direction. This resistance increases in intensity when the examiner increases the force of moving the arm or leg. The patient cannot prevent these counteracting movements, although they may be interpreted as being deliberate. Patients with frontal lobe lesions may have an abnormal gait that appears short-stepped and magnetic, as if the patient's feet are stuck to the floor. These patients often exhibit postural instability when standing, leading to loss of balance and retropulsion.

The patient's medical history can alert the clinician to several other neurological abnormalities. Query the patient about an olfactory disturbance (due to direct injury of the olfactory bulbs concomitant with orbitofrontal injury) and changes in sphincter control (due to loss of inhibitory control on the spinal detrussor reflex after medial frontal lesions). Consider autonomic dysfunction because orbitofrontal stimulation evokes autonomic responses affecting respiration, blood pressure, heart rate, gastrointestinal motility, and pupillary size.[82,83]

CLINICAL–ANATOMICAL RELATIONSHIPS IN FRONTAL LOBE FUNCTION

In 1934, Kleist[84] observed that components of the frontal lobe syndrome result from specific regional involvement; subsequent studies supported Kleist's original observation.[85] The heterogeneous morphology and connectivity patterns within the prefrontal cortex can be resolved into three functional circuits: dorsolateral frontal, orbitofrontal, and medial frontal.[85] There is no unitary "frontal lobe syndrome," despite the popularity of this concept among clinicians.

Anatomically, five parallel frontal–subcortical circuits link the frontal lobes and subcortical structures.[86] Two of these circuits originate outside the prefrontal cortex, primarily in motor areas (see Chapter 7). The first is a motor circuit that originates in the primary sensorimotor cortex, premotor cortex, and supplementary motor area. The second, oculomotor, circuit originates in the frontal eye fields (as

well as prefrontal and parietal cortex). The other three circuits, dorsolateral frontal, orbitofrontal, and medial frontal, when damaged, produce signature behavioral or cognitive syndromes (Fig. 9–6). All three circuits originate in the prefrontal cortex and project to striatal structures, which in turn project to the globus pallidus and substantia nigra, which feed to the thalamus and then complete a loop back to the prefrontal cortex (Fig. 9–7). The dorsolateral, orbital, and medial prefrontal regions project to unique regions of the basal ganglia and thalamus and create segregated parallel circuits.

Dorsolateral Frontal Circuit

The dorsolateral frontal circuit originates in the lateral convexity of the frontal lobes, specifically BAs 9, 46, and 10 (Fig. 9–8). This region projects to the dorsolateral head of the caudate nucleus, then to the dorsomedial globus pallidus interna and substantia nigra, which project to the ventral anterior and medial dorsal thalamic nuclei before returning to lateral prefrontal cortex. Damage to the dorsolateral prefrontal circuit impairs executive function, causing inflexibility of thought in generating solutions to novel problems, planning, and regulating adaptive and goal-directed behavior.

Orbitofrontal Circuit

The orbitofrontal circuit originates in both heteromodal inferolateral prefrontal cortex (BAs 10, 11) and limbic caudal–medial orbital cortex (BAs 11, 12), giving rise to the lateral and medial subcircuits (Figs. 9–8 and 7–9). The lateral region projects to the ventromedial head of the caudate nucleus, and the medial region projects to the ventral striatum. Both orbital subcircuits then send fibers to the dorsomedial globus pallidus interna and substantia nigra, which project to the ventral anterior and medial dorsal thalamic nuclei before returning to lateral or medial orbitofrontal cortex. Damage to the orbitofrontal circuit causes significant affective and social changes (disinhibition of motor activity [hyperactivity] and instinctual behaviors), failure to appreciate the consequences of one's actions, emotional lability with euphoria or dysphoria, and increased aggressiveness. These patients may be uncon-

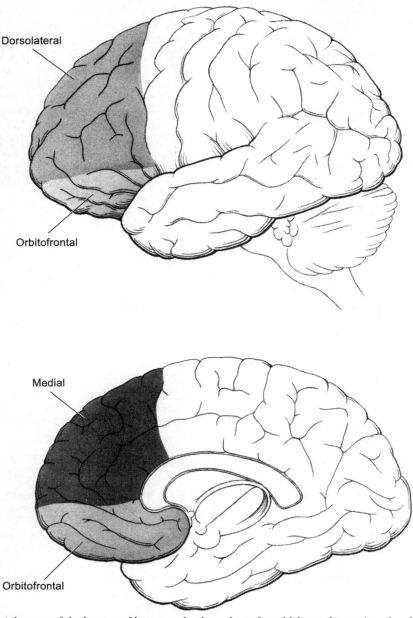

Figure 9–6. Schematic of the location of lesions in the three classic frontal lobe syndromes (e.g. dorsolateral, medial, orbitofrontal).

cerned over responsibilities or careless actions, be tactless, or laugh inappropriately, with silly and childish behavior. Patients with orbitofrontal lesions may fail to recognize their violent tendencies (i.e., impaired self-monitoring), which are often provoked by family conflicts. Patients may show anxiety and obses-sive–compulsive symptoms.[87–89] Patients with orbitofrontal damage are frequently impulsive, hyperactive, labile, and lacking in proper social skills despite reasonable performance on cognitive tasks typically impaired in patients with damage to lateral prefrontal cortex.[90–92]

There may be functional subdivisions of the

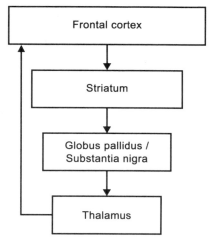

Figure 9–7. General organization of the frontal subcortical circuits.

orbitofrontal cortex. The ventromedial portion has been associated with the perception of internal autonomic states in the guidance of goal-directed behavior and involved in inhibitory processing of emotional stimuli. The ventrolateral portion of the orbitofrontal cortex may facilitate reward–punishment associations (for a review of these current ideas, see Elliott et al.[14]).

Medial Frontal Circuit

The medial frontal circuit originates in the ACC and projects to the ventral striatum (i.e.,

nucleus accumbens, olfactory tubercle) (Figs. 9–8 and 7–9). Hippocampal and amygdalar neurons also project to the ventral striatum, which pro-jects to the rostrolateral globus pallidus and substantia nigra. These regions in turn project to paramedian portions of the medial dorsal nucleus of the thalamus before returning to the ACC. Bilateral damage to the medial frontal circuit can cause the dramatic syndrome of akinetic mutism (see Chapters 6 and 7). The patient appears awake and may follow the examiner with his or her eyes but lacks spontaneous motor and verbal responses.[93] In addition, the patient may be incontinent and respond incompletely to noxious stimuli. Akinetic mutism is usually transient when the lesion is unilateral. Abulia is a less severe form of akinetic mutism.

The intimate relationship between the frontal lobes, basal ganglia, and thalamus explains why selective damage to the striatum, or thalamus, can cause behavioral and cognitive deficits similar to those observed in patients with frontal lobe lesions. For example, caudate strokes can cause executive function deficits.[94,95] Dorsal caudate lesions, like dorsolateral prefrontal lesions, cause confusion and disinterest, whereas ventral caudate lesions, like orbitofrontal lesions, cause disinhibition, euphoria and inappropriateness.[96] Huntington's disease, a degenerative disease primarily affecting the caudate nuclei, often causes prominent behavioral deficits (e.g., irritability, mood disorder, explosive disorder) and impairs executive function.[97,98] Bi-

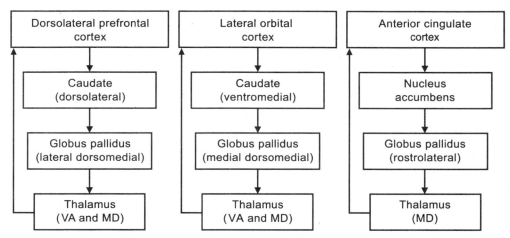

Figure 9–8. Organization of three frontal subcortical circuits in which lesions produce alterations of cognition and emotion. VA, ventral anterior; MD, medial dorsal.

lateral globus pallidus lesions from anoxia and carbon monoxide or manganese poisoning reduce spontaneous activity, impair initiative, and diminish the ability to conceive new thoughts.[99] Finally, numerous patients with thalamic strokes exhibit significant behavioral and cognitive deficits, especially when the anterior and medial thalamus are affected.[100–102]

These findings in patients with damage restricted to subcortical regions highlight the obligation of clinicians to abandon the long-held notion that subcortical lesions do not cause behavioral and cognitive deficits. In our experience, many patients have presented acutely with significant cognitive deficits, and the report of the MRI scan notes only "small vessel cerebrovascular" disease; the link between the two has not been made.

Whether prefrontal cortical function is lateralized is unclear. Historically, a traditional distinction is emphasized: language processing supported by the left hemisphere and visuospatial abilities supported by the right hemisphere. However, clear double dissociation of deficits in patients with right vs. left focal lesions is rarely observed. For example, on fluency tasks, patients with left frontal lesions perform more poorly when asked to generate verbal information (e.g., animals), whereas patients with left or right frontal lesions perform poorly when asked to generate nonverbal information (i.e., geometric designs).[103,104] Goldberg et al.[105] have proposed that hemispheric asymmetries in frontal function do exist. Rather than a linguistic–nonlinguistic distinction, it is proposed that left frontal systems are critical for guiding behavior driven by internal representations, whereas right frontal systems guide behavior driven by external representations within our environment. In this way, the right hemisphere is critical for dealing with novel situations, whereas the left hemisphere mediates well-routinized behaviors. Functional neuroimaging studies have found that the right frontal lobe shows greater activity when healthy subjects must learn novel rules and concepts, whereas the left frontal lobe is more active after such information is learned.[106,107]

From a clinical perspective, bilateral frontal lesions usually cause the most severe deficit. The fully developed "prefrontal syndrome," whether lateral, orbital, or medial, usually occurs only after bilateral lesions. As for behavioral disturbances, left frontal lobe strokes may more often cause depression than right frontal lobe strokes.[108] Patients with right prefrontal lesions show more blunted or labile affect, motor impersistence, disinhibition, excessive talkativeness, confabulation, and the alien hand sign.[109]

ROLE OF DOPAMINE IN FRONTAL LOBE FUNCTION

The cortex is strongly modulated by diffuse inputs from brain stem systems rostrally transmitting dopamine, acetylcholine, and serotonin. Keys to understanding prefrontal cortex function are deciphering its relationship with other brain regions and learning how it is modulated by such brain stem projections. Fuster[57] writes: "certain neural structures and pathways have been grouped and characterized as forming separate functional systems because they share a prevalent neurotransmitter . . . none of them can have more functional specialization than the system of interconnected brain structures in which it operates." Thus, a specific neurotransmitter's role in cognition can be derived by understanding the function of the brain regions that receive input from neurons producing that neurotransmitter.

The anatomical distribution of dopaminergic projections strongly implicates dopamine in higher-level cognitive abilities, specifically in prefrontal cortical function (for reviews, see Nieoullon[110] and Arnsten[111]). Midbrain dopaminergic neurons are organized into several major subsystems: mesocortical, mesolimbic, and nigrostriatal. The mesocortical and mesolimbic dopaminergic systems originate in the ventral tegmental area and project to the prefrontal cortex, ACC, anterior temporal structures (e.g., amygdala, hippocampus, entorhinal cortex), and basal forebrain.[112] There is an anterior–posterior gradient in brain dopamine concentration, which is highest in the prefrontal cortex.[113] Thus, the distribution of the mesocortical dopaminergic fibers suggests a greater influence on anterior brain structures.

Several lines of evidence confirm the role of dopamine in prefrontal function. First, in monkeys, depletion of dopamine in the prefrontal cortex or pharmacological blockade of dopamine receptors impaired working memory tasks.[114,115] This working memory impairment was as severe as the deficit in monkeys with prefrontal lesions and was not observed in monkeys when serotonin or norepinephrine was depleted. Dopaminergic agonists administered to these same monkeys reversed their working memory impairments.[114,116] Thus, impaired prefrontal function can result from dopamine deficiency and improve with dopamine replacement.

Another method of assessing dopamine's influence on cognitive function is testing patients with Parkinson's disease (PD) while "on" and "off" their dopaminergic replacement medication. Although the motor symptoms of PD are caused by degeneration of the nigrostriatal dopaminergic system, many PD patients also have degeneration of the dopaminergic neurons in the ventrotegmental area comprising the mesocortical system.[117] Thus, PD is an excellent model for investigating dopamine's role in prefrontal function. Since the half-life of some dopaminergic replacement drugs (e.g., levodopa) is short, brain dopamine levels can be manipulated over brief periods and monitored by observing a deterioration in the patient's motor status.

Several groups used this method to assess tasks sensitive to frontal lobe dysfunction.[118–120] In all studies, PD patients were impaired on these tasks when they were off their dopaminergic medications. In one study, the tasks that PD patients performed poorly while off their medications (Tower of London, a spatial working memory task, and a test of attentional set shifting) were specifically impaired in patients with frontal lobe lesions.[120] The evidence for a specific role of dopamine in prefrontal function is strengthened by concurrent findings that PD patients perform similarly in on/off states on long-term memory tasks sensitive to medial temporal lobe function. These studies provide evidence that dopaminergic input influences certain prefrontal functions.

Administration of dopamine receptor agonists to healthy young subjects is also a method for examining the role of dopaminergic systems in higher cognitive functions. Most dopamine receptor agonists are relatively selective for a particular receptor subtype, the two most common being D_1 and D_2 dopamine receptors. Two such drugs, approved for human use, are bromocriptine, which is relatively selective for the D_2 receptor subtype, and pergolide, which affects D_1 and D_2 receptor subtypes. Since both drugs are relatively safe for healthy volunteers and have well-understood agonist properties, they offer a useful probe of how dopamine influences prefrontal cortical function.

Healthy young subjects performed better on working memory tasks when given bromocriptine[121–124] or pergolide[125,126] than when given a placebo. In these studies, the dopaminergic medication specifically affected working memory, with no effect on other cognitive abilities such as attention or sensorimotor function. Converging on these findings, normal subjects given sulpiride, a D_2 receptor antagonist, were impaired on several tasks sensitive to frontal lobe function. Nonspecific sedative or motoric effects could not account for the impairments.[127]

Interestingly, bromocriptine's effects on prefrontal function are not the same for all subjects but interact with the subject's working memory capacity.[124,125] For example, subjects with lower baseline working memory abilities tended to improve on bromocriptine, while those with higher baseline working memory abilities worsened. A similar relationship between dopamine and prefrontal function was observed in monkeys given dopaminergic agonists and antagonists. The U-shaped dose–response curve shows that a specific dosage produces optimal performance on working memory tasks.[111] This observation suggests that "more" is not "better" and that an optimal dopamine concentration is necessary for optimal function of the prefrontal cortex.

The cognitive effect of dopamine agonists on patients with frontal lobe lesions also provides insight into the relationship between dopamine and executive function. Patients who had traumatic prefrontal damage performed measures of executive function (e.g., Stroop Task, Wisconsin Card Sorting Test, Trailmaking Task, a dual-task) and were assessed while on and off bromocriptine. Compared with placebo, bromocriptine produced significant improvement on all tasks requiring executive control processes. In contrast, bromocriptine did not improve performance on measures of minimal executive control demands, even if they were cognitively demanding, or on other simpler tasks requiring basic attentional, mnemonic, or sensorimotor processes. These findings provide evidence that the dopaminergic system may specifically modulate executive control processes and may not be critical for basic mnemonic processes.

In the cortex, D_1 receptors are more abundant than D_2 receptors, which are found mostly within the striatum.[128] However, D_2 receptors are at their highest concentrations in layer V of the prefrontal cortex, the cortical region with the highest concentration of dopamine receptors, making it especially well placed to influence behavior.[129] Future investigations may determine the relative contribution of these dopamine receptors to specific cognitive processes, as well as to synergistic interactions between these two dopamine receptor types.[130]

Knowledge about the dopaminergic system sheds light on the role of the prefrontal cortex in behavior and may help to define mechanisms underlying cognitive deficits in a wide range of disorders (e.g., attention-deficit disorder, drug addiction, and schizophrenia), in states commonly encountered by normal healthy persons (e.g., stress and sleep deprivation), and in the normal aging process. As Arnsten[111] aptly states: "the [prefrontal cortex] is extraordinarily sensitive to its neurochemical environment, and small changes in levels of dopamine . . . may contribute substantially to altered prefrontal cortical cognitive function."

NEUROLOGICAL DISORDERS AND FRONTAL LOBE DAMAGE

Several neurological disorders can cause predominantly frontal lobe damage, and in patients with these disorders, executive dysfunction is the predominant finding on examination (Table 9–2). These disorders include traumatic brain injury, vascular compromise, neoplasms, herpes encephalitis, epilepsy, and neurodegenerative disease. Thus, very different etiologies of frontal lobe damage can produce a common set of behavioral and cognitive findings.

Table 9–2. **Common Causes of Frontal Lobe Damage**

Traumatic brain injury
Anterior or middle cerebral artery stroke
Neoplasm (e.g., meningioma, glioma)
Herpes encephalitis
Epilepsy
Frontotemporal dementia

Traumatic Brain Injury

Traumatic brain injury is a common neurological disorder, with a prevalence of approximately 200 patients per 100,000 population. The pathological hallmark of traumatic brain injury is diffuse axonal injury caused by shearing forces.[131] Diffuse axonal injury is caused by significant acceleration and deceleration, as occurs in a fall from greater than 6 feet, a fall with high angular momentum (e.g., slipping on ice), or a major motor vehicle accident.[132] Such an injury stretches or tears the fragile structures in the long axes of the brain that primarily includes axons and small blood vessels. Axonal damage can be temporary or, if the axon is physically disrupted, permanent. Damage to blood vessels causes local petechial hemorrhages and edema, which may be visualized on an MRI scan. Diffuse axonal injury occurs within parasagittal white matter extending from cortex to the brain stem. The duration of coma and posttraumatic amnesia (i.e., the inability to learn new information) is strongly correlated with the extent of diffuse axonal injury; that is, the longer the coma or posttraumatic amnesia, the greater the diffuse axonal injury. Likewise, diffuse axonal injury is unlikely if the patient did not lose consciousness at the time of injury.[133]

Focal brain injury often complicates traumatic brain injury. In addition to subdural and epidural hematomas, focal brain contusions are usually located along the skull's irregular bony surfaces, affecting orbitofrontal and anterior temporal lobes (Fig. 9–9). Due to direct trauma, traumatic brain injury is a common cause of the orbitofrontal syndrome, whereas signs and symptoms of the lateral or medial prefrontal syndrome are much less common since contusions do not generally occur in these areas. Lateral and medial prefrontal syndromes typically result from anterior and middle cerebral artery infarctions, respectively.

Even mild traumatic brain injury can present a particularly difficult problem for clinicians.[134] At the time of injury, patients with a mild traumatic brain injury will lose consciousness for a period of seconds to minutes but typically not longer than 30 minutes. The score on the Glasgow Coma Scale, if performed, is 13–15, with altered mental status but no other signs. Immediately following the injury, patients are confused. Posttraumatic

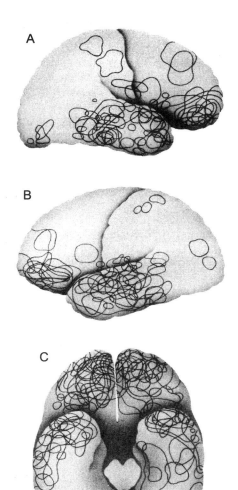

Figure 9–9. Site of cerebral contusions after traumatic brain injury. (A) Right hemisphere; (B) left hemisphere; (C) inferior view.

amnesia characterizes mild traumatic brain injury, and its duration usually ranges from minutes to hours; but even if the posttraumatic amnesia lasts up to 24 hours, the injury is still considered mild. Patients often complain of headaches, neck ache, dizziness, and nausea. There are typically no focal findings on the remainder of the neurological examination, and the results of neuroimaging studies are usually normal.

The neural injury[132] in patients with mild

traumatic brain injury results from diffuse axonal injury and causes cognitive deficits in attention, memory, and executive function. Subjectively, patients report poor concentration and forgetfulness, reflecting their attention and memory deficits. Deficits in executive function, however, may not be obvious until the patient attempts a normal routine, such as returning to work. Attention and memory deficits are usually appreciable on an office examination, if adequately assessed. However, executive function deficits are not easily captured in the typical office mental status examination.[135] Finally, early after the injury, patients may exhibit a deficit in arousal, which usually clears fairly quickly, although sleep–wake cycle disturbances may persist.

Patients with the typical mild traumatic brain injury (Glasgow Coma Scale 15, loss of consciousness <1 minute, posttraumatic amnesia 20–40 minutes) will usually recover over weeks to months. By 3 months, almost complete recovery has usually occurred.[136] When the injury is more severe (loss of consciousness >10 minutes, posttraumatic amnesia >4–6 hours), recovery may take months to years, and some patients may never recover completely. Thus, duration of coma and posttraumatic amnesia is a good indicator of the extent of neural injury, and both strongly correlate with the neurobehavioral outcome.[137] Expect recovery of older patients (>55 years) to take longer. Further, consider the patients' deficits in the context of their occupation and social circumstances. A minor physical injury that would not limit an amateur from playing softball on weekends could easily disable a professional ballplayer permanently. Likewise, a seemingly mild, persistent cognitive impairment after a mild traumatic brain injury may permanently disable a patient with a more demanding occupation (e.g., air traffic controller, surgeon).

The nonneural injury in a mild traumatic brain injury can involve the head (e.g., scalp, face), neck (e.g., soft tissue, ligaments), vestibular system, or psychological function (usually causing depression, irritability, and anxiety). Symptoms and signs of the nonneural injury typically are still present 1 month after injury but will substantially improve or recover by 3 months. Thus, by 6 months, almost all patients are completely recovered from both the neural and nonneural injuries. Nevertheless, in 10%–15% of patients with mild traumatic brain injury, symptoms persist 1 year after injury.[136] Patients with a persistent postconcussive syndrome likely suffer from an entirely different process evolving from the initial injury. The direct neural and soft tissue damage, which causes the syndrome of cognitive and neurobehavioral disorders in the majority of patients with mild traumatic brain injury, is not clearly causative in this special subset of patients.

Vascular and Neoplastic Disorders

The frontal lobes receive their blood supply from the anterior and middle cerebral arteries (ACA, MCA). The MCA supplies most of the lateral prefrontal cortex, and the ACA supplies the medial surface of the frontal lobes. Embolic or thrombotic strokes more commonly occur within the MCA distribution than the ACA distribution. A stroke within the MCA distribution, which is typically unilateral, is the most common cause of the dorsolateral prefrontal syndrome. However, it is uncommon for damage to be limited only to the prefrontal cortex (i.e., due only to frontal branches of the MCA) without involvement of the motor cortex, premotor areas, or parietal or temporal cortices. Strokes within the ACA distribution are the most common cause of the medial frontal syndrome. In addition to being embolic or thrombotic, ACA strokes can occur after rupture of an anterior communicating artery aneurysm due to vasospasm resulting from subarachnoid hemorrhage. Finally, multiple subcortical infarcts due to chronic hypertension or diabetes, affecting the basal ganglia, thalamus, or white matter projections to the frontal lobes, cause cognitive and behavioral deficits consistent with different frontal lobe syndromes.[138,139]

The frontal lobes can be the primary location of several different types of cerebral tumors. Meningiomas can arise subfrontally, impinging on orbitofrontal cortex, from the cerebral falx, impinging on the medial frontal lobes, as well as laterally compressing the dorsolateral cortex. These tumors can affect one or both frontal lobes, depending on their location. Tumors that arise from within the brain, such as gliomas, of all grades, often arise in the frontal lobes. Even though such a tumor may begin within one hemisphere, invasion across the corpus callosum can cause bilateral frontal lobe involvement. Metastases from distant neoplasms (e.g., breast, lung) can also invade the frontal lobes. Neoplastic involvement of the frontal lobes, in contrast with vascular events, causes symptoms that are usually gradual and very difficult to detect early in the course of the disease. However, primary and metastatic brain tumors may suddenly cause persistent deficits, as well as paroxysmal symptoms from seizures.

Herpes Encephalitis

Herpes simplex encephalitis is the most common cause of the sporadic encephalitis.[140] The disease shows no age, sex, or seasonal preference and is not transmissible. The most common clinical features at presentation are (in order of decreasing frequency) fever, personality change, aphasia, hemiparesis, and seizures.[141] The behavioral and cognitive changes result from infection of limbic areas of the temporal and frontal lobes, including the amygdala, hippocampus, parahippocampal gyrus, insula, and orbitofrontal and cingulate cortex. Thus, as in traumatic brain injury, an orbitofrontal syndrome occurs after this illness.

Epilepsy

Seizure foci can arise in all frontal areas, causing diverse signs and symptoms (Table 9–3).[142] Prominent early motor features help to identify frontal lobe partial seizures. Penfield and Jasper[143] made early note of head and eye version and posturing as common features of frontal lobe seizures, especially those arising from lateral premotor or supplementary motor areas. Brief (<60 seconds, often 10–20 seconds) nocturnal but often clustered seizures of motor agitation with complex automatisms affecting mainly axial (e.g., bicycling, pelvic thrusting) and vocal (e.g., screaming) musculature suggest foci in orbital or polar regions of frontal cortex but may occur with seizures arising in other areas.[144,145] Other features of frontal lobe seizures include forced thinking, fear, subjective sensations, vague cephalic feelings, and automatic behavior (e.g., laughing). Bland spells with staring accompanied by im-

Table 9–3. Clinical Features of Frontal Lobe Epilepsies

Region	Sensory, Autonomic, and Psychic	Focal Motor*	Motor Automatisms	Other
Primary motor	Paresthesia	Clonic, jacksonian march	Absent	Speech arrest
Supplementary motor	Sensations: pulling, pulsing, heaviness, tingling	Sudden, often violent posturing; head and eye version, fencer's posture, motor activity of one or more extremities, preserved awareness	Simple vocalization, complex focal motor	Speech arrest
Dorsolateral premotor	Rare	Head and eye version, focal tonic, jacksonian march, inhibition of movement	Complex focal motor: finger tapping	Speech arrest, asphasia (dominant hemisphere)
Dorsolateral prefrontal	Head sensation, mild confusion, slowed mentation	Late head and eye version, focal tonic	Simple motor	Pseudoabsence seizures
Cingulate	Autonomic, fear	Occasionally, early tonic, usually with spread, facial grimace	Appendicular, axial; laughter and other vocalization;† tongue protrusion	Urinary incontinence, pseudoabsence seizures, interictal behavioral changes
Frontopolar	Uncommon, head sensation	Rare, usually with spread	Complex motor, agitation;‡ vocalization†	Early loss of awareness, pseudoabsence seizures
Orbitofrontal	Olfactory or gustatory; hallucinations, fear, autonomic changes	Rare, usually with spread	Complex motor, agitation;‡ vocalization†	Pseudoabsence seizures, interictal behavioral changes
Opercular	Salivation, epigastric, fear, autonomic changes	Facial clonic	Chewing, swallowing	Common

The clinical features of frontal lobe epilepsies overlap, and seizures arising in one area may not produce signs or symptoms until activity spreads to another region; no specific feature definitively localizes the region of seizure onset.

*Initial and predominant motor activity is contralateral.

†Vocalization may be prominent, with intense crying or yelling, laughing, singing, or childish speech.

‡Complex motor automatisms and agitation are often marked by rapid onset, brief duration, prominent axial automatisms (e.g., bicycling, rocking, pelvic thrusting), and facial flushing or pallor.

paired consciousness and amnesia result directly from frontal lobe foci or from ictal spread to temporal areas. Compared with temporal lobe seizures, frontal lobe seizures are more frequently associated with early clonic or tonic movements, early bilateral movements, brief duration (5–30 seconds), a tendency to cluster, predominance during sleep, truncal and wild automatisms, and a minimal or absent postictal state.[146,147] Atypical features of frontal lobe seizures, such as bilateral clonic activity with preserved awareness, as well as sexual automatisms, cursing, crying, and tongue protrusion, can lead to a misdiagnosis of nonepileptic psychogenic seizures.

Three types of prefrontal seizures are reviewed here: supplementary motor seizures, ACC seizures, and orbitofrontal seizures. The localization and lateralization of prefrontal lobe foci can be extremely difficult. The frontal cortex is enormous, and large expanses lie, hidden from scalp electrodes, along the orbital floor, medial surface, and sulcal depths. When epileptiform discharges are detected, spread to contralateral or other ipsilateral regions may be falsely localizing. Even with invasive recordings, sampling bias limits precise electroclinical correlations. These issues limit surgical success rates for frontal lobe epilepsies, especially when imaging studies do not reveal a structural, epileptogenic lesion.

SUPPLEMENTARY MOTOR SEIZURES

Seizures arising from the supplementary motor area (SMA) cause sudden tonic posturing of the contralateral arm, contraversive head and eye deviation, speech arrest or vocalizations, and retention or impairment of consciousness.[143] In "fencer's posture" seizures, the eyes and head face the contralateral arm, which is elevated and flexed at the elbow, while the ipsilateral arm is tonically extended. Fencer's posture seizures strongly suggest onset or spread to the SMA but occur in only a minority of SMA seizures. Bilateral clonic activity with preserved consciousness strongly suggests a structural lesion (e.g., parasagittal tumor, arteriovenous malformation) and seizure focus in the mesial frontal region, near the SMA.[145] Contralateral ictal spread with bilateral activation of motor areas or bilateral motor activation with a unilateral focus (the SMA controls bilateral musculature) without ictal

spread to other prefrontal or temporal areas likely explains this phenomenon.[148]

ANTERIOR CINGULATE SEIZURES

Seizures arising in the ACC challenge diagnosticians. Auras are absent or nonspecific, including such symptoms as dizziness, autonomic changes (e.g., warmth, pallor, palpitations, abdominal sensation), or psychic phenomena (e.g., feeling of suffocation, fear). Arrest of motor and verbal behavior and brief staring can mimic absence seizures clinically and electrographically as the discharge spreads bilaterally over frontocentral regions (usually <3 Hz).[149] Spread to motor areas can cause contralateral or bilateral tonic or clonic movements; secondary generalized tonic-clonic seizures are common. Symptoms of isolated cingulate motor area activation are not defined but may include laughter or other "prewired" emotional vocalizations. Complex motor automatisms cause combinations of altered facial expression (fear, contortion, "haggard eyes"), appendicular behavior (repetitive touching, waving, or hitting movements), truncal motion (rocking), or vocal sounds (humming, onomatopoeia, screaming, cursing, laughter, crying). During automatisms, some patients voluntarily inhibit or modify motor behavior to blend in with ongoing activity.[148,149] (The prominent interictal behavioral changes complicating some cingulate epilepsies are reviewed in Chapter 10.)

ORBITOFRONTAL SEIZURES

Seizures arising from orbital cortex may cause early changes of altered facial expression, autonomic symptoms, fear, or olfactory or gustatory hallucinations. In many cases, however, seizures erupt suddenly from sleep with general motor agitation and complex motor automatisms and vocalization.[145,147] The motor features of orbitofrontal seizures are dramatic but can occur with seizures arising in frontopolar cortex or ACC.[145] These seizures include prominent axial automatisms such as pelvic thrusting, thrashing, rocking, and wild arm movements, as well as grunting, screaming, singing, shouting meaningless phrases, or cursing.[145,150] Autonomic features include epigastric sensation, tachycardia, tachypnea, piloerection, diaphoresis, pallor, flushing, and mydriasis.[151] Postictal symptoms are usually brief or absent.

Ictal activity can spread from orbitofrontal cortex to mesial temporal limbic areas via the uncinate fasciculus, producing a blank stare with oral and hand automatisms. As in other frontal areas, invasive electrode recordings may reveal electrographic seizures beginning a minute or more before clinical symptoms develop, indicating activation of the orbital region without behavioral change.[152] In such cases, symptoms result from ictal activation of the medial temporal lobe (e.g., dreamy state followed by lip smacking, ipsilateral hand automatism, and contralateral upper limb dystonia) or motor areas (e.g., eye and head deviation away from seizure focus).[150]

Frontotemporal Dementia

Frontotemporal dementia (FTD) is a relatively new taxonomy for a group of dementing disorders that are associated with degeneration of the anterior frontal and temporal lobes.[153,154] In 1994, guidelines for the diagnosis of FTD were established and usage of the term FTD was encouraged in order to bring together a range of diverse clinical syndromes that have similar pathology. Such syndromes include progressive subcortical gliosis,[155] frontal lobe dementia of the non-Alzheimer's type,[156] dementia of the frontal lobe type,[157] dementia lacking distinctive histological features,[158] semantic dementia,[159] primary progressive aphasia,[160] and the classic FTD, Pick's disease.[161]

The typical age at onset for FTD is in the fifth to sixth decade, which is earlier than that for Alzheimer's disease (AD). Two studies of the prevalence of FTD have estimated that 13%–22% of patients with dementia with an onset before age 65 have FTD.[157,162] The majority of patients with FTD have a positive family history for dementia, suggesting a dominant inheritance pattern,[163] although the cause of the various syndromes associated with FTD is unknown. Linkage to chromosome 17 was found in several families with FTD,[164–166] in some cases revealing mutations in the *tau* gene.

Patients with FTD present with personality changes, which typically precede any significant cognitive impairment by several years.[167] These personality changes include behavioral disinhibition, loss of judgment and insight, loss of social graces, jocularity, social withdrawal, and apathy punctuated by irritability.[157,168,169] In addition to these behavioral changes, a char-

acteristic pattern appears of cognitive deficits that are consistent with frontal and temporal degeneration. These include language and executive function impairments. For example, during the early stages of the disease, FTD patients have reduced verbal output and word-finding difficulty consistent with anomic aphasia. Patients can develop verbal stereotypes, and some patients can even become mute, suggesting significant frontal lobe involvement. If there is significant temporal lobe involvement, fluent aphasia (e.g., transcortical sensory) will develop as well as isolated semantic memory impairments (see Chapter 8). Patients with AD, in contrast, have language deficits that are more typical of parietal damage, such as problems with reading, writing, and calculations, which are not typically a problem in FTD.[157] Also, the prominent visuospatial deficits observed in AD patients secondary to parietal damage are not typically observed in FTD patients. In one behavioral study, loss of personal awareness, hyperorality, stereotyped and perseverative behavior, progressive reduction of speech, and preserved spatial orientation differentiated 100% of FTD vs. AD patients.[170]

The gross neuropathology of FTD is striking, with severe frontal and temporal lobe atrophy; gyri appear knife-like. In contrast to the predominantly cortical atrophy in AD, both cortical atrophy and white matter atrophy are observed in FTD. The distribution of predominant atrophy is highly variable across individuals. The atrophy may be symmetrical or, in more than half of cases, predominant on one side. The primary motor areas are usually spared, and atrophy may involve the basal nucleus of Meynert, caudate nucleus, and substantia nigra.[171] Microscopically, cell loss predominates in the outer cortical layers with intense astrocytic gliosis. In Pick's disease, there are abundant Pick's cells—enlarged, circular cells with intranuclear inclusions seen best with silver stains.[171] Increased amounts of tau protein are found in FTD patients compared to normal subjects.[172] The predominant neurochemical change in FTD are decreases in serotonin and postsynaptic serotonin.[173,174]

ASSESSMENT OF EXECUTIVE FUNCTION

Executive function is difficult to test at the bedside, but several tests do exist. (For in-depth coverage of this cognitive function, see Chapter 1.) Phonemic fluency (e.g., generate as many words as possible in 1 minute that start with the letter *F*) and category fluency (e.g., generate animal names) are markedly reduced in patients with executive dysfunction (<12 items in a high school–educated patient). The approach toward these tests is often quite disorganized. To assess set-shifting ability, ask the patient to recite the alphabet alternating with numbers (a–1–b–2–c–3 . . .). To assess problem solving, place a coin in one hand held behind your back and ask the patient to guess which hand it is in. By alternating the choices between hands in a sequential fashion and letting the patient know the correct answer after each guess, the patient should recognize the pattern within a few guesses. Assess response inhibition by asking the patient to put up one finger when you put up two and not to put up any fingers when you put up one finger. In an alternating, sequential motor test,[41] instruct the patient to mimic the examiner in a series of hand movements (Figure 9–10). The patient repetitively makes the sequence of three move-

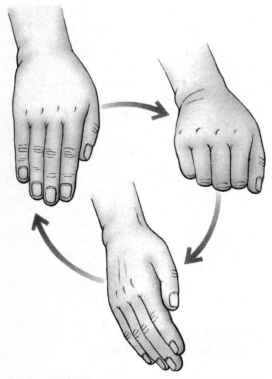

Figure 9–10. Hand sequences (i.e., knock, chop, slap) of the alternating, sequential motor test.

ments on the thigh or a counter top. The three hand positions are (1) a fist ("knock"), (2) side of open hand ("chop"), and (3) hand open with palm down ("slap"). Patients with frontal lobe lesions often fail at this task, making perseverative errors by repeating the same movement over and over or repeatedly skipping step 2 despite verbal corrections. Test perseveration by asking the patient to copy a repeating visual pattern (e.g., loops, circle–plus sign–circle).

The patient's medical history and responses to pertinent questions can elicit deficits in executive function. For example, difficulty in organization can be derived by asking the patient, spouse, or significant other about activities of daily living (e.g., "Are there problems at work or with doing chores around the house?" "Do things get started but not completed?"). Alternatively, ask the patient to describe how he or she would perform various tasks, such as planning a vacation, preparing spaghetti and meatballs, or changing a tire.

When determining if a patient has frontal lobe dysfunction, the examiner must consider the range of normal behavior in a population arising from inherent individual variability, culture, and education. For example, abstract thought is often tested with proverb interpretation. This test is often culturally biased, and a patient who is familiar with selected proverbs is at a distinct advantage. A well-to-do psychiatry resident asked an alcoholic ghetto patient the meaning of the phrase "People in glass houses shouldn't throw stones." The patient appeared puzzled and, after some hesitation, replied that they could break a window. The resident instructed the students that this was a classic concrete response, indicating frontal lobe damage. A medical student with a background similar to the patient's asked "Yo, what does it mean, what goes around comes around?" Without hesitation, the patient responded "Well, if you mess with somebody, you better look out, because either they'll come looking for you or one of their friends will." In addition, recognize that patients with frontal lobe damage are not impaired on all measures of executive function and may not necessarily show behavioral abnormalities. The remarkable heterogeneity in the cognitive and behavioral profiles of patients with frontal lobe damage highlights how much remains unknown about frontal lobe function. More knowledge about such brain–behavior relationships should produce more sensitive clinical measures and more effective therapies.

Measures of executive function are an essential element of a reliable bedside mental status examination. In our experience, this is the one cognitive domain that is commonly excluded. For example, in the widely utilized Mini-Mental Status Examination,[175] there are no true measures of executive function. Utilizing this measure in patients such as those described above may grossly underestimate their cognitive deficits.

SUMMARY

The frontal lobes constitute the largest area of cerebral cortex, and they are reciprocally connected to almost every other brain region. The frontal lobes are dedicated to multimodal processing, and their damage leads to a range of high-level behavioral and cognitive deficits. Unfortunately, these deficits may be hard to quantify on standard neuropsychological tests and may be evident only in real-life situations. The paucity of objective findings may cause clinicians to overlook the possibility of frontal lobe injuries. Moreover, frontal lobe dysfunction manifests in heterogeneous ways, depending on such factors as the site, size, laterality, nature, and temporal course of the lesion. There is no single frontal lobe syndrome. At least three signature behavioral or cognitive prefrontal syndromes may be produced by selective damage to either dorsolateral, medial, or orbitofrontal regions. Damage to the dorsolateral prefrontal circuit impairs executive function, damage to the orbitofrontal circuit causes significant affective and social changes, and damage to the medial frontal circuit reduces motivation and behavioral spontaneity with severe bilateral damage causing the dramatic syndrome of akinetic mutism. The functions of this massive and phylogenetically novel cortical region are complex, interrelated, and as yet incompletely understood. A complete picture of prefrontal function requires a full understanding of the role of the dopaminergic system. The anatomical distribution of dopaminergic projections strongly implicates the neurotransmitter dopamine in prefrontal cortical function. In 1928, the American neurologist Frederick Tilney suggested that the entire period of human evolutionary existence could be considered "the age of the frontal lobe."[176,177] Let us hope that the near future will be the age for understanding the frontal lobes.

REFERENCES

1. Ferrier D: Functions of the Brain. Smith, Elder and Company, London, 1886.
2. Hebb DO: Intelligence in man after large removals of cerebral tissue: report of four left frontal lobe cases. J Gen Psychol 21:73–87, 1939.
3. Teuber HL: The riddle of frontal lobe function in man. In Warren JM and Akert K (eds). The Frontal Granular Cortex and Behavior. McGraw-Hill, New York, 1964, pp 410–444.
4. Nauta WJH: The problem of the frontal lobe: a reinterpretation. 8:167–187, 1971.
5. Ungerleider LG and Mishkin M: Two cortical systems. In Ingle D, Goodale M, and Mansfield R (eds). Analysis of Visual Behavior. MIT Press, Cambridge, MA, 1982, pp 549–586.
6. Rao SC, Rainer G, and Miller EK: Integration of what and where in the primate prefrontal cortex. Science 276:821–824, 1997.
7. Prabhakaran V, Narayanan K, Zhao Z, et al.: Integration of diverse information in working memory within the frontal lobe. Nat Neurosci 3:85–90, 2000.
8. Arnsten AF and Goldman-Rakic PS: Selective prefrontal cortical projections to the region of the locus coeruleus and raphe nuclei in the rhesus monkey. Brain Res 306:9–18, 1984.
9. Babcock RL and Salthouse TA: Effects of increased processing demands on age differences in working memory. Psychol Aging 5:421–428, 1990.
10. Barbas H and Pandya DN: Architecture and intrinsic connections of the prefrontal cortex in the rhesus monkey. J Comp Neurol 286:353–375, 1989.
11. Hof PR, Mufson EJ, and Morrison JH: Human orbitofrontal cortex: cytoarchitecture and quantitative immunohistochemical parcellation. J Comp Neurol 359:48–68, 1995.
12. Morecraft RJ, Geula C, and Mesulam MM: Cytoarchitecture and neural afferents of orbitofrontal cortex in the brain of the monkey. J Comp Neurol 323:341–358, 1992.
13. Van Hoesen GE, Morecraft RJ, and Semendeferi K: Functional neuroanatomy of the limbic system and prefrontal cortex. In Fogel BS, Schiffer RB, and Rao SM (eds). Neuropsychiatry. Williams & Wilkins, Baltimore, 1996, pp 113–143.
14. Elliott R, Dolan RJ, and Frith CD: Dissociable functions in the medial and lateral orbitofrontal cortex: evidence from human neuroimaging studies. Cereb Cortex 10:308–317, 2000.
15. Alexander MP and Stuss DT: Disorders of frontal lobe functioning. Semin Neurol 20:427–437, 2000.
16. Stuss DT and Levine B: Adult clinical neuropsychology: lessons from studies of the frontal lobes. Annu Rev Psychol 53:401–433, 2002.
17. Harlow J: Recovery from the passage of an iron bar through the head. Proc Massachusetts Med Soc 2:725–728, 1868.

18. Benson DF: The Neurology of Thinking. Oxford University Press, New York, 1994.
19. Vijayaraghavan L, Krishnamoorthy ES, Brown RG, et al.: Abulia: a delphi survey of British neurologists and psychiatrists. Mov Disord 17:1052–1057, 2002.
20. Damasio AR and Anderson SW: The frontal lobes. In Heilman KM and Valenstein E (eds). Clinical Neuropsychology. Oxford University Press, New York, 1993, pp 409–460.
21. Stuss DT and Alexander MP: Executive functions and the frontal lobes: a conceptual view. Psychol Res 63:289–298, 2000.
22. Stuss DT: Self-awareness and the frontal lobes: a neuropsychological perspective. In Goethals GR, and Strauss J (eds). The Self: Interdisciplinary Approaches. Springer-Verlag, New York, 1991, pp 255–278.
23. Lhermitte F: Human autonomy and the frontal lobes. Part II: Patient behavior in complex and social situations: the "environmental dependency syndrome." Ann Neurol 19:335–343, 1986.
24. Lhermitte F, Pillon B, and Serdaru M: Human autonomy and the frontal lobes. Part I: Imitation and utilization behavior: a neuropsychological study of 75 patients. Ann Neurol 19:326–334, 1986.
25. Archibald SJ, Mateer CA, and Kerns KA: Utilization behavior: clinical manifestations and neurological mechanisms. Neuropsychol Rev 11:117–130, 2001.
26. Black FW: Cognitive deficits in patients with unilateral war-related lesions. J Clin Psychol 32:366–372, 1976.
27. Eslinger PJ and Damasio AR: Severe disturbance of higher cognition following bilateral frontal lobe ablation: patient EVR. Neurology 35:1731–1741, 1985.
28. Shallice T and Burgess PW: Deficits in strategy application following frontal lobe damage in man. Brain 114:727–741, 1991.
29. Lezak M: Neuropsychological Assessment, 3rd ed. Oxford University Press, New York, 1995.
30. Spreen O and Strauss E: A Compendium of Neuropsychological Tests: Administration, Norms, and Commentary. Oxford University Press, New York, 1991.
31. Berg E: A simple objective test for measuring flexibility in thinking. J Gen Psychol 39:15–22, 1948.
32. Milner B: Effects of different brain regions on card sorting. Arch Neurol 9:90–100, 1963.
33. Barcelo F and Knight RT: Both random and perseverative errors underlie WCST deficits in prefrontal patients. Neuropsychologia 40:349–356, 2002.
34. Schwartz MF, Montgomery MW, Buxbaum LJ, et al.: Naturalistic action impairment in closed head injury. Neuropsychology 12:13–28, 1998.
35. Grafman J: Plans, actions, and mental sets: managerial knowledge units in the frontal lobes. In Perceman E (ed). Integrating Theory and Practice in Neuropsychology. Lawrence Erlbaum, Hillsdale, NJ, 1989, pp 93–138.
36. Zalla T, Plassiart C, Pillon B, et al.: Action planning in a virtual context after prefrontal cortex damage. Neuropsychologia 39:759–770, 2001.
37. Partiot A, Grafman J, Sadato N, et al.: Brain activation during script event processing. Neuroreport 7:761–766, 1996.
38. Crozier S, Sirigu A, Lehericy S, et al.: Distinct prefrontal activations in processing sequence at the sentence and script level: an fMRI study. Neuropsychologia 37:1469–1476, 1999.
39. Hauser MD: Perseveration, inhibition and the pre-
frontal cortex: a new look. Curr Opin Neurobiol 9:214–222, 1999.
40. Sandson J and Albert ML: Perseveration in behavioral neurology. Neurology 37:1736–1741, 1987.
41. Luria AR: Higher Cortical Functions in Man. Basic Books, New York, 1966.
42. Stroop JR: Studies of interference in serial verbal reactions. J Exp Psychol 18:643–662, 1935.
43. Stuss DT, Floden D, Alexander MP, et al.: Stroop performance in focal lesion patients: dissociation of processes and frontal lobe lesion location. Neuropsychologia 39:771–786, 2001.
44. Perret E: The left frontal lobe of man and the suppression of habitual responses in verbal categorical behaviour. Neuropsychologia 12:323–330, 1974.
45. Skinner JE and Yingling CD: Central gating mechanisms that regulate event-related potentials and behavior. In Desmedt JE (ed). Progress in Clinical Neurophysiology, Vol 1. S Karger, Basel, 1977, pp 30–69.
46. Yingling CD and Skinner JE: Gating of thalamic input to cerebral cortex by nucleus reticularis thalami. In Desmedt JE (ed). Progress in Clinical Neurophysiology, Vol 1. S Karger, Basel, 1977, pp 70–96.
47. Barcelo F, Suwazono S, and Knight RT: Prefrontal modulation of visual processing in humans. Nat Neurosci 3:399–403, 2000.
48. Knight RT, Scabini D, and Woods DL: Prefrontal cortex gating of auditory transmission in humans. Brain Res 504:338–342, 1989.
49. Yamaguchi S and Knight RT: Gating of somatosensory inputs by human prefrontal cortex. Brain Res 521:281–288, 1990.
50. Watanabe J, Sugiura M, Sato K, et al.: The human prefrontal and parietal association cortices are involved in no-go performances: an event-related fMRI study. Neuroimage 17:1207–1216, 2002.
51. Garavan H, Ross TJ, and Stein EA: Right hemispheric dominance of inhibitory control: an event-related functional MRI study. Proc Natl Acad Sci USA 96:8301–8306, 1999.
52. Sylvester CY, Wager TD, Lacey SC, et al.: Switching attention and resolving interference: fMRI measures of executive functions. Neuropsychologia 41:357–370, 2003.
53. D'Esposito M, Postle BR, Jonides J, et al.: The neural substrate and temporal dynamics of interference effects in working memory as revealed by event-related functional MRI. Proc Natl Acad Sci USA 96:7514–7519, 1999.
54. Konishi S, Nakajima K, Uchida I, et al.: No-go dominant brain activity in human inferior prefrontal cortex revealed by functional magnetic resonance imaging. Eur J Neurosci 10:1209–1213, 1998.
55. Shimamura AP: The role of the prefrontal cortex in dynamic filtering. Psychobiology 28:207–218, 2000.
56. Baddeley A: Working Memory. Oxford University Press, New York, 1986.
57. Fuster JM: The Prefrontal Cortex: Anatomy, Physiology, and Neuropsychology of the Frontal Lobes, 3rd ed. Raven Press, New York, 1997.
58. Fuster JM and Alexander GE: Neuron activity related to short-term memory. Science 173:652–654, 1971.
59. Funahashi S, Bruce CJ, and Goldman-Rakic PS: Mnemonic coding of visual space in the monkey's dorsolateral prefrontal cortex. J Neurophysiol 61:331–349, 1989.

60. Funahashi S, Bruce CJ, and Goldman-Rakic PS: Dorsolateral prefrontal lesions and oculomotor delayed-response performance: evidence for mnemonic "scotomas." J Neurosci 13:1479–1497, 1993.

61. Bauer RH and Fuster JM: Delayed-matching and delayed-response deficit from cooling dorsolateral prefrontal cortex in monkeys. J Comp Physiol Psychol 90:293–302, 1976.

62. Goldman-Rakic PS: Circuitry of the prefrontal cortex and the regulation of behavior by representational memory. In Plum F and Mountcastle V (eds). Handbook of Physiology. The Nervous System, Sect 1, Vol 5. American Physiological Society, Bethesda, MD, 1987, pp 373–417.

63. Chao LL and Knight RT: Contribution of human prefrontal cortex to delay performance. J Cogn Neurosci 10:167–77, 1998.

64. Verin M, Partiot A, Pillon B, et al.: Delayed response tasks and prefrontal lesions in man—evidence for self generated patterns of behavior with poor environmental modulation. Neuropsychologia 31:1379–1396, 1993.

65. Pierrot-Deseilligny C, Rivaud S, Gaymard B, et al.: Cortical control of memory-guided saccades in man. Exp Brain Res 83:607–617, 1991.

66. Ptito A, Crane J, Leonard G, et al.: Visual-spatial localization by patients with frontal-lobe lesions invading or sparing area 46. Neuroreport 6:1781–1784, 1995.

67. Brandt SA, Ploner CJ, Meyer BU, et al.: Effects of repetitive transcranial magnetic stimulation over dorsolateral prefrontal and posterior parietal cortex on memory-guided saccades. Exp Brain Res 118:197–204, 1998.

68. Oliveri M, Turriziani P, Carlesimo GA, et al.: Parieto-frontal interactions in visual-object and visual-spatial working memory: evidence from transcranial magnetic stimulation. Cereb Cortex 11:606–618, 2001.

69. Mottaghy FM, Gangitano M, Sparing R, et al.: Segregation of areas related to visual working memory in the prefrontal cortex revealed by rTMS. Cereb Cortex 12:369–375, 2002.

70. D'Esposito M, Aguirre GK, Zarahn E, et al.: Functional MRI studies of spatial and non-spatial working memory. Cogn Brain Res 7:1–13, 1998.

71. D'Esposito M: Working memory. In Cabezza R and Kingstone A (eds). Handbook of Functional Neuroimaging of Cognition. MIT Press, Cambridge, MA, 2001, pp 293–327.

72. Janowsky JS, Shimamura AP, Kritchevsky M, et al.: Cognitive impairment following frontal lobe damage and its relevance to human amnesia. Behav Neurosci 103:548–560, 1989.

73. Alexander MP: Transcortical motor aphasia: a disorder of language production. In D'Esposito M (ed). Neurological Foundations of Cognitive Neuroscience. MIT Press, Cambridge, MA, 2003, pp 165–174.

74. Alexander M: Frontal lobes and language. Brain Lang 37:656, 1989.

75. Fischer CM: Left hemiplegia and motor impersistence. J Nerv Ment Dis 123:201–218, 1956.

76. Salmaso D and Denes G: Role of the frontal lobes on an attentional task: a signal detection analysis. Percept Mot Skills 55:127–130, 1982.

77. Richer F, Decary A, Lapierre MF, et al.: Target detectinon deficits in frontal lobectomy. Brain Cogn 21: 203–211, 1993.

78. Rueckert L and Grafman J: Sustained attention deficits and patients with right frontal lesions. Neuropsychologia 34:953–963, 1996.

79. Wilkins AJ, Shallice T, and McCarthy R: Frontal lesions and sustained attention. Neuropsychologia 25:359–365, 1987.

80. Watson RT, Miller BD, and Heilman KM: Nonsensory neglect. Ann Neurol 3:505–508, 1978.

81. Coslett HB, Bowers D, Fitzpatrick E, et al.: Directional hypokinesia and hemispatial inattention in neglect. Brain 113:475–486, 1990.

82. Chapman WP, Livingston RB, Livingston KE: Frontal lobotomy and electrical stimulation of orbital surface of frontal lobes: effect on respiration and on blood pressure in man. Arch Neurol Psychiatr 62: 701–716, 1949.

83. Rolls ET: The orbitofrontal cortex. Philos Trans R Soc Lond B Biol Sci 351:1433–1444, 1996.

84. Kleist K: Gehirnpathologie. JA Barth, Leipzig, 1934.

85. Cummings JL: Frontal-subcortical circuits and human behavior. Arch Neurol 50:873–880, 1993.

86. Alexander GE, DeLong MR, and Strick PL: Parallel organization of functionally segregated circuits linking basal ganglia and cortex. Annu Rev Neurosci 9:357–381, 1986.

87. Benson DF and Geschwind N: Psychiatric conditions associated with focal lesions of the central nervous system. In Arieti S and Reiser M (eds). American Handbook of Psychiatry. Basic Books, New York, 1971, pp 208–243.

88. Grafman J, Vance SC, Weingartner H, et al.: The effects of lateralized frontal lesions on mood regulation. Brain 109:1127–1148, 1986.

89. Grafman J, Schwab K, Warden D, et al.: Frontal lobe injuries, violence, and aggression: a report of the Vietnam Head Injury Study. Neurology 46:1231–1238, 1996.

90. Bechara A, Damasio H, Tranel D, et al.: Dissociation of working memory from decision making within the human prefrontal cortex. J Neurosci 18:428–437, 1998.

91. Stuss DT, Gallup GG Jr, and Alexander MP: The frontal lobes are necessary for "theory of mind." Brain 124:279–286, 2001.

92. Stone VE, Baron-Cohen S, and Knight RT: Frontal lobe contributions to theory of mind. J Cogn Neurosci 10:640–656, 1998.

93. Freemon FR: Akinetic mutism with bilateral anterior cerebral artery occlusion. J Neurol Neurosurg Psychiatry 34:693–698, 1971.

94. Bokura H and Robinson RG: Long-term cognitive impairment associated with caudate stroke. Stroke 28:970–975, 1997.

95. Petty RG, Bonner D, Mouratoglou V, et al.: Acute frontal lobe syndrome and dyscontrol associated with bilateral caudate nucleus infarctions. Br J Psychiatry 168:237–240, 1996.

96. Mendez MF, Adams NL and Lewandowski KS: Neurobehavioral changes associated with caudate lesions. Neurology 39:349–354, 1989.

97. Glosser G: Neurobehavioral aspects of movement disorders. Neurol Clin 19:535–551, 2001.

98. Butters N, Sax D, Montgomery K, et al.: Comparison of the neuropsychological deficits associated with early and advanced Huntington's disease. Arch Neurol 35:585–589, 1978.

99. Laplane D, Baulac M, Widlocher D, et al.: Pure psy-

chic akinesia with bilateral lesions of basal ganglia. J Neurol Neurosurg Psychiatry 47:377–385, 1984.

100. Graff-Radford N, Damasio H, Yamada T, et al.: Non-hemorrhagic thalamic infarction: clinical, neuropsychological, and electrophysiological findings in four anatomic groups defined by computed tomography. Brain 108:485–516, 1985.

101. Eslinger PJ, Warner GC, Grattan LM, et al.: "Frontal lobe" utilization behavior associated with paramedian thalamic infarction. Neurology 41:450–452, 1991.

102. Sandson TA, Daffner KR, Carvalho PA, et al.: Frontal lobe dysfunction following infarction of the left-sided medial thalamus. Arch Neurol 48:1300–1303, 1991.

103. Tucha OW, Smely CW, and Lange KW: Verbal and figural fluency in patients with mass lesions of the left or right frontal lobes. J Clin Exp Neuropsychol 21:229–236, 1999.

104. Baldo JV, Shimamura AP, Delis DC, et al.: Verbal and design fluency in patients with frontal lobe lesions. J Int Neuropsychol Soc 7:586–596, 2001.

105. Goldberg E, Podell K, and Lovell M: Lateralization of frontal lobe functions and cognitive novelty. J Neuropsychiatry 6:371–378, 1994.

106. Fletcher P, Buchel C, Josephs O, et al.: Learning-related neuronal responses in prefrontal cortex studied with functional neuroimaging. Cereb Cortex 9:168–178, 1999.

107. Seger CA, Poldrack RA, Prabhakaran V, et al.: Hemispheric asymmetries and individual differences in visual concept learning as measured by functional MRI. Neuropsychologia 38:1316–1324, 2000.

108. Robinson RG, Starr LB, Kubos KL, et al.: A two-year longitudinal study of post-stroke mood disorders: findings during the initial evaluation. Stroke 14:736–741, 1983.

109. Devinsky O: Right cerebral hemisphere dominance for a sense of corporeal and emotional self. Epilepsy Behav 1:60–73, 2000.

110. Nieoullon A: Dopamine and the regulation of cognition and attention. Prog Neurobiol 67:53–83, 2002.

111. Arnsten AFT: Catecholamine regulation of the prefrontal cortex. J Psychopharmacol 11:151–162, 1997.

112. Bannon MJ and Roth RH: Pharmacology of mesocortical dopamine neurons. Pharmacol Rev 35:53–68, 1983.

113. Brown RM, Crane AM, and Goldman PS: Regional distribution of monoamines in the cerebral cortex and subcortical structures of the rhesus monkey: concentrations and in vitro synthesis rates. Brain Res 168:133–150, 1979.

114. Brozoski TJ, Brown RM, Rosvold HE, et al.: Cognitive deficit caused by regional depletion of dopamine in prefrontal cortex of rhesus monkey. Science 205:929–932, 1979.

115. Sawaguchi T and Goldman-Rakic PS: D_1 dopamine receptors in prefrontal cortex: involvement in working memory. Science 251:947–950, 1991.

116. Arnsten KT, Cai JX, Murphy BL, et al.: Dopamine D_1 receptor mechanisms in the cognitive performance of young adult and aged monkeys. Psychopharmacology (Berl) 116:143–151, 1994.

117. Javoy-Agid F and Agid Y: Is the mesocortical dopaminergic system involved in Parkinson disease? Neurology 30:1326–1330, 1980.

118. Gotham AM, Brown RG, and Marsden CD: "Frontal" cognitive function in patients with Parkinson's disease "on" and "off" levodopa. Brain 111:299–321, 1988.

119. Cooper JA, Sagar HJ, Doherty M, et al.: Different effects of dopaminergic and anticholinergic therapies on cognitive and motor function in Parkinson's disease. Brain 115:1701–1725, 1992.

120. Lange KW, Robbins TW, Marsden CD, et al.: L-Dopa withdrawal in Parkinson's disease selectively impairs cognitive performance in tests sensitive to frontal lobe dysfunction. Psychopharmacology (Berl) 107:394–404, 1992.

121. Mehta MA, Swainson R, Ogilvie AD, et al.: Improved short-term spatial memory but impaired reversal learning following the dopamine D_2 agonist bromocriptine in human volunteers. Psychopharmacology (Berl) 159:10–20, 2001.

122. Luciana M, Depue RA, Arbisi P, et al.: Facilitation of working memory in humans by a D_2 dopamine receptor agonist. J Cogn Neurosci 4:58–68, 1992.

123. Luciana M and Collins PF: Dopaminergic modulation of working memory for spatial but not object cues in normal humans. J Cogn Neurosci 9:330–347, 1997.

124. Kimberg DY, D'Esposito M, and Farah MJ: Effects of bromocriptine on human subjects depend on working memory capacity. Neuroreport 8:3581–3585, 1997.

125. Kimberg DY and D'Esposito M: Cognitive effects of the dopamine receptor agonist pergolide. Neuropsychologia 41:1020–1027, 2003.

126. Muller U, von Cramon DY, and Pollmann S: D_1-versus D_2-receptor modulation of visuospatial working memory in humans. J Neurosci 18:2720–2728, 1998.

127. Mehta MA, Sahakian BJ, McKenna PJ, et al.: Systemic sulpiride in young adult volunteers simulates the profile of cognitive deficits in Parkinson's disease. Psychopharmacology (Berl) 146:162–174, 1999.

128. Camps M, Cortés R, Gueye B, et al.: Dopamine receptors in human brain: autoradiographic distribution of D_1 sites. Neuroscience 28:275–290, 1989.

129. Goldman-Rakic PS, Lidow MS, and Gallager DW: Overlap of dopaminergic, adrenergic, and serotoninergic receptors and complementarity of their subtypes in primate prefrontal cortex. J Neurosci 10:2125–2138, 1990.

130. Arnsten AFT, Cai JX, Steere JC, et al.: Dopamine D_2 receptor mechanisms contribute to age-related cognitive decline: the effects of quinpirole on memory and motor performance in monkeys. J Neurosci 15:3429–3439, 1995.

131. Gennarelli TA, Thibault LE, Adams JH, et al.: Diffuse axonal injury and traumatic coma in the primate. Ann Neurol 12:564–574, 1982.

132. Alexander MP: Minor traumatic brain injury: a review of physiogenesis and psychogenesis. Semin Clin Neuropsychiatry 2:177–187, 1997.

133. Alexander MP: In the pursuit of proof of brain damage after whiplash injury. Neurology 51:336–340, 1998.

134. Servadei F, Teasdale G, and Merry G: Defining acute mild head injury in adults: a proposal based on prognostic factors, diagnosis, and management. J Neurotrauma 18:657–664, 2001.

135. Stuss DT, Ely P, Hugenholtz H, et al.: Subtle neuropsychological deficits in patients with good recovery after closed head injury. Neurosurgery 17:41–47, 1985.

136. Levin HS, Eisenberg HM, and Benton AL. Mild

Head Injury. Oxford University Press, New York, 1989.

137. Katz DI: Neuropathology and neurobehavioral recovery from closed head injury. J Head Trauma Rehabil 7:1–15, 1992.

138. Haring HP: Cognitive impairment after stroke. Curr Opin Neurol 15:79–84, 2002.

139. Albert ML, Feldman RG, and Willis AL: The "subcortical dementia" of progressive supranuclear palsy. J Neurol Neurosurg Psychiatry 37:121–130, 1974.

140. Hinson VK and Tyor WR: Update on viral encephalitis. Curr Opin Neurol 14:369–374, 2001.

141. Whitley RJ, Soong SJ, Linneman C Jr, et al.: Herpes simplex encephalitis. Clinical assessment. JAMA 247: 317–320, 1982.

142. Shulman MB: The frontal lobes, epilepsy, and behavior. Epilepsy Behav 1:384–395, 2000.

143. Penfield W and Jasper H: Epilepsy and the Functional Anatomy of the Human Brain. Little, Brown, Boston, 1954.

144. Jobst BC, Siegel AM, Thadani VM, et al.: Intractable seizures of frontal lobe origin: clinical characteristics, localizing signs, and results of surgery. Epilepsia 41:1139–1152, 2000.

145. Manford M, Fish DR, and Shorvon SD: An analysis of clinical seizure patterns and their localizing value in frontal and temporal lobe epilepsies. Brain 119:17–40, 1996.

146. Laskowitz DT, Sperling MR, French JA, et al.: The syndrome of frontal lobe epilepsy: characteristics and surgical management. Neurology 45:780–787, 1995.

147. Williamson PD, Spencer DD, Spencer SS, et al.: Complex partial seizures of frontal lobe origin. Ann Neurol 18:497–504, 1985.

148. Geier S, Bancaud J, Talairach J, et al.: The seizures of frontal lobe epilepsy. A study of clinical manifestations. Neurology 27:951–958, 1977.

149. Devinsky O, Morrell MJ, and Vogt BA: Contributions of anterior cingulate cortex to behaviour. Brain 118:279–306, 1995.

150. Williamson PD and Jobst BC: Frontal lobe epilepsy. Adv Neurol 84:215–242, 2000.

151. Munari C and Bancaud J: Electroclinical symptomatology of partial seizures of orbital frontal origin. Adv Neurol 57:257–265, 1992.

152. Niedermeyer E: Frontal lobe epilepsy: the next frontier. Clin Electroencephalogr 29:163–169, 1998.

153. Hodges JR: Frontotemporal dementia (Pick's disease): clinical features and assessment. Neurology 56:S6–S10, 2001.

154. Miller BL: Alzheimer's disease and frontotemporal dementia. In Coffey CE and Cummings JL (eds). Textbook of Geriatric Psychiatry. American Psychiatric Press, Washington DC, 2000, pp 511–529.

155. Neumann MA and Cohn R: Progressive subcortical gliosis, a rare form of presenile dementia. Brain 90:405–418, 1967.

156. Brun A: Frontal lobe degeneration of non-Alzheimer type. I. Neuropathology. Arch Gerontol Geriatr 6:193–208, 1987.

157. Neary D, Snowden JS, Northen B, et al.: Dementia of frontal lobe type. J Neurol Neurosurg Psychiatry 51:353–361, 1988.

158. Knopman DS, Mastri AR, Frey WH 2nd, et al.: Dementia lacking distinctive histologic features: a common non-Alzheimer degenerative dementia. Neurology 40:251–256, 1990.

159. Snowden JS, Neary D, Mann DM, et al.: Progressive language disorder due to lobar atrophy. Ann Neurol 31:174–183, 1992.

160. Mesulam MM: Slowly progressive aphasia without generalized dementia. Ann Neurol 11:592–598, 1982.

161. Cherrier MM and Mendez MM: Pick's disease, an introduction and review of the literature. Neurologist 5:55–62, 1999.

162. Gustafson L, Brun A, and Risberg J: Frontal lobe dementia of non-Alzheimer type. Adv Neurol 51:65–71, 1990.

163. Gustafson L: Clinical picture of frontal lobe degeneration of non-Alzheimer type. Dementia 4:143–148, 1993.

164. Petersen RB, Tabaton M, Chen SG, et al.: Familial progressive subcortical gliosis: presence of prions and linkage to chromosome 17. Neurology 45:1062–1067, 1995.

165. Foster NL, Wilhelmsen K, Sima AA, et al.: Frontotemporal dementia and parkinsonism linked to chromosome 17: a consensus conference. Ann Neurol 41:706–715, 1997.

166. Wilhelmsen KC, Lynch T, Pavlou E, et al.: Localization of disinhibition–dementia–parkinsonism–amyotrophy complex to 17q21–22. Am J Hum Genet 55:1159–1165, 1994.

167. Miller BL, Cummings JL, Villanueva-Meyer J, et al.: Frontal lobe degeneration: clinical, neuropsychological, and SPECT characteristics. Neurology 41:1374–1382, 1991.

168. Gustafson L: Frontal lobe degeneration of non-Alzheimer type. II. Clinical picture and differential diagnosis. Arch Gerontol Geriatr 6:209–223, 1987.

169. Cummings JL and Duchen LW: Kluver-Bucy syndrome in Pick disease: clinical and pathologic correlations. Neurology 31:1415–1422, 1981.

170. Miller BL, Ikonte C, Ponton M, et al.: A study of the Lund-Manchester research criteria for frontotemporal dementia: clinical and single-photon emission CT correlations. Neurology 48:937–942, 1997.

171. Dickson DW: Neuropathology of Pick's disease. Neurology 56:S16–S20, 2001.

172. Lee VM, Goedert M, and Trojanowski JQ: Neurodegenerative tauopathies. Annu Rev Neurosci 24: 1121–1159, 2001.

173. Francis PT, Holmes C, Webster MT, et al.: Preliminary neurochemical findings in non-Alzheimer dementia due to lobar atrophy. Dementia 4:172–177, 1993.

174. Sparks DL, Danner FW, Davis DG, et al.: Neurochemical and histopathologic alterations characteristic of Pick's disease in a non-demented individual. J Neuropathol Exp Neurol 53:37–42, 1994.

175. Folstein M, Folstein S, and McHugh P: "Mini mental state:" a practical method for grading the cognitive state of patients for the clinician. J Psychiatr Res 12:189–198, 1975.

176. Tilney F: The Brain, from Ape to Man. Hoeber, New York, 1928.

177. Stuss DT and Benson DF: Neuropsychological studies of the frontal lobes. Psychol Bull 95:3–28, 1984.

Chapter 10

Emotion and the Limbic System

The limbic system helps to regulate emotion, memory, motivation, drive, instinct, and social relations. The subcortical and cortical components of the limbic system strongly interconnect with other limbic areas, as well as with the brain stem and diencephalic and neocortical association areas. These connections allow limbic areas to balance and mediate drive functions, such as hunger, thirst, sex, aggression, and defense, as well as cognitive functions modulated by personal history and environment, such as social interactions.

Emotion and memory formation (see Chapter 8) are the core limbic functions. In humans, "hard-wired," instinctive sensory perceptions of certain things, such as snakes, wasps, or objects of sexual interest, elicit strong emotional experiences and expressions without prior learning. Brain stimulation can evoke preprogrammed, instinctive responses. For instance, stimulation of the amygdala or periaqueductal gray may elicit the "freezing response" to frightening stimuli,[1,2] and hypothalamic stimulation may trigger defensive rage.[3] More elaborate neural systems evolved to endow personal significance and emotional valence to

arbitrary stimuli and settings, such as faces and places. Information with emotional meaning has the highest priority for storage and retrieval. Throughout primate phylogeny, most sensory and cognitive information stored in long-term memory has had emotional content or was conditioned to an emotional stimulus.

THEORIES AND SYSTEMS OF EMOTION

Emotions can be intense, sudden waves of experience or more persistent, tidal states. Emotional states can reflect the tone of subjective feeling (*mood*) and the tone of expression of feeling (*affect*). Emotion is influenced by phylogenetically derived behavioral patterns (*instinct*) and acquired affective forces that underlie feelings and actions. These forces include learned patterns triggered by internal states (e.g., hunger) and environmental stimuli (e.g., a snake), as well as motivation, which ignites willful, planned actions with anticipated gratification.

Primary emotions, which are often negatively biased, include fear, anger, panic, sorrow, surprise, joy, and disgust. These primary-process affective experiences, so-called raw feelings, are internal states that guide behavior. Thus, learned associations could activate simple affective experiences coding for a generalized adaptive response.[4] These emotions display remarkably similar stereotypic expressions among disparate human cultures and primate species.[5] Many primary emotions are evoked by amygdala stimulation and attenuated or extinguished by amygdala lesions in humans and other animals.[4,6] The amygdala–hypothalamic axis is critical for experiencing and expressing primary emotions. The right hemisphere dominates the cortical modulation of primary emotions.[7]

Secondary emotions, known as social emotions, are more recent in their evolution and include guilt, embarrassment, and love. Social emotions, which are often positively biased, reflect the rules of social display; that is, be agreeable, cheerful, and interested, not disapproving and unpleasant.[8] The repertoire of secondary (social) emotions expanded in parallel with social behaviors. Social emotions form a diverse species- and person-specific palette containing genetically hard-wired and experientially derived emotions. We learn social emotions through experience, family, and peers. We may feel "unwelcome at someone else's home," "picked on unfairly at work," "unappreciated," "teased," or "proud." The anatomical substrate for secondary emotions includes limbic orbitofrontal and anterior cingulate cortices and prefrontal cortex.[7,9,10] Much neurological disability results from impaired social emotions and social cognition, functions that remain poorly understood.

Mood, affect, drive, and motivation influence personality. Social learning and cognitive, verbal, self-reflective, and nonconscious processes contribute to who we are and how we present ourselves to the world. Personality is the perceptual, cognitive, and behavioral response characteristics that make individuals unique. Despite the consistency of personality after adolescence, an individual's response patterns vary depending on intrinsic factors (e.g., hormonal fluctuations, pain, or emotional changes) and external influences (e.g., recent experiences or neuroactive drugs). Neuroanatomical systems underlying personality overlap with limbic and prefrontal areas controlling emotional and social functions.

The emotion network integrates attentional, perceptual, cognitive, and motor components. Organisms must focus on a behavioral task while simultaneously surveying internal and external environments for stimuli relevant to drive and social function. Sensory phenomena (e.g., seeing an uncaged lion, smelling a familiar scent) can alter the emotional state ("bottom–up" processing), and the emotional state can alter the perception of a stimulus ("top–down" processing) (see Chapter 5, Fig. 5–4). Emotional motor (expressive) systems include motivation systems for response to drive-related or socially relevant stimuli; orienting responses, such as eye and head deviation to bring peripheral stimuli into foveal view; skeletomotor responses such as flight or attack; autonomic and endocrine responses, such as increased cardiac output and glucocorticoid release during stress or copulation; and responses to communicate affective status. Drive-related behaviors are balanced against the environmental setting (e.g., satisfying hunger vs. the risk of attack by predators, the social consequences of eating someone else's sandwich). Drive behavior is modulated by social rules. Socialization integrates instinct and emotion with learned rules for prioritizing actions. Psychological problems arise when primary drives clash with social rules. A devastating behavioral consequence of limbic disorders, such as traumatic brain injury or stroke, is disruption of the balance between primary drives, emotion, and social functions.

Peripheral and Central Theories of Emotion

In 1872, Darwin[5] observed that the full expression of emotional states intensifies feelings and that the suppression of emotional displays diminishes feelings. Self-analysis led William James,[11] in 1884, to suggest a feedback mechanism by which peripheral changes, such as tremor and tachycardia, are perceived by the brain and evoke feelings. He concluded that you "feel" nervous because your body displays the physical manifestations of fear. James postulated that "bodily changes follow directly the PERCEPTION of the exciting fact, and that our feeling of the same changes as they occur IS the emotion." He recognized, however, that some emotions are not associated with bodily changes and cannot be explained by this mechanism. Carl Lange,[12] in 1885, suggested a similar but more restricted formulation related to vasomotor activity.

In 1927, Cannon[3] challenged the James-Lange theory of peripheral feedback by proposing an alternative central theory suggested by the "sham" rage phenomenon. Cannon observed that cortical transection failed to prevent coordinated emotional displays, which were considered sham because the motor and autonomic activity was dissociated from feeling. Thus, the rage behavior was nondirected, was bound to stimulus duration with rapid return to prior activity, and could not be conditioned. Because sham rage was eliminated by midbrain transection,[13] the diencephalon was thought to mediate emotional expression.[3,14] The Cannon–Bard central theory posited that after emotional sensations reach the diencephalon, brain stem and spinal cord projections downstream produce autonomic and skeletomotor responses, while neocortical projections upstream produce feelings.

Later studies show that both peripheral and central processes modulate emotion in a complex network (Fig. 10–1). Bodily sensations influence limbic and cortical activity. In nonhuman animals, sympathectomy impairs aversive conditioning.[15] In humans, vagus nerve stimulation activates the brain stem and diencephalic and cortical limbic areas.[16] Subjects who produce facial muscle patterns mimicking emotions report feeling the associated emotions.[17] Following spinal cord transection, patients continue to experience emotions, but the intensity is lower with transection at the higher levels.[18] However, since most visceral afferents pass through the vagus nerve, spinal cord transection does not disconnect the brain from all internal stimuli. In addition, environmental context strongly modulates the emotional reaction to central and peripheral stimuli.[19]

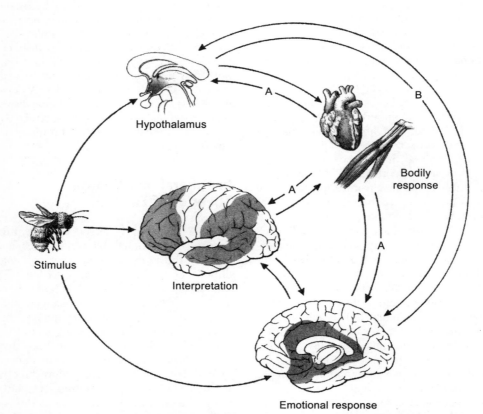

Figure 10–1. A model of how complex neural interrelations contribute to emotional experience and affective consciousness. This model integrates the principal pathways involved in the James-Lange *(A)* and Cannon-Bard *(B)* theories with other pathways and connections.

In humans, functional neuroimaging and electrical stimulation studies show that activation of mesial temporal, anterior cingulate, insular, and orbitofrontal cortices evokes negative and positive emotional feelings with or without associated autonomic and skeletomotor responses.[20,21] Thus, just as peripheral stimuli can affect cortical activity, cortical changes can alter peripheral targets (Fig. 10–1).

Relation of Emotion and Limbic Systems

The limbic system is the emotion system. In 1878, Broca[22] coined the term *limbic lobe* for the ring of gray matter separating the cortical mantle from deep structures (Fig. 10–2). Papez,[23] in 1937, conceived a circuit of interconnected structures comprising the emotion system: hippocampus (via the fornix bundle) to the hypothalamus and mamillary bodies (via the mamillothalamic tract) to the anterior thalamic nuclei (via the thalamocingulate fibers) to the cingulate cortex (via the cingulum) to the amygdala and hippocampus (Fig. 10–3). This emotion circuit theory was based on anatomical connections, sham rage studies, and lesion studies. For example, the severe anxiety and rage exhibited by rabid patients with hippocampal lesions (the pathognomonic Negri bodies are most abundant in hippocampal pyramidal cells, but brain lesions are widespread) suggested the hippocampus as a critical emotional node, although amygdala lesions probably caused these behaviors.

Later, Yakovlev[24] conceived a basolateral circuit modulating emotional behavior, including the amygdala, insula, orbitofrontal cortex, and

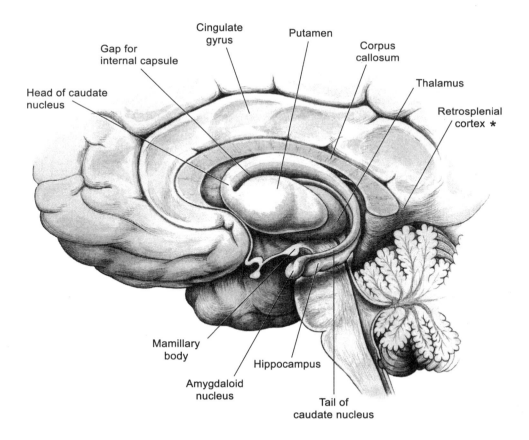

* Located in the banks of the callosal sulcus

Figure 10–2. Principal subcortical and cortical components of the striatum and limbic system.

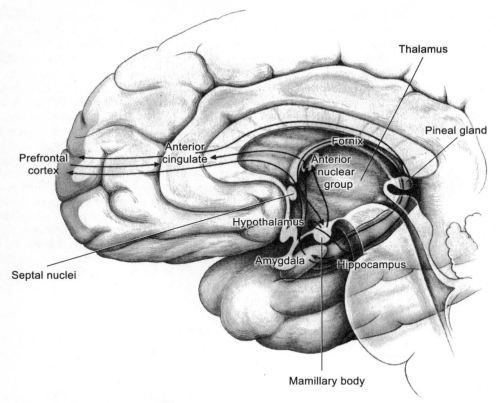

Figure 10–3. Principal structures of the limbic circuit (Papez circuit) and connections with prefrontal cortex.

dorsomedial thalamic nucleus. MacLean[25] added the septum and nucleus accumbens to the Papez–Yakovlev emotion circuits to form the limbic system. Extensive studies in humans and other species confirmed the limbic system's role in emotion. The hippocampus is mainly concerned with declarative memory for extrapersonal sensory stimuli[26] and with mnemonic processing of complex stimuli.[27] The amygdala serves as an emotion-evaluative node, endowing sensory data with emotional valence.[28] Projections from the amygdala to the hippocampus strengthen the hippocampal imprinting of an emotionally valent sensory stimulus in the neocortex.

The peripheral (James–Lange) and central (Cannon-Bard) theories of emotion are concatenated systems. The processes that perceive and evaluate a stimulus operate separately but overlap with the internal and external states that respond to a stimulus. The peripheral accompaniments of emotion, such as fear or anxiety, are probably triggered by programmed stimulus codes in the amygdala and brain stem

and then perceived by neocortical limbic areas that recognize discomfort or dangerous stimuli. Cortical areas can guide behavior based on peripheral changes in the somatic state and social perceptions. The amygdala generates the autonomic and motor expressions of fear. Where in the brain fear is "experienced" and "perceived" remains less certain, but it is likely the anterior cingulate, anterior insula, and orbitofrontal regions, as well as the amygdala. The thalamus and cortical areas process sensory information and then signal the amygdala to trigger peripheral fear responses. The peripheral somatic and neocortical cognitive loops of emotional experience overlap.

ANATOMY AND FUNCTION OF THE LIMBIC SYSTEM

Subcortical Limbic Areas

Subcortical limbic areas include the brain stem and hypothalamic, thalamic, and striatal sites

(Table 10–1), with their strong connections to each other and to cortical limbic areas. The subcortical limbic areas mediate aspects of reflexive, primitive instinct, and drive-related behaviors. These areas process and react to internal and simple environmental stimuli, such as moving peripheral visual stimuli. These evolutionarily older structures profoundly influence affective behavior, including endocrine, autonomic, arousal, and skeletomotor responses.

NUCLEUS ACCUMBENS

The nucleus accumbens (ventral striatum) forms the ventral–medial union of the caudate and putamen (Fig. 10–4) (see Chapter 8, Fig. 8–1). The accumbens comprises two regions: an inner core, with connections to dorsomedial and lateral prefrontal cortex and the globus pallidus, and an outer shell, with strong limbic connections.[29] Linked areas of prefrontal cortex and the nucleus accumbens share convergent inputs. For example, cell groups in both the basolateral amygdala and the midline thalamic nuclei project to regions of prefrontal cortex and the nucleus accumbens that are interconnected.[30] In addition, the midline thalamic nuclei project to the basolateral amygdala. Thus, this subcortical–cortical network influences multiple limbic sites.

Dopaminergic fibers from the ventral tegmental area to the nucleus accumbens are implicated in incentive and motivational reward and conditioned reinforcement.[31] Hyperactivity in this localized dopaminergic projection may contribute to psychosis,[32] and hypoactivity may contribute to abulia, as well as decreased initiative and motivation. In contrast, dopaminergic projections to the dorsal striatum regulate motor and cognitive activity, with altered dopaminergic activity causing hyperkinetic (e.g., tremor), hyperactive (e.g., recurrent intrusive thoughts), and hypoactive (e.g., diminished spontaneity and fluidness of thought) cognitive states.

BASAL FOREBRAIN

The basal forebrain comprises the septal nuclei, diagonal band of Broca, and substantia innominata. These regions provide cholinergic input to limbic and neocortical regions. They are predominantly involved in attention and memory. (Their anatomy and connectivity are shown in Fig. 10–4 and Table 10–1). However,

the septal nuclei are also implicated in positive components of drive and motivation. The medial septal nucleus provides cholinergic input to the hippocampus[33] and reinforces behavior associated with positive affective experiences, an integral component of the reward system. In monkeys, septal cells fire in response to motivational and rewarding stimuli, such as favorite food items when the animals are hungry.[34] Septal lesions cause diverse behavioral effects in animals, although the involvement of adjacent fiber tracts may contribute. The most consistent effects are hyperdypsia, a preference for sweet foods, impaired reactions to punishment (mimicked by injection of anticholinergic agents into the septum), and difficulty shifting from one reinforcing condition to the opposite (i.e., perseveration). Septal lesions also alter social behavior, causing rats to remain in contact with each other in an open field. Despite appearing fearful, the rats, if left alone, will approach cats; the need for social or physical contact overrides programmed fear.[35]

The septum's role in human behavior is poorly defined because selective lesions are rare and stimulation studies are limited. Septal tumors, rarely confined to the septum, cause amnesia, irritability, and aggressive behavior.[36] In contrast with the predominantly negative affective states evoked by stimulating other limbic areas, human septal stimulation evokes analgesia, pleasure, and sexual sensations.[37,38] The septal nuclei are part of the reward system, which includes the lateral hypothalamus, medial forebrain bundle, posterior orbitofrontal cortex, and other limbic sites.[39] The septal nuclei help to link motivation and positive affective experience for drive-related behaviors (e.g., eating, drinking) and aspects of socialization (e.g., affiliative behavior).

Amygdala

The amygdala processes and funnels emotionally relevant sensory data from diverse neocortical and limbic areas and outputs to the hypothalamus and brain stem, evoking autonomic, endocrine, and affective motor responses (Figs. 10–2, 10–3). (The orbitofrontal area and hypothalamus independently connect to autonomic and brain stem motor sites.) The amygdala consists of a central and basolateral nucleus and receives large cholinergic and monoaminergic inputs.[40] The effects of these

Table 10–1. **Connections and Functions of the Limbic Areas**

Area	Main Afferent Connections	Main Efferent Connections	Functions	Neurotransmitter Systems
Brain Stem				
Ventral tegmental	Striatonigral fibers from ventral globus pallidus	Prefrontal area and nucleus accumbens	Mental activation, emotion, mood, reward	Sends DA fibers
Periaqueductal gray	Prefrontal, cingulate, hippocampus, septum, habenula, brain stem reticular formation, spinal cord	Ventral midbrain tegmentum, ventral tegmental area, pretectal area, hypothalamus, thalamus	Pain, aggression, vocalization, reproduction, up-gaze	Enkephalin
Diencephalic				
Hypothalamus	Hippocampus, amygdala, septal nuclei, midbrain tegmentum	Anterior nucleus of thalamus, septal nuclei, midbrain tegmentum, pituitary, brain stem reticular formation and autonomic nuclei, spinal cord	Endocrine, autonomic, drive (appetite, thirst, aggression, sex), "fight or flight" response, sleep	Sends DA fibers to hypophyseal portal system; histamine; neuropeptides
Dorsomedial thalamic nucleus	Thalamic nuclei (CM, IL, lateral group), ventral pallidum, amygdala, prefrontal cortex, temporal lobe	Dorsolateral prefrontal, orbitofrontal and anterior cingulate, medial prefrontal	Memory, emotional responsiveness	—
Anterior thalamic nucleus	Hippocampal formation, mamillary bodies	Cingulate	Alertness, attention, memory	Receives 5-HT and ACh fibers
Midline thalamic nuclei	Hypothalamus	Hypothalamus, amygdala, ventral striatum, medial prefrontal	Arousal, emotional responsiveness	—
Striatal/Basal Forebrain				
Ventral striatum (nucleus accumbens)	Hippocampus, entorhinal cortex, amygdala, ventral tegmental area	Ventral pallidum, ventral tegmental area, hypothalamus, substantia innominata, septal nuclei	Goal-directed behavior, emotion, motivation	Receives DA fibers, modulates ACh activity

Structure	Inputs	Outputs	Function	Fibers
Substantia innominata	Hypothalamus, amygdala, other limbic areas	Thalamic reticular nucleus	Attention and memory	Sends ACh fibers
Septal nuclei	Hippocampus	Hippocampus, hypothalamus, midbrain tegmentum	Memory and emotion	Sends ACh fibers
Cortical				
Amygdala	Neocortical sensory association (often later stages) areas and limbic areas, thalamus	Hypothalamus, limbic areas, cortical sensory association areas, insula, prefrontal cortex	Attaches emotional significance to sensory input, fear, "fight or flight" response, autonomic	Receives 5-HT, ACh, DA, NE fibers
Hippocampus	Parahippocampus (entorhinal cortex and subiculum), septum	Subcortical–cortical association areas of memory network; fornix, bundle with most efferents	Explicit (declarative or episodic) memory consolidation and retrieval, spatial memory	Receives 5-HT, ACh, NE fibers; sends glutaminergic fibers to mamillary bodies, thalamus, and limbic areas
Parahippocampus (subiculum and entorhinal)	Neocortical association areas, hippocampus	Midline thalamic, limbic, neocortical association areas	Explicit (declarative or episodic) memory consolidation and retrieval, spatial memory	Receives 5-HT, ACh, NE fibers
Anterior cingulate cortex	Anterior nucleus of thalamus, cortical association areas	Entorhinal cortex, amygdala, septum, thalamus, prefrontal and parietal association cortex, brain stem	Motivation, attention, pain, motor, autonomic, response selection	Receives 5-HT, ACh, DA, NE fibers
Temporal pole	Inferotemporal visual association area, anterior insula	Amygdala, perirhinal cortex	Recall of specific names of persons or objects, visceral	Receives 5-HT, ACh, NE fibers
Anterior insula	All nonvisual sensory areas, amygdala	Orbitofrontal, prefrontal, amygdala, lateral hypothalamus	Autonomic, emotional response to sensory stimuli	Receives 5-HT, ACh, NE fibers
Posterior orbitofrontal cortex	Hypothalamus, olfactory cortex, amygdala, hippocampus, parahippocampal gyrus, ventral striatum, nucleus basalis, gustatory cortex	Hypothalamus, amygdala, entorhinal cortex	Modulates social and drive behavior in response to environmental stimuli	Receives 5-HT, ACh, DA, NE fibers

ACh, acetylcholinergic; CM, centromedian; DA, dopaminergic; 5-HT, serotoninergic (5-hydroxytryptamine); IL, intralaminar; NE, noradrenergic.

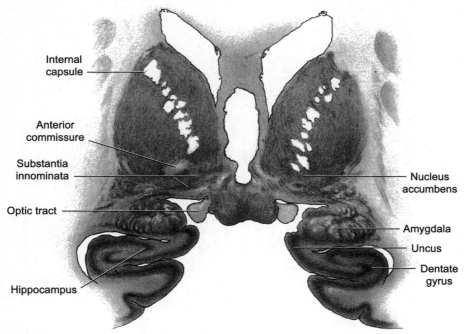

Figure 10–4. Coronal section showing nucleus accumbens, basal forebrain, and medial temporal lobe.

neurotransmitter systems (and psychotropic drugs) on mood are partially mediated by the amygdala. The main amygdala input is sensory, arising from neocortical and limbic areas.[41] The amygdala sends efferents to widespread neocortical limbic, sensory, and cognitive association areas.[41] Amygdalar projections to neocortex can provide top–down affective influences on perception. For example, fear of attack in a dangerous area leads to misinterpretation of a harmless stimulus (see Chapter 5, Fig. 5–4).

As a key interface between cortical and subcortical areas, the amygdala regulates emotion and affective expression. The amygdala helps to store semipermanent associations that drive simple behaviors such as fright and flight. Cortically processed sensory data are primarily endowed with emotional and motivational significance by the amygdala.

The amygdala responds predominantly to negative stimuli that evoke fear or defensive reactions[42] but also responds to positive stimuli such as positive emotional words,[43] sexual activity, and eating.[41,44] Stimulation of the amygdala most often causes fear.[20] Recordings from the amygdala of socially active monkeys showed the greatest activity when social communications included aversive stimuli, such as

a threating face, chasing, or other aggressive and sexual encounters.[45] In contrast, the least activity occurred with grooming and other tension-reducing behaviors.[46] Functional neuroimaging studies in normal subjects and observations in patients with amygdalar lesions support its primary role in regulating negative emotional states. Blood flow in the amygdala increases during sadness, viewing fearful faces, and perceiving aversive olfactory stimuli but can increase or decrease while viewing a happy face.[47,48] A patient with bilateral amygdalar damage could perceive only smiling or neutral faces and was unable to perceive negative emotional facial expressions, such as anger or fright, despite intact visual function.[49]

Social communication requires the assessment of sensory input to generate an appropriate response. The amygdala is the main limbic area that attaches emotional significance to sensory input and mediates the response to dangerous stimuli. The increasing size of the amygdala in primate evolution[50] supports its growing role in social behavior. After amygdalectomy, monkeys are socially isolated and survive only weeks in a natural environment,[51] and deficient maternal behavior in amygdalectomized monkeys causes infant deaths.[52]

KLÜVER-BUCY SYNDROME

In 1888, Brown and Schafer[53] described the transformation of a fierce monkey into a docile but hypersexual animal following bilateral temporal lobectomy. Although the special senses appeared intact, the monkey approached objects repetitively, as if they were strange:

He no longer clearly understands the meaning of the sounds, sights, and other impressions that reach him. His food is devoured greedily, the head being dipped into the dish, instead of the food being conveyed to the mouth by the hands. He reacts to all kinds of noises, even slight ones—such as the rustling of a piece of paper—but shows no consequent evidence of alarm or agitation and displays tyrannizing proclivities towards his mate.

When Klüver and Bucy[6,54] resected the bilateral anterior temporal lobes in male rhesus monkeys, they observed a symptom complex, later named the Klüver-Bucy syndrome, comprising *(1)* "psychic blindness" (visual agnosia); *(2)* a marked tendency to examine all objects orally (hyperorality), sometimes associated with hyperphagia and obesity; *(3)* an irresistible impulse to attend and react to visual stimuli (hypermetamorphosis, or distractibility); *(4)* emotional changes (loss of aggressive and fearful responses); and *(5)* hypersexuality.

This syndrome results mainly from bilateral amygdalectomy, which obliterates the emotional metropolis linking neocortex and hypothalamus. In neonatal monkeys, amygdala lesions increase social fear and decrease fear of objects.[55] In adult monkeys, unilateral lesions of the optic chiasm, commissures, and amygdala result in a single, intact amygdala receiving visual input from only the ipsilateral eye.[56] The normally aggressive response of caged rhesus monkeys to human experimenters occurs only when the eye ipsilateral to the preserved amygdala is open. Thus, cortically processed visual input must reach the amygdala to acquire emotional significance. Bilateral destruction of projections from sensory association cortex to limbic areas causes sense-specific amnesia and hypoemotionality syndromes.[55,57,58] For example, disconnecting temporal visual association projections to the amygdala impairs emotional reactivity to visual stimuli.[58,59] However, results from animal experiments cannot be extrapolated to native animal behavior and human disease because hypersexuality and hyperorality are uncommon among amyg-

dalectomized monkeys in naturalized settings but usually occur only in small group cages.[60]

In humans, the Klüver-Bucy syndrome occurs after bilateral mesial temporal lesions from various causes, including temporal lobectomy, herpes simplex encephalitis, head trauma, anoxia, Alzheimer's disease, Pick's disease, and adrenoleukodystrophy.[36] Humans usually have only one or two features of the Klüver-Bucy syndrome, often along with such other symptoms as amnesia, aphasia, aggressiveness, or paranoia.[61,62] Human diseases usually destroy the amygdala only partially, often leaving irritative foci and accounting for the response of some symptoms to carbamazepine or other antiepileptic drugs.[61] The human Klüver-Bucy syndrome is often associated with hyperorality, hyperphagia, and obesity. Hypersexuality is rare, but inappropriate sexual gestures and comments may occur. Anterior temporal lobectomy, with resection of one amygdala, is rarely complicated by hypersexuality or other features of the Klüver-Bucy syndrome.[63]

Bilateral lesions of the amygdala in humans cause placidity, with reduced perception and expression of aggressive and defensive behaviors.[49] Bilateral amygdalectomy reduces pathological aggression.[64] Although patients who have had an amygdalectomy experience muted emotions, they do not lack emotion or motivation.[65] The famous amnesic H.M., who underwent bilateral anterior temporal lobectomy, was content and placid nearly all the time, never complaining even when unwell. He rarely displayed anger, and when he did it dissipated quickly.[66]

CONDITIONED FEAR AND PHOBIAS

The pathological effects of amygdala hyperactivity likely contribute to unconditioned and conditioned fear, anxiety, and possibly phobic responses.[67,68] Conditioned fear utilizes direct thalamoamygdala projections for undifferentiated, nonlocalized stimuli, such as a loud noise or sudden peripheral movement (Fig. 10–5). Conditioned fear relies on indirect thalamic–neocortical–amygdala projections for more complex sensory stimuli that require neocortical recognition, such as faces.[69,70] Amygdala outputs to the subcortex can activate the arousal, autonomic, respiratory, somatic, neuroendocrine, and behavioral components of fear and anxiety (Fig. 10–6).

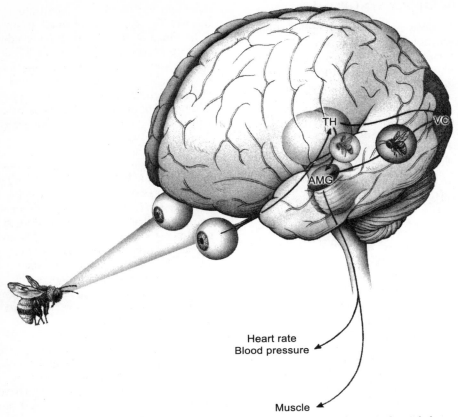

Figure 10–5. Direct and indirect sensory (visual) pathways to the amygdala (AMG). Direct pathways link incoming sensory information from the thalamus (TH, lateral geniculate nucleus) to the amygdala: data are transmitted rapidly, but the image is imprecise. Indirect pathway links sensory information from the thalamus to the visual cortex (VC) and then to the amygdala: data are transmitted slowly, but the image is precise. Both pathways can stimulate a sympathetic response.

The amygdala bonds a stimulus with its emotional connotation but cannot alter this association. The orbitofrontal or anterior cingulate cortex can change the emotional valence assigned to a sensory stimulus,[70] but amygdalar input to these cortical limbic areas is essential for them to detect the change in the emotional value of a stimulus.[69,70] For example, the amygdala is needed to condition an autonomic and motor response to a red ball presented with an electrical shock. After orbital and cingulate lesions, the conditioned reponse fails to extinguish when the red ball is no longer associated with the shock. Disruption of fibers from amygdala to orbital cortex also impairs extinction.

Following unilateral medial temporal lobectomy, acquisition of conditioned fear is impaired.[71] In humans, acquisition and extinction of conditioned fear are associated with amygdala activation that correlates with autonomic activity.[68] Conditioned fear may provide a model of traumatic memories and phobias, disorders with functional pathology likely extending to cortical limbic areas.

Stimulation studies confirm the role of the amygdala in emotional experience and expression. In animals, the fully developed and stereotypic defensive and aggressive reactions mimic the effects of hypothalamic or periaqueductal gray stimulation.[72] In humans, amygdala stimulation causes mild to moderate anxiety, terror, anger, a feeling of "someone is behind me," paranoia, and visceral sensations.[73]

EMOTIONAL MEMORIES

The amygdala is critical in forming long-term emotional memories,[74] although it lacks a general role in memory. The amygdala projects to many cortical areas, influencing attention, per-

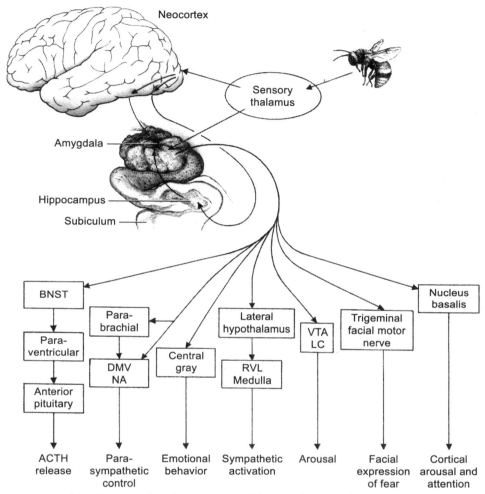

Figure 10–6. Amygdala efferents to the subcortex. Direct thalamic and indirect thalamocortical inputs stimulate the amygdala. In turn, the amygdala signals subcortical sites that mediate endocrine, autonomic, and motor responses. BNST, bed nucleus of stria terminalis; ACTH, adrenocorticotropic hormone; DMV, dorsal motor nucleus of vagus; NA, nucleus ambiguus; LH, lateral hypothalamus; RVL, rostral ventral lateral nucleus of medulla; VTA, ventral tegmental area; LC, locus ceruleus.

ception, and memory in emotional settings, especially those associated with fear. Emotional arousal activates the amygdala, which in turn facilitates memory storage in other brain regions.[75] In animals, stress-related hormones (e.g., glucocorticoids and epinephrine) and neurotransmitters (e.g., norepinephrine) enhance memory primarily through effects on the amygdala.[75]

The amygdala mediates the influence of emotional valence on learning and encodes the emotional valence of an experience. A patient with selective bilateral amygdala lesions did not acquire conditioned autonomic responses to visual or auditory stimuli.[76] However, the patient acquired the declarative facts concerning which visual or auditory stimuli were paired with the unconditioned stimulus. By contrast, another patient with selective bilateral hippocampal lesions failed to learn the facts but developed the conditioned autonomic responses.

The role of the amygdala in emotional memories helps to explain the central place of limbic structures in learning and memory. In mammalian phylogeny, linking sensory stimuli with emotion was essential (e.g., locations associated with danger or food, smells with predatory animals or food, and sexual objects).

Survival mandates that sensory stimuli with emotional or motivational value hold a preferential position in the memory queue. Hemispheric specialization may extend to the amygdala and emotional memories. In humans, functional neuroimaging studies suggest that the right amygdala predominates in nonconscious emotional learning and that the left amygdala predominates in conscious emotional learning.[77]

Hippocampus and Parahippocampal Gyrus

The hippocampal formation (hippocampus and dentate gyrus) and adjacent parahippocampal gyrus (subiculum and entorhinal cortex) are critical nodes in the memory network (Fig. 10–3) (see Chapter 8). These regions are neither repositories nor memory banks. They consolidate information into memory and revive these patterns during retrieval. Explicit (declarative or episodic) memory, the recording of specific arbitrary relationships (e.g., the name of an animal), requires these regions. Recently acquired information and associations are evanescent and require these regions to bond solidly with the matrix of prior knowledge.[78] Information learned long ago and rehearsed frequently (e.g., language) becomes densely woven into the fabric of cortical associations; it can be recalled without medial temporal lobe regions. However, these regions help to edit the incoming stream of sensory data, using amygdalar signals to prioritize data with greater emotional valence. Thus, hippocampal–parahippocampal regions are archival editors, helping to determine what information is worth encoding in neocortical memory banks.

Temporal Pole

The temporal pole, an agranular limbic area, receives strong input from other limbic areas and the inferotemporal association cortex and projects mainly to the amygdala.[79] Connectivity patterns suggest that different areas of the temporal pole are associated with different behaviors: the medial area with visceral, olfactory, and gustatory functions; the ventral area with visual functions; the dorsal area with auditory functions; and the lateral area with integrating sensory, emotional, and cognitive functions. Stimulation of the temporal pole evokes complex motor and visceral responses in nonhuman animals but not in humans.[80,81] Temporal pole lesions in monkeys disrupt social behavior, reducing affiliative behavior and leading to social isolation.[82]

In humans, the temporal pole may have naming and emotional functions. Extensive experience with temporal pole resections in patients with intractable epilepsy provides some clues to this area's role in behavior, but these observations are clouded by the effects of chronic epilepsy and by the removal of additional limbic and neocortical temporal regions. After dominant hemisphere resections, recall of persons' names, names of other living things, words acquired in late childhood and adulthood, and infrequently used words is often impaired.[83,84] Linking faces with names may be especially impaired.[85] Nondominant hemisphere resections restricted to the temporal pole are not associated with known deficits but may contribute to the occasional psychopathology that occurs more often with nondominant anterior temporal resections.[86]

Functional neuroimaging studies suggest that the temporal pole links symbols (e.g., a name) to specific sensory stimuli. For example, this area is involved in detecting stimulus familiarity,[87] learning new visual patterns,[88] and recalling proper names.[89] Functional neuroimaging studies suggest a role of the nondominant temporal pole in the diverse activities of processing abstract words, possibly reflecting the nondominant hemisphere's role in perceiving nonformed, abstract stimuli,[90] perceiving sad faces,[91] and experiencing anger.[92] The temporal poles, as well as the orbitofrontal gyri, are activated during recall of traumatic events.[93]

Anterior Cingulate Cortex

The anterior cingulate cortex (ACC) is the largest limbic structure, extending above the anterior corpus callosum on the medial hemisphere (Fig. 10–7). The ACC encircles the rostrum of the corpus callosum, continuing inferiorly as subcallosal area 25. The ACC together with other cortical limbic areas forms the upper layer of the emotional brain, providing motivational context; attending to, evaluating, and reacting with novel and complex behavior; and monitoring behavioral output.

The ACC functions in affective, autonomic, cognitive, social, and motor behavior. It is part of the network that initiates and motivates goal-directed behaviors. This system assesses the motivational content of internal and external stimuli and regulates context-dependent behaviors. Among the primary components of the ACC (Fig. 10–7) are affect and cognition areas and a cingulate motor area. The affect division (areas 25, 33, and rostral area 24) extensively connects with the amygdala, periaqueductal

gray, and autonomic brain stem motor nuclei. These areas help to assess the emotional valence of internal and external stimuli and scenarios, thereby modulating the motivational state, and may emotionally color motor actions (via the cingulate motor area).[94] The cognition division (caudal areas 24c′ and 32′) helps to select motor responses and responses to noxious stimuli. The cingulate motor area (see Chapter 7) receives a convergence of limbic input;[95] connects with primary areas, the supplementary motor area (SMA), and the basal ganglia; and sends out corticospinal fibers. The cingu-

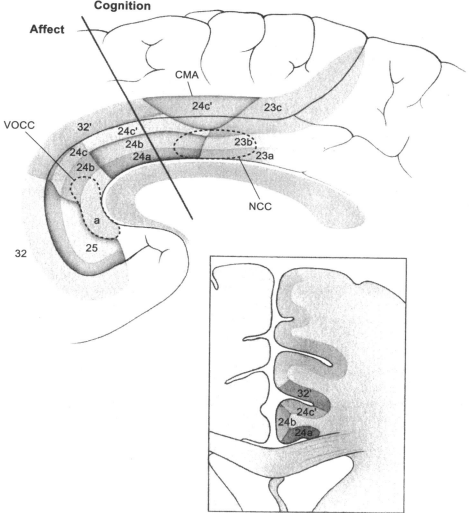

A

Figure 10–7. The cingulate cortex and its limbic and behavioral functions. Medial view of the cytoarchitectural regions in the human brain (*A*) and the macaque monkey (*B*); Flat map shows cortex buried in cingulate sulcus and the macaque monkey (*B*). VOCC, vocalization control cortex; NCC, nociceptive cortex; CMA, cingulate motor area (M3). VOCC, vocalization control cortex; NCC, nociceptive cortex; CMA, cingulate motor area (M3). (*continued*)

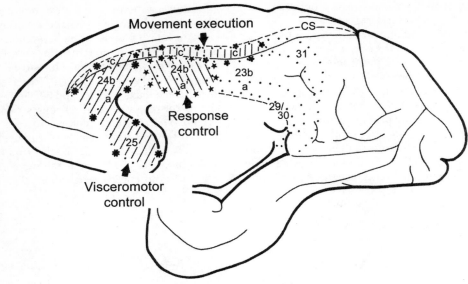

Figure 10–7. *(Continued).*

late motor area may contain programs for stereotyped "preprogrammed" behaviors, such as laughter, as well as learned emotional behaviors.

Bilateral cingulate lesions, in their most severe expression and often in association with bilateral SMA lesions (see Chapter 7), produce akinetic mutism. These lesions extinguish motivation, spontaneous motor or vocal responses, and responsiveness to internal or external states. Cingulate lesions can alter personality and individual preferences, diminish volition, impair motor initiation, cause motor neglect, reduce responses to pain, and disrupt social behavior.[94] However, paradoxically, as in other prefrontal areas, the effects of cingulate lesions are not readily identified by standard tests. Extensive neuropsychological studies after cingulectomy (bilateral cingulate resection) and cingulumotomy (bilateral cingulum bundle destruction) reveal no consistent cognitive or personality changes.[96,97]

NEGLECT SYNDROMES

The attentional and motor intentional contributions of the ACC are evident in neglect syndromes (see Chapter 4). Unilateral visual and somesthetic neglect follows ACC lesions in monkeys and humans.[98,99] Hypokinesia and hypometria can develop in the limbs con-

tralateral to ACC and SMA lesions.[100] Hypokinesia improves when the affected arm moves into the opposite hemispace, suggesting hemispatial motor neglect. Infarcts of the bilateral ACC extending to the fornices and prefrontal cortex can cause a severe attentional deficit.[101]

EMOTIONAL–SOCIAL BEHAVIOR

Sadness or happiness[102] and recognizing the emotional content in a facial expression[103] correlate with increased blood flow in the ACC. Electrical stimulation of the ACC can evoke fear, pleasure, and agitation.[94] Cingulectomy and cingulumotomy reduce the affective component of pain and can improve obsessive–compulsive and possibly depressive disorders.[104,105]

Seizures arising in ACC commonly evoke such emotional feelings or expressions as fear or laughter. Interictally, patients with cingulate seizures may exhibit irritability, anxiety, emotional lability, heightened or deviant sexual behavior, disinhibition, placidity, depression, aggressiveness, obsessive–compulsiveness, bulimia, and social problems.[94,106,107] Adjacent frontal regions are often affected, and these problems can develop into disabling personal and social behavioral disorders that blunt affect and social judgment and cause psychosis and sexually deviant behavior. In some cases, a "sociopathic personality disorder" leads to criminal acts or institutionalization.[94,108] The following case report is illustrative:

A 42-year-old man had medically intractable complex partial seizures and sociopathic behavior for more than a decade. Frequent nocturnal seizures caused grotesque facial contortions, tongue thrusting, a strangulated yell, neck and trunk flexion, bilateral arm and leg extension, and side-to-side thrashing. Interictally, he was very irritable, with poor impulse control, and sexual preoccupation and deviancy. For example, he propositioned women on the medical staff and attempted to lick a nurse's face. He had been dismissed from the police force because of excessive brutality, and then from the Drug Enforcement Agency because of brutality and the use of confiscated drugs. Following resection of the right anterior cingulate gyrus (and anterior corpus callosotomy), his seizure frequency and interictal behavior markedly improved.

Devinsky et al. (1995)[94]

The ACC is part of the prefrontal network for personal and social behavior together with the orbitofrontal and dorsolateral regions. In rodents, early cingulate damage impairs playful behavior, a marker of the evolutionary transition from reptiles to mammals.[109] Cingulectomy may reduce motivation for previously enjoyable activities. For example, patients who had voraciously read good literature read only sporadically after cingulectomy, consuming "poorer light magazines."[94] One patient gave up carpentry, gardening, reading, and his passion for sports. Other patients became less meticulous in their habits, slower in thoughts and actions, less self-conscious and timid, and more irritable and had a shallower and less sustained affect as well as impaired judgment in personal and social situations.[110]

RESPONSES TO NOXIOUS STIMULI

The ACC codes the affective content of stimuli associated with noxious events, a cognitive code for "pain." Metabolism in the ACC increases when nociceptive input is processed.[111] Cingulumotomy improves chronic pain. According to Foltz and White,[112] the pain perception is not modified, but the patient's total reaction to pain is markedly modified: "Most . . . patients . . . continued to have pain but it was 'not particularly bothersome, doesn't worry me.' "

RESPONSE SELECTION AND COGNITION

Information processing by the ACC helps to determine whether a "mental or motor" action is needed prior to the act itself and monitors performance by detecting errors and selecting responses when there are conflicting choices.[94,113] When evaluating sensory stimuli, the ACC helps to select novel responses.[114] When suspending activity while waiting for low-probability signals, reduced ACC activity can enhance signal detection, possibly by keeping "nothing in mind." [115]

Lesion studies suggest that the ACC is critical in motivated attention, as already mentioned. The ACC may allocate attentional resources when behavioral scenarios elicit incompatible response tendencies that must be reconciled to respond correctly.[116] The ACC also monitors performance and detects response errors.[117,118] This self-monitoring function is an extension of the ACC's role in resolving incongruent choices since many behavioral responses can only be judged correct or incorrect based on the subsequent response of other organisms. Self-monitoring provides on-line assessment of past and future actions in behaviorally ambiguous settings.

Blood flow in the ACC increases during difficult cognitive tasks, such as the Stroop Interference Task,[46,119] tasks generating verbs to novel nouns (mainly in the left area 32'),[120] target detection tasks,[115] and willed actions (blood flow in the dorsolateral prefrontal cortex also increases prominently).[121] In patients with dorsolateral lesions, the error-related event potential recorded from the ACC is markedly reduced, supporting a critical interaction between dorsolateral and cingulate regions in monitoring actions for errors and conflicting response choices.[122]

Posterior Orbitofrontal Cortex

The orbitofrontal cortex is divided into a posterior agranular limbic region and an anterior granular region, with a transitional dysgranular segment in between.[123] The posterior agranular and dysgranular cortices strongly connect to the limbic areas (e.g., ACC, amygdala, entorhinal cortex, olfactory cortex), midline thalamic nuclei, and brain stem reticular formation. The anterior granular orbitofrontal cortex is continuous with dorsolateral prefrontal cortex, with connections predominantly to neocortical association areas and association thalamic nuclei.[124] Anterior orbital cortex bridges the limbic posterior orbital cortex and dorsolateral heteromodal prefrontal cortex.

The posterior orbitofrontal cortex modulates arousal and responsiveness of social and drive behaviors to environmental stimuli. Connections and functions of the posterior orbitofrontal cortex parallel those of the ACC, influencing motor and visceral activity and evaluating the social–emotional context of stimuli and behavior. The posterior orbitofrontal cortex, more than the ACC, directly modulates social behavior. The posterior orbitofrontal cortex is involved in olfaction, autonomic activity, appetite, emotional responsiveness, social behavior, and inhibition of behavior. The role of the posterior orbitofrontal cortex in cognition, relative to other frontal regions, is discussed in Chapter 9.

OLFACTION, AUTONOMIC ACTIVITY, AND APPETITE

The posterior orbitofrontal cortex receives olfactory input from the mesial temporal cortex. The posterior orbitofrontal cortex and entorhinal cortex are strongly activated by pleasant and unpleasant olfactory stimuli.[125] Convergent inputs for olfactory, gustatory, and visual modalities in the posterior orbitofrontal cortex help to link a visual stimulus to its smell and taste and, thus, its hedonic value.[126] The posterior orbitofrontal cortex's role in olfactory processing may extend to sexual attraction and mate selection. Like mice, humans may differentiate body odors of the opposite sex based on immune response genes, preferring those with human leukocyte antigen (HLA) haplotypes different from their own.[127] Within a relatively inbred group, the Hutterites, fetal loss rates are higher when the HLAs between parents are closely related.[128] Further, as in mice, Hutterites tend to avoid mating with someone who has HLA genes that resemble their own, especially those that resemble their mother's.[129,130] Thus, the posterior orbitofrontal cortex integrates smell, attraction, and social behavior.

Autonomic activity frequently accompanies affective behavior. The anterior cingulate, posterior orbitofrontal, and anterior insular cortices and amygdala regulate autonomic activity. Electrical stimulation of these limbic areas elicits visceromotor changes, including alterations in respiratory and cardiac rate and blood pressure, pupil size, piloerection, facial flushing, gastrointestinal motility, nausea, vomiting, visceral sensations, salivation, and bowel or bladder evacuation.[131]

Orbitofrontal damage may "release" the autonomic nervous system from cortical control, lowering blood pressure and skin temperature, causing increased sweating, gastrointestinal disorders, aberrant micturition (i.e., in inappropriate settings), and lowering the threshold for erection.[132,133] Orbitofrontal dysfunction, possibly responding to social stresses or other factors, may excessively stimulate autonomic systems and contribute to peptic ulcer disease,[134] irritable bowel syndrome, accelerated atherosclerosis or vasospasm, and labile hypertension.

Animals and patients with bilateral orbital lesions can become hyperphagic and hyperoral.[135,136] Food and fluid intake can abnormally increase, causing a weight gain of 200 pounds or more.[137] Patients may orally explore or eat nonnutritive objects such as cigarette butts,[137] which is similar to the behaviors of monkeys with Klüver-Bucy syndrome, described earlier.

EMOTIONAL PERCEPTION AND RESPONSIVENESS

In primates, orbitofrontal lesions increase aversive reactions and reduce aggressiveness and emotional responsiveness.[136] After combined orbitofrontal and anterior cingulate lesions, a transient reduction in spontaneous and reactive behaviors is followed by emotional disinhibition.[138] Orbitofrontal lesions impair the ability to change the emotional meaning of a sensory stimulus. The orbitofrontal cortex rapidly responds to changes in stimulus–reinforcement associations,[139] and orbitofrontal lesions impair extinction of conditioned fear responses.[140] Thus, the perseverative emotional behavior following orbitofrontal lesions is analogous to the perseverative cognitive and motor responses following prefrontal lesions.[141,142] Perseverative, nonmalleable emotional reactions to stimuli that were once, but are no longer, associated with a negative emotional valence can result from the strength of the initial association (e.g., a vicious dog attack), aberrant reinforcement mechanisms (e.g., epileptogenic processes),[143] or orbitofrontal dysfunction. Abnormalities in the orbital cortex on magnetic resonance imaging (MRI) are reported in patients with obsessive–compulsive disorder.[144]

In humans, orbital lesions can cause motor hyperactivity, impulsiveness, extroversion, euphoria, talkativeness, perseveration, and socially inappropriate behavior. Affected patients may be unconcerned about responsibilities, laugh inappropriately, and exhibit careless, tactless, silly, and childish behavior. In other patients, paranoia, grandiosity, irritability, and aggressiveness punctuate their behavior.[108,137,145] Bilateral orbital lesions increase aggressive and violent behaviors.[137,146,147] Because of impaired self-monitoring, patients with orbital lesions often fail to recognize their violent tendencies, which are often provoked by family conflicts. Following orbital resections, some patients neglect or beat their children with minimal provocation.[148] The compassion and social consequences that prevent aggressive behavior fail to inhibit these patients. Thus, orbital lesions disrupt the interface between emotional and social behaviors. Pathological hyperactivity in orbitofrontal–cingulate circuits may contribute to anxiety and obsessive–compulsive symptoms.

SOCIAL AND PERSONALITY CHANGES

The orbitofrontal cortex is less developed in orangutans, largely solitary animals, than in other anthropoid apes.[149,150] Monkeys with orbital, but not dorsolateral, frontal lesions are socially devastated; they fail to show the aggressive and submissive displays and grooming behaviors that make up the fabric of their social life, with a corresponding fall in the dominance hierarchy.[151] Emotional vocalizations and maternal behavior are impoverished, and the monkeys become socially isolated.[151] After orbitofrontal resection in monkeys, the social changes mimic those following amygdalotomy and differ from those following dorsolateral frontal resections; in the latter case, the animals fail to submit to the more dominant monkey (decreased aversion) and display increased aggression.[152]

The disconnection of social and emotional networks may be the fundamental mechanism of altered behavior after posterior orbitofrontal cortex damage. In an alternative, overlapping mechanism, the posterior orbitofrontal cortex may be a critical node that generates response patterns reflecting, for example, personal history, a biological tendency toward risk-taking behavior, introvertedness versus extrovertedness, and mood. The personality changes can also be viewed from the narrower perspective of specific mechanisms, such as loss of inhibition or failure to generate or interpret autonomic and skeletomotor changes associated with affective behavior.

A hallmark of adult primate and human behavior is the inhibition of immediately attractive or reflexive responses that are less favorable in the long run. Frontal lobe lesions impair the ability to inhibit behaviors triggered by environmental stimuli. This alters personality, prominently affecting behaviors that require continued inhibition. Patients may become childish and display inappropriate language, jocularity, and other behavior. Libido and sexual activity may increase, causing marital conflicts, consorting with prostitutes, or, rarely, rape or beatings for refusal to have sex.[137] Disinhibited behaviors may impair monitoring of social behaviors and self-monitoring to determine appropriate patterns of subsequent behaviors and cause impersistence (failure to sustain an action or action plan). Patients with orbital lesions typically have some awareness of the personality changes, which can dominate family life. Thus, they can partly understand explanations of their inappropriate behavior, but this knowledge rarely changes their future behavior.

Social behavior is severely disrupted in patients with orbital lesions, with prominent antisocial traits occurring even after unilateral injury.[153] Patients become excessively dependent on, and responsive to, environmental stimuli in guiding behavior, a formula for social disaster (see Chapter 9 for a discussion of imitation and utilization behavior). The orbital cortex partly acts as our conscience and superego. The orbitofrontal cortex helps to censor, self-monitor, and incorporate social experience into behavioral decisions. The impairments in performance of laboratory-based gambling paradigms in patients with orbitofrontal lesions and activation of this area by gambling decisions in normal subjects may reflect its role in making social and other decisions.[154] The orbitofrontal cortex also appears critical for making inferences about others' mental states ("theory of mind").[155] Such inferences are a foundation for social reasoning and impaired in patients with orbitofrontal lesions, as well as such developmental disorders as Asperger's syndrome.[156]

The network for making emotional and social decisions includes the amygdala, ACC, orbitofrontal cortex, and dorsolateral prefrontal cortex.[156–158] The following case report illustrates the social consequences of orbital lesions:

Bilateral anterior cingulate and orbitofrontal damage caused a successful accountant to lose his job, finances, and marriage despite preserved "intelligence and memory" on standardized tests.[159] Impaired judgment caused devastating social behavior. He failed "in real life" because he could not interpret and adapt to social cues or prioritize among different options. Simple decisions of where to eat out, which required an "intuitive" weighting of the advantages and disadvantages of different restaurants,

became paralyzing. Although he described normal patterns of social behavior when questioned about a hypothetical setting, he failed to execute such patterns in life. His disastrous actions were often labeled "sociopathic." Exposure to emotional visual images of mutilation, nudity, and social disaster failed to evoke an electrodermal skin response,[160] indicating emotional—or at least autonomic—detachment from the images.

Partly on the basis of this case study, Damasio[161] theorized that the orbital cortex endows "gut" feelings about situations, stimuli, and decisions. These feelings, largely generated through autonomic effects such as heart rate, visceral feelings, and facial expression, can act overtly or covertly to influence behavior.[162]

The experiences of two of our patients further highlight the effects of orbitofrontal damage:

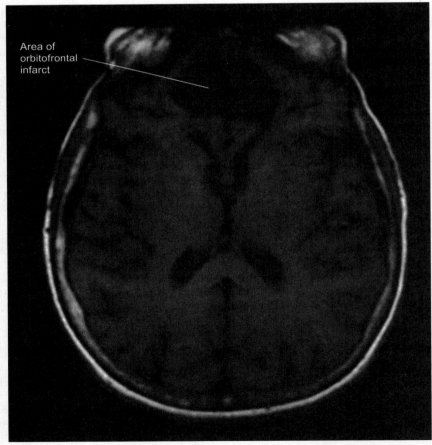

Area of orbitofrontal infarct

A

Figure 10–8. Magnetic resonance image of a 45-year-old man with bilateral orbitofrontal infarction after a ruptured aneurysm. (A) Axial view.

Patient 1

A 45-year-old former policeman had bilateral or-bitofrontal infarcts following the rupture of an aneurysm of the anterior communicating artery 8 years earlier (Fig. 10–8). He became irritable and ag-gressive, changes, his wife noted, that had improved only slightly over time. While still a police officer, he casually described severely beating people "for look-ing at me the wrong way." Now retired from the po-lice force, his wife reports that he is extremely diffi-cult to live with. He yells at her and explodes over trivial matters. His emotional reactivity is intact. For example, after his stroke, when investigating a mur-der, he was sickened upon viewing a child's mutilated body and pursued the case for several years, eventu-ally catching the killer. However, his autonomic re-sponsiveness to emotionally powerful videos of vio-lence and sexual activity was markedly attenuated.

Patient 2

A 51-year-old woman had an arteriovenous mal-formation in the right orbitofrontal cortex. Through-out her adult life, she was hypersexual and recog-nized that her enormous sexual appetite was aber-rant—for either a man or a woman. Her husband was unable to fulfill her needs, although they often had intercourse more than 10 times a week through more than two decades of marriage. She noted "I would be sitting with my girlfriends and they would all say how they wished their husbands would leave them alone at night. I just listened—I knew I was-n't normal." After successful resection of her lesion, she became hyposexual and displayed minimal in-terest in sexual activities. Now, she says, she has in-tercourse largely for her husband but experiences no pleasure or orgasm.

Combined anterior cingulate and orbito-frontal lesions disconnect intellectual under-standing of provocative images and the auto-nomic response. The lack of physiological emotional cues may impair appreciation of emotionally significant stimuli. Sociopathic in-dividuals may have blunted autonomic re-

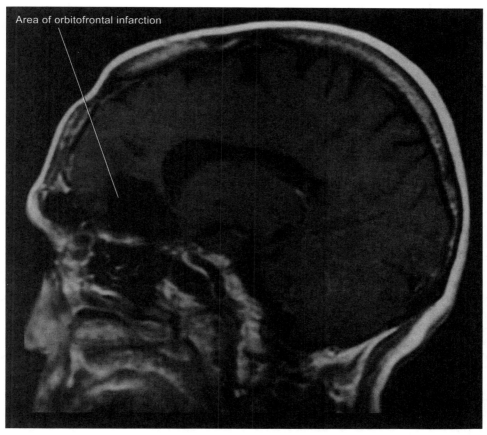

Area of orbitofrontal infarction

B

Figure 10–8. *(Continued). (B)* Sagittal view.

sponses to emotional stimuli.[163] Combined anterior cingulate and orbitofrontal lesions may attenuate the emotional changes that trigger the autonomic changes and impair perception of autonomic changes that signal emotion to other central sites. Interrupting the link between autonomic changes and emotional stimuli is one mechanism by which anterior cingulate and orbitofrontal lesions disrupt social behavior.

Insula (the "Island")

The insula, buried in the sylvian fissure, is a "fifth" lobe of the cortex, with up to six gyri that merge into opercular regions of the frontal, parietal, and temporal lobes. The anterior insula cortex has predominantly limbic connections, serving as a limbic integrative center for autonomic and sensory functions.[131,164,165] The posterior insula has mainly neocortical connections and sensory and cognitive functions (see Chapters 5 and 6, respectively). The limbic anterior insular cortex receives input from gustatory cortex (anterior portion of peri-insula frontoparietal operculum contains the gustatory area) and olfactory cortex (peri-insula anterior temporal lobe contains piriform olfactory area).[166] The posterior insula receives input from primary somatosensory cortex (poster portion of peri-insula frontoparietal operculum contains SII) and auditory and vestibular cortices (posterior portion of peri-insula temporal lobe contains auditory and vestibular areas).

The insula has unique connections as a direct convergence site for all nonvisual sensory data. Other cortical multimodal sensory areas receive polysynaptic input from sensory association cortices, but the insula and orbitofrontal cortex receive direct input from primary sensory areas. The insular cortex integrates multimodal sensory inputs, and the anterior insular cortex links stimuli with emotional valence via intense, reciprocal amygdalar connections.[167–169] The anterior insular cortex receives input from all sensory association and multimodal association cortices and projects to orbitofrontal and prefrontal cortices.

The insula is a principal site of cortical autonomic representation.[170] Experimental and clinical studies implicate the insula and its subcortical connections (e.g., lateral hypothalamus) in generating cardiac arrhythmias after stress, stroke, and seizures.[170,171] The anterior insula may also mediate stress-induced cardiovascular and gastrointestinal responses.[167,171] In animals and humans, the right anterior insula has a dominant role over sympathetic responses, and the left anterior insula has a dominant role over parasympathetic responses.[172] The anterior insular cortex modulates autonomic and somatomotor output through its connections with cortical motor areas, the amygdala, and the nucleus of the solitary tract. Blood flow in the anterior insular cortex is markedly increased by voluntary swallowing,[173] and infarcts in the area cause dysphagia.[174]

The anterior insular cortex is activated during integration and processing of the sensory aspects of emotion. When words evoke color images, the anterior insula, as well as language and higher visual integration areas and prefrontal heteromodal cortices, is activated.[175] Visualizing aversive stimuli enhances blood flow in the anterior insular cortex, visual areas, and midfrontal cortex on the left side.[176] Interfacing between the primary gustatory area and the amygdala, the anterior insular cortex responds to tastes with emotional valence.[166] The anterior insular cortex may have a special role in processing emotional vocalizations.[177] It is strongly activated by perceiving facial expressions of disgust[178,178a] and by unpleasant and pleasant smells.[179] Recalled sadness activates the anterior insular cortex, and happiness activates the ventromedial frontal cortex.[180] When an aversive tone is conditioned to a face, functional MRI reveals differential evoked responses in the ACC and anterior insular cortex, consistent with their role in emotional processing of sensory stimuli.[181] Finally, anticipatory fear activates several limbic areas, but the anterior insular cortex most prominently.[182]

The posterior insula, in addition to providing some specific sensory functions, such as detection of sound and movement of auditory stimuli,[183] auditory processing, and tactile learning, may link Wernicke's and Broca's areas[184] (see Chapter 6).[184] Lesions of the posterior insula are associated with conduction aphasia[185] and dysarthria.[186]

HEMISPHERIC CONTRIBUTIONS TO EMOTION

Perceptual, expressive, and cognitive elements of emotion emerge from the functional–anatomical networks linking the peripheral and central nervous systems, cortical and subcortical systems, and both cerebral hemispheres.

There is robust evidence of right hemisphere dominance for emotion,[187–189] extending to receptive, productive, and experiential emotional functions. The degree of right hemispheric specialization for emotion, in general, and for specific elements of emotional function varies between subjects and eludes a simplistic explanation (see Chapter 3). Further, studies of dichotic listening, facial asymmetry, and other characteristics in patients with unilateral cerebral injury and in normal subjects as well as neuroimaging studies refute simple left–right theories of hemispheric roles in emotion.[7,189–191]

The valence hypothesis offers another simplified model for hemispheric control of emotion: the right hemisphere mediates negative emotions, and the left hemisphere mediates positive emotions.[9,192,193] This hypothesis arose from the observation of emotional changes after unilateral lesions. Right hemisphere lesions and anesthetization (intracarotid amobarbital) cause emotional flattening, indifference, euphoria, and mania.[189,192,194] Left hemisphere lesions, especially frontal lesions, more often cause depression and anxiety.[195] Many studies in normal subjects and patients with focal brain deficits support the valence theory,[7,187–189,191,192,196] but many others do not.[197–199] Hemispheric processing modes may be related to emotional valence. Primary emotions such as fear and anger (see Chapter 3) and negative emotions are more closely tied to survival behaviors, such as fighting or fleeing in a threatening encounter. These behavioral patterns are predominantly served by right hemisphere systems specialized for attention to peripheral space, arousal, and gestalt perception.[187] Secondary or social emotions (e.g., pride) and positive emotions have greater linguistic, communicative, and social components, features that are served by left or bilateral hemispheric processes.[9,187] These models of emotion modulation by the cerebral hemispheres (right-dominant, valence-negative vs. -positive, primary vs. social) are not mutually exclusive. No current model accounts for the diversity, complexity, or subtlety of the neural systems underlying emotion.

BRAIN DISORDERS AND EMOTIONAL CHANGES

Disorders of the emotional state profoundly impact the organism. Limbic disorders alter affect, mood, and personality as well as social, cognitive,

and drive functions. Tumors, strokes, trauma, infections, or other pathological processes affecting the limbic system cause devastating emotional changes, psychiatric disorders, and amnesia (Table 10–2).[23,28,44,62,94,108,189] Limbic lesions are highly epileptogenic, and epilepsy

Table 10–2. **Disorders Associated with Limbic Lesions and Dysfunction**

Autoimmune–inflammatory
  Systemic lupus erythematosus
  Sydenham's chorea
  Multiple sclerosis
Dementia
  Alzheimer's disease
  Frontotemporal
  Traumatic
  Multi-infarct
Epilepsy
  Partial (e.g., hippocampus, amygdala, anterior cingulate, posterior orbitofrontal)
  Generalized
Infection
  Herpes simplex encephalitis
  Acquired immunodeficiency syndrome
  Lyme disease
Motor disorders (see Chapter 7)
  Degenerative disorders (e.g., Parkinson's disease, Huntington's disease)
  Tourette's syndrome
Psychiatric disorders
  Anxiety (panic attack, phobia, generalized anxiety)
  Mood (dysphoria, depression, bipolar disorder)
  Schizophrenia
Tumor
  Primary
  Metastatic
  Paraneoplastic limbic encephalitis
Vascular
  Anterior cerebral artery: anterior cingulate, posterior orbitofrontal cortex
  Medial striate (Heubner artery): nucleus accumbens, substantia innominata
  Anterior communicating artery rupture (aneurysm): bilateral infarct of orbitofrontal cortex and substantia innominata
  Posterior cerebral artery: middle to posterior hippocampus
  Middle cerebral artery: amygdala, anterior insula
  Anteromedial arteries (arise from anterior cerebral, anterior communicating, and proximal internal carotid): anterior hypothalamus
  Posterior circulation: brain stem, thalamic, and posterior hypothalamic areas

arising in limbic areas may cause diverse, usually pathological behavioral changes.[200–202] Two disorders with a predilection for limbic areas are paraneoplastic limbic encephalitis and epilepsy.

Paraneoplastic Limbic Encephalitis

Paraneoplastic limbic encephalitis is rare but causes mental deterioration with hallucinations, depression, anxiety, agitation, amnesia, and partial seizures.[203,204] Memory and behavioral problems progress over 2–20 months before the carcinoma (e.g., oat cell carcinoma of the lung, ovarian or breast cancer) is discovered. Cerebrospinal fluid analysis may reveal a mild lymphocytic pleocytosis and elevated protein. The MRI often reveals an increased T_2-weighted signal, maximal in mesial temporal regions.[204,205] Pathological changes include neuronal loss, gliosis, and perivascular cuffing in mesial temporal and orbitofrontal cortices and subcortical areas. Anti-Hu antibodies may be detected in cerebrospinal fluid.[206] Treatment of the carcinoma may improve behavior and memory.

Epilepsy

From antiquity to recent times, epilepsy has been mistakenly linked with curses, demonic possession, prophetic powers, and ubiquitous mental disorders. Although these misconceptions were exposed, false "facts" persist. For example, many physicians still incorrectly hold that (1) absence epilepsy and juvenile myoclonic epilepsies are not associated with higher rates of cognitive and behavioral changes, (2) behavioral changes are largely restricted to patients with temporal lobe epilepsy (TLE), (3) recurrent complex partial and tonic-clonic seizures cannot injure neuronal and cognitive function, and (4) frequent interictal epileptiform discharges cannot adversely affect behavior.

Epileptic seizures are paroxysmal electrical events in which excessive neuronal synchrony changes behavior. Behavior can also change during preictal (premonitory), interictal, and postictal periods (Table 10–3). Transitions between these periods are fluid, with overlapping neurophysiological and mental states. No specific cog-

Table 10–3. Periods of Behavioral Changes in Epilepsy

Premonitory°
  Affective: depression, irritability, aggression
  Cognitive: confusion, impaired memory
  Behavioral: withdrawal
  Headache
Ictal
  Sensory: illusions, hallucinations
  Autonomic
  Affective: depression, fear, anxiety, elation, laughing, crying, religiosity, altered familiarity (déjà vu, jamais vu)
  Cognitive: confusion, dreamy state, derealization, depersonalization, forced thoughts, distortion of time or body image
  Sexual: stereotypic ideation, genital sensations, pelvic thrusting
Postictal
  Headache
  Affective: depression, mania, aggression†
  Cognitive: confusion, amnesia, anomia, aphasia
  Psychosis
Interictal
  Affective: depression, anxiety, irritability, hypomania, increased or decreased emotionality, aggression
  Cognitive: amnesia, anomia, psychomotor slowing, impaired executive and social functions
  Sexual: reduced libido, impotence, anorgasmia
  Personality: circumstantiality, hypergraphia, hypermoralism, obsessionalism, paranoia, religiosity, viscosity
  Psychosis

°Hours or days before a seizure.
†Especially if the patient is restrained.

nitive or behavioral syndrome is associated with epilepsy. Patients with epilepsy manifest a wide diversity of behaviors, with the behavioral spectrum skewed toward cognitive impairment and psychopathology. Cognitive and behavioral changes are more frequent in children and adults with either partial or generalized epilepsies than in healthy subjects[207–209] and patients with medical or neurological disorders.[202,210,211] Psychiatric disorders such as depression, anxiety, psychosis, somatization, and dissociation occur more frequently in patients with epilepsy than in the general population.[200,202,212–214] Although some psychiatric disorders are expressed differently in patients with epilepsy than in those with primary psychiatric disorders (e.g., greater preservation of affect in interictal psychosis than in schizophrenia),[200,213] overlap is considerable.[215]

Recognizing specific epilepsy syndromes and disorders helps to define the clinical features of and biology underlying the behavioral changes. For example, TLE is often caused by mesial temporal sclerosis (Fig. 10–9), a hippocampal "scar" associated with cell loss, gliosis, and aberrant neural connections. Mesial temporal sclerosis is associated with increased risk of medical intractability, interictal amnesia, and postictal psychosis.[216,217] In patients with TLE, an abnormal T_2 signal on the MRI of the amygdala correlates with an increase in simple partial seizure symptoms and more frequent *déjà vu* and fear.[218] Ictal fear is associated with higher rates of interictal psychopathology, as discussed below. Further, animal models and human studies demonstrate selective vulnerability in certain temporolimbic areas to apoptosis and epileptogenesis in hypoxic, neurotoxic, viral, and traumatic injuries. This predilection for epileptogenic foci to develop in certain areas influences the behavioral patterns observed during, after, and between seizures.

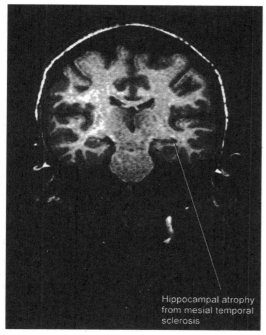

Hippocampal atrophy from mesial temporal sclerosis

Figure 10–9. Magnetic resonance image showing mesial temporal sclerosis in a patient with medically refractory partial epilepsy.

ICTAL BEHAVIOR

Among the different types of seizure, simple partial seizures (auras) provide the most information about cortical involvement in sensorimotor as well as cognitive and behavioral functions (Table 10–4). In many cases, however, the initial clinical features result from ictal spread rather than activation or inhibition of the normal functions supported by the seizure focus. This accounts for the persistence of typical auras after the primary focus is successfully removed, but residual epileptogenic cortex remains. Partial seizures can cause motor, sensory (illusions and hallucinations), autonomic, affective, and cognitive symptoms. The evoked subjective mental states are often complex and indescribable. Unusual experiential phenomena often go unreported and are identified only with questions combining open-ended and directed elements, for example, "Have you had bizarre experiences, such as feeling unreal or feeling the world is unreal?" These feelings represent, respectively, depersonalization and derealization. Other unusual phenomena are autoscopy, the experience of seeing one's double or having an out-of-body experience,[219] embarrassment,[220] religious experiences,[221] racing or involuntary thoughts,[20] paranoia, and multiple personalities.[20,222]

Ictal emotions mimic normal experiences or psychiatric symptoms. These paroxysmal feelings almost always occur spontaneously but rarely are triggered by environmental stimuli (e.g., jazz music, smell of jasmine). The sudden onset and typically brief (10–180 seconds) duration of partial seizures helps to distinguish them from psychiatric disorders such as panic attacks, which usually last more than 10 minutes. Negative affect is more common than positive emotions, paralleling the typically unpleasant ictal olfactory and gustatory hallucinations. Ictal emotion may occur in isolation or color an ongoing experience or other ictal symptoms. Ictal emotions result from altered activity in frontotemporal limbic areas. Fear and anxiety occur with activation of the amygdala, ACC, or insula. Seizure foci in the right hemisphere are more likely to evoke ictal emotions, especially negative ones (e.g., fear), and experiential phenomena (e.g., *déjà vu*, seeing a series of film clips of one's life, or religious experience)[223,224] (Table 10–4).

Table 10–4. **Localization and Lateralization of Ictal Cognitive and Behavioral Phenomena**

Psychic Phenomenon	Lateralization	Localization
Cognitive	—	—
Attention	L, R	F, T, P
Unilateral neglect	R>L	F, T, P
Memory lapse	L>R	T>F
Cognitive–language	L	—
Anomia	L>>R	T, P, F
Dysfluency	L	F
Impaired articulation	L, R	F
Impaired prosody	L, R	F, T
Receptive deficits	L	T, P
Apraxia	L	P, F
Visuospatial	R	T, P
Geographic orientation	R	T, P
Altered sense of time	L, R	F, T
Experiential–emotional	R>L	T>F
Altered sense of familiarity (*déjà vu, jamais vu*)	R>L	T
Viewing scenes from one's life	R>L	T
Dissociative phenomena	—	—
Derealization	?R>L	T>P, F
Depersonalization	?R>L	T>P, F
Autoscopy	?R>L	T>P, F
Negative emotions	—	—
Anxiety, fear	R>L	T>F
Sadness, depression, guilt	R>L	T
Embarrassment	?R>L	?F>T
Positive emotions	?	T
Joy	?R>L	T>F
Religious ecstasy	R>L	T

F, frontal lobe; L, left; P, parietal lobe; R, right; T, temporal lobe; ?, possible lateralized or localized predominance; >, higher frequency of this phenomenon with seizures arising from specific hemisphere or area.

Alterations of Familiarity

Déjà vu is a feeling of familiarity, which commonly occurs in the general population, but the feeling can occur as an aura (e.g., preceding the onset of a seizure). Ictal *déjà vu* may be accompanied by clairvoyance, "knowing" exactly what will occur next. *Jamais vu* is the feeling that familiar things appear strange, foreign, or remote. *Déjà entendu* and *jamais entendu* are familiar or unfamiliar auditory experiences, respectively.

Fear

Fear is the most frequent ictal emotion, occurring in approximately 15% of TLE patients. The intensity of fear varies from mild uneasiness to intense panic. Ictal fear must be differentiated from the reactive fear of a patient recognizing an impending seizure. Patients with ictal fear are more likely than other partial seizure patients to undergo psychiatric hospitalization, develop interictal anxiety, and score higher on psychopathology rating scales.[225,226] Disease or recurrent activation of the amygdala may contribute to increased psychopathology.

Depression

Pure ictal depression is rare. More often, depression occurs during the prodromal or postictal period.[20] Guilt, embarrassment, and loneliness rarely occur as auras. When depression accompanies a seizure, it can merge into the postictal state, persisting for hours or days.

Anger, Aggression, and Pleasure

Anger, irritability, and aggression are rare during seizures, more frequently complicating the postictal confusional state. Ictal aggression usually consists of spontaneous, nondirected, stereotypic aggressive behavior involving objects or individuals, such as throwing a glass against a wall. The low frequency of ictal aggression in studies at epilepsy centers may reflect bias against admitting violent patients and the hospital setting itself. Serious ictal violence does occur[227] and has been documented with depth electrode recording.[228] Ictal hatred or a compulsion to attack others is extremely rare. Pleasure, an uncommon ictal emotion, involves feelings such as tranquility, joy, sexual fulfillment, and ecstastic religious illumination, as discussed below.

Laughter and Crying

Ictal laughter (gelastic seizures) and crying (dacrystic seizures) are motor seizures occurring with or without preserved consciousness or concomitant mood state, despite the apparent emotional expression. The dissociation of emotional feeling (mood) and expression (affect) reflects their distinct anatomical circuits, similar to pseudobulbar palsy. The stereotypical attacks of laughter are brief and usually occur without environmental or mental provocation. Gelastic seizures occur with anterior cingulate, basal temporal, and hypothalamic seizure foci. Ictal crying may include tearing and most often occurs in patients with right-sided TLE.[229]

POSTICTAL BEHAVIOR

Postictal symptoms cause disabling deficits but offer clues about the seizure focus. Postictal symptoms can last from minutes to days, but prolonged postictal symptoms (>12 hours) often occur in patients with (a) status epilepticus or a cluster of seizures, or (b) structural lesions such as tumors or old stroke. A new postictal symptom suggests a different pattern of ictal spread, a more intense seizure, or a recent structural change. The mechanisms underlying postictal dysfunction include neuronal exhaustion or depletion of neurotransmitters (Todd–Jackson theory) and active inhibition (Gower's theory).[230]

Todd's Paralysis

Postictal (Todd's) paralysis, originally named "reversible hemiplegia after seizures,"[231] can affect sensory, language, or mental functions such as memory, verbal or visual learning, emotion, judgment, and geographic orientation.[232,233]

Postictal Psychosis

John Hughlings Jackson[234] described postictal psychosis as "epileptic mania." Psychosis can follow a series of tonic-clonic or complex partial seizures, after a lucid or delirious interval of 6–48 hours.[235–237] Mood alterations, delusional ideas, religious ideation, prolonged *déjà vu*, hallucinations, and aggressive behavior are frequent symptoms. Spontaneous recovery occurs, but the psychosis can be prolonged unless treated, usually with an antipsychotic drug and a benzodiazepine. Risk factors include bilateral seizure foci, bilateral limbic lesions, mesial temporal sclerosis, and temporal neocortical lesions.[238] Prophylaxis of recurrent postictal psychosis with psychotropic medications before or during the seizure cluster can be effective. In some patients, recurrent postictal psychosis may evolve into a chronic interictal psychosis.[237] This model of recurrent postictal symptoms evolving into interictal symptoms may extend to cognitive (e.g., memory) and behavioral (e.g., loss of social judgment) disorders.

Aggression and Other Symptoms

Postictal aggression is often provoked by restraint but also occurs during postictal psychoses.[239] Other postictal symptoms include headache, lethargy, anxiety, panic, and impaired attention.

INTERICTAL BEHAVIOR

The interictal period comprises more than 99% of most patients' lives. Interictal cognitive and behavioral disorders profoundly impair the quality of life. These disorders encompass a wide spectrum, often fitting awkwardly into neuropsychiatric categories. Interictal changes range from subtle alterations in personality, motivation, and mood to life-threatening psychiatric illness. Therapeutic opportunities are often lost when clinicians fail to diagnose or treat interictal behavioral disorders. In many cases, fears of the seizure-provoking effects of psychotropic medications are overestimated,[240] and disabling mental disease goes undertreated or untreated (see Chapter 11).[241] Finally, in some patients, epilepsy is associated with positive behavioral changes, such as deepening of emotions, hypergraphia, religious experience, intense philosophical interest, and artistic creativity.[201,202,242.243]

Memory and Other Cognitive Deficits

Romberg,[244] in 1853, recognized memory impairment as a common interictal disorder. Patients often complain of difficulty recalling recently learned information, especially names and details. A left-sided temporal lobe seizure focus impairs mainly verbal memory, and a right-sided focus impairs recently acquired visual, spatial, and geographic information. In patients with TLE, standard tests with 30–minute delays reveal significant memory impairment and longer delays reveal even greater impairment.[245] Like other cognitive disorders, several factors contribute to interictal amnesia, including structural lesions,[246] neuronal dysfunction or loss, interictal epileptiform discharges,[247] recurrent seizures, and antiepileptic drugs.[246,248,249]

Interictal hypometabolism around a seizure focus in the hippocampus, a critical site for memory, is a correlate of neuronal hypofunction.[250] Seizure control may or may not reverse interictal hypometabolism, but better seizure control improves memory in some patients. Prolonged and possibly recurrent tonic-clonic or complex partial seizures can destroy hippocampal neurons.[249,251] Neurologists often assure patients that intermittent, brief, complex partial or tonic-clonic seizures are "benign" and "do not damage the brain;" but these seizures may permanently alter cognition, especially memory.[252] Further, in susceptible individuals, kindling with strengthening of synaptic connections, as well as selective vulnerability of inhibitory interneurons to neurotoxic injury from prolonged seizures, may contribute to refractory epilepsy. Other interictal impairments affect mental processing speed, attention, language, visuospatial, executive (e.g., planning, changing mental set, abstraction), and praxis functions.

Psychosis

Interictal psychosis occurs in approximately 7% of all epilepsy patients. Rarely, a partial seizure may cause psychosis. The interictal psychoses are clinically pleomorphic.[200,215,216,253,254] Among patients with TLE, psychoses are closer to nuclear schizophrenia than in those with generalized epilepsy, whose disorders are more variable, with fewer first-rank symptoms but more manic and depressive features.[255] In contrast to schizophrenia, interictal psychosis is associated with more preserved affect and personality; a predominance of visual, rather than auditory, hallucinations; as well as less formal thought disorder, incoherent thought, emotional withdrawal, catatonia, and negative symptoms.[200,215] The outcome is more favorable in epileptic than in schizophrenic psychosis.

Chronic epilepsy probably contributes to the development of psychosis in some patients. When psychosis develops, it typically presents more than a decade after the onset of epilepsy. Risk factors for interictal psychosis include early age at onset of epilepsy, female sex, severe epilepsy, left-sided temporal lobe focus, and a structural lesion (Table 10–5).[256]

Forced normalization refers to the uncommon association between improved control of seizures or epileptiform activity and the onset or exacerbation of psychosis.[257] Forced normalization occurs with partial and generalized epilepsies, usually when seizures are controlled with antiepileptic drugs[258] or surgery.[259] When

Table 10–5. **Risk Factors for Interictal Psychosis**

Clinical and epilepsy-related
  Sex: female
  Left handedness
  Borderline intellectual function
  Onset of epilepsy before 20 years of age
  Epilepsy duration of more than a decade
  Left temporal lobe or bilateral seizure foci
  Complex partial or tonic-clonic seizures
  Postictal psychosis
Pathological and radiological
  Bilateral temporal lesions
  Large cerebral ventricles
  Periventricular gliosis
  More focal cerebral damage (greater extent of
    multifocal lesions)

psychosis develops de novo after temporal lobectomy, it is more often after a right-sided resection.[86,260] Forced normalization remains controversial and is most often reported in Europe. Of historical interest, poor epidemiological data and anecdotal observations that epilepsy and psychosis were inversely related provided the theoretical basis of convulsive therapy for schizophrenia.[261]

Depression

Interictal depression is common, with dysphoria observed in nearly half of adult patients,[262] depression in 25%–55%,[262,263] and a suicide rate 2–5 times as high as that of control groups.[262,264,265] Most depressed epilepsy patients can be successfully treated with antidepressants without increasing the seizure frequency or severity.[241] Interictal depression has biological and psychosocially reactive mechanisms.[243,256,262,263,266] Biological factors include a family history of depression;[267] a left-sided seizure focus;[268,269] mesial temporal sclerosis;[269] barbiturate, phenytoin, vigabatrin, levetiracetam, topiramate, or zonisamide therapy (see Chapter 11); and bifrontal[270] or left temporal[271] hypometabolism.

Anxiety Disorders

Anxiety, panic, and phobic symptoms can complicate interictal states in both limbic and idiopathic generalized epilepsies.[272,273] Anxiety disorders may be more frequent in patients with left than right temporal lobe epilepsy.[268] Antianxiety agents that enhance serotonin activity are usually effective and well tolerated. Benzodiazepines must be used cautiously since they are habit-forming and lead to tolerance and variations in dosage or dose reductions can provoke seizures.

Aggression

Interictal irritability and aggression are more frequent in children and adults with epilepsy than in the general population.[243,256,274,275] Several lines of evidence link TLE and aggressive behavior, although most clinical studies deny the relationship.[212] However, most of these studies found that the incidence of aggression among all patient groups was higher

than the expected rate in the general population. Experimental temporal lobe seizure foci increase aggressive behavior in animal models.[276]

Clinical and postsurgical studies support an association between interictal aggression and TLE, although data from epidemiological or controlled studies are lacking. The large majority of patients with epilepsy are not aggressive. Aggression is most often found in younger patients with epilepsy.[277,278] Rage episodes occurred in 36% of children with TLE studied prospectively.[275] Risk factors included male sex, hyperactivity, disordered homes, low intelligence quotient (IQ), and first seizure before 1 year of age.[212,256,275] Consecutive but highly selected neurosurgical and residential series, including referrals from psychiatric facilities, showed aggression in 27%–36% of patients with TLE.[278–280] Aggression may first occur after the development of limbic seizures in adults without risk factors for aggression.[281] Amygdalotomy in humans and animals reduces aggressive behavior.[6,64] Aggression improved in more than 35% of violent patients after temporal lobectomy, supporting the notion that amygdalar dysfunction contributes to aggressive behavior.[279] Almost 30% of epilepsy patients report intense, paroxysmal irritability or moodiness during the interictal period compared with 2% of normal subjects or subjects with other neurological disorders.[282]

Dissociative Disorders

Interictal dissociative disorders include conversion symptoms, especially nonepileptic seizures; multiple personality; and Ganser syndrome, in which patients make only approximate answers to questions. [Conversion symptoms were considered a dissociative disorder in the *Diagnostic and Statistical Manual of Mental Disorders* (DSM-III-R) but a somatoform disorder in the DSM-IV.] Rarely, conversion symptoms emerge during or immediately after a seizure, usually from right frontotemporal limbic foci,[283] or when seizures and interictal epileptiform activity are controlled, as a possible variant of forced normalization.[284] Patients with epilepsy who exhibit conversion (nonepileptic) seizures often have a history of physical or sexual abuse[285] or minor traumatic brain injury.[286] However, when patients with epilepsy or structural brain lesions have nonepileptic seizures, cerebral dysfunction usually involves the right frontotemporal areas.[287]

PSYCHOPATHOLOGICAL CHANGES IN DIFFERENT EPILEPSIES

Gastaut et al.[288] reported that most patients with psychomotor (complex partial) seizures had a global reduction in motor, intellectual, affective, and sexual functions, although many of them would suddenly shift into irritability without serious provocation. These behaviors were the opposite of those produced by bilateral temporolimbic lesions in the Klüver-Bucy syndrome (Table 10–6).

Temporal Lobe Epilepsy

The various positive and negative interictal personality changes often observed in patients with TLE led Waxman and Geschwind[242] to define

a syndrome of deepened emotions, circumstantiality, altered religious and sexual concerns, and hypergraphia. Deepening of emotions, characterized by intense interpersonal contact and sustained intense affect, was central. Since the features were not necessarily maladaptive or negative, they emphasized a behavioral change rather than a behavioral disorder.[242] Bear and Fedio[201] studied 18 behavioral traits and had them rated by TLE patients and observers. All 18 self-rated traits and 14 of the18 proxy-rated traits were increased in the TLE patients compared with the neuromuscular disorder patients and normal subjects. In subsequent studies, scores were increased in epilepsy patients compared with normal subjects or patients without behavioral problems, but there were no consistent differences between epilepsy patients and psychiatric patients or between patients with TLE and patients with frontal lobe or generalized epilepsies.[202,289,290]

Bear and Fedio[201] also found that TLE patients with right-sided foci displayed more

Table 10–6. **Interictal Behavior in Selected Partial Epilepsies and Related Neurological Disorders**

Anatomical Area	Interictal Human Behavior*	Interictal Animal Behavior	Behavioral Effects of Lesions
Mesial temporal	—	—	Klüver-Bucy syndrome[†]
	Increased and labile emotions, anxiety, irritability, aggressiveness, paranoia, guilt, viscosity (stickiness, tendency for prolonged interpersonal contact), obsessiveness, hypergraphia, religiosity	Lower threshold to hypothalamic stimulation-induced aggression —	Diminished fear, anxiety, aggression Hypermetamorphosis (increased distractibility), changes in social cohesion
	Hyposexuality	Hyposexuality	Hypersexuality
	No hyperorality	—	Hyperorality, weight gain
	Increased emotional response to sensory stimuli	—	Visual agnosia
Dorsolateral prefrontal	Poorly defined: impaired executive functions	Unknown	Impaired executive functions
Anterior cingulate	Sociopathic behavior, psychosis, aggression, obsessiveness	Unknown	Reduced motivation
Orbitofrontal	Sociopathic behavior, aggression	Unknown	Sociopathic behavior, aggression, disinhibition

*Observed in only a minority of individuals.
[†]Behavior observed in both humans and other species.

emotional traits and tended to deny their abnormal behavior, that is, polished their image. Patients with left-sided foci displayed more ideational traits and tended to overemphasize their behavioral problems, that is, tarnished their image. Right hemisphere lesions cause denial and neglect syndromes, and left hemisphere lesions more often cause depression.[189,192] Studies do not support consistent lateralized personality changes in TLE patients.[202,291] The interictal behavioral traits associated with TLE and other epilepsy syndromes are summarized in Tables 10–3 and 10–6.

Frontal Lobe Epilepsy

The behavioral consequences of lesions and seizure foci in the frontal lobe limbic areas are described earlier and in Chapter 9. Wieser[291] found a greater, but nonsignificant, increase in all Bear-Fedio Inventory behavioral traits in patients with frontal lobe epilepsy than in patients with TLE. In the Vietnam Head Injury Study, the frequency of psychiatric treatment was higher in patients with tonic-clonic seizures than in those with complex partial seizures,[210] possibly reflecting greater frontal lobe involvement in the former group. Even among patients with TLE, frontal dysfunction appears to contribute to affective, personality, and cognitive disorders.[270,292,293] The cognitive and behavioral changes associated with idiopathic generalized epilepsies may largely result from frontal lobe involvement.[294,295] The social disorders, such as failure to monitor ongoing behavior and comprehend other people's reactions to one's own actions, cause tremendous behavioral disability for patients with epilepsy. Frontal lobe dysfunction likely contributes to these disorders.

Idiopathic Generalized Epilepsy

Behavioral changes may occur in patients with idiopathic generalized epilepsy syndromes, such as juvenile myoclonic epilepsy (JME) and absence epilepsy. In patients with JME, Janz[296] reported irresponsibility and impaired impulse control, neglect of duties, self-interest, emotional instability, exaggeration, inconsiderateness, quick temper, and distractibility. Many of these behaviors, as well as recurrent sleep deprivation and noncompliance leading to break-through seizures, may partly reflect adolescence, not JME. Other studies found a high incidence of psychiatric disorders among patients with JME[297,298] or other idiopathic generalized epilepsies.[273]

Absence epilepsy, long considered benign, is associated with increases in behavioral problems. Wirrell et al.[211] compared patients with typical absence epilepsy and patients with juvenile rheumatoid arthritis (JRA), diagnosed over an 11–year period, who were aged 18 years or older at follow-up (mean age 23 years). Remission occurred in 57% of absence epilepsy patients and 28% of JRA patients. Patients with absence epilepsy had greater difficulties in the academic, personal, and behavioral categories ($P < 0.001$) than those with JRA. Those with ongoing seizures had the least favorable outcome. Even patients whose epilepsy had remitted had a significantly poorer outcome than the JRA patients in the academic, personal, and behavioral domains. Caplan et al.[299] found that 54% of children with idiopathic generalized epilepsy had psychiatric disorders and that early age at onset and poor seizure control were associated with the severity of illogical thinking.

SELECTED PERSONALITY TRAITS IN EPILEPSY

Although certain behavioral traits are more common in epilepsy than in comparison populations, none is specific for epilepsy, epilepsy syndromes, or localized seizure foci. Nevertheless, certain traits are related to neurological as well as other variables.

VISCOSITY

Viscosity is a tendency for prolonged interpersonal contact, such as talking repetitively, circumstantially, and pedantically and failing to end conversations or visits after a socially appropriate interval. Such individuals are socially "sticky" or "adhesive." On rating scales, viscosity scores are elevated in TLE patients with left-sided foci[201,300,301] or with left- or right-sided foci,[201] as well as in patients with generalized epilepsy.[302] A longer duration of epilepsy correlates with increased viscosity in patients with left-sided TLE.[301]

Viscosity as a personality trait may reflect a desire for interpersonal closeness, a need for affiliation with another being, although linguistic impairment causing circumstantiality and psychological dependence may also contribute. Limbic lesions profoundly alter how animals seek contact with others.[35] For example, rats with septal lesions show a dramatic increase in social cohesion with other rats, as well as predatory cats.[35]

Alterations in Sexual Function

Patients with epilepsy may experience changes in sexual behavior. Hyposexuality, including reduced libido and impotence, is common.[202,300,303] Anecdotal reports describe hyper-sexuality[304] and deviant sexual behavior, including exhibitionism, transvestism, transsexualism, and fetishism.[305] In many cases, especially when seizures begin before puberty, the patients do not marry or regard their sexuality as a problem.

Higher rates of hyposexuality and sexual dysfunction are usually found in patients with TLE than in those with other types of epilepsy. Five of six men with epilepsy and erectile dysfunction had evidence of neurogenic, not vasogenic, dysfunction.[306] Women with partial epilepsy report more dyspareunia, vaginismus, arousal insufficiency, and sexual dissatisfaction. Women with idiopathic generalized epilepsy experience more anorgasmia and sexual dissatisfaction.[307]

The pathogenetic role of temporal lobe seizures in hyposexuality is supported by animal studies[308] and reports of increased sexual activity with medical and surgical[309] control of seizures. Rarely, marked hypersexuality, similar to that in the Klüver-Bucy syndrome, develops after temporal lobectomy.[36,309] Among the antiepileptic drugs, barbiturates most often impair libido and sexual function.[310]

Religiosity

The historic association between epilepsy and mystical or religious phenomena highlights the discord between dramatic anecdotes and clinical studies. Hippocrates refuted the relation between epilepsy and the divine: patients with epilepsy do not have mystical powers; epilepsy is not a curse of the gods. Despite his wisdom and influence, religious and magical treatments of epilepsy predominated for several millenia. Moreover, observations linking epilepsy and religious experience persist into the modern

era. A classic monograph on religious mysticism[311] stated that "among the dread diseases . . . there is only one that interests us quite particularly; that disease is epilepsy."

William James[312] contrasted religious feelings of the common person with rare ecstatic experiences. Many prominent religious figures, including prophets and founders of many religions, allegedly had epilepsy.[243] Intense religious experiences may occur during or after seizures and appear more often in patients with right-sided TLE. Dostoyevsky documented eloquently his own ictal religious experience:

> The air was filled with a big noise, and I thought that it had engulfed me. I have really touched God. He came into me myself, yes, God exists, I cried, and I don't remember anything else. You all, healthy people, he said, can't imagine the happiness which we epileptics feel during the second before our attack. I don't know if this felicity lasts for seconds, hours, or months, but believe me, for all the joys that life may bring, I would not exchange this one. . . . Such instants were characterized by a fulguration of the consciousness and by a supreme exaltation of emotional subjectivity.
>
> Alajouanine (1963)[313]

Dewhurst and Beard,[314] reporting on six patients with TLE who underwent sudden religious conversions, found increased seizure activity in five patients and decreased seizure activity prior to conversion in one patient (she attributed her improved seizure disorder to the "Almighty"). One woman we care for converted to a different religion after a peri-ictal religious experience (Fig. 10–10). Notably, some,[243,315] but not all,[201,316] questionnaire surveys on religion failed to differentiate patients with epilepsy or different epilepsy syndromes from control subjects.

Hypergraphia

Hypergraphia, a tendency toward extensive and sometimes compulsive writing, occurs in a minority of TLE patients. Such patients often have a striking preoccupation with detail (words are defined and redefined and underlined) and the importance of their material, which is often focused on moral and religious concerns.[317] Patients with TLE respond more frequently and extensively to mailed questionnaires than patients in other groups.[243,318] The duration of epilepsy, hypomania, and number of recent significant life events correlate with

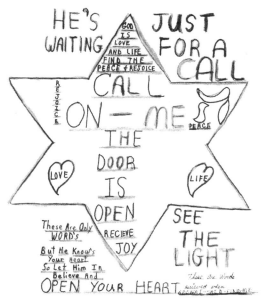

Figure 10–10. This drawing, originally done in many different colors, was created by a patient with epilepsy. Originally Jewish, she converted to Catholicism after a peri-ictal religious experience.

hypergraphia, which occurs in 7%–10% of TLE patients.[318,319] Dostoevsky,[320] in a letter dated August 27, 1849, related his writing and epilepsy in this way: ". . . whenever formerly I had such nervous disturbances, I made use of them for writing; in such a state I could write much more and much better than usual."

CAVEATS ON NEUROBEHAVIOR IN EPILEPSY

As with many neurobehavioral areas, unless they are sought, many interictal behavioral changes are overlooked. Without specific inquiry, behaviors such as hypergraphia or increased religious interests often go undetected. On rounds, a resident informed the neurologist Norman Geschwind that a young man with TLE "was not particularly religious." Geschwind asked the patient if he was religious, to which the patient responded "Nope." Geschwind asked "Why not?" The patient said "Because the rabbi in my congregation is not theological." He refused to go to temple because the rabbi did not share his profound interest in religion! Traditional neuropsychiatric categories do not encompass the diverse range of behavioral changes in epilepsy.

No personality trait or psychopathological disorder is pathognomonic of epilepsy. Although specific constellations of behavioral features may suggest epilepsy, interictal behavioral traits cannot establish the diagnosis of epilepsy. Further, paroxysmal psychosensory symptoms are common among patients with such psychiatric illnessess as major depression, bipolar disorder, schizophrenia, panic, and somatization disorders.[321] Thus, paroxysmal symptoms suggesting partial seizures frequently occur in patients with nonepileptic behavioral disorders.

FACTORS INFLUENCING BEHAVIOR IN LIMBIC EPILEPSY

Many biological, therapeutic, and psychosocial factors influence behavior in epilepsy. The causes of aberrant interictal behavior overlap with the causes of epilepsy and epileptic seizures: abnormalities in ion channel and receptor function, synaptic connectivity, neural networks, thalamocortical synchronicity, neurotransmitter activity, neuroendocrine function, cerebral metabolism, and cortical structure (e.g., neuronal loss, dysplasia). Medical and surgical therapies and the response to a psychologically life-altering single seizure or a chronic stigmatizing disorder profoundly impact patients with epilepsy. The diversity of mechanisms underlying interictal behavioral changes partly explains our failure to delineate well-defined syndromes. Indeed, in a patient with epilepsy, the contrasting effects of hypofunction and hyperfunction may produce simultaneous behavioral changes. Interictal hypometabolism and neuronal loss in patients with epilepsy correlate with cognitive deficits such as amnesia[250,293] and behavioral disorders such as depression,[270] supporting hypofunction as the mechanism. In contrast, Gastaut et al.[288] observed that certain behaviors in TLE patients were the opposite of those in patients with temporal lobe lesions, as in the Klüver-Bucy syndrome, supporting hyperfunction (e.g., sensory–limbic hyperconnection) as the mechanism.[143] In support of this mechanism is the observation that specific sensory stimuli are rarely linked with powerful and persistent affective valence, as exemplified by a patient who experienced sexual auras when he viewed a safety pin but was not aroused by his wife.[305] Further, in a model of TLE in the cat, abnormal, high-frequency neuronal activity in the temporal lobe suppressed sexual behavior.[308]

The association of certain behavioral constellations with specific epilepsy syndromes remains unproven. Alterations in cognitive and social functions, personality, affect, and drive-related behaviors like libido or aggression develop in some patients with partial and generalized epilepsies. The pathogenetic roles of biological and psychological factors interact and vary among patients and for different disorders. For example, antiepileptic drugs can cause both positive and negative behavior in patients with epilepsy (see Chapter 11). Further, irritability and aggression are associated with multiple factors, including sociodevelopmental issues; adverse medication effects, as with barbiturates; limbic seizure foci, as in the amygdala or anterior cingulate cortex; or impaired inhibitory functions, as from an orbitofrontal lesion.

An insightful hypothesis, "the epileptogenic disorder of function," was offered by Sir Charles Symonds.[322] Pondering the pathophysiological origin of interictal psychosis in patients with TLE, he stated:

> If then neither the fits nor the temporal lobe damage can be held directly responsible for the psychosis, what is the link? . . . Epileptic seizures and epileptiform discharge in the EEG are epiphenomena. They may be regarded as occasional expressions of a fundamental and continuous disorder of neuronal function. The essence of this disorder is loss of the normal balance between excitation and inhibition at the synaptic junctions. From moment to moment there may be excess either of excitation or inhibition—or even both at the same time in different parts of the same neuronal system. The epileptogenic disorder of function may be assumed to be present continuously but with peaks at which seizures are likely to occur.
>
> Symonds (1962)[322]

The role of seizures in the progressive structural, cognitive, and behavioral changes in patients with epilepsy remains controversial. The nineteenth century view that recurrent seizures may cause cell loss and progressive mental changes is supported by modern clinical and neuroimaging studies.[249,251,252,323,324] Nevertheless, in balancing seizure control with the adverse effects of medication, Lennox's admonishment, "Many physicians in attempting to extinguish seizures only succeed in drowning the finer intellectual processes of their patients," is as relevant now as it was in 1942.[325]

SUMMARY

The limbic system's core functions are to govern emotion and memory, but it also helps to regulate instinct, motivation, and social function. The limbic system includes diverse subcortical and cortical areas, which interface between phylogenetically older systems that regulate autonomic, endocrine, and drive-related behaviors and newer systems that mediate cognition. Limbic areas are richly connected with each other, as well as with diencephalic, brain stem, and neocortical areas.

The hippocampus and parahippocampal gyrus are critical nodes in the memory network; they are not a memory bank but enable consolidation of new information into memory and revive these patterns during retrieval. The amygdala regulates emotional expression and experience and endows sensory information with emotional significance. Bilateral amydagla lesions contribute to many symptoms of the Klüver-Bucy syndrome: hyperorality, loss of aggressive and fearful responses, hypersexuality, visual distractibility, and visual agnosia. The ACC provides motivational context to behavior, evaluating and reacting to novel and complex behavioral stimuli. The posterior orbitofrontal cortex is involved with olfaction, autonomic activity, emotional and drive responsiveness, social behavior, and inhibition of behavior. Lesions in this area predominantly affect personality and social interactions.

Limbic dysfunction underlies many primary psychiatric and neurobehavioral syndromes. Many diseases and disorders (e.g., inflammatory autoimmune diseases, vascular disease, tumors, and trauma) affect limbic structures. Selective limbic involvement is uncommon and represented by paraneoplastic limbic encephalitis and partial epilepsy of temporal lobe origin. Both disorders cause memory, emotional, and other behavioral problems. Neuronal dysfunction causing the diverse interictal cognitive and behavioral changes results from structural lesions, interictal epileptiform discharges, recurrent seizures, medications, and other factors. Behavioral changes are not restricted to patients with TLE, but also occur in patients with frontal lobe and generalized seizure foci.

REFERENCES

1. Kaada BR: Stimulation and regional ablation of the amygdaloid complex with reference to functional representations. In Eleftherious BE (ed). The Neurobiology of the Amygdala. Plenum, New York, 1972, pp 205–281.
2. Fanselow MS: Neural organization of the defensive behavior system responsible for fear. Psychonom Bull Rev 1:429–438, 1994.
3. Cannon WB: The James-Lange theory of emotions: a critical examination and an alternative theory. Am J Psychol 39:106–124, 1927.
4. Panksepp J: Affective Neuroscience. Oxford University Press, New York, 1998, p 26.
5. Darwin C: The Expression of Emotions in Animals and Man. John Murray, London, 1872.
6. Klüver H and Bucy P: Preliminary analysis of functions of the temporal lobes in man. Arch Neurol Psychiatry 42:979–1000, 1939.
7. Ross ED, Homan RW, and Buck R: Differential hemispheric lateralization of primary and social emotions. Neuropsychiatry Neuropsychol Behav Neurol 7:1–19, 1994.
8. Buck R, Losow JI, Murphy MM, and Costanzo P: Social facilitation and inhibition of emotional expression and communication. J Personal Social Psychol 63:962–968, 1992.
9. Tucker DM, Luu P, and Pribram KH: Social and emotional self-regulation. Ann NY Acad Sci 769: 213–239, 1995.
10. Hariri AR, Bookheimer SY, and Mazziotta JC: Modulating emotional responses: effects of a neocortical network on the limbic system. Neuroreport 11:43–48, 2000.
11. James W: What is an emotion? Mind 9:188–205, 1884.
12. Lange CG and James W: The Emotions. Williams & Wilkins, Baltimore, 1922.
13. Bazett HC and Penfield WG: A study of the Sherrington decerebrate animal in the chronic as well as the acute condition. Brain 45:185–265, 1922.
14. Bard P: A diencephalic mechanism for the expression of rage with special reference to the sympathetic nervous system. Am J Physiol 84:490–515, 1928.
15. Di Giusto EL and King MG: Chemical sympathectomy and avoidance learning in the rat. J Comp Physiol Psychol 81:491–500, 1972.
16. Henry TR, Votaw JR, Pennell PB, et al.: Acute blood flow changes and efficacy of vagus nerve stimulation in partial epilepsy. Neurology 52:1166–1173, 1999.
17. Laird JD: Self-attribution of emotion: the effects of expressive behavior on the quality of emotional experience. J Pers Soc Psychol 29:475–486, 1974.
18. Hohmann G: Some effects of spinal cord lesions on experimental emotional feelings. Psychophysiology 3:143–156, 1966.
19. Schachter S and Singer JE: Cognitive, social, and physiological determinants of emotional state. Psychol Rev 69:379–399, 1962.
20. Devinsky O and Luciano D: Psychic phenomena in partial seizures. Semin Neurol 11:100–109, 1991.
21. Davidson RJ, Abercrombie H, Nitschke JB, and Putnam K: Regional brain function, emotion and disorders of emotion. Curr Opin Neurobiol 9:228–234, 1999.
22. Broca P: Anatomie comparee des circonvolutions cerebrales. Le grand lobe limbique et las scissure limbique dans la serie des mammiferes. Rev Anthropol 1:385–498, 1878.
23. Papez JW: A proposed mechanism of emotion. Arch Neurol Psychiatry 38:725–743, 1937.
24. Yakovlev PI: Motility, behavior and the brain: stereodynamic organization and neural coordinates in behavior. J Nerv Ment Dis 107:313–335, 1948.
25. MacLean PD: The Evolution of the the Triune Brain. Plenum, New York, 1990.
26. Zola-Morgan S, Squire LR, Alvarez-Royo P, and Clower RP: Independence of memory functions and emotional behavior: separate contributions of the hippocampal formation and the amygdala. Hippocampus 1:207–220, 1991.
27. Papanicolaou AC, Simos PG, Castillo EM, Breier JI, Katz JS, and Wright AA: The hippocampus and memory of verbal and pictorial material. Learn Mem 9:99–104, 2002.
28. LeDoux J: Fear and the brain: where have we been, and where are we going? Biol Psychiatry 44:1229–1238, 1998.
29. Haber SN, Kunishio K, Mizobuchi M, et al.: The orbital and medial prefrontal circuit through the primate basal ganglia. J Neurosci 15:4851–4867, 1995.
30. Wright CI and Groenewegen HJ: Patterns of convergence and segregation in the medial nucleus accumbens of the rat: relationships of prefrontal cortical, midline thalamic and basal amygdaloid afferents. J Comp Neurol 361:383–403, 1995.
31. Schultz W: Getting formal with dopamine and reward. Neuron 36:241, 2002.
32. Deutch AY: Prefrontal cortical dopamine systems and the elaboration of functional corticostriatal circuits: implications for schizophrenia and Parkinson's disease. J Neural Transm Gen 91:197–221, 1993.
33. Mesulam M-M, Mufson EJ, Levey AI, and Wainer BH: Cholinergic innervation of cortex by the basal forebrain: cytochemistry and cortical connections of the septal area, diagonal band nuclei, nucleus basalis (substantia innominata) and hypothalamus in the rhesus monkey. J Comp Neurol 214:170–197, 1983.
34. Rolls ET, Sanghera MK, and Roper-Hall A: The latency of activation of neurones in the lateral hypothalamus and substantia innominata during feeding in the monkey. Brain Res 164:121–135, 1979.
35. Meyer DR, Ruth RA, and Lavond DG: The septal social cohesiveness effect: its robustness and main determinants. Physiol Behav 21:1027–1029, 1978.
36. Devinsky O: Behavioral Neurology: 100 Maxims. Edward Arnold, London, 1992, pp. 226–228.
37. Heath RG, Monroe RR, and Mickle WA: Stimulation of the amygdaloid nucleus in a schizophrenic patient. Am J Psychiatry 111:862–863, 1955.
38. Gol A: Relief of pain by electrical stimulation of the septal area. J Neurol Sci 5:115–120, 1967.

39. Zaborszky L: The modular organization of brain systems. Basal forebrain: the last frontier. Prog Brain Res 136:359–372, 2002.

40. Amaral DG, Price JL, Pitkanen A, and Carmichael ST: Anatomical organization of the primate amygdaloid complex. In Aggleton JP (ed). The Amygdala: Neurobiological Aspects of Emotion, Memory, and Mental Dysfunction. Wiley-Liss, New York, 1992, pp 1–66.

41. Rolls ET and Stringer SM: A model of the interaction between mood and memory. Network 12:89–109, 2001.

42. Schaefer SM, Jackson DC, Davidson RJ, Aguirre GK, Kimberg DY, and Thompson-Schill SL: Modulation of amygdalar activity by the conscious regulation of negative emotion. J Cogn Neurosci 14:913–921, 2002.

43. Hamann S and Mao H: Positive and negative emotional verbal stimuli elicit activity in the left amygdala. Neuroreport 13:15–19, 2002.

44. Davis M and Whalen PJ: The amygdala: vigilance and emotion. Mol Psychiatry 6:13–34, 2001.

45. Kling A, Steklis HD, and Deutsch S: Radiotelemetered activity from the amygdala during social interactions in the monkey. Exp Neurol 66:88–96, 1979.

46. George MS, Ketter TA, Parekh PI, et al.: Regional brain activity when selecting a response despite interference: an $H_2^{15}O$ PET study of the Stroop and an emotional Stroop. Hum Brain Mapp 1:1–16, 1994.

47. Morris JS, Frith CD, Perrett DI, et al.: A differential neural response in the human amygdala to fearful and happy facial expressions. Nature 383:812–815, 1996.

48. Yang TT, Menon V, Eliez S, et al.: Amygdalar activation associated with positive and negative facial expressions. Neuroreport 13:1737–1741, 2002.

49. Rosen HJ, Perry RJ, Murphy J, et al.: Emotion comprehension in the temporal variant of frontotemporal dementia. Brain 125:2286–2295, 2002.

50. Stephan H, Frahm HD, and Baron G: Comparison of brain structure volume in insectivora and primates. III. Amygdaloid components. J Hirnforsch 28:571–584, 1984.

51. Kling A, Lancaster J, and Benitone J: Amygdalectomy in a free-ranging vervet. J Psychiatr Res 7:191–199, 1970.

52. Steklis HD and Kling A: Neurobiology of affiliative behavior in non-human primates. In Reite M and Field T (eds). The Psychobiology of Attachment and Separation. Academic Press, New York, 1985, pp 93–129.

53. Brown S and Schafer EA: An investigation into the functions of the occipital and temporal lobes of the monkey's brain. Philos Trans Soc Lond 179:303–327, 1888.

54. Bucy PC and Klüver H: An anatomic investigation of the temporal lobe in monkeys. J Comp Neurol 103:151–252, 1955.

55. Prather MD, Lavenex P, Mauldin-Jourdain ML, et al.: Increased social fear and decreased fear of objects in monkeys with neonatal amygdala lesions. Neuroscience 106:653–658, 2001.

56. Downer JDC: Changes in visual gnostic function and emotional behavior following unilateral temporal lobe damage in the "split-brain" monkey. Nature 191:50–51, 1961.

57. Ross ED: Sensory-specific and fractional disorders of recent memory in man. II. Unilateral loss of tactile recent memory. Arch Neurol 37:267–272, 1980.

58. Bauer RM: Visual hypoemotionality as a symptom of visual–limbic disconnection in man. Arch Neurol 39:702–708, 1982.

59. Horel JA and Misantone LJ: Visual discrimination impaired by cutting temporal lobe connections. Science 193:336–338, 1976.

60. Kling A and Dunne K: Social–environment factors affecting behavior and plasma testosterone in normal and amygdala lesioned *Macaca speciosa*. Primates 17:23–42, 1976.

61. Goscinski I, Kwiatkowski S, Polak J, Orlowiejska M, and Partyk A: The Kluver-Bucy syndrome. J Neurosurg Sci 41:269–272, 1997.

62. Lilly R, Cummings JL, Benson DF, and Frankel M: The human Kluver-Bucy syndrome. Neurology 33: 1141–1145, 1983.

63. Ghika-Schmid F, Assal G, De Tribolet N, and Regli F: Kluver-Bucy syndrome after left anterior temporal resection. Neuropsychologia 33:101–113, 1995.

64. Ramamurthi B: Stereotactic operation in behaviour disorders. Amygdalotomy and hypothalamotomy. Acta Neurochir Suppl (Wien) 44:152–157, 1988.

65. Devinsky O and Bear D: Kluver-Bucy syndrome in Pick's disease. Neurology 33: 956–957, 1983.

66. Corkin S: Lasting consequences of bilateral medial temporal lobectomy: clinical course and experimental findings in H.M. Semin Neurol 4:249–259, 1984.

67. Birbaumer N, Grodd W, Diedrich O, et al.: fMRI reveals amygdala activation to human faces in social phobics. Neuroreport 9:1223–1226, 1998.

68. LaBar KS, Gatenby JC, Gore JC, LeDoux JE, and Phelps EA: Human amygdala activation during conditioned fear acquisition and extinction: a mixed-trial fMRI study. Neuron 20:937–945, 1998.

69. Barros M and Tomaz C: Non-human primate models for investigating fear and anxiety. Neurosci Biobehav Rev 26:187–201, 2002.

70. LeDoux JE: Emotion and the amygdala. In Aggleton JP (ed). The Amygdala: Neurobiological Aspects of Emotion, Memory, and Mental Dysfunction. Wiley-Liss, New York, 1992, pp 339–351.

71. LaBar KS, LeDoux JE, Spencer DD, and Phelps EA: Impaired fear conditioning following unilateral temporal lobectomy in humans. J Neurosci 15: 6846–6855, 1995.

72. Bandler RJ: Induction of "rage" following microinjection of glutamate into midbrain but not hypothalamus of cats. Neurosci Lett 30:183–188, 1982.

73. Gloor P: Role of the amygdala in temporal lobe epilepsy. In Aggleton JP (ed). The Amygdala: Neurobiological Aspects of Emotion, Memory, and Mental Dysfunction. Wiley-Liss, New York, 1992, pp 505–538.

74. Packard MG and Cahill L: Affective modulation of multiple memory systems. Curr Opin Neurobiol 11: 752–756, 2001.

75. McGaugh JL, Cahill L, and Roozendaal B: Involvement of the amygdala in memory storage: interaction with other brain systems. Proc Natl Acad Sci USA 93:13508–13514, 1996.

76. Bechara A, Tranel D, Damasio H, Adolphs R, Rockland C, and Damasio AR: Double dissociation of conditioning and declarative knowledge relative to the amygdala and hippocampus in humans. Science 269:1115–1118, 1995.

77. Morris JS, Ohman A, and Dolan RJ: Conscious and unconscious emotional learning in the human amygdala. Nature 393:467–470, 1998.

78. Mesulam M-M: From sensation to cognition. Brain 121:1013–1052, 1998.

79. Moran MA, Mufson EJ, and Mesulam MM: Neural inputs into the temporopolar cortex of the rhesus monkey. J Comp Neurol 256:88–103, 1987.

80. Kaada BR, Pribram KH, and Epstein JA: Respiratory and vascular responses in monkeys from temporal pole, insula, orbital surface and cingulate gyrus. J Neurophysiol 12:347–356, 1949.

81. Schwartz TH, Devinsky O, Doyle W, and Perrine K: Preoperative predictors of anterior temporal language areas. J Neurosurg 89:962–970, 1998.

82. Kling A and Steklis HD: A neural substrate for affiliative behavior in nonhuman primates. Brain Behav Evol 13:216–238, 1976.

83. Bell BD, Davies KG, Hermann BP, and Walters G: Confrontation naming after anterior temporal lobectomy is related to age of acquisition of the object names. Neuropsychologia 38:83–92, 2000.

84. Strauss E, Semenza C, Hunter M, et al.: Left anterior lobectomy and category-specific naming. Brain Cogn 43:403–406, 2000.

85. Gauthier I, Anderson AW, Tarr MJ, Skudlarski P, and Gore JC: Levels of categorization in visual recognition studied using functional magnetic resonance imaging. Curr Biol 7:645–651, 1997.

86. Bromfield EB, Devinsky O, Fricchione GL, et al.: Psychosis after epilepsy surgery. Epilepsia 40(Suppl 7):242, 1999.

87. Vandenberghe R, Dupont P, Bormans G, et al.: Blood flow in human anterior temporal cortex decreases with stimulus familiarity. Neuroimage 2:306–313, 1995.

88. Noppeney U and Price CJ: Retrieval of visual, auditory, and abstract semantics. Neuroimage 15:917–926, 2002.

89. Grabowski TJ, Damasio H, Tranel D, Ponto LL, Hichwa RD, and Damasio AR: A role for left temporal pole in the retrieval of words for unique entities. Hum Brain Mapp 13:199–212, 2001.

90. Perani D, Cappa SF, Schnur T, et al.: The neural correlates of verb and noun processing: a PET study. Brain 122:2337–2444, 1999.

91. Blair RJ, Morris JS, Firth CD, et al.: Dissociable neural responses to facial expressions of sadness and anger. Brain 122:883–893, 1999.

92. Shin LM, McNally RJ, Kosslyn SM, et al.: Regional blood flow during script-driven imagery in childhood sexual abuse-related PTSD: a PET investigation. Am J Psychiatry 156:575–584, 1999.

93. Kimbrell TA, George MS, Parekh PI, et al.: Regional brain activity during transient self-induced anxiety and anger in healthy adults. Biol Psychiatry 46:454–465, 1999.

94. Devinsky O, Morrell M, and Vogt B: Contributions of anterior cingulate cortex to behavior. Brain 118:279–306, 1995.

95. Morecraft RJ and Van Hoesen GW: Convergence of limbic input to the cingulate motor cortex in the rhesus monkey. Brain Res Bull 45:209–232, 1998.

96. Corkin S, Twitchell TE, and Sullivan EV: Safety and efficacy of cingulotomy for pain and psychiatric disorders. In Hitchcock ER, Ballantine HT, and Meyerson BA (eds): Modern Concepts in Psychiatric Surgery. Elsevier, New York, 1979, pp 253–272.

97. Ballantine HT, Bouckoms AJ, Thomas EK, and Giriunas IE: Treatment of psychiatric illness by stereotactic cingulotomy. Biol Psychiatry 22:807–817, 1987.

98. Heilman KM and Valenstein E: Frontal lobe neglect in man. Neurology 22:660–664, 1972.

99. Watson RT, Cauthen JC, and King FA: Neglect after cingulectomy. Neurology 23:1003–1007, 1973.

100. Meador KJ, Watson RT, Bowers D, et al.: Hypometria with hemispatial and limb motor neglect. Brain 109:293–305, 1986.

101. Laplane D, Degos JD, Baulac M, and Gray F: Bilateral infarction of the anterior cingulate gyri and or the fornices. J Neurol Sci 51:289–300, 1981.

102. George MS, Ketter TA, et al.: Brain activity during transient sadness and happiness in healthy women. Am J Psychiatry 152:341–351, 1995.

103. Veit R, Flor H, Erb M, et al. Brain circuits involved in emotional learning in antisocial behavior and social phobia in humans. Neurosci Lett 328:233–236, 2002.

104. Ballantine HT, Cassidy WL, Flanagan NW, and Marino R: Stereotaxic anterior cingulotomy for neuropsychiatric illness and intractable pain. J Neurosurg 26:488–495, 1967.

105. Mazars G: Criteria for identifying cingulate epilepsies. Epilepsia 11:41–47, 1970.

106. Levin B and Duchowny M: Childhood obsessive–compulsive disorder and cingulate epilepsy. Biol Psychiatry 30:1049–1055, 1991.

107. Tow PM and Whitty CWM: Personality changes after operations of the cingulate gyrus in man. J Neurol Neurosurg Psychiatry 16:186–195, 1953.

108. Damasio AR and Van Hoesen GW: Focal lesions of the limbic frontal lobe. In Heilman KM and Satz P (eds). Neuropsychology of Human Emotion. Guilford Press, New York, 1983, pp 85–110.

109. MacLean PD: Perspectives on cingulate cortex in the limbic system. In Vogt BA and Gabriel M (eds). Neurobiology of Cingulate Cortex and Limbic Thalamus: A Comprehensive Handbook. Birkhauser, Boston, 1993, pp 1–15.

110. Whitty CWM, Duffield JE, Tow PM, and Cairns H: Anterior cingulectomy in the treatment of mental illness. Lancet 1:475–481, 1952.

111. Derbyshire SW, Jones AK, Gyulai F, et al.: Pain processing during three levels of noxious stimulation produces differential patterns of central activity. Pain 73:431–445, 1997.

112. Foltz EL and White LE: Pain "relief" by frontal cingulotomy. J Neurosurg 19:89–100, 1962.

113. Hadland KA, Rushworth MF, Gaffan D, and Passingham RE: The anterior cingulated and reward-guided selection of actions. J Neurophysiol 89:1161–1164, 2003.

114. Barch DM, Braver TS, Akbudak E, Conturo T, Ollinger J, and Snyder A: Anterior cingulate cortex and response conflict: effects of response modality and processing domain. Cereb Cortex 11:837–848, 2001.

115. Posner MI and Petersen SE: The attention system of the human brain. Annu Rev Neurosci 13:25–42, 1990.

116. Carter CS, Botvinick MM, and Cohen JD: The contribution of the anterior cingulate cortex to executive processes in cognition. Rev Neurosci 10:49–57, 1999.

117. Botvinick M, Nystrom LE, Fissell K, Carter CS, and Cohen JD: Conflict monitoring versus selection-for-action in anterior cingulate cortex. Nature 402:179–181, 1999.

118. MacDonald AW III, Cohen JD, Stenger VA, and Carter CS: Dissociating the role of the dorsolateral prefrontal and anterior cingulate cortex in cognitive control. Science 288:1835–1838, 2000.

119. Paus T, Koski L, Caramanos Z, and Westbury C: Regional differences in the effects of task difficulty and motor output on blood flow response in the human anterior cingulate cortex: a review of 107 PET activation studies. Neuroreport 9:R37–R47, 1998.

120. Raichle ME, Fiez JA, Videen TO, et al.: Practice-related changes in human brain functional anatomy during nonmotor learning. Cereb Cortex 4:8–26, 1994.

121. Frith CD, Friston K, Liddle PF, and Frackowiak RSJ: Willed action and the prefrontal cortex in man: a study with PET. Proc R Soc Lond B Biol Sci 244:241–246, 1991.

122. Gehring WJ and Knight RT: Prefrontal–cingulate interactions in action monitoring. Nat Neurosci 3:516–520, 2000.

123. Hof PR, Mufson EJ, and Morrison JH: Human orbitofrontal cortex: cytoarchitecture and quantitative immunohistochemical parcellation. J Comp Neurol 359:48–68, 1995.

124. Carmichael ST and Price JL: Limbic connections of the orbital and medial prefrontal cortex in macaque monkeys. J Comp Neurol 363:615–641, 1995.

125. Levy LM, Henkin RI, Hutter A, Lin CS, Martins D, and Schellinger D: Functional MRI of human olfaction. J Comput Assist Tomogr 21:849–856, 1997.

126. Rolls ET, Critchley HD, Mason R, and Wakeman EA: Orbitofrontal cortex neurons: role in olfactory and visual association learning. J Neurophysiol 75:1970–1981, 1996.

127. Wedekind C and Furi S: Body odour preferences in men and women: do they aim for specific MHC combinations or simply heterozygosity? Proc R Soc Lond B Biol Sci 264:1471–1479, 1997.

128. Ober C, Hyslop T, Elias S, et al.: Human leukocyte antigen matching and fetal loss: results of a 10 year prospective study. Hum Reprod 13:33–38, 1998.

129. Ober C, Weitkamp LR, Cox N, et al.: HLA and mate choice in humans. Am J Hum Genet 61:497–504, 1997.

130. Smith MF: Love with the proper stranger. Nat Hist 107:14–19, 1998.

131. Weusten BL, Franssen H, Wieneke GH, and Smout AJ: Multichannel recording of cerebral potentials evoked by esophageal balloon distension in humans. Dig Dis Sci 39:2074–2083, 1994.

132. Delgado JMR and Livingston RB: Some respiratory, vascular, and thermal response to stimulation of frontal lobe. J Neurophysiol 11:39–55, 1948.

133. Rinkel M, Greenblatt M, Coon GP, and Solomon HC: Relations of the frontal lobe to autonomic nervous system in man. In Greenblatt M, Arnot M, and Solomon HC (eds). Studies in Lobotomy. Grune & Stratton, New York, 1950. pp 338–349.

134. Freeman W and Watts JW: Psychosurgery. Charles C Thomas, Springfield, IL, 1942.

135. Greenblatt M: Studies in Lobotomy. Grune & Stratton, Orlando, FL, 1950.

136. Butter CM and Snyder DR: Alterations in aversive and aggressive behaviors following orbital frontal lesions in rhesus monkeys. Acta Neurobiol Exp 32:525–565, 1972.

137. Joseph R: Neuropsychiatry, Neuropsychology, and Clinical Neuroscience. Williams & Wilkins, Baltimore, 1996, pp. 428–431.

138. Butter CM, Snyder DR, and McDonald JA: Effects of orbital frontal lesions on aversive and aggressive behaviors in rhesus monkeys. J Comp Physiol Psychol 72:132–144, 1970.

139. Schoenbaum G and Setlow B: Integrating orbitofrontal cortex into prefrontal theory: common processing themes across species and subdivisions. Learn Mem 8:134–147, 2001.

140. Morgan MA and LeDoux JE: Differential contributions of dorsal and ventral medial prefrontal cortex to the acquisition and extinction of conditioned fear in rats. Behav Neurosci 109:681–688, 1995.

141. LaBar KS and LeDoux JE: Emotion and the brain: an overview. In Feinberg TE and Farah MJ (eds). Behavioral Neurology and Neuropsychology. McGraw-Hill, New York, 1996, pp 675–689.

142. Fuster JM. Executive frontal functions. Exp Brain Res 133:66–70, 2000.

143. Bear DM: Temporal lobe epilepsy: a syndrome of sensory–limbic hyperconnection. Cortex 15:357–384, 1979.

144. Brambilla P, Barale F, Caverzasi E, and Soares JC: Anatomical MRI findings in mood and anxiety disorders. Epidemiol Psichiatr Soc 11:8–99, 2002.

145. Tekin S and Cummings JL: Frontal-subcortical neuronal circuits and clinical neuropsychiatry: an update. J Psychosom Res 53:647–654, 2002.

146. Blair RJ: Neurocognitive models of aggression, the antisocial personality disorders, and psychopathy. J Neurol Neurosurg Psychiatry 71:727–731, 2001.

147. Grafman J, Schwab K, Warden D, et al.: Frontal lobe injuries, violence, and aggression: a report of the Vietnam Head Injury Study. Neurology 46:1231–1238, 1996.

148. Broffman M: The lobotomized patient during the first year at home. In Greenblatt M, Arnot R, and Solomon HC (eds). Studies in Lobotomy. Grune & Stratton, Orlando, FL, 1950, pp 200–214.

149. Van Hoesen GE, Morecraft RJ, and Semendeferi K: Functional neuroanatomy of the limbic system and prefrontal cortex. In Fogel BS, Schiffer RB, and Rao SM (eds). Neuropsychiatry. Williams & Wilkins, Baltimore, 1996, pp 113–143.

150. Semendeferi K, Armstrong E, Schleicher A, et al.: Limbic frontal cortex in hominoids: a comparative study of area 13. Am J Phys Anthropol 106:129–155, 1998.

151. Kling A and Mass R: Alterations of social behavior with neural lesions in nonhuman primates. In Holloway B (ed). Primate Aggression, Territoriality, Zenophobia. Academic Press, New York, 1974, pp 361–386.

152. Brody EB and Rosvold HE: Influence of prefrontal lobotomy on social interaction in a monkey group. Psychosom Med 14:406–415, 1952.

153. Meyers CA, Berman SA, Scheibel RS, and Hayman A: Case report: acquired antisocial personality disorder associated with unilateral left orbital frontal lobe damage. J Psychiatry Neurosci 17:121–125, 1992.

154. Rogers RD, Owen AM, Middleton HC, et al.: Choosing between small, likely rewards and large, unlikely rewards activates inferior and orbital prefrontal cortex. J Neurosci 19:9029–9038, 1999.

155. Wellman HM and Cross D: Theory of mind and conceptual change. Child Dev 72:702–707, 2001.

156. Stone VE, Baron-Cohen S, and Knight RT: Frontal lobe contributions to theory of mind. J Cogn Neurosci 10:640–656, 1998.

157. Stone VE, Cosmides L, Tooby J, Kroll N, and Knight RT: Selective impairment of reasoning about social exchange in a patient with bilateral limbic system damage. Proc Natl Acad Sci USA 99:11531–11536, 2002.

158. Bechara A, Damasio H, and Damasio AR: Emotion, decision making and the orbitofrontal cortex. Cereb Cortex 10:295–307, 2000.

159. Eslinger PJ and Damasio AR: Severe disturbance of higher cognition after bilateral frontal lobe ablation: patient EVR. Neurology 35:1731–1741, 1985.

160. Damasio AR, Tranel D, and Damasio H: Individuals with sociopathic behavior caused by frontal damage fail to respond autonomically to social stimuli. Behav Brain Res 41:81–94, 1990.

161. Damasio AR: Descartes' Error. Putnam, New York, 1994.

162. Tranel D and Damasio H: Neuroanatomical correlates of electrodermal skin conductance responses. Psychophysiology 31:427–438, 1994.

163. Van Honk J, Hermans EJ, Putman P, Montagne B, and Schutter DJ: Defective somatic markers in subclinical psychopathy. Neuroreport 13:1025–1027, 2002.

164. Habib M, Daquin G, Milandre L, et al.: Mutism and auditory agnosia due to bilateral insular damage—role of the insula in human communication. Neuropsychologia 33:327–339, 1995.

165. Shimojo S and Shams L: Sensory modalities are not separate modalities: plasticity and interactions. Curr Opin Neurobiol 11:505–509, 2001.

166. Ogawa H: Gustatory cortex of primates: anatomy and physiology. Neurosci Res 20:1–13, 1994.

167. Mufson EJ, Mesulam MM, and Pandya DN: Insular interconnections with the amygdala in the rhesus monkey. Neuroscience 6:1231–1248, 1981.

168. Cechetto DF: Identification of a cortical site for stress-induced cardiovascular dysfunction. Integr Physiol Behav Sci 29:362–373, 1994.

169. Rauch SL, Savage CR, Alpert NM, et al.: A positron emission tomographic study of simple phobic symptom provocation. Arch Gen Psychiatry 52:20–28, 1995.

170. Oppenheimer S: Forebrain lateralization of cardiovascular function: physiology and clinical correlates. Ann Neurol 49:555–556, 2001.

171. Oppenheimer SM: Neurogenic cardiac effects of cerebrovascular disease. Curr Opin Neurol 7:20–24, 1994.

172. Hilz MJ, Deutsch M, Perrine K, Nelson PK, Rauhut U, and Devinsky O: Hemispheric influence on autonomic modulation and baroreceptor sensitivity. Ann Neurol 49:575–584, 2001.

173. Zald DH and Pardo JV: The functional neuroanatomy of voluntary swallowing. Ann Neurol 46:281–286, 1999.

174. Daniels SK and Foundas AL: The role of insular cortex in dysphagia. Dysphagia 12:146–156, 1997.

175. Walsh V: Perception: the seeing ear. Curr Biol 6:389–391, 1996.

176. Kosslyn SM, Shin LM, Thompson WL, et al.: Neural effects of visualizing and perceiving aversive stimuli: a PET investigation. Neuroreport 7:1569–1576, 1996.

177. Morris JS, Scott SK, and Dolan RJ: Saying it with feeling: neural responses to emotional vocalization. Neuropsychologia 37:1155–1163, 1999.

178. Kettenmann B, Hummel C, Stefan H, and Kobal G: Multiple olfactory activity in the human neocortex identified by magnetic source imaging. Chem Senses 22:493–502, 1997.

178a. Krolak-Salmon P, Hénaff M-A, Isnard J, et al: An attention modulated response to disgust in human ventral anterior insula. Ann Neurol 53:446–453, 2003.

179. Phillips ML, Young AW, Senior C, et al.: A specific neural substrate for perceiving facial expressions of disgust. Nature 389:495–498, 1997.

180. Lane RD, Reiman EM, Ahern GL, et al.: Neuroanatomic correlates of happiness, sadness, and disgust. Am J Psychiatry 154:926–933, 1997.

181. Buchel C, Morris J, Dolan RJ, and Friston KJ: Brain systems mediating aversive conditioning: an event-related fMRI study. Neuron 20:947–957, 1998.

182. Chua P, Krams M, Toni I, Passingham R, and Dolan R: A functional anatomy of anticipatory anxiety. Neuroimage 9:563–571, 1999.

183. Griffiths TD, Bench CJ, and Frackowiak RS: Human cortical areas selectively activated by apparent sound movement. Curr Biol 4:892–895, 1994.

184. Mesulam M-M and Mufson EJ: The insula of Reil in man and monkey. In Peters A and Jones EG (eds).: Cerebral Cortex, Vol 4. Plenum Press, New York, 1985 pp 179–226.

185. Marshall RS, Lazar RM, Mohr JP, Van Heertum RL, and Mast H: "Semantic" conduction aphasia from a posterior insular cortex infarction. J Neuroimaging 6:189–191, 1996.

186. Dronkers NF: A new brain region for coordinating speech articulation. Nature 384:159–161, 1996.

187. Borod JC, Bloom RL, Brickman AM, Nakhutina L, and Curko EA: Emotional processing deficits in individuals with unilateral brain damage. Appl Neuropsychol 9:23–36, 2002.

188. Heilman KM and Gilmore RL: Cortical influences in emotion. J Clin Neurophysiol 15:409–423, 1998.

189. Devinsky O: Right cerebral hemisphere dominance for a sense of corporeal and emotional self. Epilepsy Behav 1:60–73, 2000.

190. Efron R: The Decline and Fall of Hemispheric Specialization. Lawrence Erlbaum, Hillsdale, NJ, 1990.

191. Gainotti G: Emotional disorders in relation to unilateral brain damage. In Feinberg TE and Farah MJ (eds). Behavioral Neurology and Neuropsychology. McGraw-Hill, New York, 1996, pp 691–698.

192. Gainotti G: Emotional behavior and hemispheric side of the lesion. Cortex 8:41–55, 1972.

193. Anderson AK, Spencer DD, Fulbright RK, and Phelps EA: Contribution of the anteromedial temporal lobes to the evaluation of facial emotion. Neuropsychology 14:526–536, 2000.

194. Ahern GL, Herring AM, Tackenberg JN, et al.: Affective self-report during the intracarotid sodium amobarbital test. J Clin Exp Neuropsychol 16:372–376, 1994.

195. Starkstein SE and Robinson R: Depression following cerebrovascular lesions. Semin Neurol 10:247–253, 1990.

196. Sackheim HA, Greenberg MS, Weiman AL, et al.: Hemispheric asymmetry in the expression of positive and negative emotion: neurologic evidence. Arch Neurol 39:210–218, 1982.

197. Weddell R, Miller R, and Trevarthen C: Voluntary emotional facial expressions in patients with focal cerebral lesions. Neuropsychologia 28:49–60, 1990.

198. Kurthen M, Linke DB, Reuter BM, et al.: Severe negative emotional reactions in intracarotid sodium amytal procedures: further evidence for hemispheric asymmetries? Cortex 27:333–337, 1991.

199. Borod JC, Rorie KD, Pick LH, et al.: Verbal pragmatics following unilateral stroke: emotional content and valence. Neuropsychology 14:112–124, 2000.

200. Slater E and Beard AW: The schizophrenia-like psychoses of epilepsy. Br J Psychiatry 109:95–150, 1963.

201. Bear DM and Fedio P: Quantitative analysis of interictal behavior in temporal lobe epilepsy. Arch Neurol 34:454–467, 1977.

202. Devinsky O and Najjar S: Evidence against the existence of a temporal lobe epilepsy personality syndrome. Neurology 53(Suppl 2):S13–S25, 1999.

203. Newman NJ, Bell IR, and McKee AC: Paraneoplastic limbic encephalitis: neuropsychiatric presentation. Biol Psychiatry 27:529–542, 1990.

204. Ahern GL, O'Connor M, Dalmau J, et al.: Paraneoplastic temporal lobe epilepsy with testicular neoplasm and atypical amnesia. Neurology 44:1270–1274, 1994.

205. Lacomis D, Khoshbin S, and Schick RM: MR imaging of paraneoplastic limbic encephalitis. J Comput Assist Tomogr 14:115–117, 1990.

206. Dalmau J, Graus F, Rosenblum MK, and Posner JB: Anti-Hu associated paraneoplastic encephalomyelitis/sensory neuronopathy: a clinical study of 71 patients. Medicine 71:59–72, 1992.

207. Whitman S, Hermann BP, and Gordon A: Psychopathology in epilepsy: how great is the risk? Biol Psychiatry 19:213–216, 1984.

208. Haverkamp F, Hanisch C, Mayer H, and Noeker M: Evidence of a specific vulnerability for deficient sequential cognitive information processing in epilepsy. J Child Neurol 16:901–905, 2001.

209. Helmstaedter C and Kurthen M: Memory and epilepsy: characteristics, course, and influence of drugs and surgery. Curr Opin Neurol 14:211–216, 2001.

210. Swanson SJ, Rao SM, Grafman J, Salazar AM, and Kraft J: The relationship between seizure type and interictal personality. Results from the Vietnam Head Injury Study. Brain 118:91–103, 1995.

211. Wirrell EC, Camfield CS, Camfield PR, Dooley JM, Gordon KE, and Smith B: Long-term psychosocial outcome in typical absence epilepsy. Sometimes a wolf in sheeps' clothing. Arch Pediatr Adolesc Med 151:152–158, 1997.

212. Hermann BP and Whitman S: Behavioral and personality correlates of epilepsy: a review, methodological critique, and conceptual model. Psychol Bull 95:451–497, 1984.

213. Getz K, Hermann B, Seidenberg M, et al.: Negative symptoms in temporal lobe epilepsy. Am J Psychiatry 159:644–651, 2002.

214. Ettinger AB and Kanner AM: Psychiatric Issues in Epilepsy: A Practical Guide to Diagnosis and Treatment. Lippincott-Williams & Wilkins, Baltimore, 2001.

215. Sachdev P: Schizophrenia-like psychosis and epilepsy: the status of the association. Am J Psychiatry 155:325–336, 1998.

216. Kanemoto K, Takeuchi J, Kawasaki J, and Kawai I: Characteristics of temporal lobe epilepsy with mesial temporal sclerosis, with special reference to psychotic episodes. Neurology 47:1199–1203, 1996.

217. Hermann BP, Seidenberg M, Schoenfeld J, and Davies K: The characteristics of the syndrome of mesial temporal lobe epilepsy. Arch Neurol 54:369–376, 1997.

218. Van Paesschen W, King MD, Duncan JS, and Connelly A: The amygdala and temporal lobe simple partial seizures: a prospective and quantitative MRI study. Epilepsia 42:857–862, 2001.

219. Devinsky O, Feldmann E, Burrowes K, and Bromfield EB: Autoscopic phenomena with seizures. Arch Neurol 46:1080–1088, 1989.

220. Devinsky O, Hafler DA, and Victor J: Embarrassment as the aura of a complex partial seizure. Neurology 32:1264–1265, l983.

221. Cirignotta F, Todesco CV, and Lugaresi E: Temporal lobe epilepsy with ecstatic seizures (so-called Dostoevsky epilepsy). Epilepsia 21:705–710, 1980.

222. Schenk L and Bear D: Multiple personality and related dissociative phenomena in patients with temporal lobe epilepsy. Am J Psychiatry 138:1131–1316, 1981.

223. Penfield W and Perot P: The brain's record of auditory and visual experience: a final summary and discussion. Brain 86:595–696, 1963.

224. Hermann BP, Wyler AR, Blummer D, and Richey ET: Ictal fear. Neuropsychiatry Neuropsychol Behav Neurol 5:205–210, 1992.

225. Hermann BP, Dikmen S, Schwartz MS, and Karnes WE: Interictal psychopathology in patients with ictal fear: a quantitative investigation. Neurology 32:7–11, 1982.

226. Devinsky O, Witt E, Cox C, Fedio P, and Theodore WH: Ictal fear in temporal lobe epilepsy: association with interictal behavioral changes. J Epilepsy 4:231–238, 1991.

227. Ashford JW, Schulz SC, and Walsh FO: Violent automatism in a partial complex seizure. Arch Neurol 37:120–122, 1980.

228. Saint-Hilaire JM, Gilbert M, and Bouner G: Aggression as an epileptic manifestation: two cases with depth electrodes. Epilepsia 21:184, 1980.

229. Luciano D, Devinsky O, and Perrine K: Crying seizures. Neurology 43:2113–2117, 1993.

230. Schacter SC and Fisher RS: Postical state: a neglected entity in the management of epilepsy. Epilepsy Behav 1:52–59, 2000.

231. Todd RB: Clinical Lectures on Paralysis, Diseases of the Brain, and Other Affections of the Nervous System. Lindsay & Blakiston, Philadelphia, 1855, pp 196–210.

232. Devinsky O, Kelley K, Yacubian EM, et al.: Postictal behavior. A clinical and subdural electroencephalographic study. Arch Neurol 51:254–259, 1994.

233. Helmstaedter C, Elger CE, and Lendt M: Postictal courses of cognitive deficits in focal epilepsies. Epilepsia 35:1073–1078, 1994.

234. Jackson JH: On post-epileptic states: a contribution to the comparative study of insanities. J Ment Sci 34:349–365, 1888.

235. Logsdail SJ and Toone BK: Post-ictal psychoses. A clinical and phenomenological description. Br J Psychiatry 152:246–252, 1988.

236. Devinsky O, Abramson H, Alper K, et al.: Postical psychosis: a case control series of 20 patients and 150 controls. Epilepsy Res 20:247–253, 1995.

237. Tarulli A, Devinsky O, and Alper K: Progression of postictal to interictal psychosis. Epilepsia 42:1468–1471, 2001.

238. Kanemoto K, Takeuchi J, Kawasaki J, and Kawai I: Characteristics of temporal lobe epilepsy with mesial temporal sclerosis, with special reference to psychotic episodes. Neurology 47:1199–1203, 1996.

239. Gerard ME, Spitz MC, Towbin JA, and Shantz D: Subacute postictal aggression. Neurology 50:384–388, 1998.

240. Gross A, Devinsky O, Westbrook LE, Wharton AH, and Alper K: Psychotropic medication use in patients with epilepsy: effect on seizure frequency. J Neuropsychiatry Clin Neurosci 12:458–464, 2000.

241. Devinsky O, Kanner AM, Ettinger AB (ed). Therapy for Cognitive and Behavioral Disorders in Epilepsy. Epilepsy Behav (Suppl 5): 2002

242. Waxman SG and Geschwind N: The interictal behavior syndrome in temporal lobe epilepsy. Arch Gen Psychiatry 32:1580–1586, 1975.

243. Devinsky O: Interictal changes in behavior. In Devinsky O and Theodore WH (eds). Epilepsy and Behavior. Wiley-Liss, New York, 1991, pp 1–21.

244. Romberg MD: A Manual of the Nervous Diseases of Man. Translated by Sieveking. Sydenham Society, London, 1853.

245. Blake RV, Wroe SJ, Breen EK, and McCarthy RA: Accelerated forgetting in patients with epilepsy: evidence for an impairment in memory consolidation. Brain 123:472–483, 2000.

246. Pulliainen V, Kuikka P, and Jokelainen M: Motor and cognitive functions in newly diagnosed adult seizure patients before antiepileptic medication. Acta Neurol Scand 101:73–78, 2000.

247. Aarts JHP, Bimmin CD, Smit AD, and Wilkins AJ: Selective cognitive impairment during focal and generalized epileptiform EEG activity. Brain 107:293–308, 1984.

248. Loring DW and Meador KJ: Cognitive and behavioral effects of epilepsy treatment. Epilepsia 42(Suppl 8):24–32, 2001.

249. Lado FA, Laureta EC, and Moshe SL: Seizure-induced hippocampal damage in the mature and immature brain. Epileptic Disord 4:83–97, 2002.

250. Salanova V, Markand O, and Worth R: Focal functional deficits in temporal lobe epilepsy on PET scans and the intracarotid amobarbital procedure. Epilepsia 42:198–203, 2001.

251. O'Brien TJ, So EL, Meyer FB, et al.: Progressive hippocampal atrophy in chronic intractable temporal lobe epilepsy. Ann Neurol 45:526–529, 1999.

252. Kalvianen R, Salmenpera T, Partanen K, et al.: Recurrent seizures may cause hippocampal damage in temporal lobe epilepsy. Neurology 50:1377–1382, 1998.

253. Adachi N, Onuma T, Hara T, et al.: Frequency and age-related variables in interictal psychoses in localization-related epilepsies. Epilepsy Res 48:25–31, 2002.

254. Mendez MF, Grau R, Doss RC, and Taylor JL: Schizophrenia in epilepsy: seizure and psychosis variables. Neurology 43:1073–1077, 1993.

255. Bredkjaer SR, Mortensen PB, and Parnas J: Epilepsy and non-organic non-affective psychosis. National epidemiologic study. Br J Psychiatry 172:235–238, 1998.

256. Devinsky O and Vazquez B: Behavioral changes associated with epilepsy. Neurol Clin 11:127–149, 1993.

257. Landolt H: Serial electroencephalographic investigations during psychotic episodes in epileptic patients and during schizophrenic attacks. In Lorentz de Haas AM (ed). Lectures on Epilepsy. Elsevier, Amsterdam, 1958, pp 91–133.

258. Pakalnis A, Drake ME Jr, John K, and Kellum JB: Forced normalization. Acute psychosis after seizure control in seven patients. Arch Neurol 44:289–292, 1987.

259. Reutens DC, Savard G, Andermann F, Dubeau F, and Olivier A: Results of surgical treatment in temporal lobe epilepsy with chronic psychosis. Brain 120:1929–1936, 1997.

260. Callender JS and Fenton GW: Psychosis de novo following temporal lobectomy. Seizure 6:409–411, 1997.

261. Von Meduna L: General discussion of the cardiozol therapy. Am J Psychiatry 94(Suppl):40–50, 1938.

262. Mendez MF, Cummings JL, and Benson DF: Depression in epilepsy: significance and phenomenology. Arch Neurol 43:766–770, 1986.

263. Kanner AM and Balabanov A: Depression and epilepsy: how closely related are they? Neurology 58(Suppl 5):S27–S39, 2002.

264. Nilsson L, Ahlbom A, Farahmand BY, Asberg M, and Tomson T: Risk factors for suicide in epilepsy: a case control study. Epilepsia 43:644–651, 2002.

265. Matthews WS and Barbaras G: Suicide and epilepsy: a review of literature. Psychosomatics 22:515–524, 1981.

266. Moore PM and Baker GA: The neuropsychological and emotional consequences of living with intractable temporal lobe epilepsy: implications for clinical management. Seizure 11:224–230, 2002.

267. Lambert MV and Robertson MM: Depression in epilepsy: etiology, phenomenology, and treatment. Epilepsia 40(Suppl 10):S21–S47, 1999.

268. Altshuler LL, Devinsky O, Post RM, and Theodore W: Depression, anxiety and temporal lobe epilepsy: laterality of focus and symptomatology. Arch Neurol 47:284–288, 1990.

269. Quiske A, Helmstaedter C, Lux S, and Elger CE: Depression in patients with temporal lobe epilepsy is related to mesial temporal sclerosis. Epilepsy Res 39:121–125, 2000.

270. Bromfield EB, Altshuler L, Leiderman DB, Balish M, Ketter TA, and Devinsky O: Cerebral metabolism and depression in patients with complex partial seizures. Arch Neurol 49:617–623, 1992.

271. Victoroff JI, Benson F, Grafton ST, Engel J Jr, and Mazziotta JC: Depression in complex partial seizures. Electroencephalography and cerebral metabolic correlates. Arch Neurol 51:155–163, 1994.

272. Scicutella A: Anxiety disorders in epilepsy. In Ettinger AB and Kanner AM (eds). Psychiatric Issues in Epilepsy. Lippincott Williams & Wilkins, Philadelphia, 2001 pp 95–110.

273. Cutting S, Lauchheimer A, Barr W, and Devinsky O: Adult-onset idiopathic generalized epilepsy: clinical and behavioral features. Epilepsia 42:1395–1398, 2001.

274. Schachter SC: Aggression in epilepsy. In Ettinger AB and Kanner AM (eds). Psychiatric Issues in Epilepsy. Lippincott Williams & Wilkins, Philadelphia, 2001, pp 201–214.

275. Lindsay J, Ounsted C, and Richards P: Long term outcome in children with temporal lobe epilepsy: III. Psychiatric manifestations in adult life. Dev Med Child Neurol 21:630–636, 1979.

276. Griffith N, Engel J, and Bandler R: Ictal and enduring interictal disturbances in emotional behavior in an animal model of temporal lobe epilepsy. Brain Res 400:360–364, 1987.

277. Hermann BP, Schwartz MS, Whitman S, and Karnes WE: Aggression and epilepsy: seizure-type comparisons and high-risk variables. Epilepsia 21:691–698, 1980.

278. Bogdanovic MD, Mead SH, and Duncan JS: Aggressive behaviour at a residential epilepsy centre. Seizure 9:58–64, 2000.

279. Falconer MA: Reversibility by temporal-lobe resection of the behavioral abnormalities of temporal-lobe epilepsy. N Engl J Med 289:451–455, 1973.

280. Taylor DC: Aggression and epilepsy. J Psychosom Res 13:229–236, 1969.

281. Devinsky O and Bear D: Varieties of aggressive behavior in temporal lobe epilepsy. Am J Psychiatry 141:651–656, 1984.

282. Devinsky O, Feldmann E, Bromfield E, et al.: Structured interview for partial seizures: clinical phenomenology and diagnosis. J Epilepsy 4:107–116, 1991.

283. Devinsky O and Gordon E: Epileptic seizures progressing into nonepileptic conversion seizures. Neurology 51:1293–1296, 1998.

284. Benson DF, Miller BL, and Signer SF: Dual personality associated with epilepsy. Arch Neurol 43:471–474, 1986.

285. Rosenberg HJ, Rosenberg SD, Williamson PD, and Wolford GL II: A comparative study of trauma and posttraumatic stress disorder prevalence in epilepsy patients and psychogenic nonepileptic seizure patients. Epilepsia 41:447–452, 2000.

286. Barry E, Krumholz A, Bergey GK, Chatha H, Alemayehu S, and Grattan L: Nonepileptic posttraumatic seizures. Epilepsia 39:427–431, 1998.

287. Devinsky O, Mesad, S, and Alper K: Nondominant hemisphere lesions and coversion nonepileptic seizures. J Neuropsychol Clin Neurosci 13:367–373, 2001.

288. Gastaut H, Morin G, and Leserve N: Study of the behavior of psychomotor epileptics during the interval between seizures. Ann Med Psychol 113:1–27, 1955.

289. Sorensen AS, Hansen H, Andersen R, et al.: Personality characteristics and epilepsy. Acta Psychiatr Scand 80:620–631, 1989.

290. Csernansky JG, Leiderman DB, Mandabach M, and Moses JA: Psychopathology and limbic epilepsy: relationship to seizure variables and neuropsychological function. Epilepsia 31:275–280, 1990.

291. Wieser HG: Selective amygdalohippocampectomy: indications, investigative technique and results. Adv Tech Stand Neurosurg 13:39–133, 1986.

292. Schmitz EB, Moriarty J, Costa DC, et al.: Psychiatric profiles and patterns of cerebral blood flow in focal epilepsy: interactions between depression, obsessionality, and perfusion related to the laterality of the epilepsy. J Neurol Neurosurg Psychiatry 62:458–463, 1997.

293. Jokeit H, Seitz RJ, Markowitsch HJ, Neumann N, Witte OW, and Ebner A: Prefrontal asymmetric interictal glucose hypometabolism and cognitive impairment in patients with temporal lobe epilepsy. Brain 120:2283–2294, 1997.

294. Levav M, Mirsky AF, Herault J, Xiong L, Amir N, and Andermann E: Familial association of neuropsychological traits in patients with generalized and partial seizure disorders. J Clin Exp Neuropsychol 24:311–326, 2002.

295. Devinsky O, Gershengorn J, Brown E, Perrine K, Vazquez B, and Luciano D: Frontal functions in juvenile myoclonic epilepsy. Neuropsychiatry Neuropsychol Behav Neurol 10:243–246, 1997.

296. Janz D: Die epilepsien. George Thieme, Stuttgart, 1969.

297. Perini GI, Tosin C, Carraro C, Bernasconi G, Canevini MP, Canger R, et al.: Interictal mood and personality disorders in temporal lobe epilepsy and juvenile myoclonic epilepsy. J Neurol Neurosurg Psychiatry 61:601–605, 1996.

298. Vasquez B, Devinsky O, Luciano D, et al.: Juvenile myoclonic epilepsy: clinical features and factors related to misdiagnosis. J Epilepsy 6:233–238, 1993.

299. Caplan R, Arbelle S, Guthrie D, et al.: Formal thought disorder and psychopathology in pediatric primary generalized and complex partial epilepsy. J Am Acad Child Adolesc Psychiatry 36:1286–1294, 1997.

300. Blumer D: Evidence supporting the temporal lobe epilepsy personality syndrome. Neurology 53(Suppl 2):S9–S12, 1999.

301. Rao SM, Devinsky O, Grafman J, et al.: Viscosity in complex partial seizures: relationship to cerebral laterality and seizure duration. J Neurol Neurosurg Psychiatry 55:149–152, 1992.

302. Brandt J, Seidman LJ, and Kohl D: Personality characteristics of epileptic patients: a controlled study of generalized and temporal lobe cases. J Clin Exp Neuropsychol 7:25–38, 1985.

303. Lambert MV: Seizures, hormones and sexuality. Seizure 10:319–340, 2001.

304. Geschwind N, Shader RI, Bear D, et al.: Behavioral changes with temporal lobe epilepsy: assessment and treatment. J Clin Psychiatry 41:89–95, 1980.

305. Mitchell W, Falconer MA, and Hill D: Epilepsy with fetishism relieved by temporal lobectomy. Lancet 2:626–636, 1954.

306. Morrell MJ and Guldner GT: Self-reported sexual function and sexual arousability in women with epilepsy. Epilepsia 37:1204–1210, 1996.

307. Guldner GT and Morrell MJ: Nocturnal penile tumescence and rigidity: evaluation in men with epilepsy. Epilepsia 37:1211–1214, 1996.

308. Feeney DM, Gullotta FP, and Gilmore W: Hyposexuality produced by temporal lobe epilepsy in the cat. Epilepsia 39:140–149, 1998.

309. Blumer D: Hypersexual episodes in temporal lobe epilepsy. Am J Psychiatry 126:1099–1106, 1970.

310. Mattson RH, Cramer JA, Collins JF, et al.: Comparison of carbamazepine, phenobarbital, phenytoin, and primidone in partial and secondarily generalized tonic-clonic seizures. N Engl J Med 313:145–151, 1985.

311. Leuba JH: The Psychology of Religious Mysticism. Kegan, Paul, Trench, Trubner & Co, London.

312. James W: The Varieties of Religious Experience. Longmans, Green, New York, 1902.

313. Alajouanine T: Dostoiewski's epilepsy. Brain 86: 209–218, 1963.

314. Dewhurst K and Beard AW: Sudden religious conversions in temporal lobe epilepsy. Br J Psychiatry 117:497–507, 1970.

315. Tucker DM, Novelly RA, and Walker PJ: Hyperreligiosity in temporal lobe epilepsy: redefining the relationship. J Nerv Ment Dis 175:181–184, 1987.

316. Hayton T, Boylan LS, Jackson SC, and Devinsky O: Religious/spiritual beliefs and behavior in epilepsy. Ann Neurol 52:520, 2002. (Abstract)

317. Waxman SG and Geschwind N: Hypergraphia in temporal lobe epilepsy. Neurology 24:629–631, 1974.

318. Hermann BP, Whitman S, and Arntson P: Hypergraphia in epilepsy: is there a specificity to temporal lobe epilepsy? J Neurol Neurosurg Psychiatry 46:848–853, 1983.

319. Hermann BP, Whitman S, Wyler AR, Richey ET, and Dell J: The neurological, psychosocial and demographic correlates of hypergraphia in patients with epilepsy. J Neurol Neurosurg Psychiatry 51:203–208, 1988.

320. Dostoevsky FM: Letters of Fyodor Michaelovitch Dostoevsky to his Family and Friends. Mayne EC (translator). Macmillan, New York, 1914, p 50.

321. Silberman EK, Post RM, Nurnberger J, Theodore W, and Boulenger JP: Transient sensory, cognitive and affective phenomena in affective illness. A comparison with complex partial epilepsy. Br J Psychiatry 146:81–89, 1985.

322. Symonds C: Discussion. Proc R Soc Med 55:314–315, 1962.

323. Lansberg MG, O'Brien MW, Norbash AM, et al.: MRI abnormalities associated with partial status epilepticus. Neurology 52:1021–1027, 1999.

324. Tasch E, Cendes F, Li M, et al.: Neuroimaging evidence of progressive neuronal loss and dysfunction in temporal lobe epilepsy. Ann Neurol 45:568–576, 1999.

325. Lennox WG: Brain injury, drugs, and environment as causes of mental decay in epilepsy. Am J Psychiatry 99:174–180, 1942.

Chapter 11

Therapy for Cognitive and Neurobehavioral Disorders

Therapy for cognitive and behavioral disorders remains unsatisfactory. Encompassing the fields of neurology, psychiatry, and psychology, neurobehavioral therapies usually treat symptoms, not the disease process. Unraveling of the genetic, metabolic, and chemical mechanisms underlying neurobehavioral disorders outpaces therapeutic advances. Symptom-based therapy, however, reflects a limited understanding of disease origin and progression

(e.g., Parkinson's disease, Alzheimer's disease, schizophrenia) and of ways to translate known mechanisms into therapy (e.g., Huntington's disease) and to reverse the physiological or structural changes that underlie all neurobehavioral disorders.

In addition to the classic syndromes of behavioral neurology (e.g., aphasia, apraxia, alexia without agraphia, agnosia), a wide array of cognitive and behavioral problems result from brain

372

dysfunction. Rating scales and inventories are invaluable for their diagnosis and the assessment of their clinical outcome, as well as research purposes.[1,2] More measures are needed to assess specifically the cognitive and behavioral disorders complicating neurological diseases. These problems are common in a wide group of neurological disorders, including stroke, multiple sclerosis, traumatic brain injury, brain tumor, Parkinson's disease, Huntington's disease, epilepsy, dementia, and encephalitis. Treating the underlying disorder, such as removing a brain tumor or controlling seizures, often improves the cognitive and behavioral sequelae. However, the primary neurological disorder is often not treatable, or therapy does not reduce the burden of behavioral symptoms.

The treatment of cognitive and neurobehavioral symptoms is remarkably consistent across neurological disorders. Anxiety, depression, aggression, and psychosis appear to respond similarly regardless of whether the patient has multiple sclerosis, a hemispheric or subcortical stroke, epilepsy, or dementia. Clinical features such as the patient's age, comorbid disorders (e.g., cardiac arrhythmia, migraine), concurrent medications, and response to prior therapies are often more important therapeutic guides than the specific neurological disorder.

Therapeutic challenges are illustrated by the symptom cluster of irritability, personality change, and amnesia that can complicate epilepsy, encephalitis, Alzheimer's disease, and traumatic brain injury. While epilepsy and certain encephalitides can be successfully treated, traumatic brain injuries cannot be reversed, and the clinical deterioration in Alzheimer's disease can be slowed only slightly. For all these disorders, chronic problems respond variably to therapy. Irritability is managed with environmental changes, psychotherapy, or medications. Personality changes are relatively immutable but often modified with behavioral approaches, treating psychiatric disorders such as depression, and eliminating behaviorally toxic medications (e.g., phenobarbital). The impact of amnesia can be diminished by teaching compensatory strategies and possibly by pharmacological agents (e.g., donepezil, ginkgo biloba). For chronic symptoms, therapy must be individualized, with consideration of the efficacy, toxicity, and cost in time, energy, and affordability.

THERAPY: THE BIG PICTURE

Therapy for cognitive and neurobehavioral problems is summarized in Table 11–1. Effective therapy rests on an accurate diagnosis. Diagnosing cognitive and behavioral disorders requires localizing central nervous system (CNS) dysfunction, identifying the pathological process, classifying the syndrome, and never losing sight of the person behind the signs and symptoms of the disorder. Directing attention toward the mechanism of disease and the patient complements the usual focus on localization, diagnosis, and treatment of problematic symptoms. For example, in addition to prescribing medication for a depressed patient, it is helpful to explore psychosocial stressors and consider

Table 11–1. **Therapies for Cognitive and Neurobehavioral Disorders**

Inpatient and outpatient rehabilitation
Speech therapy
Physical and occupational therapy
Cognitive therapy
Vocational rehabilitation
Pragmatic approaches
Psychotherapy
Psychopharmacology
  Antidepressants
    Tricyclics
    Tetracyclics
    Selective serotonin reuptake inhibitors
    Novel antidepressants: trazodone, nefazodone, bupropion, mirtazapine, venlafaxine
  Mood stabilizers and antimanic agents
    Lithium
    Antiepileptics
  Anxiolytics
    Benzodiazepines
    Buspirone
  Antipsychotics
    Typical
    Atypical
  Antiepileptics
  Central nervous system stimulants
  Cognitive enhancers
  Sedative-hypnotics
Electroconvulsive therapy
Potential therapies
  Transcranial magnetic stimulation
  Vagus nerve stimulation

other factors (e.g., hypothyroidism, side effects of cardiac medications).

Disorders straddling the fence between neurology and psychiatry often defy simple diagnostic criteria. The *Diagnostic and Statistical Manual of Mental Disorders-IV* (DSM-IV) provides rigor and clarity but uses somewhat arbitrary criteria for diagnosing psychiatric disorders. The DSM-IV emphasizes reliability, not validation by treatment outcome. Further, the DSM-IV was not intended to diagnose behavioral disorders that complicate neurological disease. For instance, dysphoric and major depressive disorders complicating stroke or brain tumors are pleomorphic, resulting from the concomitance of multiple factors: concurrent therapy (e.g., glucocorticoid withdrawal), structural pathology, metabolic disturbances, as well as the psychological reaction to a devastating illness. Neurobehavioral disorders span a diverse range, evolve over time, and may not be constrained by inclusionary or exclusionary features. The rigid application of DSM-IV criteria restricts diagnostic accuracy, promoting "clean" but artificial "pigeonholes" that cannot accommodate many patients' disorders.

Lesion localization, the foundation of neurological diagnosis, provides more clues about therapy for acute than for chronic neurobehavioral problems. For example, fever, hallucinations, and emotional changes suggest a limbic encephalitis and treatment with acyclovir. However, the treatment of long-term sequelae, such as amnesia and aggressiveness, is influenced little by the pathogen or lesion site. No data differentiate pharmacological therapy for depression, whether associated with a right frontal lobe tumor, a left temporal lobe stroke, mesial temporal lobe epilepsy, or Parkinson's disease. Current neurobehavioral therapy is blind to lesion localization and etiology. However, there are exceptions. Anxiety resulting from a partial seizure, hyperthyroidism, pheochromocytoma, or Cushing's syndrome responds to specific interventions. In contrast, anxiety associated with a stroke or brain tumor may respond to general behavioral and pharmacological approaches. Parkinson's disease with relatively selective involvement of the substantia nigra responds well to dopaminergic therapies. Atypical parkinsonian syndromes respond little, if at all, to dopaminergic therapies.

The therapeutic approach to neurobehavioral disorders leans far to the biological side. Behavioral, humanistic, and practical approaches are relatively neglected. Stress aggravates most medical and neurobehavioral disorders. The impacts of stressors, environment, family, and fears are often underestimated, leaving therapeutic windows unopened. Listening to a patient's story, understanding a family's dynamic, and examining the patient in his or her world are too often neglected in favor of molecular biology, functional imaging, and psychopharmacology. It is as limiting to explain a disorder of the mind with an aberrant nucleotide sequence or a single neurochemical deficiency as with a dysfunctional childhood. Diagnosis and therapy must be balanced, with emphasis on the patient and his or her mental world, as well as neurobiology.

Neurobehavioral disorders often escape recognition. Symptoms and disorders are reported and noted, but their significance may remain unacknowledged. The diagnosis may be buried at the end of a neuropsychological report. A stroke patient's report that he or she "has nothing to live for" may be attributed to "normal adjustment" or a cry for attention, and a disabling depression goes untreated. Omissions and misconceptions limit the diagnosis and therapy of behavioral disorders. Furthermore, effective management of complex neurobehavioral disorders requires expertise and coordinated care, as illustrated by the following case:

A 67-year-old man with progressive supranuclear palsy suffered from falls, anxiety, and depression. He was taking levodopa, to which his internist added fluoxetine, a selective serotonin reuptake inhibitor (SSRI), 20 mg/day. The symptoms persisted, and 10 days later the dose was increased to 40 mg/day. Akathisia and ataxia developed within days, and the fluoxetine was discontinued. His neurologist recommended a trial of another SSRI with a more gradual dose escalation, but the patient refused. Six months later, as his anxiety worsened and may have contributed to a mild myocardial infarction, a psychopharmacologist prescribed buspirone, with excellent results.

A core element of behavioral medicine is simply asking a patient how he or she truly feels. This requires looking him or her in the eye as he or she responds, assessing hesitation, directness, body language, and comfort with the answer. Many psychological and neurological disorders lead a patient to deny or fail to recognize feelings and problems. Family members, friends, and caretakers must also be questioned.

NONPHARMACOLOGICAL THERAPY

Therapy for cognitive and neurobehavioral disorders extends over a wide range of measures, but randomized controlled studies and consensus are often lacking. While therapy focuses on psychopharmacology, other approaches are often safer and more effective.

Rehabilitation

Following the acute stages of traumatic brain injury, stroke, multiple sclerosis, or other CNS insults, inpatient and outpatient rehabilitation programs provide coordinated care of psychological, psychiatric, cognitive, and neurological problems.[3] The assessment, treatment, and outcome evaluation of subacute and long-term care are often fragmented. Therapists, nurses, doctors, and families must communicate to identify and respond consistently to the patient's problems that impede functional recovery (e.g., inappropriate sexual comments, agitation). The response to speech and physical therapies may plateau after many months. However, new problems, such as anxiety or depression, can develop, and old problems, such as spasticity, can become more disabling. Rehabilitation benefits not only patients with acute CNS disorders but also those with chronic CNS disorders such as multiple sclerosis, parkinsonism, brain tumors, and other neuropsychiatric disorders.

In all rehabilitation and medical venues, patients must be viewed as unique individuals with strengths and preserved capacities, not as clusters of deficits. Physicians are often ill-prepared to interact with severely impaired patients: they may be uncertain how to help and may prescribe medication too quickly; they may be uncomfortable with the patient's emotional needs and unfamiliar with the rehabilitation process. Dissecting the disorder—understanding its anatomy, physiology, and process—is fundamental but often fosters emotional isolation from the patient.

Speech Therapy

Speech therapy strives to maximize functional communication in disorders ranging from autism to stroke. Speech–language patholo-gists use assessment tools to devise individual treatment protocols. The approach is based on three major therapy models: classic language-oriented, functional/pragmatic, and cognitive neuropsychology. Each model uses different techniques; therapists often mix the most helpful ones from each model. Meta-analyses support the efficacy of therapy for aphasia but also highlight its limitations.[4,5]

The traditional language-oriented model is most often used. Standard assessment tools, such as the Boston Diagnostic Aphasia Examination[6] and the Minnesota Test for Differential Diagnosis of Aphasia,[7] quantify the range and severity of deficits. Therapies are combined eclectically. For example, intensive multimodal stimulation evokes language in different contexts (situational, linguistic) and with different tasks (phonemic cueing, repetition),[7] or behavioral learning theory is applied therapeutically.[8]

Functional or pragmatic models use spared functions and compensatory strategies to improve verbal or nonverbal communication. For example, a patient may be taught the effective use of head nods, pointing, or short overlearned phrases to communicate needs or feelings.

Cognitive neuropsychology analyzes the language deficit as a disorder of information processing, targeting the impaired architecture of language function. This model can tap different therapeutic approaches but relies on defining the fundamental disorder in neural processing to select a treatment. For example, patients with anomia resulting from disorders in semantic coding may benefit from repetitively matching pictures to semantically related words.[9] In contrast, patients with anomia resulting from impaired phonological processing may respond to such sound-based techniques as repeating a name.[10]

Physical and Occupational Therapy

Physical therapists treat disorders of gross movement, coordination, and sensation resulting from disorders of the CNS and peripheral nervous system, as well as non-neurological systems. Stretching, exercise, and skills development are used to enhance function. Although outside the traditional bounds of behavioral neurology, sensorimotor disorders profoundly influence quality of life and mood.

Occupational therapists treat disorders of fine motor control, such as that used in writing, buttoning clothes, and picking up objects. Problems of spasticity, unsteadiness, weakness, lack of proprioceptive input to guide movement, apraxia, and others require tailored therapy. Occupational therapists often help to assess functional capacities, such as driving a motor vehicle.[11]

Cognitive Therapy

Cognitive remediation develops more adaptive strategies and routines to accommodate and overcome functional limitations. These solutions, which often fall outside the realm of other therapists, tackle problems with sustained and complex attention, learning and memory, abstracting and integrating information, executive function, and behavior (e.g., impulsivity, inability to handle stress, aggressiveness, poor motivation, and disturbed social interactions at home or work). Cognitive remediation can range from completing a paper-and-pencil task to improving visual attention and suppressing impulsive responses to taking clients on shopping trips for systematically approaching issues such as list making, cost, transportation, and item location.[12] Cognitive therapy should begin early after a CNS insult and may continue for years as a person moves from inpatient to outpatient rehabilitation, to community reentry programs, transitional living, and long-term structured programs.

Randomized controlled studies and clinical series support specific recommendations for remediation of language and perception after a stroke in the left and right hemispheres, respectively, and for remediation of attention, memory, functional communication, and executive functioning after traumatic brain injury.[13] Interventions to improve cognition include (1) reinforcing, strengthening, or relearning previously acquired behavioral patterns; (2) establishing or creating new patterns of compensatory cognitive activity by tapping preserved brain functions or external mechanisms (e.g., environmental structuring and support); and (3) enabling persons to understand long-term deficits and adapt to them despite the inability to directly or indirectly compensate for the functional losses.[13] For many patients, this "acceptance of loss" is a critical step in moving forward and letting go of negative emotions. Cognitive rehabilitation develops activities in

naturalistic settings to achieve successful transition into social and occupational roles.[14]

Vocational Rehabilitation

Neurobehavioral disorders compromise the capacity to work. A broad spectrum of behavioral and cognitive problems, such as medication side effects, fatigue, depression, distractibility, impulsivity, inappropriate social interactions, and problems with language and memory, limit employment. Vocational counselors and rehabilitation services can help persons who have never held a job or those who have been out of the work force to train for and get employment that meets their individual needs. Specialized training helps to develop skills, confidence, and strategies to enhance their chances for employment.

The Rehabilitation Act of 1973 provides employment rights for people with disabilities. Vocational services available under this act include diagnostic evaluation; counseling to set goals and determine job-skill training needs; psychological, physical, occupational, and other therapies; training for specific and general job skills; referral to training programs and job experiences; transportation; job placement; postemployment services to help maintain employment and identify needed accommodations; and assistance in working with such agencies as the Social Security Administration, the Department of Social Services, and the Office of Mental Health. States are also required to establish "one-stop shopping" centers so that individuals can have access to job training, education, and related employment services.

Pragmatic Therapeutic Approaches

Simple and practical interventions can be some of the most effective for patients with cognitive or neurobehavioral disorders. In many cases, time, listening, and empathy represent simple but helpful measures. For instance, the physician may recommend a therapist for a patient or the family or prescribe a shoe orthotic to facilitate ambulation. A patient's quality of life may be improved by educating a relative about the disorder. Pragmatic approaches are often helpful in managing aphasia, amnesia, or insomnia (Table 11–2). Taking a detailed sleep history and counseling about sleep hygiene

Table 11–2. **Pragmatic Therapeutic Approaches for Patients and Families**

Aphasia	Amnesia	Insomnia
Eliminate loud noises and other distractions during communication	Use visual imagery (?efficacy in amnesia)	Treat stress or teach stress-reduction methods
Speak slowly	Use lists and schedules, display them prominently	Use relaxation techniques
Use brief sentences and phrases	Use small, portable notepads, organized by topic	Exercise regularly but at least 3–4 hours before bedtime
Avoid complex grammatical constructions	Carry important telephone numbers and addresses	Avoid alcohol, caffeine, cigarettes, diet pills, daytime naps
Look for verbal signs of understanding; do not be fooled by smiles or nods	Teach patient simple, clear note taking	Establish regular sleeping and waking times
Use nonverbal signs to support verbal communication	Date notes only meaningful for short periods	May read but not watch TV before sleep
Use repetition to ensure comprehension	Use a clock or watch alarm as a reminder of certain routines (e.g., when alarm sounds, check time, check notepad for activity scheduled for that time)	Avoid extraneous light and sound in bedroom (e.g., use shades and earplugs)
Use yes-or-no questions to confirm comprehension or to probe incomplete expressions	Avoid ineffective techniques, such as memory exercises and drills (as if memory were a "muscle" or cognitive retraining software packages)	
Offer choices vs. open-ended questions (e.g., ask "Would you like steak or fish for dinner?" but not "What would you like for dinner?")		
Be patient in awaiting a response		

Table 11–3. Guidelines for History Taking in Patients with Sleep Disorders

The problem (as described by the patient, bed partner, or parent)
  Insomnia: disorders of falling asleep and maintaining sleep
  Disorder of excessive somnolence
  Disorder of the sleep–wake cycle
  Dysfunctional sleep, sleep stages, or partial arousal (parasomnia)
The 24-hour sleep–wake cycle: inquire about daytime naps
Onset and duration of the disorder
Life situation: inquire about stress, bedtime anxiety, and ruminations
Medical, neurological, and psychiatric history
Current medications: prescribed and over-the-counter
Alcohol, sedative-hypnotic, or illicit drug use
Family history of sleep disorder

(Table 11–3) may be helpful in combating insomnia, which exacerbates cognitive and behavioral disorders.

COEXISTING PSYCHIATRIC AND NEUROLOGICAL DISORDERS

Depression, anxiety, psychosis, impulsiveness, and aggression commonly complicate neurological disease. These problems also exist as primary psychiatric disorders, often with hereditable components that interface with acquired brain disorders. Defining the anatomical sites and physiological mechanisms underlying psychiatric problems in neurological disorders may advance the understanding of primary psychiatric disorders and guide therapy.

Therapy for behavioral symptoms may improve the speed of recovery, cognitive function, quality of life, independence, and survival.[15–19] For example, stroke is the third leading cause of death in America and injures 600,000 brains each year. Many classic syndromes, such as the aphasias and apraxias, were originally described in stroke patients. Therapy for these syndromes remains elusive, while common behavioral complications—depression, anxiety, apathy, psychosis, pathological affect, and fatigue—are treatable.

Depression

Depression impairs quality of life in many patients with neurological diseases.[20–22] Depression is highly treatable and often underdiagnosed. Many medical and most brain disorders are associated with depression (Table 11–4). Among these are brain stem disorders (e.g., Parkinson's disease, progressive supranuclear palsy, narcolepsy), diencephalic disorders (e.g., stroke, tumor), and cortical disorders (e.g., stroke, tumor, Alzheimer's disease). Depression results from biological, psychological, and genetic factors.

Clinicians and patients often falsely accept depression as a normal response to disease. Identifying and addressing situational contributors to depression is essential, but pharmacological therapy is warranted for patients with reactive as well as endogenous depression. The goal of treatment is full remission of depressive symptoms.

The physician should see the "big picture" of the patient's life, that is, know the patient's living and family circumstances, educational and occupational status, and how his or her days are spent in routine and leisure activities. The context of a patient's day-to-day life helps to target symptoms; it is also therapeutic for a patient to know that the physician cares about his or her life. For instance, patients who are depressed, anxious, in pain, physically disabled, apathetic, or chronically fatigued may become socially isolated. Social isolation may also reflect the withdrawal of social support due to a patient's irritability, aggressiveness, or other inappropriate behavior. In this case, familiarity with the patient's circumstances enables the physician to address the social isolation by prescribing a drug to control the aggression rather than an antidepressant. Referral to social services and patient advocacy or support groups is also important.

To assess depression, start by asking about vegetative symptoms (Table 11–5). For many patients (and clinicians), it is easier to discuss sleep and eating changes and loss of interest in formerly pleasurable activities than to talk about mood and internal feelings. Knowledge of specific vegetative signs also may influence the choice of first-line treatment. However, vegetative symptoms are nonspecific and found in patients with medical and neurological disorders. Inquire about affective, cognitive–psy-

Table 11–4. **Disorders Associated with Depression**

Medical Disorders	Neurological Disorders	Adverse Effect of Drugs	Nutritional Deficiencies
Cancer	Brain tumor	Antiepileptics	Folate
Lung	Degenerative disease	Antihypertensives	Iron
Pancreatic	Alzheimer's disease,	β-blockers	Pyridoxine
Cardiovascular disorders	other dementias	Clonidine	(vitamin B_6)
Congestive heart failure	Parkinson's disease	Reserpine	Thiamine (vitamin B_1)
Myocardial infarction	Progressive	Cytotoxic drugs	Vitamin B_{12}
Endocrine disorders	supranuclear palsy	Drugs of abuse	
Addison's disease	Encephalitis	Alcohol	
Cushing's syndrome	Epilepsy	Phencyclidine	
Diabetes mellitus	Huntington's disease	Marijuana	
Glucocorticoid withdrawal	Migraine	Amphetamines	
Hyperparathyroidism	Multiple sclerosis	Cocaine	
Hyperthyroidism	Sleep disorders	Opiates	
Hypoglycemia	Sleep apnea	Glucocorticoids	
Hypoparathyroidism	Narcolepsy	Levodopa	
Hypothyroidism	Stroke	Oral contraceptives	
Ovarian failure	Wilson's disease	Phenothiazines	
Testicular failure		Sedative-hypnotics	
Immune system disorders		Benzodiazepines	
Acquired immunodeficiency		Barbiturates	
syndrome			
Hepatitis			
Infectious diseases			
Influenza			
Lyme disease			
Mononucleosis			
Rheumatoid arthritis			
Sjögren syndrome			
Systemic lupus			
erythematosus			
Tuberculosis			

chological, and somatic symptoms. Ask about suicidal feelings or past suicide attempts. Social isolation, poor social support, substance abuse, and recent stressful life events all increase a patient's suicide risk. The actively suicidal patient may need immediate hospitalization. Since psychosis can complicate depression, inquire about hallucinations and somatic or paranoid delusions.

Depression frequently complicates subcortical and cortical disorders. The correlation of cortical lesion location and depression frequency and severity is unclear. Many studies report a significant correlation between poststroke depression and left anterior hemispheric or basal ganglia strokes.[15,23–26] However, other studies and meta-analyses clearly do not support either the left-sided or the anterior local-

ization of poststroke depression.[27,28] Lesion location does not appear to influence the efficacy or tolerability of therapy for poststroke depression. Sexual dysfunction in stroke patients may occur more frequently with left-sided lesions and is often associated with depression.[29] Treatment of poststroke depression improves sexual function in many patients.

The relation between stroke and depression may be bidirectional. Depression predicts a greater risk of stroke in both sexes and different ethnic groups.[30] Many older persons with depression beginning in later life may have subclinical strokes that spare sensorimotor areas; the ischemic brain changes may contribute to depression.[31] However, the existence of a "vascular depression" resulting from small vessel disease remains unproven.

Table 11–5. Clinical Manifestations of Depression

Affective	Cognitive–Psychological	Psychotic	Somatic	Vegetative
Anxiety	Guilt	Delusions (somatic, paranoid)	Gastrointestinal complaints	Appetite decreased or increased; weight decreased or increased
Feeling "blue"	Helplessness	Hallucinations (usually auditory)	Pain	
Inability to enjoy life (anhedonia)	Hopelessness		Headache	
Irritability	Impaired attention		Back pain	Constipation
Sadness	Impaired memory, concentration, or decisiveness		Other	Fatigue or lack of energy (anergia)
	Obsessive thoughts			Libido decreased
	Social withdrawal			Psychomotor retardation or, occasionally, agitation
	Suicidal ideation			Sleep decreased or increased
	Worthlessness			Morning worsening of mood

TYPES OF DEPRESSION

Depression may be unipolar or bipolar. Unipolar disorders are subcategorized into major depression (severe depression lasting at least 2 weeks), dysthymic disorder (a lower-grade depression lasting at least 2 years), and depression not otherwise specified ("clinically significant" depression that does not fit into another category). In DSM-IV, mood disorders are segregated into "primary" psychiatric disorders and those due to a "general medical condition" when there is evidence "that the disturbance is the direct physiological consequence of a general medical condition." Since primary depression has a substantial biological basis and the etiology of psychiatric manifestations of neurological diseases is poorly understood, such a distinction is of uncertain meaning for neuropsychiatric conditions.

There are few differences in response to therapy between the different types of primary psychiatric depression. Notably, depressed patients with bipolar disorder may exhibit mania with antidepressant medication, particularly without a mood-stabilizing agent (e.g., lithium, carbamazepine, lamotrigine, or valproate). Antiepileptic drugs can benefit patients with bipolar depression, but antiepileptic drugs have no established role in unipolar depression.[32] Benzodiazepines have limited antidepressant[33] and antimanic[34] properties. Dysthymia can be more difficult to treat than severe depression. Patients with "atypical depression" are distinguished by greater mood reactivity and a tendency to overeat, gain weight, and oversleep. These patients may respond to monoamine oxidase inhibitors (MAOIs) when other treatments fail.[35]

PSYCHOLOGICAL THERAPY FOR DEPRESSION

Various psychological therapies, including supportive counseling, cognitive–behavioral therapy, interpersonal therapy, or dynamic psychotherapy, may help depressed patients, particularly in preventing relapse. Randomized controlled trials show the efficacy of short-term, focused psychotherapy for mildly to moderately depressed patients.[36] However, antidepressant medication should be a part of treatment for severely depressed patients. The beneficial effect of offering the patient encouragement, support, and a sympathetic ear is immeasurable.

PHARMACOLOGICAL THERAPY FOR DEPRESSION

The use of antidepressant medications to treat neurological disorders is based mainly on data from primary mood disorders since there are few well-designed randomized controlled trials in neurological populations. Antidepressants from multiple classes are effective at treating depression in dementia,[37,38] traumatic brain injury,[39] Parkinson's disease,[40] and stroke.[41,42] The response rate to antidepressants does not differ between demented and nondemented elderly.[43]

Stroke provides a well-studied model of depression complicating a neurological disorder. Depression occurs in 20%–50% of stroke patients and often goes undiagnosed.[15,19,44] The prevalence of poststroke depression varies in different settings: in acute stroke (major depression, 22%; minor depression, 17%), rehabilitation (major depression, 23%; minor depression, 35%), and the community (major depression, 13%; minor depression, 10%).[19,41,44] Although most often recognized in the acute or subacute setting, a new peak incidence of depression may occur 2–3 years after a stroke.[45]

The first line of therapy for most patients with poststroke depression is an SSRI, but the efficacy and safety of any specific SSRI have not been proven.[42] Drug interactions are more likely with fluoxetine, fluvoxamine, and paroxetine than with citalopram, ascitalopram, or sertraline. Fluoxetine's long half-life (>24 hours) is an advantage during tapering off since it reduces the frequency of withdrawal symptoms. However, a long half-life is a disadvantage if the patient cannot tolerate the drug or experiences an adverse drug interaction. Tricyclic antidepressants are effective for poststroke depression,[46] but their anticholinergic properties and potential cardiac toxicity make them second-line agents (Table 11–6). Trazodone is also effective but may cause sedation, hypotension, or priapism.[47]

Initial therapy for poststroke depression should be based on the specific neurological disorder, comorbid medical disorders, and the patient's tolerance of side effects. In most cases, a favorable profile of side effects and safety in overdosage makes an SSRI the first-

Table 11–6. **Effects of Tricyclic Antidepressants**

	MODE OF ACTION	
Effect	**Receptor Blockade**	**Reuptake Inhibition**
Beneficial Effect		
Antidepressant	$5\text{-}HT_1$, $5\text{-}HT_{2A}$, $?\alpha_1$	NE, 5-HT, DA
Anxiolytic	$5\text{-}HT_1$, $5\text{-}HT_{2C}$	5-HT
Antiobsessive–compulsive		5-HT
Antipsychotic	D_2, $5\text{-}HT_2$	
Improved sleep	H_1, α_1, $5\text{-}HT_2$	
Antiaggressive	$5\text{-}HT_1$	
Antimigraine	$5\text{-}HT_2$	
Adverse Effect		
Cardiac		
Contraindicated with heart block or post-myocardial infarction		
Tachycardia	ACh, α_1	NE
Arrhythmia and QRS changes, most frequent in elderly, children, or overdosage; obtain EKG before use in elderly and children°	ACh	
Orthostatic hypotension, mainly in elderly	α_1, H_1	
Visual		
Dry eyes, most bothersome to contact lens wearers	ACh	
Blurred vision	ACh	
Increased intraocular pressure in unsuspected narrow-angle glaucoma	ACh	

(*Continued on following page*)

Table 11–6.—*continued*

| Effect | MODE OF ACTION | |
	Receptor Blockade	Reuptake Inhibition
Gastrointestinal		
Discomfort, nausea		5-HT
Dry mouth, may lead to tooth decay, often resolves after weeks, sugarless lozenges offer symptomatic relief	ACh	
Constipation	ACh	
Urinary		
Difficulty initiating and maintaining urinary stream and retention, especially in men with enlarged prostate	ACh	
Weight gain	H_1, 5-HT_2	
?From carbohydrate craving and slowed metabolism; desipramine and protriptyline are least likely to cause weight gain		
Anorexia		5-HT
Sexual		
Variable effects, common with clomipramine and imipramine; buproprion and mirtazapine are unlikely to cause sexual dysfunction and may be used for long-term therapy		
Decreased libido		5-HT
Impotence	5-HT_2, α_2, D_2	NE, 5-HT
Inability to ejaculate or painful ejaculation	α_2	NE
Central nervous system		
Sedation	H_1, α_1, 5-HT_2	
Dizziness	α_1, H_1, ACh	
Tremor	D_2	NE
Memory impairment	ACh	
Can cause delirium when combined with other drugs, especially in the elderly		
Anxiety		5-HT
Seizures		
Rare, usually with high doses in predisposed persons	?H_1, ?ACh, ?D_2	
Insomnia		NE
Sweating		NE
Headache		5-HT
Psychomotor activation, aggravation of psychosis		DA
Overdosage		
Dangerous in patients with cardiac arrhythmias or seizures; a week's supply of full-dose amitriptyline is potentially lethal		
Blocks Na^+ channels	ACh	

α, adrenergic receptor; ACh, acetylcholine (muscarinic receptor); D, dopamine receptor; DA, dopamine; 5-HT, 5-hydroxytryptamine (serotonin); H_1, histamine receptor type 1; EKG, electrocardiogram; ?, possible effect.
*Desipramine is most cardiotoxic in children.

line treatment (Table 11–7). However, a tricyclic antidepressant is the medication of choice for patients with nocturia, insomnia, and comorbid headaches who are not at risk for suicide and have no cardiac disease. The patient's or a first-degree family member's history of treatment for depression is important. The patient's historic response to or the efficacy of a specific antidepressant in a first-degree relative supports the use of that agent. Assess the adequacy of the patient's previous medication trials. Ideally, in a minimally adequate trial, medication is taken for 6 weeks in at least the maximum dose specified in the *Physician's Desk Reference*. Elderly patients often require lower doses. When depression is moderate to severe and little or no response is seen after 3–4 weeks, another agent may be considered. Unpleasant side effects such as dizziness, nausea, or sweating often precede therapeutic effects and frequently subside in the first weeks of treatment; counsel patients to assure adequate trials. Starting medication at a low dose may reduce the frequency or severity of side effects. If psychosis develops in a depressed patient, use both an antidepressant and an antipsychotic.

If the patient's depression is only partially relieved after 4–6 weeks of taking a standard dose of an antidepressant, consider increasing the dose or adding another agent. An antidepressant from another class may be added to the initial agent. In refractory cases, an atypical antipsychotic agent may be used. Lithium and thyroid hormone may be used as adjunctive treatments. However, minimize polypharmacy and taper off ineffective agents.

If the depression shows no response to the combination therapy, try another medication. It is advisable to select another antidepressant from a different class, although depression may respond to one agent but not another from the same class. Successful treatment of depression may involve serial trials of multiple agents alone or in combination.

Apathy, a common symptom of depression, may occur without depression. In patients with neurodegenerative disorders, apathy correlates with cognitive dysfunction rather than depression.[48] Dopaminergic agents may improve apathy in Parkinson's disease and akinetic mutism. Stimulants are used to treat amotivational states, but their efficacy is unproven.

ELECTROCONVULSIVE THERAPY

Electroconvulsive therapy (ECT) is the most rapid and effective treatment for mood disorders with or without psychosis.[49] Results of ECT in schizophrenia are variable.[50] It is used from adolescence to senescence and in patients with diverse medical and neurological disorders (e.g., during pregnancy, after stroke or traumatic brain injury, Parkinson's disease, progressive supranuclear palsy). More than 60% of depressed patients who have not responded to medications respond to ECT. However, in spite of its efficacy in depression, ECT is limited by its cognitive side effects.[51]

The overall safety of ECT is very good, especially when the risk–benefit ratio is considered in treatment-refractory patients (e.g., high risk of suicide). Common side effects of ECT are a transient retrograde amnesia during the course of treatment, headache, and muscle aches. Major limitations are high relapse rates, treatment-emergent delirium, and sometimes severe retrograde amnesia. Unilateral, right-sided ECT has fewer effects on memory and is probably as efficacious as bilateral ECT.[52] Serious cardiovascular effects are rare.

POTENTIAL THERAPIES FOR DEPRESSION

Transcranial magnetic stimulation (TMS) is a noninvasive technique in which a pulsed magnetic field creates current flow in cortical neurons and temporarily excites or inhibits specific areas.[53] This current flow influences neuronal activity locally and at distant sites.[54] In the motor cortex, TMS may evoke a muscle twitch or inhibit movement; TMS of the occipital cortex may produce visual phosphenes or scotomas.[53] This technique is used extensively to study sensorimotor and cognitive physiology.[53,55] The prolonged alteration of neuronal activity by TMS offers the potential for therapy. Preliminary studies suggest a therapeutic effect of repetitive TMS in depression, epilepsy, and other neuropsychiatric disorders. Most research has focused on depression. Although controlled clinical studies have reported some benefit of repetitive TMS for depression,[54] its antidepressant efficacy is not established.

Another therapy with antidepressant potential is vagus nerve stimulation, in which the

Table 11–7. Guidelines for Selecting Antidepressants

Depression Type/Comorbid Disorder	First-Line Agent	Comments
Dysthymia	SSRIs	MAOIs are as effective as SSRIs, but their safety profile is poorer; antidepressants may be less effective for dysthymia than major depression
Major depression	SSRIs	All other antidepressants are as effective as SSRIs, so the profile of adverse effects largely determines the medication choice; family or personal history of response to antidepressants may guide selection
Atypical depression*	SSRIs	MAOIs may be more effective than SSRIs, but their safety profile is poorer
Delusional depression	Antidepressant plus low doses of an antipsychotic	Electroconvulsive therapy is an effective alternative
Bipolar disorder	Mood stabilizer (lithium, carbamazepine, valproate, lamotrigine) with or without atypical antipsychotic (e.g., olanzapine)	An antidepressant may be added to mood stabilizer to treat depression and is often discontinued when depressive symptoms abate; all antidepressants can provoke mania, but the risk is presumably lower with bupropion
Mania	Lithium, carbamazepine, valproate, lamotrigine, or atypical antipsychotic	—
Refractory depression	MAOIs, electroconvulsive therapy	Determine if the original diagnosis is correct, standard antidepressants were maximized, and compliance is good; consider trying another antidepressant augmented with a combination of antidepressants, lithium, or thyroid hormone
Comorbid psychiatric disorders		
OCD	SSRIs	—
Eating disorders	SSRIs	Amitriptyline, desipramine, imipramine
Social phobia	SSRIs	—
Anxiety, panic disorder	SSRIs	Clomipramine, desipramine, doxepin, imipramine; bupropion and trazodone are not effective for panic disorder
Comorbid neurological disorders		
Epilepsy	SSRIs	Venlafaxine, mirtazapine, and tricyclic antidepressants are alternatives (avoid

Condition	Recommended	Notes / Alternatives
		bupropion, clomipramine, maprotiline)
Parkinson's disease	SSRIs	Tricyclic antidepressant, bupropion
Stroke	SSRIs	Nortriptyline, trazodone, CNS stimulants
Migraine (prophylaxis)	Amitriptyline, nortriptyline	SSRIs are effective alternatives for associated depression but do not improve headache
Chronic pain (fibromyalgia)	Amitriptyline, doxepin, desipramine, nortriptyline, or imipramine	SSRIs are effective alternatives for associated depression but do not improve pain
Cataplexy	Protriptyline, clomipramine, desipramine, or imipramine	—
Other comorbid disorders		
Cardiovascular disease	Fluoxetine, sertraline, paroxetine, bupropion, nortriptyline, or desipramine	—
Cancer		
Normal appetite and weight	SSRIs or bupropion	—
Anorexia and weight loss	Nortriptyline or other tricyclic antidepressant	—
Nausea with chemotherapy	Nortriptyline	—
Chronic diarrhea	Doxepin or trimipramine	—
Peptic ulcer	Doxepin, nortriptyline, imipramine	—
Urticaria, pruritis	Doxepine, nortriptyline	—
Angle-closure glaucoma	SSRIs or bupropion	Nefazodone is an alternative
Erectile dysfunction	Bupropion	Mirtazapine is an alternative
Anorgasmia	Bupropion or desipramine	Mirtazapine is an alternative

MAOIs, monoamine oxidase inhibitors; OCD, obsessive–compulsive disorder; SSRIs, selective serotonin reuptake inhibitors; CNS, central nervous system.

[a] Atypical depression is marked by a transient improvement in mood with environmental stimuli and two of the following: weight gain or increased appetite, leaden "paralysis," hypersomnia, oversensitivity.

vagus nerve on the left side is repetitively stimulated electrically by a programmable stimulator implanted in the left upper chest. In an open pilot study of vagus nerve stimulation in treatment-resistant depression,[56] approximately one-third of patients improved and patients who had never received ECT were 3.9 times more likely to respond. A randomized blinded study found no significant benefit for low-current vagus nerve stimulation in depressed patients (J.B. Bruins, Cyberonics, personal communication, 2001).

Anxiety

Anxiety and fear are common emotions in response to such physical symptoms as muscle tension, tremor, difficulty breathing, increased heart and respiratory rate, diaphoresis, and abdominal sensations. Anxiety naturally results from distressing experiences. Situational anxiety is short-lived and related to stressful stimuli. Knowledge of a potentially stressful situation can reduce its negative impact. Phobic anxiety is a form of situational anxiety where avoidance is the primary method of coping. Systematic desensitization (i.e., progressive exposure to stimuli) may be helpful. Anticipatory anxiety may exist before actual exposure to a feared stimulus or setting. Posttraumatic anxiety occurs in those who survive intense and uncontrollable natural (e.g., earthquake) or human-made (e.g., rape, war) disasters. Anxiety complicates medical, neurological, and psychiatric disorders and may be a side effect of pharmacological therapy (Table 11–8).

Therapeutic listening and supportive psychotherapy may help patients vent their feelings and understand the biological and environmental causes of their anxiety disorder. Dynamic or behavioral psychological therapy can identify provocative factors and help to target therapy. Cognitive–behavioral therapies improve self-confidence and coping by reducing mental and physical tension and avoidance. Education and systematic desensitization with a hierarchy of exposure to feared sensations with imaginary and real stimuli, as well as breathing and relaxation techniques, are mainstays of treatment. Medi-

Table 11–8. **Disorders Associated with Anxiety**

Medical Disorders	Neurological Disorders	Adverse Effect of Drugs
AIDS	Alzheimer's disease	CNS stimulants
Angina	Brain tumor	Caffeine
Asthma	Epilepsy	Methylphenidate
Carcinoid	Ictal	Akathisia
Cardiac arrhythmia	Postictal	Dopamine receptor
Congestive heart failure	Interictal	blockers
Hypercalcemia, parathyroid disease	Huntington's disease	CNS depressant
Hypercortisolism, Cushing's syndrome	Meniere's disease	withdrawal
Hyperglycemia, diabetes mellitus	Parkinson's disease	Alcohol
Hyperthyroidism	Stroke	Barbiturates
Hypothyroidism		Benzodiazepines
Hypoglycemia		
Hypoxia		
Mitral valve prolapse		
Pain		
Pheochromocytoma		
Porphyria		
Premenstrual symptoms		
Pulmonary embolism		
Systemic lupus erythematosus		

AIDS, acquired immunodeficiency syndrome; CNS, central nervous system.

tation, biofeedback, exercise, and yoga are also helpful. The role of nonpharmacological therapies for anxiety disorders associated with neurological disease has not been well studied.

A dangerous cycle can develop when a benzodiazepine is used for the long-term treatment of anxiety or insomnia. Initially, the drug works extremely well, but as tolerance develops, symptoms recur and the dose is further increased. As further tolerance develops, patients want to increase the dose as this invariably improves symptoms. Eventually, a high dose is reached, and cognitive and behavioral toxicity are severe but difficult to trace to the benzodiazepine because it is often combined with other psychotropic medications and because other disorders (e.g., depression) that cause similar problems may coexist.

Anxiety disorders are the most common psychiatric illnesses and often complicate neurological disorders affecting limbic areas or stressing a patient's physical and emotional well-being. Anxiety symptoms comprise four broad categories: panic attacks, phobias, obsessive–compulsive symptoms, and generalized anxiety.

PANIC DISORDER

Panic attacks are discrete episodes of intense fear, dysphoria, and physical discomfort (e.g., palpitations, tachycardia, sweating, tremor, numbness, chest discomfort, dizziness, shortness of breath, choking), typically lasting 5–30 minutes. The attacks may be spontaneous or situational. Fear in a simple partial seizure typically lasts less than 3 minutes, which helps to distinguish the seizure from a panic attack. Panic disorder is characterized by recurrent panic attacks.

The first-line therapy for panic disorder is an SSRI.[57] A very low dose of an SSRI is used initially and gradually increased to control the "jitteriness" that can complicate early therapy. The tricyclic imipramine is the drug most extensively studied for panic disorder. The usual starting dose of 25–50 mg/day is gradually increased to 100–300 mg/day. Other tricyclic antidepressants and benzodiazepines also may be effective. Often, a benzodiazepines (e.g., clonazepam, lorazepam) is used briefly until the optimal antidepressant dose is achieved. Panic symptoms also respond to MAOIs. Buspirone does not prevent panic attacks.

PHOBIAS

A *phobia* is a persistent and irrational fear of a specific object, situation, or activity that leads to a strong desire to avoid the feared stimulus. Phobic disorders include specific phobias (e.g., a certain type of animal, blood, heights, crowded public places) and social phobias, persistent and intense situational anxiety regarding social settings (e.g., performance in the presence of strangers or when closely observed by others). Disorders such as Tourette's syndrome or temporal lobe epilepsy, as well as lesions of the frontal or temporal lobes, basal ganglia, or thalamus, are associated with phobias.[58–60] Social phobias often improve with SSRIs and benzodiazepines; MAOIs are effective but more toxic. Gabapentin may be effective in some patients.

OBSESSIVE–COMPULSIVE DISORDER

Obsessive–compulsive disorder (OCD) is characterized by recurrent and troublesome thoughts and actions. *Obsessions* are undesired and often disturbing thoughts or images that cannot be excluded from awareness. Obsessive thoughts often relate to themes of contamination, morality/religion, health/illness, orderliness, sex/shameful acts, and aggression. Compulsive acts are repetitive, stereotyped, anxiety-reducing ritualistic behaviors that are driven from within and often linked to obsessive thoughts. Compulsive acts commonly relate to cleaning, counting, checking, and dressing (particular sequence, laying out, or appearance of clothing). Attempts to control the obsessions and compulsions often fail and cause anxiety. While the DSM-IV criteria require patients' insight into the dysfunctional nature of their symptoms, patients with brain diseases and secondary OCD may have less insight than other patients.

Primary OCD is associated with hypermetabolism in the orbitofrontal cortex, caudate, and anterior cingulate cortex.[61] Obsessions and compulsions often exist in neurological disorders affecting the prefrontal, anterior cingulate, and temporal cortex and the basal ganglia.[62,63] These include inflammatory and autoimmune disorders such as pediatric autoimmune neuropsychiatric disorders associated with streptococcal infection[64] as well as dementias,[65] Parkinson's and Huntington's diseases, tics, Tourette's syndrome (see Chapter 7),[66] and stroke. While patients with primary OCD often obsess on contamination, Tourette's patients often focus on symmetry and getting things "just right."[67]

Initially, OCD is treated with SSRIs or clomipramine. In patients with comorbid neurological disorders, SSRIs are preferred owing to the anticholinergic and other side effects of tricyclic antidepressants. The dosage of SSRIs for OCD is higher than that for depression. If initial therapy fails, another SSRI or clomipramine should be tried. Buspirone or low-dose antipsychotics can augment the response to these agents.

Behavioral and cognitive approaches to OCD are effective for some patients.[68] Therapeutic approaches may be combined, as in exposure procedures to reduce anxiety in obsessions and response prevention to reduce the frequency of obsessions and compulsions.

GENERALIZED ANXIETY DISORDER

Generalized anxiety disorder is characterized by excessive worry or anxiety that is difficult to control volitionally and occurs on a majority of days for 6 months or longer. Common symptoms are nervousness, easy fatigability, impaired concentration, irritability, muscle tension, and sleep difficulties. Shortly after a stroke, nearly one-third of patients experience generalized anxiety disorder, and the incidence declines only modestly after 3 years.[24] Major depression is often a comorbid disorder, and generalized anxiety disorder worsens the prognosis of depression. Acutely, the incidence of generalized anxiety disorder with depression may be higher in patients with left hemispheric strokes, while anxiety occurs more often with right hemispheric lesions.[24]

Buspirone is effective for generalized anxiety disorder and causes less sedation, psychomotor slowing, and addiction than benzodiazepines. The onset of buspirone action is delayed for 1–3 weeks, while benzodiazepines work within hours. Paroxetine, sertraline, and venlafaxine are also approved for treating generalized anxiety disorder. Imipramine or an SSRI other than paroxetine or sertaline helps some patients. Depression or panic disorder is often comorbid with generalized anxiety disorder and should be treated first.

Benzodiazepines prevent and treat generalized and anticipatory anxiety, as well as panic attacks and phobias. Alprazolam is the drug most extensively studied, but other benzodiazepines are effective and have a longer half-life than alprazolam and, therefore, less abuse potential and fewer withdrawal symptoms.

Benzodiazepines (e.g., chlorazepate, clobazam, clonazepam, diazepam, lorazepam) are anxiolytic and sedative-hypnotic agents. The sedation, cognitive impairment (attention, memory, executive functions), ataxia, tolerance, and dependence associated with benzodiazepines limit their usefulness. Children are more subject than adults to the adverse psychotropic effects of benzodiazepines, including hyperactivity, restlessness, irritability, disruptiveness, depression, and aggressiveness. However, a randomized controlled trial found similar cognitive function among children receiving clobazam or carbamazepine alone.[69] Rapid withdrawal of benzodiazepines, especially after long-term use, may produce severe behavioral reactions, including anxiety, insomnia, delirium, psychosis, and seizures.[70]

Psychosis

Psychosis encompasses a broad and elusive mental expanse. Common features include impaired content and coherence of thought, reduced connection to reality, hallucinations, delusions, disorganized speech and behavior, and extremes of affect and motivation. The diagnosis of psychosis can be difficult as many patients actively hide their aberrant behavior and delusional beliefs and others are "quietly psychotic," showing only quirky mannerisms. Psychotic symptoms are divided into positive and negative categories. John Hughlings Jackson viewed positive symptoms as "release phenomena" generated by preserved brain areas and negative symptoms as "dissolution" or loss of function.[71] Positive symptoms include hallucinations; delusions; aggression; tangential, incoherent speech and thought; as well as exaggerated, bizarre, or disorganized behaviors. Negative symptoms include *alogia* (poverty of speech or speech content), flattened affect, social withdrawal, anhedonia, apathy, and impaired attention and self-monitoring.

Psychosis occurs in patients with such pri-

Table 11–9. **Disorders Associated with Psychosis**

Medical Disorders	Neurological Disorders	Adverse Effect of Drugs
Autoimmune disease	Brain tumor	Alcohol
Systemic lupus erythematosus	Dementia	Anticholinergics
Paraneoplastic limbic encephalitis	Alzheimer's disease	CNS stimulants
Hyperthyroidism	Frontotemporal dementia	Cocaine
Hypothyroidism	Encephalitis	Hallucinogens
Cushing's syndrome	AIDS	Lysergic acid diethylamide
Addison's disease	Neurosyphilis	Phencyclidine
	Epilepsy	Psilocybin
	Ictal (rare)	Levodopa
	Interictal	
	Postictal	
	Huntington's disease	
	Parkinson's disease	
	Stroke	

AIDS, acquired immunodeficiency syndrome; CNS, central nervous system.

mary psychiatric disorders as schizophrenia and major depression and complicates many neurological disorders. Psychosis may coexist with endocrine disorders or arise secondary to the side effects of medications (Table 11–9). Identifying and treating the underlying cause are critical. Regardless of the cause, however, psychosis is associated with a higher incidence of suicide, mortality, and violent behavior.[72]

Psychosis is treated primarily with dopamine receptor blockers; i.e., the conventional and atypical antipsychotic drugs. The dopamine receptor blockers are most effective for positive symptoms such as hallucinations and delusions. The atypical antipsychotic drugs are more effective than conventional agents for negative symptoms. Although blockade of D_2 dopamine receptors occurs within hours, antipsychotic action takes days or weeks, which suggests that changes in dopamine receptor affinity or secondary effects are important. For acutely psychotic and agitated patients, the combination of a high-potency antipsychotic agent and a benzodiazepine is often effective. Lack of insight, denial of illness, and disorganized thought often lead to noncompliance. The role of ECT in refractory psychosis is controversial, unless the psychosis complicates major depression.[73] Psychosocial intervention is essential since high stress levels exacerbate psychosis. Social skills training and promotion of vocational and independent living skills help to restore a patient's reentry into the community.

Impulsivity

Impulsive actions are poorly conceived, prematurely expressed, unduly risky, or inappropriate to the situation; they often result in undesirable outcomes.[74] Frontal lobe dysfunction impairs the capacity to inhibit stimulus-bound behavior and assess long-term consequences of actions, leading to impulsivity.[75] Impulsivity is prominent in psychiatric disorders with prefrontal dysfunction, including disorders of impulse control (e.g., intermittent explosive disorder, pyromania, kleptomania, pathological gambling, and trichotillomania), paraphilias, sexual compulsions and addictions, personality disorders (e.g., borderline, antisocial, histrionic, and narcissistic behavior), substance use disorders, and bipolar disorder.[76,77]

Impulsive actions may be physically dangerous and socially disabling. After a right hemispheric stroke, impulsivity accounted for more than 75% of the risk for falls in an inpatient rehabilitation study. Impaired attention or perception, hemispatial neglect, and other factors accounted for less than 25% of the risk.[78] Just as impulsivity can cause a patient to get out of bed too quickly and fall, it can also foster dangerous driving, alcohol and drug consumption, and failure to use such precautions as wearing a bicycle helmet or a condom. Impulsivity also has social consequences, as exemplified by the following incident:

A 30-year-old man was shot in the frontal region, and after prolonged rehabilitation, the only sequelae were behavioral changes. After extensive vocational training, he was hired as a department store sales clerk. A frustrated woman finally made it through the checkout line to the cash register and voiced her displeasure. The patient replied that she would "be better off exercising your fat body than your fat mouth." He was fired. After additional counseling and taking buspirone, he is employed.

Impulsivity results from abnormalities in serotonergic,[76] dopaminergic, and noradrenergic[79] activity, as well as orbitofrontal dysfunction. Cognitive–behavioral therapies reduce impulsive tendencies. Impulsivity may be improved by SSRIs,[75,76] stimulants,[79] α_2-adrenergic blockers (e.g., clonidine),[80] antipsychotic drugs (e.g., olanzapine),[81] and anxiolytics (e.g., buspirone).[82] Drug selection is directed by the underlying disorder. When impulsivity complicates OCD, SSRIs are used. Stimulants and α_2-adrenergic blockers are used when impulsivity complicates attention-deficit hyperactivity disorder (ADHD). Antipsychotics are used in refractory cases of impulsivity and to treat psychosis or aggressive behavior.

Aggression

Therapy for aggressive behavior must address interacting biological and environmental causes. Environmental factors include physical abuse or witnessing intrafamily violence in childhood,[83] lower socioeconomic status, physical crowding, and higher environmental temperature. Biological factors include genetics; hormones (e.g., hypercortisolism, hyperthyroidism, hyperandrogenemia), low serotonin levels in the CNS, limbic disorders (e.g., postictal state, see Chapter 10), mental retardation, stroke, delirium, dementia, brain tumor, encephalitis, psychiatric disorders (e.g., schizophrenia, mania), and legal or illegal drugs (e.g., alcohol, phencyclidine, amphetamines, cocaine). Pathological aggression is a long-standing response pattern that often occurs at home or work, settings with strong emotional valence. Counseling and behavioral therapies are helpful. Behavior modification techniques may reduce aggression in patients with pervasive developmental delay, mental retardation, personality disorder, conduct disorder, and dementia.[84–86] Music diminishes aggression in dementia.[87]

Pharmacological therapy reduces aggression in neurological and psychiatric patients (Table 11–10). The comparative efficacy of the different antipsychotic agents for treating aggressive behavior is unexplored, but the atypical antipsychotics have a more favorable side-effect profile, including a reduced likelihood of adverse extrapyramidal effects. Randomized controlled trials often limited in size and power support the efficacy of risperidone, olanzapine, carbamazepine, estrogen, and metrifonate for dementia;[85,88–92] clonidine and CNS stimulants for ADHD with comorbid aggressive, oppositional, defiant behavior or conduct disorder;[79] risperidone for conduct disorder;[93,94] risperidone, buspirone, and lithium for mental retardation;[95–97] valproate for borderline personality disorder;[98] pindolol for violence in schizophrenia;[99,100] risperidone and fluvoxamine for pervasive developmental delay and autism;[101,102] fluoxetine for impulsive aggression in personality disorders;[103] and propranolol for traumatic brain injury.[104] Valproate and carbamazepine are often used in patients with dementia, organic brain syndromes, and mental retardation,[105] with dosages and plasma drug levels similar to those required for the treatment of epilepsy. Although benzodiazepines are often useful in managing acute agitation and aggression and may benefit some patients with chronic aggressive tendencies, these drugs may cause disinhibition and increased aggression, an effect similar to that of alcohol.[106]

PHARMACOLOGICAL THERAPY

Tricyclic Antidepressants

Tricyclic antidepressants were the most commonly prescribed antidepressant drugs for three decades but recently have been displaced by SSRIs. Tricyclic antidepressants effectively treat major depression, whether primary or secondary to neurological disorders (e.g., stroke, Parkinson's disease). They also effectively treat migraine, neuropathic and chronic pain syndromes, panic attacks, generalized anxiety disorder, anorexia, bulimia nervosa,

Table 11–10. **Therapy for Agitation and Aggression**

Drug Class	Adult Dose, Oral (mg/day)	Adverse Effects
Antiepileptics		
Carbamazepine (Tegretol, 100, 200 mg; Tegretol XR, 100, 200, 400 mg; Carbatrol, 200, 300 mg)	600–1600	Nausea, dizziness, blurred or double vision, tiredness, headache, hyponatremia, dysarthria, rash, fever, bone loss, low white blood cell count
Valproate (Depakote, 125, 250, 500; 250, 500 mg ER)	750–3000	Nausea, dizziness, tiredness, tremor, weight gain, hair loss, rash (rare), low platelet count, polycystic ovarian syndrome, bone loss, liver damage (rare)
Antimania Agent		
Lithium (Eskalith, 300, 450 mg ER)	1200–2400 (acute) 600-1200 (chronic)	Conduction defects, leukocytosis, nephrogenic diabetes insipidus, renal failure, goiter and hypothyroidism, teratogenic effects, psoriasis, weight gain, GI effects, tremors, acne
Atypical Antipsychotics°†		
Risperidone (Risperdal, 0.25, 0.5, 1, 2, 3, 4 mg)	2–6	Insomnia, agitation, dizziness, orthostatic hypotension, tachycardia; causes greatest prolactin elevation of the atypical agents
Olanzapine (Zyprexa, 2.5, 5, 7.5, 10, 15, 20 mg)	5–20	Somnolence, dry mouth, insomnia, weight gain
Quetiapine (Seroquel, 25, 100, 200, 300 mg)	50–800 (higher dose range in schizophrenics)	Dizziness, orthostatic hypotension, dry mouth, constipation, dyspepsia, somnolence, mild weight gain
Aripiprazole (Abilify, 10, 15, 20, 30 mg)	10–30	Dizziness, nausea, vomiting, orthostatic hypotension, insomnia, akathisia; no prolactinemia or weight gain
Ziprasidone (Geodon, 20, 40, 60, 80 mg)	20–160	Somnolence, GI effects, neuroleptic malignant syndrome, tardive dyskinesia, seizures (rare), syncope (rare), rash, priapism, sexual dysfunction, mild weight gain; use with caution in patients with prolonged QT
Clozapine† (Clozaril, 25, 100 mg) l	50–900	Seizures, leukopenia, agranulocytosis, deep vein thrombosis (rare), pericarditis, myocarditis; no prolactinemia
β-Blockers		
Propranolol (Inderal, 10, 20, 40, 60, 80 60 LA, 120 LA mg)	160–320 (>500 with careful monitoring)	Bradycardia, depression, dizziness, bronchospasm, agranulocytosis, fatigue, insomnia, GI effects, alopecia, impotence
SSRI		
Fluoxetine (Prozac, 10, 20, 40 mg)	10–60	Nausea, loose stools, dizziness, headache, decreased libido, impotence, insomnia, tiredness, dry mouth, sweating, weight gain
Sertraline (Zoloft, 25, 50, 100 mg)	25–200	As above
Paroxetine (Paxil, 10, 20, 30, 40 mg)	10–50	As above

The antiepileptics lamotrigine, topiramate, and gabapentin are used as mood stabilizers. Calcium channel blockers, neuroleptics, anxiolytics, antidepressants, and benzodiazepines are also used to treat agitation and aggression.

°Neuroleptic malignant syndrome can occur with typical antipsychotic drugs and, according to case reports, atypical antipsychotic drugs; the syndrome is very rarely reported with clozapine; tardive dyskinesia can occur with all dopamine receptor antagonists, but the incidence is not yet defined for atypical antipsychotics with dopaminergic and serotonergic activity.

†Upper dose ranges are usually used only in patients who partially respond to moderate doses.

‡Clozapine is rarely used to treat aggression owing to the risk of agranulocytosis.

ER, extended release; LA, long-acting; GI, gastrointestinal.

enuresis, cataplexy (associated with narcolepsy syndrome), and emotional incontinence in pseudobulbar palsy.

Tricyclic antidepressants affect multiple neurotransmitter systems (Table 11–11), including serotonin (5- hydroxytryptamine [5–HT], norepinephrine (NE), dopamine (D), acetylcholine (ACh), and histamine (H). Most tricyclic antidepressants block both 5–HT and NE reuptake; some, such as clomipramine, have predominant 5–HT effects, and others, such as desipramine, maprotilene, nortriptyline, and protriptyline, have predominant NE effects. Tricyclic antidepressants also block muscarinic, H_1–histaminergic, and α_1- adrenergic receptors. Most tricyclic antidepressants block serotonin2A receptors (strongest blocker is amoxapine, weakest blockers are desipramine and maprotiline), which may contribute to their efficacy. The serotonin$_{2A}$ receptor density decreases with chronic antidepressant therapy.

Tricyclic antidepressants and SSRIs are equally effective for major depression, but the former are most often second-line choices owing to their anticholinergic side effects and potential for cardiac toxicity. The adverse effects of tricyclic antidepressants (Table 11–6) limit the maximally tolerated dose and patient compliance, which together reduce the drugs' efficacy and increase the need for patient and doctor interaction. In selected circumstances, however, the sedative or analgesic effects of tri-

cyclic antidepressants may be beneficial as co-morbidity of headaches, pain disorders, and insomnia is common in depression. An important advantage of tricyclic antidepressants over SS-RIs is that sexual side effects are much less common. The response to tricyclic antidepressants and SSRIs typically lags 5–21 days after treatment is begun. Unlike SSRIs, a 2–week supply of a tricyclic antidepressant may be fatal in overdosage.

Selective Serotonin Reuptake Inhibitors

Serotonin is an ancient neurotransmitter, modulating motility and aggressive behavior in invertebrates and aggressive, sexual, and affective behavior in vertebrates.[107,108] Neuromodulatory effects depend on dose as well as rate and duration of serotonin exposure.[109] Blockade of serotonin reuptake at presynaptic axon terminals is the principal mechanism of SSRI action, but the downstream consequences of this effect are not fully understood. Down-regulation (desensitization) of somatodendritic serotonin$_{1A}$ autoreceptors is also important. Initial treatment increases serotonin levels mainly in the median raphe (serotonin neuron soma), not at the axon terminal regions. These acute effects correlate more with adverse than therapeutic effects. After several weeks, down-regulation of the serotonin$_{1A}$ autoreceptors

Table 11–11. Neurochemical Effects of Tricyclic Antidepressants

Drug	RECEPTOR BLOCKADE					REUPTAKE INHIBITION		
	ACh-M	H_1	α_1	α_2	D_2	NE	5-HT	DA
Amitriptyline	++++	++++	+++	+	±	+	++	±
Amoxapine	+	++	++	±	++	+++	+	±
Clomipramine	++	++	++	±	+	++	+++	±
Desipramine	+	+	+	±	±	++++	+	±
Doxepin	++	++++	++	±	±	++	+	±
Imipramine	++	++	++	±	±	++	++	±
Maprotiline	+	+++	++	±	+	+++	±	±
Nortriptyline	++	++	++	±	±	+++	+	±
Protriptyline	++	++	+	±	±	++++	+	±
Trimipramine	++	++++	++	±	+	+	±	±

ACh-M, acetycholine muscarinic; H_1, histamine-1 receptor; α_1, α_1-adrenergic receptor; α_2, α_2-adrenergic receptor; D_2, dopamine-2 receptor; NE, norepinephrine; 5-HT, 5-hydroxytryptamine (serotonin); DA, dopamine; +/++++, active to strongly active; ±, weakly active.

correlates with therapeutic effects and tolerance to adverse effects.[110] However, the role of these autoreceptors on these effects remains uncertain.

The SSRIs effectively treat major depression, dysphoria, OCD, panic disorder, generalized anxiety disorder, social phobia, premenstrual syndrome, bulimia, and anorexia nervosa. They may also help behavioral symptoms in autism, impulsive aggressive behavior, intermittent explosive disorder, and pedophilia. They significantly improve major depression in 70% of patients but completely resolve the symptoms in less than 30%. Antidepressant action usually begins within 5–21 days, but maximal benefit often takes months. Escitalopram appears to have an earlier onset of antidepressant action.[110a] When depression and anxiety coexist, SSRIs remain the treatment of choice over more sedating antidepressants (e.g., amitriptyline). However, the paradoxical effect of SSRI-induced anxiety in some patients must be monitored. Although the half-lives of the different SSRIs vary (Table 11–12), their times to onset of antidepressant action are similar.

The side effects of SSRIs cause 30% of patients to discontinue therapy, 20% within 6 weeks, and 10% over the next year. Common problems include nausea, loose stools, decreased appetite, headache, weight gain, nervousness and anxiety, insomnia, drowsiness, and sexual dysfunction. The side effects are often dose-related, and bothersome effects can be managed by reducing or dividing the dose or increasing the dose in smaller increments. Nervousness and anxiety (20%), nausea (25%), and headache (30%) often resolve within 2–6 weeks. Nausea is reduced by taking the medication with meals. Insomnia (20%) often improves with a single, early-morning dose. Persistent insomnia may result from the underlying depression or drug-induced mania or akathisia.[111] Drowsiness (20%), if not a product of insomnia, improves when the SSRI is taken at bedtime.

Sexual dysfunction afflicts 30%–40% of patients taking SSRIs. Sexual disorders include diminished libido, delayed or painful orgasm, failure to achieve orgasm, and erectile dysfunction. Escitalopram may have fewer sexual side effects than other SSRIs.[110a] Several strategies are helpful: with a short half-life drug, such as sertraline or paroxetine, hold the dose a day or two before sexual activity; change to another antidepressant, such as a tricyclic antidepressant, bupropion, nefazodone, or mirtazapine (α_2-adrenoceptor and $5\text{-}HT_2$/$5\text{-}HT_3$ receptor antagonist); or reverse the side effects of the SSRI with another medication (e.g., yohimbine, dopamine agonists, sildenafil, cyproheptadine).

The SSRIs have few other adverse effects. Hyponatremia is most common in elderly patients who take other sodium-depleting medications.[112] Hair loss is infrequent and more common in women. Easy bruising and bleeding are infrequent. A reversible parkinsonism rarely complicates long-term or short-term SSRI therapy.[113] Combining an SSRI with an MAOI or other serotonin enhancer may produce the serotonin syndrome of abdominal pain, diarrhea, tachycardia, increased blood pressure, diaphoresis, fever, myoclonus, irritability, delirium, and, very rarely, cardiovascular shock and death. After withdrawal of an SSRI, wait at least 2 weeks before starting an MAOI.

Among the SSRIs, paroxetine clearance is most significantly reduced by renal impairment. The half-lives of all SSRIs are prolonged in elderly patients. Diminished metabolism in the elderly may be the most problematic for paroxetine, citalopram, and escitalopram.[114,115]

The safety of SSRIs during pregnancy remains uncertain. Preliminary studies show no definite risk from SSRIs of major congenital malformations or developmental delays.[116,117] There may be an increased risk of minor perinatal complications[118] or later neurodevelopmental abnormalities. The most safety data are available for fluoxetine; there are less for paroxetine and sertraline and even less for other SSRIs.[119,120] Breast-feeding during SSRI therapy appears safe, but closely monitor breast-fed babies for irritability, sedation, or poor feeding.

Discontinuation of SSRIs may cause mild and self-limited withdrawal symptoms, which usually emerge within several days and resolve within a week. Symptoms include dizziness, nausea, fatigue, aches, insomnia, anxiety, irritability, and crying. Paroxetine and fluvoxamine and related drugs (e.g., venlafaxine) with short half-lives should be tapered as their discontinuation often causes such symptoms. Overdosage of SSRIs is generally well tolerated.

The SSRIs inhibit the cytochrome P-450

Table 11–12. **Pharmacological Properties of Selective Serotonin Reuptake Inhibitors (SSRIs) and Other Drugs with Serotonergic Properties**

Drug class	Starting Dose, Oral (mg/day)	Adult Dose, Oral* (mg/day)	Mean Half-Life (hours)	Protein Binding (%)	Adverse Effect Profile Compared with Other SSRIs
SSRI					
Fluoxetine (Prozac, 10, 20, 40 mg C, T, L, ER)	10–20	10–80 q.d.	60 (48–72) (120–380)†	94	⇑⇑⇑ Activation and insomnia
Sertraline (Zoloft, 25, 50, 100 mg T, L)	25–50	50–200 q.d.	26 (62–104)†	99	⇑ GI effects; ⇑ Activation and insomnia
Paroxetine (Paxil, 10, 20, 30, 40 mg T, L)	10–20	20–60 q.d.	20 (3–65)	95	⇓ Activation and insomnia; ⇑ Anticholinergic†
Fluvoxamine (Luvox, 25, 50, 100 mg T)	25–50	100–300 b.i.d.	15 (9–28)	77	⇑ Sedation
Citalopram (Celexa, 10, 20, 40 mg T, L)	10–20	20–60 q.d.	32 (23–45)	80	—
Escitalopram (Lexapro, 10 mg T)	10	10–20	30	55	⇓ Incidence of diminished libido
Related Drugs					
Venlafaxine (Effexor, 25, 37.5, 50, 75, 100 mg T; 37.5, 75, 150 mg C-XR)	25–75; 37.5–75 XR	75–375 b.i.d., t.i.d 75–225 XR q.d.	4 (3–7) (9–13)†	27	⇑ GI effects; ⇑ Activation and insomnia; ⇑ Orthostatic hypotension; ⇑ Sexual dysfunction

Trazodone (Desyrel, 50, 100, 150, 300 mg T)	150–200	150–600 b.i.d., t.i.d.	7 (4–9)	90	⇓⇓ Sexual dysfunction ⇓⇓ GI effects ⇑⇑ Orthostatic hypotension ⇑⇑ Sedation
Nefazodone (Serzone, 50, 100, 150, 200, 250 mg T)	100–200	100–600 b.i.d.	3.5 (2–4) (1.5–18)†	99	*"Black box" warning*: hepatic toxicity ⇓⇓ Sexual dysfunction ⇓⇓ GI effects ⇑ Sedation
Bupropion (Wellbutrin, Zyban; 100, 150 mg T; 100, 150 mg SR)	100–200	225–450 b.i.d 150–400 SR	14 (20–27)†	85	⇑ Activation and insomnia ⇓⇓ Sexual dysfunction ⇓⇓ GI effects
Mirtazapine (Remeron, 15, 30 mg T)	15 h.s.	15–45 h.s.	30 (20–40)	85	⇓⇓ Sexual dysfunction, GI effects, activation ⇑⇑ Sedation

T, tablet; C, capsule; L, liquid; XR, extended release; SR, sustained release; OCD, obsessive–compulsive disorder; GI, gastrointestinal.
Adverse effect relative to average SSRI: ⇑, increased; ⇑⇑, strongly increased; ⇓, decreased; ⇓⇓, strongly decreased.
aTotal (maximal) daily dose, which may be administered in one or three daily doses. For most SSRIs, the lower dose is usually adequate for depression and the higher dose is needed for some cases of OCD.
†Half-life of major active metabolite.
‡Anticholinergic effects, although greater than with other SSRIs, are slight.

isoenzyme 2D6 and increase the blood level of drugs metabolized by this isoenzyme. These drugs (e.g., carbamazepine, tricyclic antidepressants, several antipsychotics, flecainide) have a narrow therapeutic index and, when combined with an SSRI, may cause toxicity to develop. Similarly, if these concomitant medications are added to an SSRI and their blood levels are in the therapeutic range, withdrawal of the SSRI may cause the blood drug levels to become subtherapeutic. Inhibition of isoenzyme 2D6 varies for the SSRIs, with paroxetine, fluoxetine, sertraline, fluvoxamine, and citalopram ranging in order of potency from the most to the least.

Venlafaxine

Venlafaxine, a bicyclic phenylethylamine, is a serotonin and NE reuptake inhibitor (Table 11–12). Its major action is on serotonin, with NE effects clinically relevant at higher doses. Venlafaxine weakly inhibits dopamine reuptake but has no substantial effect on other neurotransmitter systems. Venlafaxine's psychotropic effect may begin sooner than that of the SSRIs. Venlafaxine is indicated for depression and generalized anxiety disorder. Nausea is the most common side effect; others include headache, insomnia, tiredness, dizziness, sexual dysfunction, tremor, dry mouth, constipation, sweating, and anxiety. A dose-related increase in blood pressure occurs, usually at doses exceeding 225 mg/day, and is clinically significant in a minority of patients. Abrupt discontinuation of venlafaxine may cause serotonin withdrawal symptoms within 8 hours (see Selective Serotonin Reuptake Inhibitors, above). Drug interactions are rare except with MAOIs.

Trazodone

Trazodone is a 5–HT$_{2A}$ receptor antagonist and serotonin reuptake inhibitor (Table 11–12). Antihistamine (sedation) and α_1-antagonist (orthostatic hypotension) properties limit tolerability to the drug. For depressed patients with prominent agitation, anxiety, or insomnia, sedation can be beneficial. Other adverse effects include dizziness, dry mouth, nausea, constipation, and priapism (~1 in 6000 men).

Drug interactions are limited to MAOIs and the potentiating effects of CNS depressants and antihypertensives.

Nefazodone

Nefazodone, also a 5-HT$_{2A}$ receptor antagonist and serotonin reuptake inhibitor, is much better tolerated than trazodone, with minimal α_1 antagonism and no effect on muscarinic receptors (Table 11–12). Common side effects include dizziness, drowsiness, weakness, weight gain, and lack of energy. Advantages of nefazodone over SSRIs, venlafaxine, and bupropion are less anxiety, insomnia, and diaphoresis. Sexual dysfunction is less likely to occur with nefazodone than with SSRIs but occurs more often than with bupropion. Nefazodone may increase blood carbamazepine levels and should not be used with MAOIs. In 2001, the Food and Drug Administration (FDA) issued a "black box" warning about rare cases of potentially fatal hepatic toxicity caused by nefazodone.

Bupropion

Bupropion is a unicyclic aminoketone that acts primarily as an NE reuptake blocker (Table 11–12). It weakly inhibits dopamine reuptake but has no effect on serotonin. Bupropion effectively treats major depression and anxiety but not panic attacks or OCD. A major advantage of bupropion over SSRIs is the absence of sexual side effects and less fatigue, but it causes more nervousness and palpitations. Bupropion may be less likely than other antidepressants to provoke a manic episode in depressed bipolar patients. Bupropion's activating properties may improve the fatigue associated with depression. It is often given twice daily in a sustained-release form.

Common side effects include nausea, dry mouth, insomnia, anxiety, and tremor. Weight loss and agitation may occur. Menstrual irregularities develop in 5%–10% of women. In an early study, tonic-clonic seizures developed in 4 of 55 bulimic patients, leading the manufacturer to withdraw bupropion from the market from 1986 to 1989. The frequency of seizures was related to a maximal single dose (patients should not double up on missed doses) and the total daily dose. In doses of up to 450 mg/day, the incidence of seizures during an 8–week trial in patients with eating disorders was approximately 0.35% and the cumulative 2-year risk was approximately 0.50%.[121,122] Since the efficacy of 300 mg/day of a sustained-release formulation is similar to that of higher doses of an immediate-release preparation, the daily dose of bupropion should not exceed 300 mg in patients with neurological disorders. Although never a first-line drug for depression in epilepsy patients, we have safely used doses of up to 300 mg/day.

Overdosage of bupropion is rarely fatal. Drug interactions are infrequent. The MAOIs are absolutely contraindicated. In parkinsonism patients taking levodopa preparations, bupropion may produce troublesome gastrointestinal and CNS stimulatory effects. Use bupropion cautiously with other drugs that can lower the seizure threshold (e.g., alcohol, antihistamines).

Mirtazapine

Mirtazapine is a tetracyclic antidepressant with potent α_2-adrenergic antagonistic effects and modest antagonistic effects on 5–HT$_2$ and 5–HT$_3$ receptors (Table 11–12). Blockage of the presynaptic α_2 autoreceptors increases NE release, and blockage of the α_2 heteroreceptors increases serotonin release. The net effect on serotonergic activity is an increase in 5–HT$_1$ transmission. Mirtazapine also has a high affinity for blocking H$_1$ receptors, which paradoxically leads to sedation at lower doses (H$_1$ blockade predominates) and activation at moderate to high doses (NE release predominates).

Common adverse effects of mirtazapine include sedation, dry mouth, asthenia, increased appetite, and weight gain. These effects are usually mild and transient. Starting at <15 mg/day decreases sedation. Sexual side effects are rare. Mild increases in serum cholesterol occur in up to 20% of patients. Liver transaminases are elevated as much as three times the upper limit of normal in 2% of patients. Agranulocytosis (<500 white blood cells/mm^3) occurs in 0.11% of patients. Obtain a white blood cell count if there is a fever or other signs of infection; routine monitoring is controversial. Toxicity limits the clinical usefulness of mirtazapine.

Monoamine Oxidase Inhibitors

The MAO isoenzymes A and B are present in specific neuronal populations: MAO-A is found in NE and dopamine neurons, and MAO-B is found mainly in serotonergic neurons.[122a] Monoamine oxidase occurs on the outer side of the mitochondrial membrane, deaminating cytoplasmic amines. Treatment with MAOIs rapidly increases cytoplasmic amine concentrations and, after several weeks, reduces the number of β and α adrenoceptors and 5-HT$_1$ and 5-HT$_2$ receptors, which is similar to the action of tricyclic antidepressants and other antidepressants.

Pharmacotherapeutic advances have largely relegated the MAOIs to specialized psychopharmacologists. They are effective for atypical depression (excessive mood reactivity with some combination of overeating, oversleeping, extreme fatigue, and oversensitivity to rejection), major depression, dysthymia, panic disorder, bulimia, atypical facial pain, and treatment-resistant depression. The efficacy of MAOIs is less well documented in OCD, narcolepsy, headache, chronic pain syndromes, and generalized anxiety disorder. The MAOIs are comparable to tricyclic antidepressants in efficacy for major depression.

The side effects of MAOIs are more severe and frequent than those of most other antidepressants. Common side effects include headache, dry mouth, dizziness, orthostatic hypotension, constipation, nausea, and weight gain. Less commonly, MAOIs produce insomnia, sexual dysfunction (anorgasmia, decreased libido, impotence, delayed ejaculation) peripheral edema, weakness, syncope, urinary hesitancy, and myoclonic jerks. Approximately 4% of patients have elevated levels of hepatic transaminases. Dietary interactions are a major concern and limit the use of MAOIs; foods containing tyramine provoke headache and, with larger exposure, a hypertensive crisis. Counsel patients who take MAOIs to avoid cheese (except cream cheese and cottage cheese), wine, beer, sherry, liquors, pickled fish, sausage, overripe aged fruit, and liver. Patients may need to moderate consumption of chocolate, colas, caffeine, yogurt, soy sauce, and other foods. In addition to foods, patients taking MAOIs along with other medications, including tricyclic antidepressants, SSRIs, stimulants, and carbamazepine, must be made aware of the potential for adverse reactions. Use intravenous phentolamine or sublingual nifedipine to treat a hypertensive crisis induced by the combination of an MAOI and a tyramine-containing food or certain drugs.

The major MAOIs include hydrazines (phenelzine and isocarboxazid) and nonhydrazines (tranylcypromine and selegiline). While selegiline is used mainly in Parkinson's disease (low doses do not require dietary restrictions), the others are used mainly to treat psychiatric disorders. Except for selegiline, MAOIs are contraindicated during levodopa therapy. The hydrazines often cause troublesome orthostatic hypotension. Tranylcypromine may lead to the syndrome of inappropriate antidiuretic hormone release, as well as physical dependence with withdrawal symptoms such as nervousness and depression.

Lithium

Lithium is a monovalent cation that stabilizes mood in patients with bipolar disorder. Lithium's mechanism of action remains uncertain, but it influences neural membranes and signal transduction, as well as neurotransmitter activity. Lithium is approved to treat acute mania and for long-term prophylaxis of bipolar disorder (Table 11–10). It is also used to potentiate a response to antidepressants and antipsychotics and to treat aggression. Lithium is used to treat cluster headache and may have antiviral properties.[123]

Lithium has a narrow therapeutic index. Therapeutic serum lithium levels are 0.8–1.2 mEq/l, with higher levels increasing the frequency of side effects. Frequent and clinically significant side effects include excessive thirst, polyuria, tremor, weight gain, memory problems, tiredness, and diarrhea. Other possible complications are hypothyroidism, cognitive problems (e.g., impaired concentration and slowed thinking), impaired renal tubular concentrating ability, and teratogenic effects. Lithium also interacts with diuretics, nonsteroidal anti-inflammatory drugs, neuroleptics, antiarrhythmics, antidepressants, and antiepileptic drugs.

Antipsychotic Drugs

Antipsychotic drugs (neuroleptics, major tranquilizers) are used to treat psychotic disorders resulting from psychiatric and neurological causes. Positive symptoms of psychosis, including disordered thinking, anxiety, delusions, hallucinations, aggression, and insomnia, respond best to antipsychotic drugs. Negative symptoms, such as apathy, aspontaneity, social withdrawal, and catatonia, are more difficult to treat and respond better to the newer, atypical antipsychotics. Antipsychotic drugs are also used to treat symptoms in nonpsychotic patients such as delusions, hallucinations, agitation, aggression, tics, severe anxiety, nausea, and sedation. Disabling borderline or schizotypal personality disorders and severe OCD are also treated with antipsychotic drugs.

Antipsychotic drugs are grouped into two major classes: conventional, older agents (e.g., chlorpromazine, haloperidol) and atypical, newer agents (e.g., risperidone, olanzapine, quetiapine, aripiprazole) (Table 11–13). Antipsychotic drugs are also divided into "low-potency" (e.g., chlorpromazine, thioridazine) and "high-potency" (e.g., fluphenazine, haloperidol) groups. Potency is determined mainly by clinically effective dosages and affinities for the D_2 receptor. Among the conventional antipsychotic drugs, high-potency agents are less sedating, hypotensive, and anticholinergic but have more acute extrapyramidal side effects.

Tardive dyskinesia, a potential complication of antipsychotic therapy, may be irreversible even if diagnosed promptly. The incidence of tardive dyskinesia is similar for low- and high-potency conventional antipsychotic drugs. The rate varies: a meta-analysis showed a 24.2% overall rate, but the incidence approached 50% in elderly patients.[124,125]

The conventional antipsychotic drugs act mainly on D_2 receptors, without selectivity between striatal and limbic/mesocortical sites. In contrast, the atypical antipsychotics are relatively selective for the limbic/mesocortical D_2 site.[126] In addition, the $5\text{-}HT_2$ receptor antagonist properties may account for their greater efficacy and lower extrapyramidal toxicity. The binding of atypical antipsychotics to D_4 receptors, found in limbic and frontal but not striatal areas, may also contribute to their efficacy and toxicity profiles.[127] Aripiprazole is a partial agonist at D_2 and $5\text{-}HT_{1A}$ receptors and an antagonist at $5\text{-}HT_2$ receptors. This drug acts as a functional antagonist at D_2 receptors under hyperdopaminergic states but functional agonism in hypodopaminergic conditions.[127a]

Table 11–13. Therapy for Psychosis and Delusions

Drug Class	Adult Dose, Oral* (mg/day)	Adverse Effects
Typical Antipsychotics		
Chlorpromazine (Thorazine, 10, 25, 50, 100, 200 [tabs]; 30, 75, 150 [capsules] mg)	25–2000	Sedation, postural hypotension, weight gain, rash, intermediate risk of extrapyramidal symptoms (EPS; parkinsonism, dystonia, motor restlessness), tardive dyskinesia, neuroleptic malignant syndrome, anticholinergic, α_1-adrenergic and antihistaminic side effects (see Table 11–6), sexual dysfunction, seizures, fetal toxicity, agranulocytosis, jaundice, prolonged QT interval, pigmentary retinopathy
Thioridazine (Mellaril, 10, 15, 25, 50, 75, 100, 150, 200 mg)	50–800	As above (pigmentary retinopathy at >900 mg/day), lower incidence of EPS, greater risk of prolonged QT interval, impaired ejaculation
Haloperidol† (Haldol, 0.5, 1, 2, 5, 10, 20 mg)	1–40	As above, less sedation, hypotension, anticholinergic and cardiovascular effects, liver toxicity, ocular damage, blood disorders, and photosensitivity
Molindone† (Moban, 5, 10, 25, 50, 100 mg)	15–225	As above, less anticholinergic effects, hypotension, seizures, and weight gain.
Atypical Antipsychotics		
Risperidone (Risperdal, 0.25, 0.5, 1, 2, 3, 4 mg)	2–6	Lower incidence of EPS and tardive diskinesia
Olanzapine (Zyprexa, 2.5, 5, 7.5, 10, 15, 20 mg)	5–20	Sedation, agitation, dizziness, orthostatic hypotension, tachycardia, constipation, weight gain, impotence
Quetiapine (Seroquel, 25, 100, 200, 300 mg)	50–800	Somnolence, dry mouth, insomnia, weight gain, dizziness, orthostatic hypotension, nausea
Aripiprazole (Abilify, 10, 15, 20, 30 mg)	10–30	Dizziness, orthostatic hypotension, dry mouth, constipation, dyspepsia, somnolence, mild weight gain
Ziprasidone (Geodon, 20, 40, 60, 80 mg)	20–160	Dizziness, nausea, vomiting, orthostatic hypotension, insomnia, akathisia; no prolactinemia or weight gain
Clozapine (Clozaril, 25, 100 mg)	50–900	Somnolence, gastrointestinal effects, neuroleptic malignant syndrome, tardive dyskinesia, mild weight gain, seizures (rare), syncope (rare), rash, priapism, sexual dysfunction
		Seizures, leukopenia, agranulocytosis, neuroleptic malignant syndrome, tardive dyskinesia, hyperglycemia, deep vein thrombosis, pericarditis, myocarditis

*Lowest effective dose shown may be lower than that found in standard psychiatry references, but such doses may be effective in neuropsychiatric and elderly populations. Maximal doses for many antipsychotic agents are used only for patients with a partial response to lower doses; high doses are more likely to cause sedation, seizures, or other adverse effects.

†These drugs have a higher rate of extrapyramidal side effects and a lower rate of anticholinergic side effects than other typical antipsychotic drugs.

The atypical antipsychotics have fewer acute and tardive extrapyramidal side effects and cause less hyperprolactinemia than conventional antipsychotics. Aripiprazole appears less sedating and less likely to cause weight gain, extrapyramidal side effects, and hyperprolactinemia than other atypical antipsychotic agents.[127a] With the exception of clozapine, which can cause agranulocytosis in 1% of patients, atypical antipsychotics are considered first-line agents. However, their cost is much higher than that of conventional antipsychotics. The low incidence of extrapyramidal side effects makes atypical antipsychotics the preferred medications for patients with Parkinson's disease and dementia syndromes.

Side effects of antipsychotic drugs are largely attributable to receptor-blocking properties. Blockade of striatal dopamine receptors leads to extrapyramidal side effects of acute dystonic reactions, parkinsonism, rabbit syndrome (fine, rapid lip movements), and tardive dyskinesia. Among the atypical antipsychotics, these side effects are most common with risperidone. Antipsychotic drugs also impair motivation and energy, leading some sedated patients to report a "zombielike" state that fosters noncompliance. Other adverse effects include weight gain (aripiprazole and ziprasidone are the least and quetiapine is the third least provocative of the atypical antipsychotics), dia-betes mellitus, hypertriglyceridemia, hypercholesterolemia, anticholinergic effects, hypotension and infrequently seizures (clozapine is most provocative of the atypical antipsychotics).

Central Nervous System Stimulants

Central nervous system stimulants are used to treat ADHD and narcolepsy. They are also used to treat resistant depression, and neurological causes of impaired attention and hyperactivity; to ameliorate somnolence induced by other medications (e.g., opioids); to augment analgesia; and to improve cognitive function in patients with medical and neurological disorders (e.g., cancer, traumatic brain injury).[128] The stimulants increase central noradrenergic and dopaminergic activity. The choice of stimulant is influenced by its duration of action and side-effect profile (Table 11–14), although an individual's response to a specific agent is variable. A major advance is the introduction of several extended-release preparations, allowing longer duration of action and less variation between peak (adverse effect) and trough (lack of efficacy) blood drug levels. Dosage is based on clinical response and tolerability; body mass does not reliably predict the dosage. Because their effectiveness usually occurs within days or weeks, when the

Table 11–14. **Therapy for Impaired Attention and Hyperactivity**

Drug class	Adult Dose, Oral (mg/day)	Adverse Effects
CNS Stimulants		
Methylphenidate (Ritalin,° 5, 10; 20 mg SR; 20, 30, 40 mg LA)	10–90	*Common:* nervousness, insomnia, anorexia, dizziness, weight loss, dysphoria, headache *Infrequent:* rash, drowsiness, mood changes, tremor, palpitations, tachycardia, hypertension, dyskinesia, tics, diarrhea, GI effects, impotence, drug abuse and dependence *Rare:* exacerbation of seizure disorder, growth retardation, arrhythmia, angina, blood dyscrasias, psychosis, Tourette's syndrome *Overdose:* agitation, tremor, confusion, seizures, hallucinations, cardiovascular
Methylphenidate SR (Ritalin SR, Metadate ER; 10, 20 mg)	10–60	As above

(*Continued on following page*)

Table 11–14.—*continued*

Drug class	Adult Dose, Oral (mg/day)	Adverse Effects
CNS Stimulants		
Methylphenidate ER (Concerta, 18, 36, 54 mg; Metadate CD, 20 mg)	18–54	As above
Dextroamphetamine (Dexedrine, Dextrostat; 5, 10 mg)	5–60	As above
Dextroamphetamine SR (Dexedrine Spansules, 5, 10, 15 mg SR)	10–45	As above
Amphetamine+dextro-amphetamine (Adderall, 5, 7.5, 10, 12.5, 15, 20, 30 mg)	5–40	As above
Dexmethylphenidate (Focalin, 2.5, 5, 10 mg)	2.5–20	As above
Pemoline (Cylert, 18.75, 37.5, 75 mg)	37.5–112.5	As above *"Black box" warning:* hepatic failure (must monitor liver function tests)
Modafinil (Provigil, 100, 200 mg)	200–400	*Common:* headache, nausea, nervousness, anxiety, insomnia, mood change
Propylamine		
Atomoxetine (Strattera, 10, 18, 25, 40, 60 mg)		Fatigue, nausea, dizziness, decreased appetite, mood swings, rash, sexual dysfunction
Antidepressants		
Tricyclics		
Imipramine (Tofranil, 75, 100, 125, 150 mg)	100–300	See Table 11–6; very strong anticholinergic effects (e.g., sedation, orthostatic hypotension EKG changes), frequent sexual dysfunction, infrequent GI effects
Desipramine (Norpramin, 10, 25, 50, 75, 100, 150 mg)	100–300	See Table 11–6; less anticholinergic effects than other tricyclic antidepressants, frequent sexual dysfunction, infrequent GI effects
Heterocyclic		
Bupropion (Wellbutrin, 75, 100 mg; 100, 150 mg SR)	150–450 150–400 SR	*Common:* agitation, dry mouth, insomnia, headache, nausea, vomiting, constipation, tremor, blurred vision *Infrequent:* rash, seizures (~0.4% at 450 mg/day), mania, "spaciness," weight loss
α_2-*agonists*		
Clonidine (Catapres, 0.1, 0.2, 0.3 mg)	0.2–0.5	Dry mouth and eyes, drowsiness, dizziness, nausea, nervousness, orthostatic hypotension
Guanfacine (Tenex, 1, 2 mg)	2–3	As above, less sedating and shorter half-life

*Ritalin LA is a mixture of rapidly acting and sustained-release medication and may be better tolerated and more effective throughout the day than Ritalin or Ritalin SR.

CNS, central nervous system; GI, gastrointestinal; SR, sustained release; LA, long-acting; ER, extended release; CD, extended release.

dose is gradually increased, different stimulants are easily tried. If adverse effects persist and are bothersome or benefits are minimal or lacking, discontinue the medication. All CNS stimulants can cause tolerance and lead to abuse and dependence.

All stimulants share rapid absorption and metabolism and low protein binding. They also share similar side effects, which are usually mild and transient. If bothersome side effects do not improve, dose reduction is often helpful. Stimulants commonly cause decreased appetite and weight loss, irritability, abdominal discomfort, headache, and increased emotional sensitivity. Less common side effects include insomnia, dysphoria, social withdrawal, anxiety, tics, and nervous habits (e.g., picking at skin, pulling hair). Rare side effects include depression, growth retardation, hypertension, tachycardia, hallucinations, psychosis, stereotypic compulsions, and seizures (with methylphenidate).

Modafanil (Table 11–14) is a racemic compound that promotes wakefulness. Its mechanism of action is unknown but may be blockage of dopamine reuptake. The effective half-life is approximately 15 hours. The drug is metabolized by the liver and reversibly inhibits the isoenzyme CYP2C19. Therefore, coadministration with diazepam, phenytoin, or propranolol increases blood levels of these compounds. Modafanil effectively treats excessive daytime somnolence in narcolepsy. Pilot data suggest a role for modafanil in treating fatigue and ADHD.[129] Side effects include headache, nausea, anxiety, insomnia, diarrhea, dry mouth, and anorexia. Modafinil produces psychoactive and euphoric effects similar to those of methylphenidate, suggesting a similar potential for abuse and dependence.

Atomoxetine (Table 11–14) is a selective norepinephrine reuptake inhibitor approved to treat ADHD. We have not found it as effective as stimulants. The drug is metabolized by the CYP2D6 pathway, and half-life (5–21 hours) depends on an individual's genetics as a normal or slow metabolizer (7% of Caucasians and 2% of African Americans are slow metabolizers). Drugs that inhibit this pathway (e.g., fluoxetine, paroxetine) cause increased atomoxetine levels. The drug is not classified as a controlled substance like the traditional stimulants (e.g., methyl-phenidate, dextroamphetamine). It does not cause euphoria and is not associated with abuse or dependence. Dosing is usually once a day, starting with 0.5 mg/kg/d in children and increasing to a maximum of 1.4 mg/kg/d or a maximum of 100 mg/d (whichever is less). It can be given in two divided doses or at bedtime. The most common side effects are fatigue, nausea, decreased appetite, dizziness, mood swings, and sexual dysfunction. Atomoxetine can be discontinued without tapering.

α_2-Adrenergic Agonists

The α_2–adrenergic agonist clonidine (Table 11–14) is used to treat ADHD, Tourette's syndrome, impulsivity, insomnia induced by stimulant drugs, and behavioral problems (e.g., hyperarousal) in autistic children. In ADHD, clonidine is a second-line medication that improves cooperation, frustration tolerance, and impulsivity. In Tourette's syndrome, clonidine slightly reduces tics, but also reduces distress associated with tics and improves hyperactivity and impulsivity.

Sedation, a bothersome side effect of clonidine, may diminish over the first 2–4 weeks of therapy. Taking clonidine at bedtime promotes sleep and helps to reduce daytime sedation. Other adverse effects, common at higher doses, include low blood pressure, dizziness, dry mouth, and decreased glucose tolerance (most often in patients at risk for diabetes mellitus). When the skin patch is used, a localized pruritic reaction may develop. Measure the patient's blood pressure before clonidine is started. A baseline electrocardiogram and a fasting blood glucose test may be performed as well.

Although reports of sudden death in several children treated with clonidine and methylphenidate were of considerable concern, there is no clear evidence that this combination of drugs is unsafe. However, good compliance and clear clinical indications are important; consider cardiovascular screening and monitoring when these drugs are used together.

Guanfacine is another α_2–adrenergic agonist that causes less sedation than clonidine and may improve attention in children with ADHD (Table 11–14). Few controlled studies have examined the safety and efficacy of guanfacine.

Sedative–Hypnotic and Anxiolytic Drugs

Insomnia is treated with the sedative-hypnotic benzodiazepines and nonbenzodiazepines (Table

11–15). Zolpidem, a commonly used sedative, is an imidazopyridine approved for short-term (<4 weeks) treatment of insomnia. It selectively acts at the ω-1 benzodiazepine receptor. Zolpidem has a half-life of 2.5 hours. Its hypnotic efficacy is comparable to that of the benzodiazepine (e.g., flurazepam, triazolam) and nonbenzodiazepine (e.g., zopiclone and trazodone) hypnotic agents. Adult doses are 5–10 mg/day and no more than 5–7.5 mg/day in elderly patients or patients with hepatic dysfunction. Tolerance to the hypnotic effects of zolpidem does not develop after 6 months of therapy with the usual dosage but may develop at high dosages taken longer than 1 year. When zolpidem is used at doses of no more than 10 mg daily for less than 6 months, discontinuation causes only occasional and mild rebound insomnia or withdrawal symptoms. The most common side effects are nausea, dizziness, and drowsiness. Zolpidem has few next-morning effects on ease of arousal, cognition, or coordination.[130] It has a low potential for abuse, although patients with chronic insomnia may become dependent.

Buspirone, an anxiolytic, is an azapirone, an agonist at 5-HT_{1A} receptors, approved for generalized anxiety disorder. Its half-life is 3–7 hours. Efficacy for generalized anxiety disorder may be delayed 2–3 weeks after the start of therapy. Limited evidence supports the efficacy of buspirone for anxiety and agitation in dementia, aggression, social phobia, SSRI-induced adverse events, and tobacco dependence. It is used to augment therapy for panic disorder, major depressive disorder, OCD, body dysmorphic disorder, and posttraumatic stress disorder.[131] Side effects, including nausea, headache, insomnia, dizziness, and nervousness, are infrequent and usually mild. Unlike the benzodiazepines, buspirone does not cause dependence or memory or motor impairment. For generalized anxiety disorder, buspirone is started at 15–20 mg/day and increased to 45–75 mg/day. Patients with neurological disorders associated with anxiety often benefit from lower doses (10–40 mg/day).

Table 11–15. **Therapy for Insomnia**

Drug Class	Generic Name (Brand Name) Strength (mg)	Adult Dose, Oral (mg/day)
Benzodiazepines		
Long-acting	Clonazepam (Klonopin) 0.5, 1, 2	0.5–2
	Diazepam (Valium) 2, 5, 10	2–10
	Quazepam (Doral) 7.5, 15	7.5–15
	Flurazepam (Dalmane) 15, 30	15–30
Medium-acting	Estazolam (ProSom) 1, 2	1–2
	Lorazepam (Ativan) 0.5, 1, 2	0.5–2
	Temazepam (Restoril) 7.5, 15, 30	15–30
Short-acting	Triazolam (Halcion) 0.125, 0.25	0.125–0.25
Nonbenzodiazepines		
Imidazopyridine	Zolpidem (Ambien) 5, 10	5–10
Pyrazolopyrimidine	Zaleplon (Sonata) 5, 10	5–10
Antidepressants		
Tricyclics	Amitriptyline (Elavil, Endep) 10, 25	10–25
	Trimipramine (Surmontil) 25, 50, 100	25–50
Triazolopyridine	Trazodone (Desyrel) 50, 100, 150	25–150
Antihistimines		
	Diphenhydramine (Benadryl) 25, 50	25–50
	Hydroxyzine (Atarax) 10, 25, 50, 100	50–100
Neurohormone	Melatonin 1, 2, 3	1–3

Antiepileptic Drugs

PSYCHOTROPIC PROPERTIES

Antiepileptic drugs are important psychotropic agents. Their meteoric rise as therapy for psychiatric disorders outpaces evidence of their efficacy. Large, randomized controlled trials on the behavioral effects of antiepileptic drugs are few. Such evidence established the efficacy of antimanic and mood-stabilizing properties of carbamazepine, valproate, and lamotrigine in bipolar disorder.[132] Gabapentin is effective for some cases of social phobia.[133] However, antiepileptic drugs are used to treat a wide spectrum of other behavioral disorders ranging from depression to aggression to binge eating. Their growing off-label use in psychiatric disorders is dangerous. For instance, despite numerous anecdotal reports on the beneficial effect of gabapentin in bipolar and unipolar depression, two randomized controlled trials showed that gabapentin is ineffective for these disorders.[134,135] Similarly, the negative cognitive effects of topiramate were shown in randomized controlled trials[136,137] and supported by clinical observations in large epilepsy practices.[138,139] Although there is no evidence from randomized controlled trials of topiramate's efficacy for any psychiatric disorder, its use in behavioral disorders is growing steadily.

The mechanisms by which antiepileptic drugs affect behavior are incompletely defined. They may affect behavior via actions that suppress seizures, such as increased γ-aminobutyric acid (GABA) activity or inhibition of fast-conducting sodium channels or both. In general, sedative antiepileptic drugs possess anxiolytic, antimanic, and hypnotic efficacy but may cause fatigue, impair attention, and depress mood.[140] These drugs, which often enhance GABA activity, include barbiturates, benzodiazepines, valproate, gabapentin, tiagabine, and vigabatrin. Activating antiepileptic drugs, such as felbamate and lamotrigine, paradoxically reduce excitatory neurotransmission. These drugs may possess antidepressant and attention-enhancing efficacy[141] but may cause anxiety, insomnia, and agitation. Topiramate, levetiracetam, and zonisamide have multiple CNS actions that straddle these categories. These generalizations are limited by the heterogeneity of clinical responses. For example, barbiturates, valproate, vigabatrin, and levetiracetam cause sedation and, in some patients, irritability, anxiety, and depression. All antiepileptic drugs can have positive or negative psychotropic properties in different patients. Atypical behavioral responses to antiepileptic drugs and other medicines are more frequent in children and the developmentally disabled. An individual's behavioral response to a specific antiepileptic drug is influenced by the neuropsychiatric disorder, drug interactions, genetic factors, and environmental aspects. While treatment concerns individual patients, studies identify group averages. More data are needed to predict individual responsiveness to antiepileptic drugs.

PRINCIPLES OF ANTIEPILEPTIC DRUG USE

Whether antiepileptic drugs are used to treat behavioral disorders or epilepsy, the principles guiding their use are the same. Use antiepileptic drugs cautiously, with careful and ongoing attention to risk–benefit analysis over time. Antiepileptic drugs may produce idiosyncratic, dose-related, chronic, and teratogenic adverse effects. Idiosyncratic reactions include rash, Stevens–Johnson syndrome, erythema multiforme, liver failure, and bone marrow failure. For most antiepileptic drugs, the chance of a life-threatening idiosyncratic reaction is approximately 1 in 40,000 patients (exceptions are listed in Table 11–16). The highest risk for most idiosyncratic reactions is in the first 6–9 months after an antiepileptic drug is prescribed. Rash usually begins 5–18 days after drug initiation (lamotrigine is an exception). When rash or skin sensitivity is a concern, the safe choice is usually gabapentin, levetiracetam, or valproate. When the concern is liver dysfunction, gabapentin or levetiracetam is usually safe.

How do we educate patients about rare life-threatening problems without provoking unproductive fears? Patients should report such unusual symptoms as excessive bleeding, abdominal pain and tenderness, hair loss, fever, or unusual infections while taking a drug, especially a new drug. Although occasional blood tests offer a sense of protection, blood tests are valuable only when done often. Since the problems are rare, it makes little sense to screen a large number of patients to identify a single case (it might take 500,000 blood tests to identify a single serious problem), and even then self-reporting of unusual symptoms might work better. When an unusual symptom is reported (e.g., fever with shaking chills), blood tests are obtained within 12–24 hours. For certain high-risk antiepileptic drugs, such as felbamate, obtain blood cell counts and liver function tests every few weeks during the first year of use.

Treatment of chronic side effects includes lowering the dose or discontinuing the offending drug, as well as introducing a medicine or vitamin to counteract the undesired effect. For example, bone loss stimulated by carbamazepine can be minimized (although lost bone cannot be replaced) with a calcium and vitamin D replacement. Aldendronate (Fosamax), an inhibitor of osteoclast-mediated bone resorption, may also be helpful for some patients. For patients at risk for valproate-induced pancreatitis, hepatotoxicity, or hair loss, anecdotal reports suggest that low doses of selenium, approximately 20 μg/day, and zinc, approximately 50 mg/day, may offer some protection.[142,143]

Dose-related side effects of antiepileptic drugs are common and usually occur during initial use or with the use of high doses or multiple antiepileptic drugs (Table 11–16). Systemic side effects include nausea and vomiting. Central nervous system side effects are the most common and include sedation, dizziness, impaired cognition and mood, tremor (mainly with valproate), blurred or double vision, and unsteadiness. Dose-related side effects of antiepileptic drugs are reduced by lowering the dosage, adjusting medication schedules, or using sustained-released preparations. For instance, the drug can be taken with food if nausea occurs when it is taken on an empty stomach, or the doses can be spread out across the day.

Unfortunately, both the patient and the physician often grow accustomed to the dose-related side effects of antiepileptic drugs; with time they seem to meld into the patient's persona. The following case exemplifies this effect:

An 18–year-old man was referred for surgical evaluation for refractory epilepsy. He was taking carbamazepine (1400 mg/day; trough blood carbamazepine level, 9.7 μg/ml) and valproate (2750 mg/day; trough blood valproate level, 93 μg/ml).

When asked if he had any troublesome side effects of his medication, he said "no." His mother reminded him that he often complained of nausea, blurred vision, and headache. Her greatest concerns were his tiredness, lack of motivation to do his schoolwork, and marked academic decline (grade point average, 2.5), which were attributed mainly to the ongoing complex partial seizures. When asked how many hours a day he slept, he said "I sleep around 12 or 13 hours every night, and then an hour or so in the afternoon." Carbamazepine and valproate were discontinued, and lamotrigine was prescribed. His seizure frequency increased by 20%, but he had no sedation (average sleep, 8.5 hours a night), nausea, blurred vision, or headache and his academic performance improved (grade point average, 3.2).

The long-term use of antiepileptic drugs can produce side effects that may be poorly recognized by practitioners who are unfamiliar with these drugs (Table 11–16). Bone loss often complicates therapy with enzyme-inducing antiepileptic drugs (e.g., barbiturates, carbamazepine, phenytoin, topiramate, valproate, zonisamide). Weight gain complicates treatment with valproate, gabapentin, and other antiepileptic drugs.[144] Valproate may cause polycystic ovarian syndrome.[145]

FREQUENTLY USED ANTIEPILEPTICS

Pharmacological properties of the most frequently used antiepileptic drugs are summarized in Table 11–17.

Barbiturates

The barbiturates (e.g., phenobarbital, mephobarbital, primidone) are rarely prescribed as psychotopic agents, although they possess anxiolytic, sedative-hypnotic, and mood-stabilizing properties in some patients.[146,147] Barbiturates can impair cognition (e.g., attention, memory, executive function) and motivation; depress mental and physical energy and mood; and cause hyperactivity, irritability, aggressive behavior, and impotence. Barbiturates are most likely to cause depression and suicidal ideation in patients with a family or personal history of affective disorder.[148] In depressed, irritable, or aggressive patients on long-term barbiturate therapy, gradual conversion to a nonbarbiturate may avoid the need for prescribing a psy-

Table 11–16. **Major Adverse Effects of Antiepileptic Drugs**

Drug	Dose-Related Effects	Rare Idiosyncratic Effects	Long-Term Effects
Barbiturates			
Phenobarbital, primidone	Tiredness, depression, hyperactivity, dizziness, memory problems, impotence, dysarthria, nausea, anemia, rash,° fever°	Liver damage, severe rash hypersensitivity reaction	Anemia, bone loss, connective tissue side effects (joint pain, frozen shoulder, soft tissue growths, Dupuytren's)
Benzodiazepines			
Clobazam, clonazepam, clorazepate, diazepam, lorazepam	Tiredness, dizziness, unsteadiness, impaired attention and memory, hyperactivity, irritability, aggressivity, drooling (children), nausea, loss of appetite	None known	None known
Other Antiepileptics			
Carbamazepine, oxcarbazepine	Nausea, vomiting, blurred or double vision, tiredness, dizziness, unsteadiness, slurred speech, hyponatremia, rash,° fever°	Very low WBC or CBC,°° liver damage,°° severe rash, other hypersensitivity reactions, heart block	Bone loss, weight gain
Ethosuximide	Nausea, vomiting, decreased appetite, weight loss, behavioral changes, tiredness, dizziness, earache	Very low WBC or CBC	None known
Gabapentin	Dizziness, tiredness	None known	Weight gain
Lamotrigine	Insomnia, nausea, unsteadiness, rash, fever	Severe rash	None

Drug	Common adverse effects	Serious adverse effects	Long-term adverse effects
Levetiracetam	Tiredness, dizziness, unsteadiness, irritability, agitation, depression	None known	Possible mild weight gain
Phenytoin	Tiredness, dizziness, rash,° fever,° gum hypertrophy, hirsutism, anemia, acne, slurred speech, low calcium, bone loss	Liver damage, severe rash,° other hypersensitivity reactions, behavioral changes	Anemia, bone loss, cerebellar atrophy, gum hypertrophy, hirsutism, coarsening of facial features, neuropathy
Tiagabine	Dizziness, tiredness, mood changes	None known	None known
Topiramate	Dizziness, tiredness, decreased appetite, paresthesias, impaired concentration and word finding, memory problems, mood changes	Kidney stones, rash, oligohydrosis, angle closure glaucoma	Possible bone loss, weight loss
Valproate	Nausea, vomiting, tiredness, weight gain, hair loss, tremor	Liver damage, very low platelet count, pancreatic inflammation, hearing loss, behavioral changes	Bone loss, polycystic, ovarian syndrome (oligomenorrhea amenorrhea, anovulation or infertility, hirsutism, acne), weight gain
Vigabatrin	Tiredness, mood disorder, psychosis	None known	Retina injury, weight gain
Zonisamide	Drowsiness, dizziness, decreased appetite, GI discomfort, rash°	Kidney stones, severe rash, oligohydrosis	Possible bone loss, weight loss

WBC, white blood cell count; CBC, complete blood cell count; GI, gastrointestinal.
Some adverse effects of antiepileptic drugs (very low blood cell or platelet count, liver damage, hypersensitivity reactions, severe rash, pancreatic inflammation) are serious and potentially fatal.

°Rash and fever are common (3%–6% of patients) but not dose-related.
°°Only reported with carbamazepine; not with oxcarbazepine.

Table 11–17. **Pharmacological Properties of Frequently Used Antiepileptic Drugs**

Drug	Adult Daily Dose	Time to Peak Blood Level* (hours)	Therapeutic Blood Level (μg/ml of blood)	Half–Life[†] (hours)
Carbamazepine[‡]	600–1600	2–12	5–12	8–20
Clonazepam[§]	0.5–5.0	1–4	20–80 (ng/ml)	15–40
Clorazepate	3.75–15	0.5–2	?	30–60
Ethosuximide[§]	500–1500	1–4	50–100	25–70
Felbamate[§]	1200–3600	1–4	30–100	14–20
Gabapentin[§]	900–2700	2–4	4–16	5–7
Lamotrigine[§]	200–500	2–4	1–20	7–60[**]
Levetiracetam	1500–3000	0.75–2.5	3–37	6–8
Oxcarbazepine	600–2400	3–6	10–35 (only MHD measured)	2 9 (MHD)
Phenobarbital	60–240	2–12	12–40	26–140
Phenytoin	250–500	4–8	10–20	14–30[††]
Primidone	375–1000	2–5	5–18	12
Tiagabine	32–56		5–70 ng/ml	4–9
Topiramate	200–400		2–25	20
Valproate[§]	750–3000	2–8 1–3[‡‡]	50–140	8–16
Zonisamide	200–600	5–6	10–40	40–60

MHD, monohydroxyderivative, an active metabolite.
*Measured after blood drug levels reach steady state.
[†]Children metabolize many drugs more rapidly than adults do, so the half–life is often shorter in children.
[‡]Active metabolite.
[§]In general, when these drugs are given together with carbamazepine, phenobarbital, phenytoin, or primidone, their blood level is lower and their half–life is shorter.
[**]Valproate prolongs the half–life of lamotrigine.
[††]The half-life of phenytoin increases as the dose or blood phenytoin level increases.
[‡‡]After oral dose of valproate.

chotropic medication, as illustrated by the following case:

> Seizures in a 52-year-old man with partial epilepsy were well controlled on a daily dose of 1000 mg of primidone for two decades, but he complained of lethargy and depression. Over a year, carbamazepine, 1200 mg/day, was substituted, and seizure control was maintained. His Beck depression score fell from 22 to 3. He and his wife and employer observed a marked improvement in his motivation and memory. His wife noted "I never realized it, but he had a terrible habit of bumping other cars. When he thought a driver cut him off or passed too closely, when he got to a red light, he would bump the other car, never bad enough to cause a dent, but there were a few fistfights. He hasn't bumped any cars now that he's off primidone."

Carbamazepine

Although carbamazepine is structurally similar to the tricyclic antidepressant imipramine, it is not an effective antidepressant. Carbamazepine effectively treats mania and stabilizes mood in bipolar disorder.[131] Many uncontrolled studies support a role for carbamazepine in treating impulse control disorders such as borderline personality disorder with aggression and episodic dyscontrol syndrome.[149] Carbamazepine is not effective at treating panic disorder[150] or cocaine dependence.[151]

Carbamazepine can cause sedation and occasionally causes behavioral problems. Ten percent of patients with mental retardation treated with carbamazepine for mood disorders developed adverse behavioral reactions.[152] Carbamazepine-induced behavioral disorders usually occur in patients with existing behavioral difficulties.

Ethosuximide

Ethosuximide, used to treat absence seizures, may cause confusion, sleep disturbances, aggressive behavior, depression, and rarely psychosis. Forced normalization (see Chapter 10) with ethosuximide, that is, normalizing an electroencephalogram showing abundant generalized epileptiform discharges, may cause behavioral abnormalities.[153]

Gabapentin

Social phobia and other forms of anxiety may be effectively treated with gabapentin.[133] In two double-blind studies, gabapentin was ineffective for bipolar or unipolar depressive disorders,[134,135] although in open-label studies gabapentin improved mania[154,155] and the depressive phase of bipolar disorder.[156,157] Preliminary studies suggest a beneficial effect of gabapentin on behavioral dyscontrol,[158] agitation in senile dementia,[159] and self-injurious behaviors in neurological syndromes.[160] In uncontrolled studies of patients with epilepsy, gabapentin appeared to improve the sense of well-being and mood dysfunction independent of seizure reduction.[136,161,162] Gabapentin has minimal cognitive side effects in patients with epilepsy.[136,163]

Gabapentin occasionally causes irritability and agitation. This problem most often occurs in children with developmental disabilities but may affect children with normal development as well as adults.[164,165]

Lamotrigine

Lamotrigine effectively treats refractory bipolar disorder, especially the depressed phase of bipolar disorder.[134,166,167] Preliminary studies suggest that lamotrigine may have a beneficial effect on unipolar depression,[134] borderline personality disorder,[168] and schizoaffective disorder.[169] Lamotrigine can cause mild stimulation that leads to insomnia. This effect may be managed by shifting most of the dose to the morning or early afternoon.

In patients with epilepsy, lamotrigine has a favorable cognitive and behavioral profile.[170] Patients with developmental disabilities and epilepsy can experience either positive or negative psychotropic effects.[171,172] Positive effects include diminished irritability, hyperactivity, and perseveration and improved energy and social function. Negative effects include irritability, hyperactivity, and stereotypic and aggressive behavior. Serum lamotrigine levels do not clearly predict a psychotropic response.

Levetiracetam

No positive psychotropic effects are established for levetiracetam, although it is chemically related to the putative nootropic drug piracetam. In our experience, approximately 10% of adults and 25% of children taking levetiracetam exhibit irritability, anxiety, depression, and other behavioral disorders. These problems may occur more often in patients with developmental delays.

Phenytoin

Once promoted as an antidepressant,[173] phenytoin is rarely used as a psychotropic agent. A controlled study found efficacy for mania.[174] Phenytoin has a cognitive and behavioral profile similar to that of carbamazepine and some other antiepileptic drugs.[175] Some patients experience sedation, psychomotor slowing, mild cognitive impairment, and depression. A chronic, cumulative encephalopathy may occur after long-term exposure to high doses of phenytoin, perhaps resulting partly from cerebellar atrophy (Fig. 11–1). An acute encephalopathy and seizures may develop with phenytoin toxicity (blood phenytoin levels >35 μg/ml).

Tiagabine

In patients with epilepsy, tiagabine may improve mood or cause irritability, emotional lability, and dysphoria.[176,177] Preliminary studies indicate that tiagabine is not effective in bipolar disorder.[178]

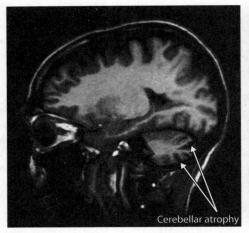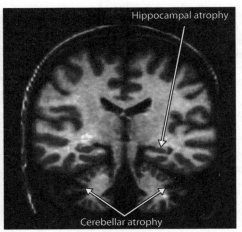

Figure 11–1. Brain magnetic resonance images (coronal sections) from a woman with temporal lobe epilepsy on long-term phenytoin therapy. Double arrows show cerebellar atrophy. Single arrow shows left-sided hippocampal atrophy.

Topiramate

Topiramate may improve mania and stabilize mood in bipolar disorder.[179,180] Topiramate may help to treat selected cases of binge-eating disorder.[181] Indeed, the weight loss often associated with topiramate is a beneficial effect in many patients, especially those who have been treated with drugs promoting weight gain (e.g., antipsychotic drugs, valproate, gabapentin, SSRIs). Cognitive and behavioral problems associated with topiramate use are a significant concern. However, both cognitive and behavioral problems are less frequent and severe when the starting dose is low and increased slowly.[137]

Cognitive disorders related to topiramate use include impaired attention, word-finding and verbal fluency, memory, and psychomotor slowing. Behavioral changes include depression, irritability, and rarely psychosis.[182] In a randomized controlled trial of topiramate, gabapentin, and lamotrigine in healthy young adults, only topiramate-treated subjects showed significant declines on measures of attention and word fluency and increases on an anger-hostility scale.[136] These changes were observed with acute doses and at 2– and 4–week visits. In patients with Lennox-Gastaut syndrome, severe adverse events included somnolence, mood problems, nervousness, personality disorder, and language problems.[183]

Valproate

Valproate effectively treats mania and stabilizes mood in patients with bipolar disorder.[184,185] It reduces the severity of acute alcohol withdrawal and minimizes the need for benzodiazepines.[186] Valproate may improve mood in patients with epilepsy, developmental disabilities, and schizoaffective disorder.[187,188] It may help treat panic disorder,[189] borderline personality disorder,[190] and OCD. Irritability, agitation, aggression, self-injurious behavior, and mood problems in patients with CNS disorders such as head trauma, seizures, or dementia may respond well to valproate therapy.[188,191]

Valproate commonly causes sedation and infrequently causes significant cognitive impairment, irritability, depression, hyperactivity, and aggressive behavior. Adverse effects include weight gain, hair loss (possibly minimized by selenium 10–20 μg/day and zinc 25–50 mg/day), hyperandrogenism, and polycystic ovary disease.

Vigabatrin

Vigabatrin is an irreversible inhibitor of GABA transaminase, which increases GABA levels in the CNS. Vigabatrin has no established positive psychotropic effects. It may cause depression and psychosis and exacerbate hyperactivity.[192,193] Retinal toxicity limits its use.

Zonisamide

Preliminary studies suggest that zonisamide has a role in the treatment of mania in patients with bipolar and schizoaffective disorders.[194,195] However, zonisamide may induce irritability, emotional lability, and rarely mania or psychosis.

Cognition Enhancers

In Alzheimer's disease, the progressive loss of basal forebrain neurons that synthesize ACh with the choline acetyltransferase enzyme produces a diffuse cortical and subcortical deficiency of ACh. The postsynaptic cholinergic receptors are normal and postsynaptic cholinergic cells are relatively spared. Cholinesterase (ChE) inhibitors increase intrasynaptic ACh, enhancing postsynaptic stimulation. In Alzheimer's disease, the efficacy of ChE inhibitors is limited by the progressive loss of basal forebrain cholinergic neurons and postsynaptic cells and the extensive involvement of other noncholinergic neuronal systems.

CHOLINESTERASE INHIBITORS

Four ChE inhibitors are approved for the treatment of Alzheimer's disease (Table 11–18). All other uses of these agents are off-label. In randomized controlled trials in patients with Alzheimer's disease, ChE inhibitors modestly improved the quality of life, activities of daily living, and behavioral, neuropsychological, and global outcomes. A large randomized controlled trial found significant benefit of ChE inhibitors in diffuse Lewy body disease, which may cause a more profound cholinergic deficit than Alzheimer disease.[196] No trials have directly compared the four ChE inhibitors, but data suggest a similar modest efficacy for all the drugs. Their main side effects are gastrointestinal, with nausea, cramping, diarrhea, and vomiting. The ChE inhibitors interact with other cholinergic and neuromuscular agents (e.g., succinylcholine).

Tacrine

Tacrine was the first ChE inhibitor approved for use in humans, but hepatic toxicity severely restricts its utility.[197] Tacrine inhibits ACh binding to ChE, increasing cholinergic activity at muscarinic and nicotinic receptors. Tacrine also increases ACh release by blocking slow potassium channels and increasing postsynaptic monoamines. Randomized controlled studies with more than 2000 patients, employing doses up to 160 mg/day for 2–12 months, showed cognitive skill improvements in 15%–30% of patients with Alzheimer's disease.[198,199] Postmarketing experience revealed significant hepatic toxicity; and now that other ChE inhibitors are available, tacrine is rarely used. If tacrine is used, liver function tests should be obtained every other week as the dose is increased and then every 3 months thereafter. Hepatic toxicity is dose-dependent and reversible in 90% of cases.

Donepezil

A reversible and noncompetitive inhibitor of ChE, donepezil dose-dependently increases brain extracellular ACh. Donepezil augments rapid eye movement (REM) sleep, possibly contributing to enhanced memory performance in healthy elderly persons.[200] In addition to common gastrointestinal symptoms, infrequent effects include muscle cramps, insomnia, fatigue, and anorexia. Adverse effects are usually mild and transient. Use donepezil cautiously in patients with active gastrointestinal disease, chronic obstructive pulmonary disease, benign prostatic hyperplasia, cardiac arrhythmias, and seizures.

An initial donepezil dose of 5 mg at bedtime is often effective. A dose of 10 mg once a day produces a statistically nonsignificant cognitive improvement but more gastrointestinal toxicity. We suggest a 4- to 6-week trial of 5 mg/day before increasing the dose to 10 mg/day. In 2-year open-label follow-up studies in patients with Alzheimer's disease, donepezil remained safe and effective.[201] Donepezil is effective for and well tolerated by patients with advanced Alzheimer's disease.[202]

Donepezil's potential role in other dementia syndromes (e.g. idiopathic and atypical Parkinson's disease, diffuse Lewy body disease, and frontotemporal dementias) remains uncertain. In patients with epilepsy-related cognitive impairment, pilot data suggest that donepezil slightly improves memory without increasing the risk of seizures.[203] In preliminary studies, donepezil improved cognition and behavior in patients with trau-

Table 11–18. **Pharmacological Properties of Cognition Enhancers**

Compound (Class), Strength (mg)	Enzyme Selectivity	Effect of Food on Absorption	Adult Total Daily Dose, Oral (mg/day)	Delay to Peak Serum Level (hours)	Half-Life (hours)	Protein Binding (%)	Hepatic Metabolism
Acetylcholinesterases							
Tacrine (acrinidine) 10, 20, 30, 40	ButyrylChE>AchE	Delays	40–160 (q.i.d.)	1–2.5	2–4	75	CYP1A2, CYP2D 6
Donepezil (piperidine) 5, 10	AchE	None	5 – 10 (q.d.)	3–5	70	95	CYP2D6, CYP3A4
Rivastigmine (carbamate) 1.5, 3, 4, 5, 6; 2 mg/ml syrup	AchE=ButyrylChE	Delays	6–12 (b.i.d.)	0.5–1.5	10	40	None
Galantamine (phenanthrene alkaloid) 4, 8, 12	AChE and modulates nicotinic Ach receptors	Delays	16–32 (b.i.d.)	0.5–1.0	5–6	15	CYP2D6, CYP3A4
MAO-B Inhibitor							
Selegiline 5	MAO-B>> MAO-A	Increases bioavailability three- to fourfold	10 (b.i.d.) (breakfast and lunch)	0.5–1.5	10	Not known	Cytochrome P-450
Cyclic GABA Inhibitor							
Piracetam (acetamide) 800 not available in US	None	?	1600–4800 (t.i.d.)	0.5–1.0	5–6	?	None

MAO, monoamine oxidase; GABA, γ-aminobutyric acid; ChE, cholinesterase; ACh, acetylcholine; AChE, acetylcholinesterase.

matic brain injuries[204] and "sundowning" symptoms.[205]

Rivastigmine

A pseudoirreversible, noncompetitive ChE inhibitor, rivastigmine is regionally selective for the hippocampus and cortex. Rivastigmine preferentially inhibits the ChE inhibitor G1 four times as much as the G4 form. The G1 form is found in high levels in the brain of patients with Alzheimer's disease. It is approved to treat mild to moderate Alzheimer's disease. Rivastigmine significantly increases REM sleep density by 50% during the first two-thirds of the night, possibly contributing to cognitive improvement.[206] Adverse effects include gastrointestinal symptoms, dizziness, fatigue, agitation, loss of appetite, asthenia, and diaphoresis. Use rivastigmine cautiously in cardiovascular or pulmonary disease, diabetes mellitus, gastrointestinal disorders, urogenital tract obstruction, and Parkinson's disease (may exacerbate motor symptoms). Doses need not be adjusted in patients with hepatic and renal impairment. Rivastigmine is metabolized primarily by ChE, not cytochrome P-450 enzymes. It has few drug interactions.

Galantamine

A reversible, competitive ChE inhibitor, galantamine also binds to nicotinic receptors, amplifying ACh effects at presynaptic and postsynaptic nicotinic ACh receptors. Galantamine's modulation of nicotinic receptors alters the concentrations of other neurotransmitters, possibly accounting for behavioral improvement.[207] Galantamine is approved to treat mild to moderate dementia. Trials in more than 3000 patients with 16–32 mg/day of galantamine improved cognition, activities of daily living, sleep quality, and behavior for up to 12 months.[208,209] There was no additional cognitive improvement with doses higher than 24 mg/day. Use galantamine cautiously in patients with gastrointestinal or cardiac disorders. Doses must be adjusted in patients with renal or hepatic impairment.

POTENTIAL COGNITION ENHANCER

Piracetam is a cyclic GABA derivative, a nootropic agent with anti-myoclonic and possible cognition-enhancing and neuroprotective properties (Table 11–18). It has not been approved for use in the United States. Its mechanism of action is unknown but may involve alterations of membrane fluidity[210,211] and increased brain adenosine triphosphate levels.[212] Piracetam is excreted unchanged in the urine. Lower doses are used in the elderly or patients with renal impairment. Piracetam inhibits platelet aggregation and may help in stroke prophylaxis.[213] Its use with warfarin increases the risk of bleeding. Piracetam achieves high concentrations in brain tissue. Adverse effects include nervousness, irritability, head-ache, agitation, dizziness, gastrointestinal effects, choreiform movements, and very rarely hepatic toxicity.

Many, but methodologically limited, studies suggest that piracetam enhances cognition in humans and other species.[212,214–216] Piracetam may be beneficial for Alzheimer's disease,[217] autism,[218] poststroke aphasia,[219] dyslexia,[220] and memory impairment from brain disorders. As yet, however, there is no firm evidence in support of piracetam for treating cognitive disorders.[217,221] Piracetam appears effective for treating some epileptic and nonepileptic myoclonic disorders.[222,223]

Antioxidants

The model of oxidative neuronal injury mediated by β-amyloid suggests that antioxidant agents could slow degeneration in Alzheimer's disease. Medicines or vitamins that increase brain catecholamines may protect against oxidative damage. In a 2–year randomized controlled trial, the antioxidants selegiline (10 mg/day) and α-tocopherol (vitamin E, 2000 IU/day) retarded the decline in cognition and ability to perform activities of daily living and prolonged survival in patients with moderately severe Alzheimer's disease.[224] Patients treated with selegiline or α-tocopherol or both improved in all clinical outcomes compared with those receiving placebo. Combined therapy had no advantage over either antioxidant alone. A meta-analysis of 15 studies showed that selegiline improves memory in Alzheimer's disease,[225] but behavioral improvements were not consistent. Estrogen replacement therapy in postmenopausal women, nonsteroidal anti-inflammatory agents, and statins have not been proven to prevent or slow the progression of Alzheimer's disease, although epidemiological studies show a lower rate of Alzheimer's disease among individuals on these therapies.[226,227]

VITAMIN E

Vitamin E is a free radical–scavenging antioxidant that may help to stabilize neural membrane phosopholipids rich in polyunsaturated fatty acids. Vitamin E deficiency can cause a rare neurological syndrome of spinocerebellar degeneration, polyneuropathy, and pigmentary degeneration. High doses of vitamin E may cause gastrointestinal upset or impair clotting mechanisms, leading to easy bruising or bleeding. Vitamin E should be stopped at least a week before elective surgery.

SELEGILINE

In addition to its use in Alzheimer's disease, selegiline is adjunctive therapy for Parkinson's disease. It may be neuroprotective in Parkinson's disease by slowing striatal dopamine metabolism. Selegiline delays the need to initiate levodopa therapy and decreases the dosages required. Response is usually seen within 1–3 days after initiation of therapy. Selegiline may improve both memory and motor functions in patients with Parkinson's disease.[228] Preliminary studies suggest a potential role for selegiline in depression[229] and ADHD.[230] In rodents, selegiline improves cognitive functions and enhances neuroplasticity after traumatic brain injury.[231]

Selegiline is an irreversible selective inhibitor of MAO-B, blocking presynaptic re-uptake of catecholamines and presynaptic dopamine autoreceptors and thereby enhancing its dopaminergic activity.[232] The usual dose is 5 mg twice daily, morning and mid-day; bioavailability is improved when the drug is consumed with food (Table 11–18). Selegiline is hepatically metabolized to active metabolites. Doses higher than 10 mg/day also inhibit MAO-A. The peripheral side effects are milder than those of nonspecific MAOIs and include nausea, dizziness, anorexia, headache, and hypotension. The CNS side effects include insomnia, anxiety, increased libido, agitation, psychosis, hallucinations, confusion, and dys-kinesias. A hypertensive crisis induced by tyramine-rich foods is rare with selegiline. Use selegiline cautiously with SSRIs, tricyclic antidepressants, or meperidine.

OTHER THERAPIES

Herbs and Dietary Supplements

Dietary supplements are widely used and generally considered nontoxic.[233] The purity and composition of nutritional supplements are not controlled by the FDA, and some supplements are potentially toxic. Many methodologically limited studies suggest that St. John's wort and S-adenosylmethionine improve depression, and one placebo-controlled trial found that ω-3 fatty acids improve symptoms in bipolar disorder.[233–235] Advise patients that reports of the risks and benefits of herbal and dietary supplements are often unreliable and that some of these agents can interact adversely with prescribed medications.[236]

ST. JOHN'S WORT

St. John's wort (*Hypericum perforatum*) has been used for centuries to treat insomnia and anxiety. Hypericin, the main active ingredient, is extracted from the flowers and leafy portions of St. John's wort. Whole-plant, but weakly active, hypericin is also available. Typical doses range from 300 to 900 mg/day of a 0.3% hypericin extract (2–4 g of dried herb). The mechanism of hypericin action is uncertain but may be biogenic amine or GABAergic activity. It is not clear whether hypericin crosses the blood–brain barrier. If it does not, another active ingredient or a placebo response seems likely.

The efficacy of hypericin compared with standard antidepressants is uncertain. In a meta-analysis of 22 randomized controlled trials, hypericin was significantly more effective than placebo at treating depression (relative risk 1.98).[237] However, in many of these studies, the rates of placebo efficacy were unusually low; and a large, double-blind study is under way in an attempt to answer unresolved questions regarding dose, efficacy, and tolerability. Hypericin has milder and fewer side effects than standard antidepressants,[237] with the main problems being dry mouth, stomach discomfort, dizziness, fatigue, and confusion. Hypericin increases the likelihood of a serotonin syndrome in patients concomitantly taking SSRIs and decreases the bioavailability of digoxin, warfarin, indinavir, amitriptyline, theophylline, cyclosporin, and phenprocoumon.[238]

KAVA

Kava, derived from the roots of the *Piper methysticum* shrub from the South Pacific, has been made into a "relaxing" beverage for centuries. α-Lactones (kavalactones) are probably the active agents, possibly affecting the GABAergic system. There are no well-controlled studies of kava. A meta-analysis showed that kava is superior to placebo at reducing anxiety.[239] Kava may diminish anxiety and tension and promote sleep without inhibiting mental concentration. Side effects of kava are rare; long-term use of 400 mg/day or more may cause skin scaling. The FDA has issued an advisory that kava-containing dietary supplements may cause severe liver injury (e.g., hepatitis, cirrhosis, liver failure).

S-ADENOSYLMETHIONINE

S-Adenosylmethionine (SAMe) is present in all cells and plays a critical role in transmethylation, transsulfuration, and aminopropylation. These pathways produce more than 100 reactions involved in diverse functions, including gene activation, repairing damaged protein, forming the phosphatidylcholine in cell membranes, and the synthesis and catabolism of monamines. The latter effect is implicated in the possible psychotropic effect as SAMe increases brain concentrations of NE and serotonin in rodents.[240] Four of five randomized double-blind studies found SAMe to be more effective than placebo at treating depression.[240] Overall, more than 45 studies in patients with depression suggest a response rate similar to that of tricyclic antidepressants, although the available data are not definitive.[240,241] It has a low incidence of side effects, which are generally mild and transient. These include anxiety, nervousness, insomnia, dizziness, jitteriness, headache, loose stools, constipation, gastrointestinal discomfort, dry mouth, and sweating. Doses for minor depression average 400 mg/day and, for major depression, 800–1600 mg/day.

GINKGO BILOBA

Ginkgo biloba is a tree whose seeds have long been used in Chinese medicine. Phytomedicinal extracts from the leaves are sold as dietary supplements in the United States and elsewhere. The main active compounds in the leaves are flavonoid glycosides and ginkgolides. The latter are unique diterpenes that are antioxidants, platelet-activating factor inhibitors, and circulatory enhancers.[242] One extract, EGb, may underlie potential cognitive and circulatory benefits.[243] Clinical studies suggest that ginkgo extracts may improve memory function in Alzheimer's disease, other dementias, and age-related memory impairment.[242,243] In some studies, 240 mg/day of EGb produced a higher rate of response than 120 mg/day.[244] However, blinded, controlled studies showed no effect on memory in healthy subjects or mildly to moderately demented patients.[245,246] Ginkgo's adverse event profile is similar to that of placebo.[244] However, ginkgo and other plant derivatives may increase the risk of bleeding in patients taking warfarin[247] and may cause intracerebral hemorrhage[248] or increase surgical bleeding.[249]

Vagus Nerve Stimulation

Vagus nerve stimulation is the repetitive electrical stimulation of the vagus nerve on the left side by a programmable stimulator implanted in the left upper chest. Vagus nerve stimulation is effective for partial and generalized epilepsies. Although complete control is achieved in less than 3% of patients with refractory epilepsy, more than a 50% reduction in seizures occurs in 25%–35% of patients. The mechanism by which vagus nerve stimulation suppresses seizures is unknown. However, vagal afferents terminating in the solitary tract nucleus may inhibit ascending outputs from this nucleus that influence forebrain and brain stem areas that modulate seizure activity.[250] Studies in animal models and humans suggest that vagus nerve stimulation enhances memory. It improves retention performance in rats[251] and possibly recognition memory in humans.[252] In uncontrolled studies, vagus nerve stimulation improved cognition and mood in some patients with epilepsy.[253,254] In contrast with standard stimulation (7– to 30–second trains), prolonged stimulation (4.5–minute trains) impairs figural memory during the stimulus train in patients with epilepsy.[255] The role of vagus nerve stimulation as a therapy for depression remains uncertain.

Vagus nerve stimulation is generally well tolerated but has a 1% risk of infection (usually requiring removal of the stimulator) and a 1% risk of recurrent laryngeal nerve injury. Common adverse reactions include hoarseness, change in voice quality, and neck paresthesias during stimulation, which usually improve after weeks or months. Psychiatric disturbances may result from this type of therapy.[256] Although vagus nerve stimulation requires a surgical procedure, it avoids the CNS side effects such as sedation and impaired cognition that may complicate antiepileptic drug use.

CONDITIONS AFFECTING COGNITION AND BEHAVIOR

Fatigue

Subjective fatigue, the feeling of early exhaustion developing during mental activity, with weariness, lack of energy, and aversion to effort, is a common symptom in many neurological disorders (e.g., brain tumor, multiple sclerosis, stroke, epilepsy). Fatigue after stroke is commonly overlooked and associated with brain stem and thalamic lesions.[257] In multiple sclerosis, fatigue is associated with reduced metabolic activity in the prefrontal cortex and basal ganglia.[258] Sedating medications (e.g., antiepileptic drugs) for the underlying disorder often cause fatigue.

The treatment of fatigue involves reduction or elimination of sedating medications, therapy for comorbid mood disorders, education about ways of conserving energy,[259] use of medications (amantadine and CNS stimulants), exercise, and stress-management techniques. Chronic fatigue is a controversial entity that may occur with depression, pain and other neurological disorders. Amantadine (200–300 mg/day) and modafinil (200 mg/day) reduce fatigue in multiple sclerosis.[260–262] Central nervous system stimulants such as methylphenidate and modafinil reduce fatigue in cancer and human immunodeficiency syndrome patients, but studies in neurological disorders are limited.

Insomnia

Sleep disturbance is a common feature and exacerbating factor in many neurobehavioral disorders. Insomnia is a subjective disorder of inadequate, nonrestorative sleep. Difficulty falling asleep is the most common problem in insomnia and often associated with awakenings throughout the night and early final awakening. Insomnia is the most common sleep disorder, afflicting one-third of adults annually, most often women, the elderly, and those with psychiatric, substance-abuse, and medical disorders. The patient's sleep history is important (Table 11–3).

On the basis of its duration, insomnia is classified as transient (lasting <3 nights), short-term (lasting 3 nights to 3 weeks), and chronic (lasting >3 weeks). This classification is key to assessing and treating insomnia. Transient and short-term insomnia are common and usually caused by stress, pain, and drug or alcohol use. Improved sleep is often achieved by addressing stressful issues; relaxation exercises; avoidance of alcohol, caffeine, cigarettes, diet pills, and daytime naps; regular, moderate daytime exercise; a bedtime routine (fairly regular sleeping and rising times, reading but no television watching before bedtime); and optimal sleep environment (shades and earplugs to minimize extraneous light and sound, comfortable room temperature). Sedative-hypnotic drugs may be an effective adjunct to these behavioral measures. These drugs should not be prescribed unless the physician has explored the nature and cause of the insomnia and should be a part of, but not the entire, therapeutic strategy.

Benzodiazepines and zolpidem are most commonly used to treat insomnia, but antihistamines, tricyclic antidepressants, zaleplon, and melatonin are also effective (Table 11–15). Benzodiazepines with short half-lives are less likely to accumulate or cause sedative or anxiolytic effects the following day but are more likely to cause rebound insomnia after discontinuation, anterograde amnesia, tolerance to hypnotic effects, and early final awakening. Neurological side effects of benzodiazepines increase with the patient's age, dose, and duration of therapy. Benzodiazepines predispose patients to falls and fractures, probably as the result of ataxia and confusion, especially in the elderly.

Chronic insomnia leads to conditioned anxiety, with bedtime provoking fear of the inability to sleep and the effects of lost sleep. The anxiety commonly leads to depression and less frequently to psychiatric disorders. Alcohol, sedative and illicit drug use, medical and neurological disorders (e.g., hyperthyroidism, dementia), chronic pain, sleep apnea, and nocturnal movement disorders (e.g., myoclonus, restless legs syndrome) may cause chronic insomnia. Nonpharmacological strategies described earlier are often helpful. Their efficacy and mild side effects make benzodiazepines and zolpidem ideal for short-term therapy, although they also are often used to treat chronic insomnia. Therapy-resistant patients may be referred to a sleep disorder center.

Pain

Pain complicates many neurological disorders, often predominating the clinical picture and disability. Pain retards cognitive, psychological, physical, and occupational therapies. Persistent pain often creates a chronic disorder, fortified by psychological processes that further impede functional recovery. Pain medications, especially opiates but also nonsteroidal anti-inflammatory agents, are habit-forming and may further limit mental and physical function. Pain must be identified and treated, but psychological factors (e.g., depression) that promote the pain cycle and medication dependence are equally important. Acupuncture can help to treat pain that complicates neurological disorders such as stroke.[263]

Sexual Dysfunction

Neurobehavioral disorders often disrupt the complex interaction of mental, nervous, vascular, and endocrine systems that produce desire, arousal, erection, and orgasm. Sexual arousal stimulates the parasympathetic nerves that increase blood flow to the penis and clitoris. Orgasm is mediated by sympathetic fibers. In the brain, arousal and orgasm are facilitated by androgenic and dopaminergic activity and inhibited by serotonergic activity.

Common behavioral factors in sexual dysfunction include performance anxiety (most common cause of erectile and orgasmic dysfunction), unconscious anxiety and guilt about sex, misinformation about sexual and social interactions, and poor communication between partners about their sexual feelings and desired sexual behaviors. Neurological causes include multiple sclerosis, stroke, epilepsy, spinal cord disease, and neuropathies. Neuropsychiatric disorders involving the limbic regions affect the appetitive and excitement stages of the sexual response. Sexual dysfunction often results from medications and illness. Drugs that may impair sexual function include antihypertensives (e.g., diuretics, β-blockers), opiates, antipsychotics, antidepressants (e.g., SSRIs, tricyclic antidepressants, trazodone [priapism], nefazodone, venlafaxine, mirtazapine), glucocorticoids, estrogens, and cimetidine, as well as alcohol and cocaine.

Hypoactive sexual desire disorder (inhibited sexual desire) is characterized by a sustained reduction in sexual fantasies and desires. This may be a primary disorder, or it may be secondary to another sexual dysfunction. In patients with epilepsy, control of seizures with antiepileptic drugs does not usually improve the disorder. Combinations of cognitive therapy, behavioral exercises to enhance sexual pleasure and communication, and marital therapy may be helpful.

Male erectile disorder is often treated with education and "behavioral assignments" to reduce performance anxiety. Premature ejaculation may improve with clomipramine, paroxetine, or fluoxetine. Sildenafil is the most effective and commonly prescribed oral medication for erectile dysfunction; others include yohimbine, trazodone, apomorphine, phentolamine, and arginine. A variety of agents (e.g., prostaglandin E_1, alprostadil, papaverine with phentolamine) are used for intracavernous self-injections for erectile disorders. Intracavernous injections may cause priapism and penile pain or fibrosis.[264] Testosterone is of uncertain benefit in men or women; masculinizing side effects are problematic in women. Testosterone is useful for pituitary or gonadal dysfunction (determined by total testosterone and sex hormone–binding globulin) but is not beneficial otherwise.

Delirium

Delirium is often caused by a life-threatening but treatable disorder (see Chapter 4, Table 4–1). The underlying cause must be identified and treated together with symptomatic and supportive care. Good nutrition, fluid and electrolyte balance, and a nonthreatening environment are essential. The room should be quiet and well lit and should contain some familiar objects, as well as a visible clock and calendar for the patient's orientation. Simplify the environment (e.g., single room, remove unnecessary objects) and keep the room temperature comfortable. The medical and nursing staff should be supportive and help to reorient the patient. Adjust medication schedules and nursing assessments to avoid interrupting the patient's sleep. Communicate with the patient clearly and concisely. Repeated verbal reminders and a chart with the day's schedule are helpful.

The use of drugs in managing delirium requires weighing the benefits of improving target symptoms and the possibility of producing adverse effects. The best course of treatment will be based on the patient's needs and not the wishes of family or staff pressures. Sedative and psychotropic drugs complicate the clinical assessment of mental function, reduce attention and comprehension, and increase the risk of falls. However, agitation can prove dangerous to the patient and others. Sleep deprivation aggravates delirium. Antipsychotic agents are the most effective treatment for agitation and severe behavioral disturbances unless the cause is withdrawal of alcohol or benzodiazepines or seizures, in which case benzodiazepines are preferred.[265,266] Haloperidol is effective and has minimal anticholinergic effects; the usual dose ranges from 0.5 to 5 mg, administered two or three times daily (orally, intramuscularly, or intravenously).[267] If the patient remains unmanageable after 20 minutes of parenterally administered medications and no adverse effects develop, the dose can be doubled and this cycle repeated with close observation for possible parkinsonism, neuroleptic malignant syndrome, and cardiac arrhythmias (e.g., QT prolongation).[268] Atypical antipsychotic agents (e.g., olanzapine, 5–10 mg; risperidone, 1–4 mg) may be effective.[269,270] Although they have fewer side effects than haloperidol, there is less experience with their use.[268]

Lorazepam, 1–2 mg (intramuscularly or intravenously), may be helpful in managing the extrapyramidal side effects of an antipsychotic by permitting dosage reduction. Respiration and blood pressure must be monitored more closely with parenteral benzodiazepines. Low doses of short-acting benzodiazepines or diphenhydramine (25–50 mg) promote sleep.

Oral as well as parenteral benzodiazepines occasionally aggravate delirium, especially when inadequate initial doses lead to behavioral disinhibition. Parenteral lorazepam doses should not exceed 2 mg every 4 hours. Benzodiazepine side effects are rapidly reversed with flumazenil, but withdrawal symptoms must be carefully monitored.

SUMMARY

Neurobehavioral therapies focus on target symptoms, not the disease process. Even when therapy is directed at the underlying disorder, it is often of limited benefit (e.g., antioxidants in Alzheimer's disease). The treatment of cognitive and behavioral symptoms is consistent across neurological disorders. In general, depression, anxiety, OCD, aggression and psychosis respond similarly regardless of whether the patient has multiple sclerosis, a hemispheric or subcortical stroke, epilepsy, or dementia. Many psychotropic medications are available for treating behavioral symptoms, often affording an opportunity to improve the patient's quality of life and reduce morbidity in disorders such as stroke, Parkinson's disease, and epilepsy. Therapy must encompass both pharmacological and nonpharmacological approaches, and respond not only to the symptoms but also to the patient as a whole person deserving to live life to the fullest extent possible.

REFERENCES

1. Bech P (ed): Rating Scales for Psychopathology, Health Status and Quality of Life. Springer-Verlag, New York, 1992.
2. Herndon RM (ed): Handbook of Neurological Rating Scales. Demos, New York, 1997.
3. Macdonell RA and Dewey HM: Neurological disability and neurological rehabilitation. Med J Aust 174:653–658, 2001.
4. Whurr R, Lorch MP, and Nye C: A meta-analysis of studies carried out between 1946 and 1988 concerned with the efficacy of speech and language therapy treatment for aphasic patients. Eur J Disord Commun 27:1–17, 1992.
5. Robey RR and Dalebout SD: A tutorial on conducting meta-analyses of clinical outcome research. J Speech Lang Hear Res 41:1227–1241, 1998.
6. Goodglass H and Kaplan E: Assessment of Aphasia and Related Disorders. Lea & Febiger, Philadelphia, 1983.
7. Schuell H: Minnesota Test for Differential Diagno-

sis of Aphasia. University of Minnesota Press, Minneapolis, 1965.

8. Shewan C and Bandur D: Treatment of Aphasia: A Language-Oriented Approach. College-Hill Press, Boston, 1986.

9. Pring T, White-Thomson M, Pound C, et al.: Picutre/word matching tasks and word retrieval: some follow-up data and second thoughts. Aphasiology 4:479–483, 1990.

10. Robson J, Marshall J, Pring T, and Chiat S: Phonological naming therapy in jargon aphasia: positive but paradoxical effects. J Int Neuropsychol Soc 4:675–686, 1998.

11. Korner-Bitensky N, Sofer S, Kaizer F, Gelinas I, and Talbot L: Assessing ability to drive following an acute neurological event: are we on the right road? Can J Occup Ther 61:141–148, 1994.

12. Kay T and Silver SM: Closed head trauma: assessment for rehabilitation. In Lezak M (ed). Assessment of the Behavioral Consequences of Head Trauma. Alan R Liss, New York, 1989, pp 145–170.

13. Cicerone KD, Dahlberg C, Kalmar K, Langenbahn DM, Malec JF, and Berquist TF: Evidence-based cognitive rehabilitation: recommendations for clinical practice. Arch Phys Med Rehabil 81:1596–1615, 2000.

14. Lee SS, Powell NJ, and Esdaile S: A functional model of cognitive rehabilitation in occupational therapy. Can J Occup Ther 68:41–50, 2001.

15. Narushima K and Robinson RG: Stroke-related depression. Curr Atheroscler Rep 4:296–303, 2002.

16. Kimura M, Robinson RG, and Kosier JT: Treatment of cognitive impairment after poststroke depression: a double-blind treatment trial. Stroke 31:1482–1486, 2000.

17. Gawronski DW and Reding MJ: Post-stroke depression: an update. Curr Atheroscler Rep 3:307–312, 2001.

18. Gainotti G, Antonucci G, Marra C, and Paolucci S: Relation between depression after stroke, antidepressant therapy, and functional recovery. J Neurol Neurosurg Psychiatry 71:258–261, 2001.

19. House A, Knapp P, Bamford J, and Vail A: Mortality at 12 and 24 months after stroke may be associated with depressive symptoms at 1 month. Stroke 32:696–701, 2001.

20. Schrag A, Jahanshahi M, and Quinn N: What contributes to quality of life in patients with Parkinson's disease? J Neurol Neurosurg Psychiatry 69:308–312, 2000.

21. Simmons Z, Bremer BA, Robbins RA, Walsh SM, and Fischer S: Quality of life in ALS depends on factors other than strength and physical function. Neurology 55:388–392, 2000.

22. Baker GA: The psychosocial burden of epilepsy. Epilepsia 43(Suppl 6):26–30, 2002.

23. Herrmann M, Bartels C, Schumacher M, and Wallesch CW: Poststroke depression. Is there a pathoanatomic correlate for depression in the postacute stage of stroke? Stroke 26:850–856, 1995.

24. Astrom M: Generalized anxiety disorder in stroke patients. A 3–year longitudinal study. Stroke 27:270–275, 1996.

25. Morris PL, Robinson RG, Raphael B, and Hopwood MJ: Lesion location and poststroke depression. J Neuropsychiatry Clin Neurosci 8:399–403, 1996.

26. Starkstein SE and Robinson RG: Mood disorders in neurodegenerative diseases. Semin Clin Neuropsychiatry 1:272–281, 1996.

27. Singh A, Herrmann N, and Black SE: The importance of lesion location in poststroke depression: a critical review. Can J Psychiatry 43:921–927, 1998.

28. Carson AJ, MacHale S, Allen K, Lawrie SM, Dennis M, House A, et al.: Depression after stroke and lesion location: a systematic review. Lancet 356:122–126, 2000.

29. Kimura M, Murata Y, Shimoda K, and Robinson RG: Sexual dysfunction following stroke. Compr Psychiatry 42:217–222, 2001.

30. Jonas BS and Mussolino ME: Symptoms of depression as a prospective risk factor for stroke. Psychosom Med 62:463–471, 2000.

31. Krishnan KR: Depression as a contributing factor in cerebrovascular disease. Am Heart J 140:70–76, 2000.

32. Calabrese JR, Bowden CL, Sachs GS, Ascher JA, Monaghan E, and Rudd GD: A double-blind placebo-controlled study of lamotrigine monotherapy in outpatients with bipolar I depression. Lamictal 602 Study Group. J Clin Psychiatry 60:79–88, 1999.

33. Rickels K, Chung HR, Csanalosi IB, Hurowitz AM, London J, Wiseman K, et al.: Alprazolam, diazepam, imipramine, and placebo in outpatients with major depression. Arch Gen Psychiatry 44:862–866, 1987.

34. Meehan K, Zhang F, David S, Tohen M, Janicak P, Small J, et al.: A double-blind, randomized comparison of the efficacy and safety of intramuscular injections of olanzapine, lorazepam, or placebo in treating acutely agitated patients diagnosed with bipolar mania. J Clin Psychopharmacol 21:389–397, 2001.

35. Nierenberg AA, Alpert JE, Pava J, Rosenbaum JF, and Fava M: Course and treatment of atypical depression. J Clin Psychiatry 59(Suppl 18):5–9, 1998.

36. Gruenberg AM and Goldstein RD: Depressive disorders. In Tasman A, Kay J, and Lieberman JA (eds). Psychiatry. WB Saunders, New York, 1997, pp 990–1016.

37. Lyketsos CG, Sheppard JM, Steele CD, Kopunek S, Steinberg M, Baker AS, et al.: Randomized, placebo-controlled, double-blind clinical trial of sertraline in the treatment of depression complicating Alzheimer's disease: initial results from the Depression in Alzheimer's Disease Study. Am J Psychiatry 157:1686–1689, 2000.

38. Petracca GM, Chemerinski E, and Starkstein SE: A double-blind, placebo-controlled study of fluoxetine in depressed patients with Alzheimer's disease. Int Psychogeriatr 13:233–240, 2001.

39. Newburn G, Edwards R, Thomas H, Collier J, Fox K, and Collins C: Moclobemide in the treatment of major depressive disorder (DSM-3) following traumatic brain injury. Brain Inj 13:637–642, 1999.

40. Hauser RA and Zesiewicz TA: Sertraline for the treatment of depression in Parkinson's disease. Mov Disord 12:756–759, 1997.

41. Robinson RG, Schultz SK, Castillo C, Kopel T, Kosier JT, Newman RM, et al.: Nortriptyline versus fluoxetine in the treatment of depression and in short- term recovery after stroke: a placebo-controlled, double-blind study. Am J Psychiatry 157: 351–359, 2000.

42. Wiart L, Petit H, Joseph PA, Mazaux JM, and Barat

M: Fluoxetine in early poststroke depression: a double-blind placebo-controlled study. Stroke 31:1829–1832, 2000.

43. Whyte EM and Mulsant BH. Post-stroke depression: epidemiology, pathophysiology, and biological treatment. Biol Psychiatry 52:253–264, 2002.

44. Astrom M, Adolfsson R, and Asplund K: Major depression in stroke patients. A 3-year longitudinal study. Stroke 24:976–982, 1993.

45. Aben I, Verhey F, Honig A, Lodder J, Lousberg R, and Maes M: Research into the specificity of depression after stroke: a review on an unresolved issue. Prog Neuropsychopharmacol Biol Psychiatry 25:671–689, 2001.

46. Gustafson Y, Nilsson I, Mattsson M, Astrom M, and Bucht G: Epidemiology and treatment of poststroke depression. Drugs Aging 7:298–309, 1995.

47. Reding MJ, Orto LA, Winter SW, Fortuna IM, Di Ponte P, and McDowell FH: Antidepressant therapy after stroke. A double-blind trial. Arch Neurol 43:763–765, 1986.

48. Levy ML, Cummings JL, Fairbanks LA, Masterman D, Miller BL, Craig AH, et al.: Apathy is not depression. J Neuropsychiatry Clin Neurosci 10:314–319, 1998.

49. Fink M: Convulsive therapy: a review of the first 55 years. J Affect Disord 63:1–15, 2001.

50. Rabheru K and Persad E: A review of continuation and maintenance electroconvulsive therapy. Can J Psychiatry 42:476–484, 1997.

51. Sackeim HA, Prudic J, Devanand DP, Kierskey JE, Fitzsimons L, Moody BJ, et al.: Effects of stimulus intensity and electrode placement on the efficacy and cognitive effects of electroconvulsive therapy. N Engl J Med 328:839–846, 1993.

52. Sackeim HA, Luber B, Moeller JR, Prudic J, Devanand DP, and Nobler MS: Electrophysiological correlates of the adverse cognitive effects of electroconvulsive therapy. J ECT 16:110–120, 2000.

53. Hallett M: Transcranial magnetic stimulation and the human brain. Nature 406:147–150, 2000.

54. Wassermann EM and Lisanby SH: Therapeutic application of repetitive transcranial magnetic stimulation: a review. Clin Neurophysiol 112:1367–1377, 2001.

55. Walsh V and Cowey A: Transcranial magnetic stimulation and cognitive neuroscience. Nat Rev Neurosci 1:73–79, 2000.

56. Sackeim HA, Rush AJ, George MS, Marangell LB, Husain MM, Nahas Z, et al.: Vagus nerve stimulation (VNS) for treatment-resistant depression: efficacy, side effects, and predictors of outcome. Neuropsychopharmacology 25:713–728, 2001.

57. Coplan JD, Pine DS, Papp LA, and Gorman JM: An algorithm-oriented treatment approach for panic disorder. Psychiatr Ann 26:192–201, 1996.

58. Kogeorgos J, Fonagy P, and Scott DF: Psychiatric symptom patterns of chronic epileptics attending a neurological clinic: a controlled investigation. Br J Psychiatry 140:236–243, 1982.

59. Kurlan R, Como PG, Miller B, et al.: The behavioral spectrum of tic disorders: a community-based study. Neurology 59:414–420, 2002.

60. Kazui H, Mori E, Hashimoto M, and Hirono N: Phobia after bilateral thalamic hemorrhage. Cerebrovasc Dis 12:283–284, 2001.

61. Micallef J and Blin O: Neurobiology and clinical pharmacology of obsessive–compulsive disorder. Clin Neuropharmacol 24:191–207, 2001.

62. Tekin S and Cummings JL: Frontal-subcortical circuits and clinical neuropsychiatry: an update. J Psychosom 53:647–654, 2002.

63. Berthier ML, Kulisevsky J, Gironell A, and Heras JA: Obsessive–compulsive disorder associated with brain lesions: clinical phenomenology, cognitive function, and anatomic correlates. Neurology 47:353–361, 1996.

64. Kurlan R: Tourette's syndrome and "PANDAS:" will the relation bear out? Pediatric autoimmune neuropsychiatric disorders associated with streptococcal infection. Neurology 50:1530–1534, 1998.

65. Ames D, Cummings JL, Wirshing WC, Quinn B, and Mahler M: Repetitive and compulsive behavior in frontal lobe degenerations. J Neuropsychiatry Clin Neurosci 6:100–113, 1994.

66. Jankovic J: Tourette's syndrome. N Engl J Med 345:1184–1192, 2001.

67. George MS, Trimble MR, Ring HA, Sallee FR, and Robertson MM: Obsessions in obsessive–compulsive disorder with and without Gilles de la Tourette's syndrome. Am J Psychiatry 150:93–97, 1993.

68. Cottraux J, Note I, Yao SN, Lafonts S, Note B, Mollard E, et al.: A randomized controlled trial of cognitive therapy versus intensive behavior therapy in obsessive compulsive disorder. Psychother Psychosom 70:288–297, 2001.

69. Bawden HN, Camfield CS, Camfield PR, Cunningham C, Darwish H, Dooley JM, et al.: The cognitive and behavioural effects of clobazam and standard monotherapy are comparable. Epilepsy Res 33:133–143, 1999.

70. Hauser P, Devinsky O, DeBellis M, Theodore WH, and Post RM: Benzodiazepine withdrawal delirium with catatonic features. Arch Neurol 46:696–699, 1989.

71. Berrios GE: Positive and negative symptoms and Jackson. A conceptual history. Arch Gen Psychiatry 42:95–97, 1985.

72. Tarulli A, Devinsky O, and Alper K: Progression of postictal to interictal psychosis. Epilepsia 42:1468–1471, 2001.

73. Sobin C, Prudic J, Devanand DP, Nobler MS, and Sackeim HA: Who responds to electroconvulsive therapy? A comparison of effective and ineffective forms of treatment. Br J Psychiatry 169:322–328, 1996.

74. Evenden JL: Varieties of impulsivity. Psychopharmacology 146:348–361, 1999.

75. Evenden J: Impulsivity: a discussion of clinical and experimental findings. J Psychopharmacol 13:180–192, 1999.

76. Hollander E and Rosen J: Impulsivity. J Psychopharmacol. 14(Suppl 1):S39–S44, 2000.

77. Moeller FG, Barratt ES, Dougherty DM, Schmitz JM, and Swann AC: Psychiatric aspects of impulsivity. Am J Psychiatry 158:1783–1793, 2001.

78. Rapport LJ, Webster JS, Flemming KL, Lindberg JW, Godlewski MC, Bress JE, et al.: Predictors of falls among right-hemisphere stroke patients in the rehabilitation setting. Arch Phys Med Rehabil 74:621–626, 1993.

79. Himelstein J, Newcorn JH, and Halperin JM: The neurobiology of attention-deficit hyperactivity disorder. Front Biosci 5:D461–D478, 2000.

80. Connor DF, Barkley RA, and Davis HT: A pilot study of methylphenidate, clonidine, or the combination in ADHD comorbid with aggressive oppositional defiant or conduct disorder. Clin Pediatr 39:15–25, 2000.

81. Schulz SC, Camlin KL, Berry SA, and Jesberger JA: Olanzapine safety and efficacy in patients with borderline personality disorder and comorbid dysthymia. Biol Psychiatry 46:1429–1435, 1999.

82. Verhoeven WM and Tuinier S: The effect of buspirone on challenging behaviour in mentally retarded patients: an open prospective multiple-case study. J Intellect Disabil Res 40:502–508, 1996.

83. Tartar RE, Kirisci L, Vanyukov M, Cornelius J, Pajer K, Shoal GD, et al.: Predicting adolescent violence: impact of family history, substance use, psychiatric history, and social adjustment. Am J Pscyhiatry 159:1541–1547, 2002.

84. Alpert JE and Spillmann MK: Psychotherapeutic approaches to aggressive and violent patients. Psychiatr Clin North Am 20:453–472, 1997.

85. Tariot PN, Jakimovich LJ, Erb R, Cox C, Lanning B, Irvine C, et al.: Withdrawal from controlled carbamazepine therapy followed by further carbamazepine treatment in patients with dementia. J Clin Psychiatry 60:684–689, 1999.

86. Gormley N, Lyons D, and Howard R: Behavioural management of aggression in dementia: a randomized controlled trial. Age Ageing 30:141–145, 2001.

87. Clark ME, Lipe AW, and Bilbrey M: Use of music to decrease aggressive behaviors in people with dementia. J Gerontol Nurs 24:10–17, 1998.

88. Devanand DP, Marder K, Michaels KS, Sackeim HA, Bell K, Sullivan MA, et al.: A randomized, placebo-controlled dose-comparison trial of haloperidol for psychosis and disruptive behaviors in Alzheimer's disease. Am J Psychiatry 155:1512–1520, 1998.

89. DeDeyn PP, Rabheru K, Rasmussen A, Bocksberger JP, Dautzenberg PL, Erikson S, et al.: A randomized trial of risperidone, placebo, and haloperidol for behavioral symptoms of dementia. Neurology 53:946–955, 1999.

90. Kyomen HH, Hennen J, Gottlieb GL, and Wei JY: Estrogen therapy and noncognitive psychiatric signs and symptoms in elderly patients with dementia. Am J Psychiatry 159:1225–1227, 2002.

91. Street JS, Clark WS, Gannon KS, Cummings JL, Bymaster FP, Tamura RN, et al.: Olanzapine treatment of psychotic and behavioral symptoms in patients with Alzheimer disease in nursing care facilities: a double-blind, randomized, placebo-controlled trial. Arch Gen Psychiatry 57:968–976, 2000.

92. Cummings JL, Nadel A, Masterman D, and Cyrus PA: Efficacy of metrifonate in improving the psychiatric and behavioral disturbances of patients with Alzheimer's disease. J Geriatr Psychiatry Neurol 14:101–108, 2001.

93. Campbell M, Adams PB, Small AM, Kanfantaris V, Silva RR, Shell J, et al.: Lithium in hospitalized aggressive children with conduct disorder: a double-blind and placebo-controlled study. J Am Acad Child Adolesc Psychiatry 34:445–453, 1995.

94. Findling RL, McNamara NK, Branicky LA, Schuchter MD, Lemon E, and Blumer JL: A double-blind pilot study of risperidone in the treatment of conduct disorder. J Am Acad Child Adolesc Psychiatry 39:509–516, 2000.

95. Ratey J, Sovner R, Parks A, and Rogentine K: Buspirone treatment of aggression and anxiety in mentally retarded patients: a multiple-baseline, placebo lead-in study. J Clin Psychiatry 52:159–162, 1991.

96. Malone RP, Delaney MA, Luebbert JF, Cater J, and Campbell M: A double-blind placebo-controlled study of lithium in hospitalized aggressive children and adolescents with conduct disorder. Arch Gen Psychiatry 57:649–654, 2000.

97. Buitelaar JK, van der Gaag RJ, Cohen-Kettenis P, and Melman CT: A randomized controlled trial of risperidone in the treatment of aggression in hospitalized adolescents with subaverage cognitive abilities. J Clin Psychiatry 62:239–248, 2001.

98. Hollander E, Allen A, Lopez RP, Beinstock CA, Grossman R, Siever LJ, et al.: A preliminary double-blind, placebo-controlled trial of divalproex sodium in borderline personality disorder. J Clin Psychiatry 62:199–203, 2001.

99. Allan ER, Alpert M, Sison CE, Citrome L, Laury G, and Berman I: Adjunctive nadolol in the treatment of acutely aggressive schizophrenic patients. J Clin Psychiatry 57:455–459, 1996.

100. Caspi N, Modai I, Barak P, Waisbourd A, Zbarsky H, Hirschmann S, et al.: Pindolol augmentation in aggressive schizophrenic patients: a double-blind crossover randomized study. Int Clin Psychopharmacol 16:111–115, 2001.

101. McDougle CJ, Naylor ST, Cohen DJ, Volkmar FR, Heninger GR, Price LH, et al.: A double-blind, placebo-controlled study of fluvoxamine in adults with autistic disorder. Arch Gen Psychiatry 53:1001–1008, 1996.

102. McDougle CJ, Holmes JP, Carlson DC, Pelton GH, Cohen DJ, and Price LH: A double-blind, placebo-controlled study of risperidone in adults with autistic disorder and other pervasive developmental disorders. Arch Gen Psychiatry 55:633–641, 1998.

103. Coccaro EF and Kavoussi RJ: Fluoxetine and impulsive aggressive behavior in personality-disordered subjects. Arch Gen Psychiatry 54:1081–1088, 1997.

104. Brooke MM, Patterson DR, Questad KA, Cardenas D, and Farrel-Roberts L: The treatment of agitation during initial hospitalization after traumatic brain injury. Arch Phys Med Rehabil 73:917–921, 1992.

105. Lindenmayer JP and Kotsaftis A: Use of sodium valproate in violent and aggressive behaviors: a critical review. J Clin Psychiatry. 61:123–128, 2000.

106. Ben-Porath DD and Taylor SP: The effects of diazepam (valium) and aggressive disposition on human aggression: an experimental investigation. Addict Behav 27:167–77, 2002.

107. Kravitz EA: Serotonin and aggression: insights gained from a lobster model system and speculations on the role of amine neurons in a complex behavior. J Comp Physiol 186:221–238, 2000.

108. Andersson KE: Pharmacology of erectile function and dysfunction. Urol Clin North Am 28:233–247, 2001.

109. Teshiba T, Shamsian A, Yashar B, Yeh SR, Edwards DH, and Krasne FB: Dual and opposing modulatory effects of serotonin on crayfish lateral giant escape command neurons. J Neurosci 21:4523–4529, 2001.

110. Stahl SM: Mechanism of action of serotonin selective reuptake inhibitors. Serotonin receptors and pathways mediate therapeutic effects and side effects. J Affect Disord 51:215–235, 1998.

110a. Burke WJ: Escitalopram. Expert Opin Investig Drug 11:1477–1486, 2002.

111. Lane RM: SSRI-induced extrapyramidal side-effects and akathisia: implications for treatment. J Psychopharmacol 12:192–214, 1998.

112. Kirby D and Ames D: Hyponatraemia and selective serotonin re-uptake inhibitors in elderly patients. Int J Geriatr Psychiatry 16:484–493, 2001.

113. Pina Latorre MA, Modrego PJ, Rodilla F, Catalan C, and Calvo M: Parkinsonism and Parkinson's disease associated with long-term administration of sertraline. J Clin Pharm Ther 26:111–112, 2001.

114. Bourin M, Chue P, Guillon Y: Paroxetine: a review. CNS Drug Rev 7:25–47, 2001.

115. Preskorn SH: Clinically relevant pharmacology of selective serotonin reuptake inhibitors. An overview with emphasis on pharmacokinetics and effects on oxidative drug metabolism. Clin Pharmacokinet 32:1–21, 1997.

116. Goldstein DJ, Corbin LA, and Sundell KL: Effects of first-trimester fluoxetine exposure on the newborn. Obstet Gynecol 89:713–718, 1997.

117. Nulman I, Rovet J, Stewart DE, Wolpin J, Gardner HA, Theis JG, et al.: Neurodevelopment of children exposed in utero to antidepressant drugs. N Engl J Med 336:258–262, 1997.

118. Misri S, Burgmann A, and Kostaras D: Are SSRIs safe for pregnant and breastfeeding women? Can Fam Physician 46:626–628, 631–633, 2000.

119. Kulin NA, Pastuszak A, Sage SR, Schick-Boschetto B, Spivey G, Feldkamp M, et al.: Pregnancy outcome following maternal use of the new selective serotonin reuptake inhibitors: a prospective controlled multicenter study. JAMA 279:609–610, 1998.

120. Masand PS and Gupta S: Selective serotonin-reuptake inhibitors: an update. Harv Rev Psychiatry 7:69–84, 1999.

121. Aubin HJ: Tolerability and safety of sustained-release bupropion in the management of smoking cessation. Drugs 62(Suppl 2):45–52, 2002.

122. Johnston JA, Lineberry CG, Ascher JA, Davidson J, Khayrallah MA, Feighner JP, et al.: A 102–center prospective study of seizure in association with bupropion. J Clin Psychiatry 52:450–456, 1991.

122a. Shih JC, Chen K, Ridd MJ: Monoamine oxidase: from genes to behavior. Annu Rev Neurosci 22:197–217, 1999.

123. Rybakowski JK: Antiviral and immunomodulatory effect of lithium. Pharmacopsychiatry 33:159–164, 2000.

124. Kane JM, Woerner M, and Lieberman J: Tardive dyskinesia: prevalence, incidence, and risk factors. J Clin Psychopharmacol 8(Suppl 4):52S–56S, 1988.

125. Yassa R and Jeste DV: Gender differences in tardive dyskinesia: a critical review of the literature. Schizophr Bull 18:701–715, 1992.

126. Gessa GL, Devoto P, Diana M, Flore G, Melis M, and Pistis M: Dissociation of haloperidol, clozapine, and olanzapine effects on electrical activity of mesocortical dopamine neurons and dopamine release in the prefrontal cortex. Neuropsychopharmacology 22:642–649, 2000.

127. Strange PG: Antipsychotic drugs: importance of dopamine receptors for mechanisms of therapeutic actions and side effects. Pharmacol Rev.53:119–133, 2001.

127a. Kane JM, Carson WH, Saha AR, McQuade RD, Ingenito GG, Zimbroff DL, et al.: Efficacy and safety of aripprazole and haloperidol versus placebo in patients with schizophrenia and schizoaffective disorder. J Clin Psychiatry 63:763–771, 2002.

128. Rozans M, Dreisbach A, Lertora JJ, and Kahn MJ: Palliative uses of methylphenidate in patients with cancer: a review. J Clin Oncol 20:335–339, 2002.

129. Rugino TA and Copley TC: Effects of modafinil in children with attention-deficit/hyperactivity disorder: an open-label study. J Am Acad Child Adolesc Psychiatry 40:230–235, 2001.

130. Holm KJ and Goa KL: Zolpidem: an update of its pharmacology, therapeutic efficacy and tolerability in the treatment of insomnia. Drugs 59:865–889, 2000.

131. Apter JT and Allen LA: Buspirone: future directions. J Clin Psychopharmacol 19:86–93, 1999.

132. DeLeon OA: Antiepileptic drugs for the acute and maintenance treatment of bipolar disorder. Harv Rev Psychiatry 9:209–222, 2001.

133. Pande AC, Davidson JRT, Jefferson JW, Janney CA, Katzelnick DJ, Weisler RH, et al.: Treatment of social phobia with gabapentin: a placebo controlled study. J Psychopharmacol 19:341–348, 1999.

134. Frye MA, Ketter TA, Kimbrell TA, Dunn RT, Speer AM, Osuch EA, et al.: A placebo-controlled study of lamotrigine and gabapentin monotherapy in refractory mood disorders. J Clin Psychopharmacol 20:607–614, 2000.

135. Pande AC, Crockatt JG, Janney CA, Werth JL, and Tsaroucha G: Gabapentin in bipolar disorder: a placebo-controlled trial of adjunctive therapy. Gabapentin Bipolar Disorder Study Group. Bipolar Disord 2:249–255, 2000.

136. Martin R, Kuzniecky R, Ho S, Hetherington H, Pan J, Sinclair K, et al.: Cognitive effects of topiramate, gabapentin, and lamotrigine in healthy young adults. Neurology 52:321–327, 1999.

137. Besag FM: Behavioural effects of the new anticonvulsants. Drug Saf 24: 513–536, 2001.

138. Crawford P: An audit of topiramate use in a general neurology clinic. Seizure 7:207–211, 1998.

139. Stephen LJ, Sills GJ, and Brodie MJ: Topiramate in refractory epilepsy: a prospective observational study. Epilepsia 41:977–980, 2000.

140. Ketter TA, Post RM, and Theodore WH: Positive and negative psychotropic effects of antiepileptic drugs in patients with seizure disorders. Neurology 53(Suppl 1):S52–S66, 1999.

141. Uvebrant P and Bauziene R: Intractable epilepsy in children. The efficacy of lamotrigine treatment, including non-seizure-related benefits. Neuropediatrics 25:284–289, 1994.

142. Hurd RW, Van Rinsvelt HA, Wilder BJ, Karas B, Maenhaut W, and De Reu L: Selenium, zinc, and copper changes with valproic acid: possible relation to drug side effects. Neurology 34:1393–1395, 1984.

143. Fatemi SH and Calabrese JR: Treatment of valproate-induced alopecia. Ann Pharmacother 29:1302, 1995.

144. Jallon P and Picard F: Bodyweight gain and anticonvulsants: a comparative review. Drug Saf 24: 969–978, 2001.

145. Duncan S: Polycystic ovarian syndrome in women with epilepsy: a review. Epilepsia 42(Suppl 3):60–65, 2001.

146. Rickels K, Pereira-Ogan JA, Chung HR, Gordon PE, and Landis WB: Bromazepam and phenobarbital in anxiety: a controlled study. Curr Ther Res Clin Exp 15:679–690, 1973.

147. Schaffer LC, Schaffer CB, and Caretto J: The use of primidone in treatment of refractory bipolar disorder. Ann Clin Psychiatry 11:61–66, 1999.

148. Brent DA, Crumrine PK, Varma R, Brown RV, and Allan MJ: Phenobarbital treatment and major depressive disorder in children with epilepsy. Pediatrics 80:909–917, 1987.

149. Stein G: Drug treatment of the personality disorders. Br J Psychiatry 161:167–184, 1992.

150. Uhde TW, Stein MB, and Post RM: Lack of efficacy of carbamazepine in the treatment of panic disorder. Am J Psychiatry 145:1104–1109, 1988.

151. Lima AR, Lima MS, Soares BG, and Farrell M: Carbamazepine for cocaine dependence. Cochrane Database Syst Rev 4:CD002023, 2001.

152. Friedman DL, Kastner T, and Plummer AT: Adverse behavioral effects in individuals with mental retardation and mood disorders treated with carbamazepine. Am J Ment Retard 96:541–546, 1992.

153. Landolt H: Serial electroencephalographic investigations during psychotic episodes in epileptic patients and during schizophrenic attacks. In deHass L (ed). Lectures on Epilepsy. Elsevier, London, 1958, pp 91–133.

154. McElroy SL, Soutullo CA, Keck PE Jr, and Kmetz GF: A pilot trial of adjunctive gabapentin in the treatment of bipolar disorder. Ann Clin Psychiatry 9:99–103, 1997.

155. Schaffer CB and Schaffer LC: Gabapentin in the treatment of bipolar disorder. Am J Psychiatry 154:291–292, 1997.

156. Ghaemi SN, Katzow JJ, Desai SP, and Goodwin FK: Gabapentin treatment of mood disorders: a preliminary study. J Clin Psychiatry 59:426–429, 1997.

157. Young LT, Robb JC, Patelis-Siotis I, MacDonald C, and Joffe RT: Acute treatment of bipolar depression with gabapentin. Biol Psychiatry 42:851–853, 1997.

158. Ryback R and Ryback L: Gabapentin for behavioral dyscontrol. Am J Psychiatry 152:1399, 1995.

159. Sheldon LJ, Ancill RJ, and Holliday SG: Gabapentin in geriatric psychiatry patients. Can J Psychiatry 43:422–423, 1998.

160. McManaman J and Tam DA: Gabapentin for self-injurious behavior in Lesch-Nyhan syndrome. Pediatr Neurol 20:381–382, 1999.

161. Dimond KR, Pande AC, Lamoreaux L, and Pierce MW: Effect of gabapentin (Neurontin) on mood and well being in patients with epilepsy. Prog Neuropsychopharmacol Biol Psychiatry 20:407–417, 1996.

162. Harden CL, Lazar LM, Pick LH, Nikolov B, Goldstein MA, Carson D, et al.: A beneficial effect on mood in partial epilepsy patients treated with gabapentin. Epilepsia 40:1129–1134, 1999.

163. Dodrill CB, Arnett JL, Hayes AG, Garafalo EA, Greeley CA, Greiner MJ, et al.: Cognitive abilities and adjustment with gabapentin: results of a multisite study. Epilepsy Res 35:109–121, 1999.

164. Lee DO, Steingard RJ, Cesena M, Helmers SL, Riviello JJ, and Mikati MA: Behavioral side effects of gabapentin in children. Epilepsia 37:87–90, 1996.

165. Ettinger AB, Barr W, and Solomon S: Psychotropic properties of antiepileptic drugs in patients with developmental disabilities. In Devinsky O and Westbrook L (eds). Developmental Disabilities. Butterworth-Heinemann, Boston, 2002, pp 219–230.

166. Hurley SC: Lamotrigine update and its use in mood disorders. Ann Pharmacother 36:860–873, 2002.

167. Muzina DJ, El-Sayegh S, and Calabrese JR: Antiepileptic drugs in psychiatry—focus on randomized controlled trial. Epilepsy 50:195–202, 2002.

168. Pinto OC and Akiskal HS: Lamotrigine as a promising approach to borderline personality: an open case series without concurrent DSM-IV major mood disorder. J Affect Disord 51:333–343, 1998.

169. Erfurth A, Walden J, and Grunze H: Lamotrigine in the treatment of schizoaffective disorder. Neuropsychobiology 38:204–205, 1998.

170. Meador KJ and Baker GA: Behavioral and cognitive effects of lamotrigine. J Child Neurol 12:S44–S47, 1997.

171. Beran RG and Gibson RJ: Aggressive behavior in intellectually challenged patients with epilepsy treated with lamotrigine. Epilepsia 39: 280–282, 1998.

172. Ettinger AB, Weisbrot DM, Saracco J, Dhoon A, Kanner A, and Devinsky O: Positive and negative psychotropic effects of lamotrigine in epilepsy patients with mental retardation. Epilepsia 39:874–877, 1998.

173. Sun M: Book touts Dilantin for depression. Science 215:951–952, 1982.

174. Mishory A, Yaroslavsky Y, Bersudsky Y, and Belmaker RH: Phenytoin as an antimanic anticonvulsant: a controlled study. Am J Psychiatry 157:463–465, 2000.

175. Devinsky O: Cognitive and behavioral effects of antiepileptic drugs. Epilepsia 36(Suppl 2):46–65, 1995.

176. Pereira J, Marson AG, and Hutton JL: Tiagabine add-on for drug-resistant partial epilepsy. Cochrane Database Syst Rev 3:CD001908, 2002.

177. Dodrill CB, Arnett JL, Shu V, Pixton GC, Lenz GT, and Sommerville KW: Effects of tiagabine monotherapy on abilities, adjustment, and mood. Epilepsia 39:33–42, 1998.

178. Carta MG, Hardoy MC, Grunze H, and Carpiniello B: The use of tiagabine in affective disorders. Pharmacopsychiatry 35:33–34, 2002.

179. Calabrese JR, Keck PE Jr, McElroy SL, and Shelton MD: A pilot study of topiramate as monotherapy in the treatment of acute mania. J Clin Psychopharmacol 21:340–342, 2001.

180. Grunze HC, Normann C, Langosch J, Schaefer M, Amann B, Sterr A, et al.: Antimanic efficacy of topiramate in 11 patients in an open trial with an on–off–on design. J Clin Psychiatry 62:464–468, 2001.

181. Shapira NA, Goldsmith TD, and McElroy SL: Treatment of binge-eating disorder with topiramate:

a clinical case series. J Clin Psychiatry 61:368–372, 2000.

182. Dohmeier C, Kay A, and Greathouse N: Neuropsychiatric complications of topiramate therapy [abstract]. Epilepsia 39(Suppl 6):189, 1998.

183. Sachdeo RC, Glauser TA, Ritter F, Reife R, Lim P, and Pledger G: A double-blind, randomized trial of topiramate in Lennox-Gastaut syndrome. Topiramate YL Study Group. Neurology 52:1882–1887, 1999.

184. Muller-Oerlinghausen B, Berghofer A, and Bauer M: Bipolar disorder. Lancet 359:241–247, 2002.

185. Post RM, Ketter TA, Denicoff K, Pazzaglia PJ, Leverich GS, Marangell LB, et al.: The place of anticonvulsant therapy in bipolar illness. Psychopharmacology 128:115–129, 1996.

186. Reoux JP, Saxon AJ, Malte CA, Baer JS, and Sloan KL: Divalproex sodium in alcohol withdrawal: a randomized double-blind placebo-controlled clinical trial. Alcohol Clin Exp Res 25:1324–1329, 2001.

187. Kastner T, Finesmith R, and Walsh K: Long-term administration of valproic acid in the treatment of affective symptoms in people with mental retardation. J Clin Psychopharmacol 13:448–451, 1993.

188. Stoll AL, Banov M, Kolbrener M, Mayer PV, Tohen M, Strakowski SM, et al.: Neurological factors predict a favorable valproate response in bipolar and schizoaffective disorders. J Clin Psychopharmacol 14:311–313, 1994.

189. Baetz M and Bowen RC: Efficacy of divalproex sodium in patients with panic disorder and mood instability who have not responded to conventional therapy. Can J Psychiatry 43:73–77, 1998.

190. Stein DJ, Simeon D, Frenkel M, Islam MN, and Hollander E: An open trial of valproate in borderline personality disorder. J Clin Psychiatry 56:506–510, 1995.

191. Gupta S, O'Connell RO, Parekh A, Krotz B, and Stockwell D: Efficacy of valproate for agitation and aggression in dementia: case reports. Int J Geriatr Psychopharmacol 1:244–248, 1998.

192. Ben-Menachem E and French J: Vigabatrin. In Engel J, Pedley TA (eds). Epilepsy: A Comprehensive Textbook. Lippincott-Raven, Philadelphia, 1997, pp 1609–1618.

193. Levinson DF and Devinsky O: Psychiatric adverse events during vigabatrin therapy. Neurology 53:1503–1511, 1999.

194. Yatham LN, Kusumakar V, Calabrese JR, Rao R, Scarrow G, and Kroeker G: Third generation anticonvulsants in bipolar disorder: a review of efficacy and summary of clinical recommendations. J Clin Psychiatry 63:275–283, 2002.

195. McElroy SL and Keck PE Jr: Pharmacologic agents for the treatment of acute bipolar mania. Biol Psychiatry 48:539–557, 2000.

196. McKeith I, Del Ser T, Spano P, Emre M, Wesnes K, Anand R, et al.: Efficacy of rivastigmine in dementia with Lewy bodies: a randomised, double-blind, placebo-controlled international study. Lancet 356:2031–2036, 2000.

197. Growdon JH: Treatment for Alzheimer's disease? N Engl J Med 327:1306–1308, 1992.

198. Knapp MJ, Knopman DS, Solomon PR, Pendlebury WW, Davis CS, and Gracon SL: A 30-week randomized controlled trial of high-dose tacrine in patients with Alzheimer's disease. JAMA 271:985–991, 1994.

199. Maltby N, Broe GA, Creasey H, Jorm AF, Christensen H, and Brooks WS: Efficacy of tacrine and lecithin in mild to moderate Alzheimer's disease: double blind trial. BMJ 308:879–883, 1994.

200. Schredl M and Weber B: Donepezil-induced REM sleep augmentation enhances memory performance in elderly, healthy persons. Exp Gerontol 36:353–361, 2001.

201. Doody RS, Geldmacher DS, Gordon B, Perdomo CA, and Pratt RD: Open-label, multicenter, phase 3 extension study of the safety and efficacy of donepezil in patients with Alzheimer disease. Arch Neurol 58:427–433, 2001.

202. Feldman H, Gauthier S, Hecker J, Vellas B, Subbiah P, and Whalen E: A 24–week, randomized, double-blind study of donepezil in moderate to severe Alzheimer's disease. Neurology 57:613–620, 2001.

203. Fisher RS, Bortz JJ, Blum DE, Duncan B, and Burke H: A pilot study of donepezil for memory problems in epilepsy. Epilepsy Behav 2:330–334, 2001.

204. Masanic CA, Bayley MT, VanReekum R, and Simard M: Open-label study of donepezil in traumatic brain injury. Arch Phys Med Rehabil 82:896–901, 2001.

205. Skjerve A and Nygaard HA: Improvement in sundowning in dementia with Lewy bodies after treatment with donepezil. Int J Geriatr Psychiatry 15:1147–1151, 2000.

206. Weinstock M, Razin M, Chorev M, and Enz A: Pharmacological evaluation of phenyl-carbamates as CNS-selective actylcholinesterase inhibitors. J Neural Transm 43(Suppl):219–225, 1994.

207. Stahl SM: The new cholinesterase inhibitors for Alzheimer's disease. Part 1: Their similarities are different. J Clin Psychiatry 61:710–711, 2000.

208. Blesa R: Galantamine: therapeutic effects beyond cognition. Dement Geriatr Cogn Disord 11(Suppl 1):28–34, 2000.

209. Lilienfeld S and Parys W: Galantamine: additional benefits to patients with Alzheimer's disease. Dement Geriatr Cogn Disord 11(Suppl 1):19–27, 2000.

210. Eckert GP, Cairns NJ, and Muller WE: Piracetam reverses hippocampal membrane alterations in Alzheimer's disease. J Neural Transm 106:757–761, 1999.

211. Muller WE, Eckert GP, and Eckert A: Piracetam: novelty in a unique mode of action. Pharmacopsychiatry 32(Suppl 1):2–9, 1999.

212. Nicholson CD: Pharmacology of nootropics and metabolically active compounds in relation to their use in dementia. Psychopharmacology (Berl) 101:147–159, 1990.

213. Grotemeyer KH, Evers S, Fischer M, and Husstedt IW: Piracetam versus acetylsalicylic acid in secondary stroke prophylaxis. J Neurol Sci 181:65–72, 2000.

214. Nicholson CD: Nootropics and metabolically active compounds in Alzheimer's disease. Biochem Soc Trans 17:83–85, 1989.

215. Noble S and Benfield P: Piracetam: a review of its clinical potential in the management of patients with stroke. CNS Drugs 9:497–511, 1998.

216. Greener J, Enderby P, and Whurr R: Pharmacological treatment for aphasia following stroke. Cochrane Database Syst Rev 4:CD000424, 2001.

217. Flicker L and Grimley Evans G: Piracetam for dementia or cognitive impairment. Cochrane Database Syst Rev 2:CD001011, 2001.

218. Paczynski M: Piracetam: a novel therapy for autism? J Autism Dev Disord 27:628–630, 1997.

219. Huber W, Willmes K, Poeck K, Van Vleymen B, and Deberdt W: Piracetam as an adjunct to language therapy for aphasia: a randomized double-blind placebo-controlled pilot study. Arch Phys Med Rehabil 78:245–250, 1997.

220. Wilsher CR, Bennett D, Chase CH, Conners CK, DiIanni M, Feagans L, et al.: Piracetam and dyslexia: effects on reading tests. J Clin Psychopharmacol 7:230–237, 1987.

221. Ackerman PT, Dykman RA, Holloway C, Paal NP, and Gocio MY: A trial of piracetam in two subgroups of students with dyslexia enrolled in summer tutoring. J Learn Disabil 24:542–549, 1991.

222. Obeso JA, Artieda J, Quinn N, Rothwell JC, Luquin MR, Vaamonde J, et al.: Piracetam in the treatment of different types of myoclonus. Clin Neuropharmacol 11:529–536, 1988.

223. Fedi M, Reutens D, Dubeau F, Andermann E, D'Agostino D, and Andermann F: Long term efficacy and safety of piracetam in the treatment of progressive myoclonus epilepsy. Arch Neurol 58:781–786, 2001.

224. Sano M, Ernesto C, Thomas RG, Klauber MR, Schafer K, Grundman M, et al.: A controlled trial of selegiline, alpha-tocopherol, or both as treatment for Alzheimer's disease. The Alzheimer's Disease Cooperative Study. N Engl J Med 336:1216–1222, 1997.

225. Birks JS, Melzer D, and Beppu H: Donepezil for mild and moderate Alzheimer's disease. Cochrane Database System Rev 4:CD001190, 2000.

226. Cummings JL: Treatment of Alzheimer's disease. Clin Corner 3:27–39, 2001.

227. Rockwood K, Kirkland S, Hogan DB, MacKnight C, Merry H, Verreault R, et al.: Use of lipid-lowering agents, indication bias, and the risk of dementia in community-dwelling elderly people. Arch Neurol 59:223–227, 2002.

228. Dixit SN, Behari M, and Ahuja GK: Effect of selegiline on cognitive functions in Parkinson's disease. J Assoc Physicians India 47:784–786, 1999.

229. Birkmayer W, Riederer P, Linauer W, and Knoll J: L-Deprenyl plus L-phenylalanine in the treatment of depression. J Neural Transm 59:81–87, 1984.

230. Wender PH: Attention-deficit hyperactivity disorder in adults. Psychiatr Clin North Am 21:761–774, 1998.

231. Zhu J, Hamm RJ, Reeves TM, Povlishock JT, and Phillips LL: Postinjury administration of L-deprenyl improves cognitive function and enhances neuroplasticity after traumatic brain injury. Exp Neurol 166:136–152, 2000.

232. Olanow CW: MAO-B inhibitors in Parkinson's disease. Adv Neurol 60:666–671, 1993.

233. Ernst E: The risk–benefit profile of commonly used herbal therapies: ginkgo, St. John's wort, ginseng, echinacea, saw palmetto, and kava. Ann Intern Med 136:42–53, 2002.

234. Stoll AL, Severus WE, Freeman MP, Reuter S, Zboyan HA, Diamond E, et al.: Omega 3 fatty acids in bipolar disorder: a preliminary double-blind, placebo- controlled trial. Arch Gen Psychiatry 56:407–412, 1999.

235. Fetrow CW and Avila JR: Efficacy of the dietary supplement S-adenosyl-L-methionine. Ann Pharmacother 35:1414–1425, 2001.

236. Fugh-Berman A: Herbs and dietary supplements in the prevention and treatment of cardiovascular disease. Prev Cardiol 3:24–32, 2000.

237. Whiskey E, Werneke U, and Taylor D: A systematic review and meta-analysis of *Hypericum perforatum* in depression: a comprehensive clinical review. Int Clin Psychopharmacol 16:239–252, 2001.

238. Izzo AA and Ernst E: Interactions between herbal medicines and prescribed drugs: a systematic review. Drugs 61:2163–2175, 2001.

239. Pittler MH and Ernst E: Efficacy of kava extract for treating anxiety: systematic review and meta-analysis. J Clin Psychopharmacol 20:84–89, 2000.

240. Brown RP, Gerbarg P, and Bottiglieri T: S-Adenosylmethionine (SAMe) for depression. Psychiatr Ann 32:29–44, 2002.

241. Bressa GM: S-Adenosyl-l-methionine (SAMe) as antidepressant: meta-analysis of clinical studies. Acta Neurol Scand Suppl 154:7–14, 1994.

242. McKenna DJ, Jones K, and Hughes K: Efficacy, safety, and use of ginkgo biloba in clinical and preclinical applications. Altern Ther Health Med 27:70–90, 2001.

243. DeFeudis FV and Drieu K: Ginkgo biloba extract (EGb 761) and CNS functions: basic studies and clinical applications. Curr Drug Targets 1:25–58, 2000.

244. LeBars PL and Kastelan J: Efficacy and safety of a ginkgo biloba extract. Public Health Nutr 3:495–499, 2000.

245. Van Dongen MC, Van Rossum E, Kessels AG, Sielhorst HJ, and Knipschild PG: The efficacy of ginkgo for elderly people with dementia and age-associated memory impairment: new results of a randomized clinical trial. J Am Geriatr Soc 48:1183–1194, 2000.

246. Moulton PL, Boyko LN, Fitzpatrick JL, and Petros TV: The effect of ginkgo biloba on memory in healthy male volunteers. Physiol Behav 73:659–665, 2001.

247. Heck AM, DeWitt BA, and Lukes AL: Potential interactions between alternative therapies and warfarin. Am J Health Syst Pharm 57:1221–1227, 2000.

248. Benjamin J, Muir T, Briggs K, and Pentland B: A case of cerebral haemorrhage—can ginkgo biloba be implicated? Postgrad Med J 77:112–113, 2001.

249. Fessenden JM, Wittenborn W, and Clarke L: Gingko biloba: a case report of herbal medicine and bleeding postoperatively from a laparoscopic cholecystectomy. Am Surg 67:33–35, 2001.

250. Walker BR, Easton A, and Gale K: Regulation of limbic motor seizures by GABA and glutamate transmission in nucleus tractus solitarius. Epilepsia 40:1051–1057, 1999.

251. Clark KB, Krahl SE, Smith DC, and Jensen RA: Post-training unilateral vagal stimulation enhances retention performance in the rat. Neurobiol Learn Mem 63:213–216, 1995.

252. Clark KB, Naritoku DK, Smith DC, Browning RA,

and Jensen RA: Enhanced recognition memory following vagus nerve stimulation in human subjects. Nat Neurosci 2:94–98, 1999.

253. Ettinger AB, Nolan E, Vitale S, et al.: Changes in mood and quality of life in adult epilepsy patients treated with vagal nerve stimulation [abstract]. Epilepsia 40:62, 1999.

254. Harden CL, Pulver MC, Nikolov B, Halper JP, and Labar DR: Effects of vagus nerve stimulation on mood in adult epilepsy patients [abstract]. Neurology 52(Suppl 2):A238, 1999.

255. Helmsteader C, Hoppe C, and Elger CE: Memory alterations during acute high-intensity vagus nerve stimulation. Epilepsy Res 47:37–42, 2001.

256. Blumer D, Davies K, Alexander A, and Morgan S: Major psychiatric disorders subsequent to treating epilepsy by vagus nerve stimulation. Epilepsy Behav 2:466–472, 2001.

257. Staub F and Bogousslavsky J: Fatigue after stroke: a major but neglected issue. Cerebrovasc Dis 12:75–81, 2000.

258. Comi G, Leocani L, Rossi P, and Colombo B: Physiopathology and treatment of fatigue in multiple sclerosis. J Neurol 248:174–179, 2001.

259. Mathiowetz V, Matuska KM, and Murphy ME: Efficacy of an energy conservation course for persons with multiple sclerosis. Arch Phys Med Rehabil 8:449–456, 2001.

260. Krupp LB and Rizvi SA: Symptomatic therapy for underrecognized manifestations of multiple sclerosis. Neurology 58 (Suppl 4):S32–S39, 2002.

261. Branas P, Jordan R, Fry-Smith A, Burls A, and Hyde C: Treatments for fatigue in multiple sclerosis: a rapid and systematic review. Health Technol Assess 4:1–61, 2000.

262. Rammohan KW, Rosenberg JH, Lynn DJ, Blumenfeld AM, Pollak CP, and Nagaraja HN: Efficacy and safety of modafinil (Provigil) for the treatment of fatigue in multiple sclerosis. J Neurol Neurosurg Psychiatry 72:179–183, 2002.

263. NIH: Acupuncture. NIH Consensus Statement Bethesda, MD. 15:1–34, 1997.

264. Meinhardt W, Kropman RF, and Vermeij P: Comparative tolerability and efficacy of treatments for impotence. Drug Saf 20:133–146, 1999.

265. Mayo-Smith MF: Pharmacological management of alcohol withdrawal. A meta-analysis and evidence-based practice guideline. JAMA 278:144–151, 1997.

266. American Psychiatric Association: Practice Guidelines for the Treatment of Patients with Delirium. American Psychiatric Association, Washington DC, 1999.

267. Hassan E, Fontaine DK, and Nearman HS: Therapeutic considerations in the management of agitated or delirious critically ill patients. Pharmacotherapy 18:113–129, 1998.

268. Meagher DJ: Delirium: optimising management. BMJ 322:144–149, 2001.

269. Sipahimalani A and Masand PS: Use of risperidone in delirium: case reports. Ann Clin Psychiatry 9:105–107, 1997

270. Sipahimalani A and Masand PS: Olanzapine in the treatment of delirium. Psychosomatics 39:422–430, 1998.

Index